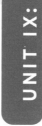

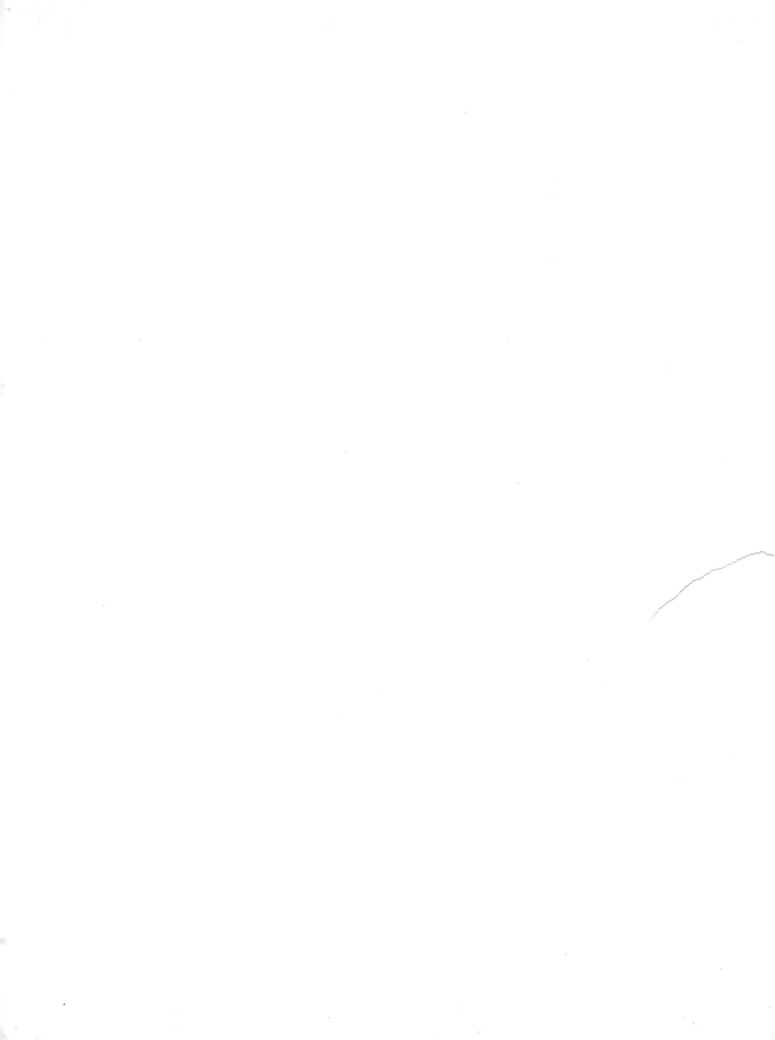

CANADIAN
Fundamentals *of* Nursing

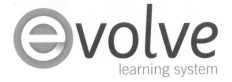

evolve
learning system

REGISTER TODAY!

Evolve provides online access to free learning resources and activities designed specifically for the textbook you are using in your class. The resources will provide you with information that enhances the material covered in the book and much more.

Visit the Web address listed below to start your learning evolution today!

http://evolve.elsevier.com/Canada/Potter/fundamentals/

Evolve® Student Learning Resources for Potter & Perry, Canadian Fundamentals of Nursing, 4th Edition, *offer the following features:*

Student Resources

- **Audio Summaries for each chapter are downloadable to an MP3 device or CD.**
- **Student Learning Activities include Hangman, Match Its, and Drag and Drop exercises.**
- **Animations feature exciting images related to various chapters in the textbook.**
- **Video Clips demonstrate important aspects of various nursing skills described in the textbook.**
- **Web links are a useful resource that allows you link to hundreds of Web sites carefully chosen to supplement the content of the textbook.**
- **Content Updates include the latest information from the authors of the textbook to help you keep abreast of recent developments in select areas of study.**

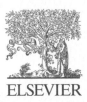

ELSEVIER

CANADIAN
Fundamentals of Nursing

FOURTH EDITION

PATRICIA A. POTTER
  RN, MSN, PhD, FAAN
Research Scientist
Barnes-Jewish Hospital
Siteman Cancer Center at Washington
  University School of Medicine
St. Louis, Missouri

ANNE GRIFFIN PERRY
  RN, EdD, FAAN
Professor and Chair
Department of Primary Care and Health
  Systems Nursing
School of Nursing, Southern Illinois University
Edwardsville, Illinois

SECTION EDITORS

AMY HALL, RN, BSN, MS, PhD
Chair
Department of Nursing and Health Sciences
Associate Professor of Nursing
University of Evansville
Evansville, Indiana

PATRICIA A. STOCKERT, RN, BSN, MS, PhD
Professor and Associate Dean
Undergraduate Program
Saint Francis Medical Center College of Nursing
Peoria, Illinois

CANADIAN EDITORS

JANET C. ROSS-KERR, RN, BScN, MS, PhD
Professor Emeritus
Faculty of Nursing
University of Alberta
Edmonton, Alberta

MARILYNN J. WOOD, BSN, MSN, DrPH
Professor Emeritus
Faculty of Nursing
University of Alberta
Edmonton, Alberta

CANADIAN SECTION EDITORS

BARBARA ASTLE, RN, PhD
Faculty of Nursing
University of Alberta
Calgary, Alberta

NICOLE LETOURNEAU, RN, PhD
Canada Research Chair in Healthy Child
  Development
Peter Lougheed/CIHR New Investigator
  (honourary)
Professor
Faculty of Nursing and Research Fellow CRISP
University of New Brunswick
Fredericton, New Brunswick

SONYA GRYPMA, RN, PhD
Associate Professor
School of Nursing
Trinity Western University
Langley, British Columbia

MOSBY

ELSEVIER

MOSBY
ELSEVIER

Notice

Knowledge and best practice in this field are constantly changing. As new research and expertise broaden our knowledge, changes in practice, treatment, and drug therapy may become necessary or appropriate. Readers are advised to check the most current information provided (i) on procedures featured or (ii) by the manufacturer of each product to be administered and to verify the recommended dose or formula, the method and duration of administration, and contraindications. It is the responsibility of practitioners, relying on their own experience and knowledge of the client, to make diagnoses, to determine dosages and the best treatment for each individual patient, and to take all appropriate safety precautions. To the fullest extent of the law, neither the Publisher nor the Authors assumes any liability for any injury and/or damage to persons or property arising out of or related to any use of the material contained in this book.

The Publisher

Library and Archives Canada Cataloguing in Publication

Potter, Patricia Ann

      Canadian fundamentals of nursing / Patricia A. Potter, Anne Griffin Perry;
Canadian editors, Janet C. Ross-Kerr, Marilynn J. Wood—4th ed.

Includes bibliographical references and index.
ISBN 978-1-926648-16-3

     1. Nursing–Textbooks. 2. Nursing–Canada–Textbooks. I. Perry, Anne Griffin
II. Kerr, Janet C., 1940– III. Wood, Marilynn J. IV. Title.

RT41.P68 2010   610.73   C2009-906645-9

ISBN-13-978-1-926648-16-3
ISBN-10-1-926648-16-1

Vice President, Publishing: Ann Millar
Developmental Editor: Toni Chahley
Managing Developmental Editor: Martina van de Velde
Managing Production Editor: Lise Dupont/Roberta Spinosa-Millman
Copy Editor: Anne Ostroff
Cover, Interior Design: Christine Rae, Interrobang Graphics, Inc.
Typesetting and Assembly: Jansom
Printing and Binding: Transcontinental

Elsevier Canada
905 King Street West, 4th Floor
Toronto, ON, Canada M6K 3G9
Phone: 1-866-896-3331
Fax: 1-866-359-9534

Printed in Canada

1 2 3 4 5   14 13 12 11 10

Contents

Preface to the Student

Canadian Fundamentals of Nursing provides you with all of the fundamental nursing concepts and skills you will need in a visually appealing, easy-to-use format. As you begin your nursing education, it is very important that you have a resource that includes all the information required to prepare you for lectures, classroom activities, clinical assignments, and examinations. We've designed this text to meet all of those needs.

Check out the following special learning aids featured in *Canadian Fundamentals of Nursing*:

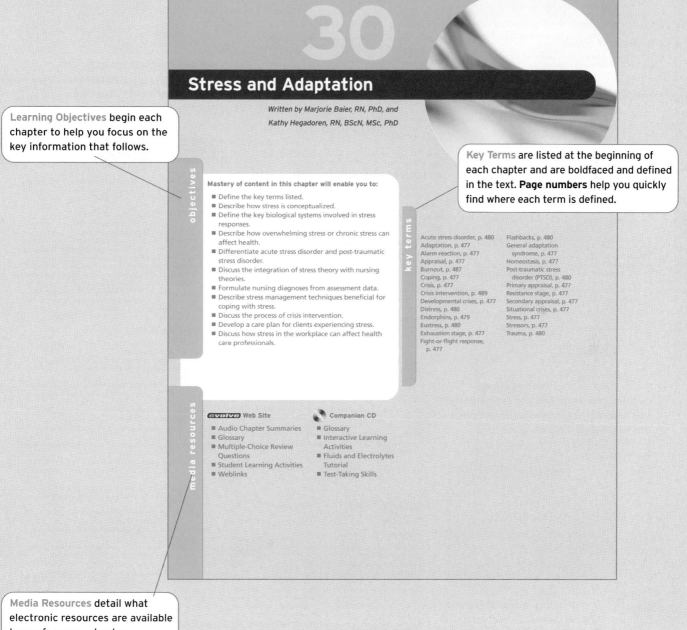

Learning Objectives begin each chapter to help you focus on the key information that follows.

Key Terms are listed at the beginning of each chapter and are boldfaced and defined in the text. **Page numbers** help you quickly find where each term is defined.

Media Resources detail what electronic resources are available to you for every chapter.

30

Stress and Adaptation

Written by Marjorie Baier, RN, PhD, and
Kathy Hegadoren, RN, BScN, MSc, PhD

objectives

Mastery of content in this chapter will enable you to:

- Define the key terms listed.
- Describe how stress is conceptualized.
- Define the key biological systems involved in stress responses.
- Describe how overwhelming stress or chronic stress can affect health.
- Differentiate acute stress disorder and post-traumatic stress disorder.
- Discuss the integration of stress theory with nursing theories.
- Formulate nursing diagnoses from assessment data.
- Describe stress management techniques beneficial for coping with stress.
- Discuss the process of crisis intervention.
- Develop a care plan for clients experiencing stress.
- Discuss how stress in the workplace can affect health care professionals.

key terms

Acute stress disorder, p. 480
Adaptation, p. 477
Alarm reaction, p. 477
Appraisal, p. 477
Burnout, p. 487
Coping, p. 477
Crisis, p. 477
Crisis intervention, p. 489
Developmental crises, p. 477
Distress, p. 480
Endorphins, p. 479
Eustress, p. 480
Exhaustion stage, p. 477
Fight-or-flight response, p. 477

Flashbacks, p. 480
General adaptation syndrome, p. 477
Homeostasis, p. 477
Post-traumatic stress disorder (PTSD), p. 480
Primary appraisal, p. 477
Resistance stage, p. 477
Secondary appraisal, p. 477
Situational crises, p. 477
Stress, p. 477
Stressors, p. 477
Trauma, p. 480

media resources

evolve Web Site
- Audio Chapter Summaries
- Glossary
- Multiple-Choice Review Questions
- Student Learning Activities
- Weblinks

Companion CD
- Glossary
- Interactive Learning Activities
- Fluids and Electrolytes Tutorial
- Test-Taking Skills

✳ CRITICAL THINKING EXERCISES

1. An 82-year-old client is admitted for surgery on a fractured hip caused by a fall. What postoperative complications are typical in the older client undergoing this type of surgery?

2. Mr. B. is a 52-year-old client who will undergo thoracic surgery. He has smoked one pack of cigarettes per day for 30 years. What type of pulmonary preventive measures would you expect Mr. B to need postoperatively?

3. Mrs. C. was admitted for ambulatory surgery for an inguinal hernia repair. What discharge criteria would be used for Mrs. C., and what discharge instructions would she require?

4. Your client is scheduled for abdominal hysterectomy at 2:00 p.m. Based on NPO guidelines, what fasting schedule should you implement in collaboration with the surgeon and the anaesthesiologist?

5. You are doing preoperative teaching for a client undergoing a minimally invasive surgical technique. Identify one advantage of this type of surgery.

✳ REVIEW QUESTIONS

1. An obese client is at risk for poor wound healing and for wound infection postoperatively because:
   1. Ventilatory capacity is reduced
   2. Fatty tissue has a poor blood supply
   3. Risk for dehiscence is increased
   4. Resuming normal physical activity is delayed

2. You should ask each client preoperatively for the name and dose of all prescription and over-the-counter medications taken before surgery because they:
   1. May cause allergies to develop
   2. Are automatically ordered postoperatively
   3. May create greater risks for complications or interact with anaesthetic agents
   4. Should be taken on the morning of surgery with sips of water

3. A client who smokes two packs of cigarettes per day is most at risk postoperatively for:
   1. Infection
   2. Pneumonia
   3. Hypotension
   4. Cardiac dysrhythmias

4. Family members should be included when you teach the client preoperative exercises so that they can:
   1. Supervise the client at home
   2. Coach the client postoperatively
   3. Practise with the client while waiting to be taken to the operating room
   4. Relieve you by getting the client to do his or her exercises every 2 hours

5. In the postoperative period, measuring input and output helps assess:
   1. Renal and circulatory function
   2. Client comfort
   3. Neurological function
   4. Gastrointestinal function

6. In the PACU, one measure taken to maintain airway patency is to:
   1. Suction the pharynx and bronchial tree
   2. Give oxygen through a mask at 10 L/minute
   3. Position the client so that the tongue falls forward
   4. Ask the client to use an incentive spirometer

7. Which one of the following measures promotes normal venous return and circulatory blood flow?
   1. Suctioning artificial airways and the oral cavity
   2. Monitoring fluid and electrolyte status during every shift
   3. Having the client use incentive spirometry
   4. Encouraging the client to perform leg exercises at least once an hour while awake

8. A client with an international normalized ratio (INR) or an activated partial thromboplastin time (APTT) greater than normal is at risk postoperatively for:
   1. Anemia
   2. Bleeding
   3. Infection
   4. Cardiac dysrhythmias

9. When the client is engaging in deep breathing and coughing exercises, it is important to have the client sitting because this position:
   1. Is more comfortable
   2. Facilitates expansion of the thorax
   3. Increases the client's view of the room and is more relaxing
   4. Helps the client to splint with a pillow

10. In the postoperative period, if a client has unexpected tachycardia and tachypnea; jaw muscle rigidity; body rigidity of limbs, abdomen, and chest; or hyperkalemia, you should suspect:
    1. Infection
    2. Hypertension
    3. Pneumonia
    4. Malignant hyperthermia

✳ RECOMMENDED WEB SITES

Canadian Anesthesiologists' Society: http://www.cas.ca
This Web site offers client information about and guidelines for using anaesthesia.

National Association of PeriAnesthesia Nurses of Canada: http://www.napanc.org
Perianaesthesia nurses are registered nurses with advanced knowledge in the care of clients during all phases of perianaesthesia, including, for example, nurses in postanaesthetic care units, same-day surgery, and diagnostic imaging.

Operating Room Nurses Association of Canada: http://www.ornac.ca
This Web site provides practice standards for Canadian operating room nurses, as well as information on certification with the Canadian Nurses Association (CNA).

Ontario PeriAnesthesia Nurses Association: http://www.opana.org
This Web site provides position statements on and standards of peri-anaesthesia nursing practice.

> **Critical Thinking Exercises** encourage you to think creatively and effectively to apply essential content.

> **Recommended Web Sites** list up-to-date online resources and are annotated to give you some information about each.

> **Review Questions** at the end of each chapter help you review and evaluate what you have learned. Answers and rationales are provided at the back of the book.

> **Key Concepts** appear at the end of each chapter to help you review important content.

to assist the client in returning to as healthy and functional a state as possible. Your evaluation also includes determining the extent to which the client and the family have learned self-care measures.

Client Expectations

With short hospital stays and ambulatory surgery, it is especially important to evaluate client expectations early in the postoperative process. Pain relief is usually a priority. Asking the client if everything possible has been done to alleviate pain, including nonpharmacological measures, can determine whether the client's needs have been met. Timeliness of response to the client's needs, such as scheduled times for pain medication and prompt answering of a call light, may increase satisfaction. The client usually wants to be discharged from acute care as soon as possible and when indicated by the physician. Ensuring that discharge plans are in place facilitates that process and enhances the client's satisfaction with care.

✳ KEY CONCEPTS

- Perioperative nursing is nursing care provided to the surgical client before, during, and after surgery.
- Surgery is classified by level of severity, urgency, and purpose.
- The preoperative period may be several days or only a few hours long.
- Preoperative assessment of vital signs and physical findings provides an important baseline with which to compare postoperative assessment data.
- Nursing diagnoses of the surgical client may pose implications for nursing care during one or all phases of surgery.
- Primary responsibility for obtaining informed consent rests with the client's surgeon.
- Structured preoperative teaching has a positive influence on a client's postoperative recovery.
- Basic to preoperative teaching is an explanation of all preoperative and postoperative routines and demonstration of postoperative exercises.
- In ambulatory surgery, nurses must use the limited time available to educate clients, assess their health status, and prepare them for surgery.
- A routine preoperative (preprocedure) checklist can be used as a guide for final preparation of the client before surgery.
- Many responsibilities of nurses within the OR focus on protecting the client from potential harm.
- All medications taken before surgery are automatically discontinued after surgery unless a physician reorders the drugs.
- Family members or other supportive networks are important in assisting clients with any physical limitations and in providing emotional support during postoperative recovery and ongoing care at home.
- Assessment of the postoperative client centres on the body systems most likely to be affected by anaesthesia, immobilization, and surgical trauma.
- Accurate pain assessment and intervention are necessary for healing
- Nurses in the postoperative surgical unit provide the discharge education required so that the client and the family can manage at home.

surgical settings, you consult with the client and the family to gather evaluation data. You can evaluate the ambulatory surgical client's outcomes via a telephone call to the client's home, asking specific questions to determine whether complications have developed and whether the client understands restrictions or medications. This call is usually placed 24 hours after surgery, which allows you to evaluate the progress of recovery.

In an acute care setting, evaluation of a surgical client is ongoing. If a client fails to progress as expected, you revise the client's care plan according to the priorities of the client's needs. Every effort is made

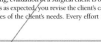

✳ BOX 49-8   FOCUS ON PRIMARY HEALTH CARE

Recovery at Home

Regardless of the length of time the client spends in hospital, it is essential that you ensure that the client and family have the appropriate information and skills needed to continue a successful recovery at home.

However, time is often very limited, especially with the move toward preadmission units and short hospital stays. A comprehensive approach is needed to ensure continuity of care from hospital to home. A client often has to continue dressing care, follow activity restrictions, continue medication therapy, and observe for signs and symptoms of complications on returning home. In addition, the client needs someone to be present for the first 24 hours to ensure that there is no delayed reaction from the anaesthesia, such as difficulty breathing. A referral to home care assists clients who are unable to perform self-care activities. Close association with home care services is required for some clients if dressing changes or physiotherapy is needed. It is useful to have a case management nurse in attendance at discharge to convey what tasks a client can perform effectively.

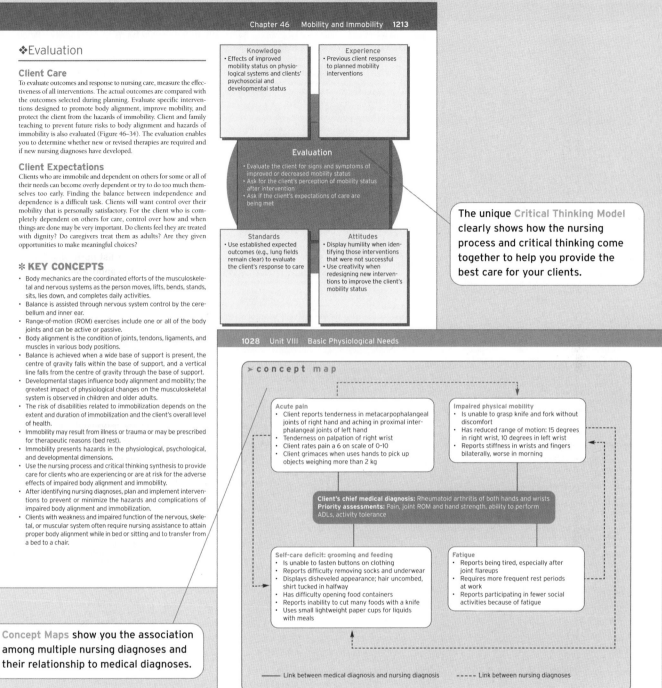

❖ Evaluation

Client Care

To evaluate outcomes and response to nursing care, measure the effectiveness of all interventions. The actual outcomes are compared with the outcomes selected during planning. Evaluate specific interventions designed to promote body alignment, improve mobility, and protect the client from the hazards of immobility. Client and family teaching to prevent future risks to body alignment and hazards of immobility is also evaluated (Figure 46–34). The evaluation enables you to determine whether new or revised therapies are required and if new nursing diagnoses have developed.

Client Expectations

Clients who are immobile and dependent on others for some or all of their needs can become overly dependent or try to do too much themselves too early. Finding the balance between independence and dependence is a difficult task. Clients will want control over their mobility that is personally satisfactory. For the client who is completely dependent on others for care, control over how and when things are done may be very important. Do clients feel they are treated with dignity? Do caregivers treat them as adults? Are they given opportunities to make meaningful choices?

✳ KEY CONCEPTS

- Body mechanics are the coordinated efforts of the musculoskeletal and nervous systems as the person moves, lifts, bends, stands, sits, lies down, and completes daily activities.
- Balance is assisted through nervous system control by the cerebellum and inner ear.
- Range-of-motion (ROM) exercises include one or all of the body joints and can be active or passive.
- Body alignment is the condition of joints, tendons, ligaments, and muscles in various body positions.
- Balance is achieved when a wide base of support is present, the centre of gravity falls within the base of support, and a vertical line falls from the centre of gravity through the base of support.
- Developmental stages influence body alignment and mobility; the greatest impact of physiological changes on the musculoskeletal system is observed in children and older adults.
- The risk of disabilities related to immobilization depends on the extent and duration of immobilization and the client's overall level of health.
- Immobility may result from illness or trauma or may be prescribed for therapeutic reasons (bed rest).
- Immobility presents hazards in the physiological, psychological, and developmental dimensions.
- Use the nursing process and critical thinking synthesis to provide care for clients who are experiencing or are at risk for the adverse effects of impaired body alignment and immobility.
- After identifying nursing diagnoses, plan and implement interventions to prevent or minimize the hazards and complications of impaired body alignment and immobilization.
- Clients with weakness and impaired function of the nervous, skeletal, or muscular system often require nursing assistance to attain proper body alignment while in bed or sitting and to transfer from a bed to a chair.

Knowledge
- Effects of improved mobility status on physiological systems and clients' psychosocial and developmental status

Experience
- Previous client responses to planned mobility interventions

Evaluation
- Evaluate the client for signs and symptoms of improved or decreased mobility status
- Ask for the client's perception of mobility status after intervention
- Ask if the client's expectations of care are being met

Standards
- Use established expected outcomes (e.g., lung fields remain clear) to evaluate the client's response to care

Attitudes
- Display humility when identifying those interventions that were not successful
- Use creativity when redesigning new interventions to improve the client's mobility status

> The unique **Critical Thinking Model** clearly shows how the nursing process and critical thinking come together to help you provide the best care for your clients.

➤ concept map

Acute pain
- Client reports tenderness in metacarpophalangeal joints of right hand and aching in proximal interphalangeal joints of left hand
- Tenderness on palpation of right wrist
- Client rates pain a 6 on scale of 0–10
- Client grimaces when uses hands to pick up objects weighing more than 2 kg

Impaired physical mobility
- Is unable to grasp knife and fork without discomfort
- Has reduced range of motion: 15 degrees in right wrist, 10 degrees in left wrist
- Reports stiffness in wrists and fingers bilaterally, worse in morning

Client's chief medical diagnosis: Rheumatoid arthritis of both hands and wrists
Priority assessments: Pain, joint ROM and hand strength, ability to perform ADLs, activity tolerance

Self-care deficit: grooming and feeding
- Is unable to fasten buttons on clothing
- Reports difficulty removing socks and underwear
- Displays disheveled appearance; hair uncombed, shirt tucked in halfway
- Has difficulty opening food containers
- Reports inability to cut many foods with a knife
- Uses small lightweight paper cups for liquids with meals

Fatigue
- Reports being tired, especially after joint flareups
- Requires more frequent rest periods at work
- Reports participating in fewer social activities because of fatigue

———— Link between medical diagnosis and nursing diagnosis   ----- Link between nursing diagnoses

Figure 42–10 Concept map for client with pain related to rheumatoid arthritis.

> **Concept Maps** show you the association among multiple nursing diagnoses and their relationship to medical diagnoses.

pain in affected areas. Occupational therapists can devise splints to support painful body parts. Clergy members can help clients resolve spiritual pain. The family should also be involved in the care plan because they may need to administer care in the home after discharge. If the pain management plan is not successful, you should talk with the physician about changing the plan. Consultation with pain experts might be necessary.

> The five-step **Nursing Process** provides a consistent framework for presentation of content in clinical chapters.

❖ Implementation

The nature of the pain and how much it affects well-being determines the choice of interventions. Pain therapy requires an *individualized* approach, perhaps more so than any other client problem. You, the client, and the family must be partners in using pain-control measures. Administer and monitor pain treatments ordered by a physician, but consider using other complementary comfort measures. Client remedies are often most successful, especially when the client

has already had experience with pain. Generally, the least invasive or safest therapy should be tried first.

Health Promotion

The Ottawa Charter for Health Promotion (https://www.who.int/healthpromotion/conferences/previous/ottawa/en/) defines health promotion as the process of enabling individuals to gain control over and to improve their health and well-being (World Health Organization, 1990). Chronic pain and suffering diminishes quality of life; thus, relieving pain and promoting self-control becomes important. Once pain is controlled to an acceptable level, provide clients and their families with education and information about pain so that they can participate in the pain care decision-making process. This will help reduce anxiety and increases a client's sense of control. For example, clients who are in hospital for the first time may know that they require tests, but do not understand them. As a result, they may become anxious and fearful. Fear increases the perception of painful stimuli. Remember, however, that health promotion goes beyond teaching. Using pain management techniques from the Ottawa

✳ BOX 23-5   RESEARCH HIGHLIGHT

Breastfeeding

Research Focus

Success in breastfeeding largely depends on the woman's self-confidence in her ability to breastfeed. You can play an important role in assisting new mothers to feel more confident in their ability to breastfeed by being aware of some of the factors that promote successful breastfeeding.

Research Abstract

Kingston et al. (2007) explored some of the factors that enhanced women's self-efficacy in breastfeeding 48 hours and 4 weeks after the birth of their babies. Kingston et al. examined such influences as previous successful breastfeeding experiences, professional assistance with breastfeeding, watching other mothers breastfeed, watching videos of other women breastfeeding, giving positive feedback and consistent advice, receiving praise from family members and friends, encouraging mothers to continue breastfeeding, and encouraging mothers to think positively about the breastfeeding experience, as well as physiological influences on breastfeeding such as pain, fatigue, and feeling overwhelmed. Self-efficacy was measured by the Breastfeeding Self-Efficacy Scale–Short Form. The study was performed with a small sample of mothers ($N = 65$) in a hos-

pital in central Canada. The researchers found that self-efficacy was significantly higher in women who had seen videotapes of women breastfeeding as part of their breastfeeding education or had received praise from their partners or own mothers. Women who reported pain or received help with breastfeeding from professionals had significantly lower scores. Women receiving more help would have a greater need for assistance, and this might affect self-efficacy.

Evidence-Informed Practice

- Assess the breastfeeding self-efficacy of new mothers.
- Examine the educational material used with clients, and show clients videos of successful breastfeeding.
- Consider the physiological condition of the mother, and address issues such as pain.
- Include the mother's partner and, if possible, the woman's own mother in supporting and offering praise to the breastfeeding mother.
- Examine other factors that increase or decrease the mother's self-confidence in her ability to breastfeed.

References: Kingston, D., Dennis, C.-L., & Sword, W. (2007). Exploring breast-feeding self-efficacy. *Journal of Perinatal and Neonatal Nursing, 21*, 207–215.

dietary habits through feeding experiences mutually satisfying for the parents and infant. Eating habits are frequently affected by the family's sociocultural background. Because some cultures consider a fat baby to be a sign of good mothering, any suggestion to limit intake or slow weight gain may be seen as a threat. It is important for you to develop an understanding of the cultural influences to develop effective nursing interventions.

Dentition. The average age at which the first tooth erupts is 7 months, but considerable variation exists among infants because of their genetic endowment. An occasional infant is born with a tooth, whereas others remain toothless at 1 year. The order of tooth eruption is fairly predictable: The lower central incisors are first to appear, closely followed by the upper central incisors. Most 1-year-olds have six teeth.

Teething may result in considerable discomfort for some infants and little or none for others. The inflammation of the gums before the tooth emerges may result in a low-grade fever and irritability. Some infants exhibit increased drooling, biting, or finger sucking. Biting on a frozen teething ring or ice cube wrapped in a washcloth may be soothing. Over-the-counter teething medications to rub on the inflamed gums and appropriate doses of acetaminophen are helpful when the infant is irritable and has difficulty eating or sleeping.

Most dentists recommend that parents cleanse their infant's teeth after each feeding. The parent can place a clean, wet washcloth or piece of gauze over a finger and use it to wipe the infant's teeth. Because of the risk of developing dental caries, discourage prolonged breast- or bottle-feeding, especially just before the infant goes to sleep because the infant is likely to leave milk in the mouth and around the teeth. The infant should never go to bed with a bottle of juice or milk (Behrman et al., 2008).

Immunizations. The widespread use of immunizations has resulted in the dramatic decline of infectious diseases since the 1950s and is therefore a most important factor in health promotion during childhood. Although most immunizations can be given to people of

any age, the Public Health Agency of Canada (2006) recommended that the administration of the primary series begin soon after birth and be completed during early childhood (Table 23–2). Minor side effects may occur, but serious reactions are rare. Parents must receive instructions regarding the potential side effects of immunizations. High fever and extreme irritability should be reported to their health care professional.

As a result of complacency and fear regarding the side effects of certain vaccines, especially diphtheria and tetanus toxoids and pertus-

---

> **Research Highlight** boxes provide abstracts of current nursing research studies and explain the implications for your daily practice.

> **Nursing Care Plans** feature a format that helps you understand the process of assessment, the relationship between assessment findings and nursing diagnoses, the identification of goals and outcomes, selection of interventions, and the process for evaluating care.

▶ BOX 14-4   NURSING CARE PLAN

Acute Pain

Assessment

Ms. Devine is a 52-year-old woman who was injured in a fall two months ago that caused rupture of a lumbar disc. She is scheduled for a lumbar laminectomy this afternoon. Ms. Devine is the office manager for a realty business she runs with her husband. She was not able to work regularly over the first month after the injury. She has sciatic pain that is sharp and burning, radiating down from her right hip to her right foot. The pain worsens when she sits. Her vital signs are as follows: temperature, 99.2°F; blood pressure, 138/82 mm Hg; pulse, 84 beats per minute; and respirations, 24 breaths per minute.

Assessment Activities	Findings and Defining Characteristics*
Observe client's body movements	Client limps **slightly with right leg. Turns** in bed **slowly.**
Observe client's facial expression	Client **grimaces** when she attempts to sit down.
Ask client to rate pain at its worst	Client **rates pain on a scale of 0 to 10 at an 8 or 9 at its worst.**

*Defining characteristics are in boldface type.

Nursing Diagnosis: Acute pain related to pressure on spinal nerves

Planning

Goal (Nursing Outcomes Classification)† Pain Control	Expected Outcomes† Knowledge of Treatment Procedures
Client will achieve improved pain control before surgery.	Client's self-report of pain will be 3 or less on a scale of 0 to 10 Client's facial expressions reveal less discomfort when turning and repositioning.

†Outcomes classification labels from Moorhead S, Johnson, M., & Maas, M. (2008). *Nursing Outcomes Classification (NOC)* (3rd ed). St. Louis, MO: Mosby.

Interventions (Nursing Interventions Classification)‡	Rationale
Analgesic Administration	
Set positive expectations regarding effectiveness of analgesics.	Optimizes client's response to medication (Bulechek et al., 2008).
Give analgesic 30 minutes before turning or positioning client and before pain increases in severity.	Medication will exert peak effect when client attempts to increase movement.
Pain Management	
Reduce environmental factors in client's room (e.g., noise, lighting, temperature extremes).	Pleasurable sensory stimuli reduce pain perception.
Offer client information about any procedures and efforts at reducing discomfort.	Information satisfies client's interests and enables client to evaluate and communicate pain (McCaffery & Pasero, 1999).
Progressive Muscle Relaxation	
Direct client through progressive muscle relaxation exercise.	Relaxation techniques enable self-control when pain develops, reversing
Coach client through exercise.	the cognitive and affective–motivational component of pain perception.

‡Intervention classification labels from Bulechek, G. M., Butcher, H. K., & Dochterman, J. M. (2008). *Nursing Interventions Classification (NIC)* (4th ed.). St. Louis, MO: Mosby.

Evaluation

Nursing Actions	Client Response and Finding	Achievement of Outcome
Ask client to report severity of pain 30 minutes after analgesic administration.	Ms. Devine reports pain at a level of 5 on a scale of 0 to 10.	Pain is reduced, necessitates further nonpharmacological intervention to achieve outcome.
Observe client's facial expressions.	Ms. Devine is observed to have a relaxed facial expression.	Client's level of comfort is improving.

> **Rationales** for each of the interventions in the care plans help you to understand why a specific step or set of steps is performed.

> **Evaluation** explains how to evaluate and determine whether the outcomes have been achieved.

Evidence-Informed Practice Guideline boxes provide examples of recent state-of-the-science guidelines for nursing practice.

Client Teaching boxes highlight what and how to teach clients and how to evaluate learning.

✳ BOX 44-13 CLIENT TEACHING

Pelvic Floor Muscle Exercises (Kegels)

Objectives

The client who is cognitively alert and motivated will achieve continence or experience fewer episodes of incontinence through increased pelvic floor muscle tone and strength.

Teaching Strategies

- Explain the method used to identify proper muscle contraction: female client sits on toilet with knees apart and tightens muscles to stop the flow of urine; male client tries to stop the flow of urine midstream.
- After muscle is identified, instruct the client to lie down with knees bent and apart, or to sit.
- Instruct the client to contract the pelvic floor muscle gradually and hold for 3 to 10 seconds without tensing muscles of legs, buttocks, back, or abdomen. Remind the client to breathe during the exercise.
- Instruct the client to relax the muscle gradually for an equal time period between each contraction.
- The client should repeat this exercise at least two or three times, and work up to 10 repetitions as it becomes easier. The client should do this exercise two or three times a day, or as often as possible.
- Explain that within the first week of exercises, the client and nurse can assess whether proper muscle contraction is occurring by placing two fingers in the vagina (or, for men, one finger in the rectum) while contracting the pelvic floor muscle. The client should feel tightening in the vagina or anus during the contraction.
- Teach the client and the caregiver to keep a 24- to 72-hour urinary diary to identify changes in patterns of urinary elimination.

Evaluation

- Ask the client if he or she has identified pelvic floor muscle via finger insertion.
- During vaginal or rectal (male) bimanual examination, ask the client to do exercises and assess muscle tone.
- Monitor the client's urinary diary.
- Ask the client and the caregiver about degree of satisfaction related to the control achieved over urinary elimination.

✳ BOX 44-14 EVIDENCE-INFORMED PRACTICE GUIDELINE

Prompted Voiding for People with Urinary Incontinence

- Approach the client at scheduled prompted voiding times.
- Wait five seconds for the client to initiate a request to toilet.
- Ask the client if he or she is wet or dry.
- Physically assess the client to determine continence status.
- Provide positive feedback if the client is dry.
- Prompt the client to toilet.
- Offer assistance with toileting.
- Provide feedback.
- Inform the client of the next scheduled prompted voiding session.
- Encourage the client to self-initiate requests to toilet.
- Record the result of the prompted voiding session.

Adapted from Wyman, J. (2008). Prompted voiding. In B. Ackley, B. Swan, G. Ludwig, & S. Tucker (Eds.), *Evidence-based nursing care guidelines. Medical–surgical interventions* (pp. 696–698). St. Louis, MO: Mosby.

The first step in bladder training is establishing a baseline. The client or caregiver completes a urinary diary to assess maximum voiding intervals. It is not uncommon for the client with frequency or an overactive bladder to void small amounts hourly or more often. An initial training schedule for such a client might involve a voiding schedule of every 75 minutes while awake, increasing every 1 to 3 weeks by 15-minute increments toward a 3-hour schedule. The rate of incremental changes will depend on the client's progress and on his or her ability to adhere to a rigid schedule. Urge-suppression techniques, such as counting backward from 100 when the urge to void is felt and performing pelvic floor muscle contractions, are helpful. You must be aware that the client who has experienced an episode of incontinence in public will be particularly hesitant to deter voiding for even brief periods.

Habit Retraining and Prompted Voiding. Habit retraining and **prompted voiding** are useful strategies for clients with cognitive or physical impairment, or both, who rely on caregiver assistance. Habit retraining involves assessment of a client's normal pattern of voiding to establish a toileting schedule that pre-empts incontinence (Ostaszkiewicz et al., 2008). Such individualized toileting schedules have demonstrated effectiveness but are labour-intensive. You should help the client to the bathroom before episodes of incontinence occur. Fluids and medications are timed to prevent interference with the toileting schedule. When combined with positive reinforcement, this approach is also called prompted voiding (Box 44–14).

Self-Catheterization. Some clients with chronic disorders such as spinal cord injury learn to perform self-catheterization. The client must be physically able to manipulate equipment and assume a position for successful catheterization. You must teach the client the structure of the urinary tract, the clean versus sterile technique, the importance of adequate fluid intake, and the frequency of self-catheterization. In general, the goal is to have clients perform self-catheterization every six to eight hours, but the schedule should be individualized.

❖Evaluation

Client Care

The client is the best source of evaluation of outcomes and responses to nursing care (Figure 44–18). However, you will also evaluate the effectiveness of nursing interventions through comparisons with baseline data. You should evaluate for changes in the client's voiding pattern, the presence of urinary tract alteration, and the client's physical condition. Actual outcomes are compared with expected outcomes to determine the client's health status. Continuous evaluation allows you to determine whether new or revised therapies are required or if any new nursing diagnoses have developed.

Client Expectations

If you have developed a trust relationship with the client, indications of the client's degree of satisfaction with his or her care will be evident. The client may smile or nod in appreciation. However, you need to confirm whether the client's expectations have been met to full satis-

Older Adults. The cardiac and respiratory systems undergo changes throughout the aging process (Box 39–3). The changes are associated with calcification of the heart valves, SA node, and costal cartilages. The arterial system develops atherosclerotic plaques. Osteoporosis leads to changes in the size and shape of the thorax.

The trachea and large bronchi become enlarged from calcification of the airways. The alveoli enlarge, decreasing the surface area available for gas exchange. The number of functional cilia is reduced, causing a decrease in the effectiveness of the cough mechanism, putting the older adult at increased risk for respiratory infections (Meiner & Leuckenotte, 2006). Ventilation and transfer of respiratory gases decline with age because the lungs are unable to expand fully, leading to lower oxygenation levels.

Lifestyle Risk Factors

Lifestyle modifications that influence cardiopulmonary functioning are frequently difficult because a client is being asked to change a habit or behaviour that may be enjoyed, such as cigarette smoking or eating certain foods; however, these changes can be achieved with encouragement, support, and time (Box 39–4). Risk factor modification is important, including smoking cessation, weight reduction, a low-cholesterol and low-sodium diet, management of hypertension, and moderate exercise. Although it may be difficult to get older adults to change long-term behaviour, developing healthy behaviours can slow or halt the progression of their cardiopulmonary disease (Meiner & Leuckenotte, 2006).

Poor Nutrition. Nutrition affects cardiopulmonary function in several ways. Severe obesity decreases lung expansion, and the increased body weight increases oxygen demands to meet metabolic needs. The malnourished client may experience respiratory muscle wasting, resulting in decreased muscle strength and respiratory excursion. Cough efficiency is reduced secondary to respiratory muscle weakness, putting the client at risk for retention of pulmonary secre-

ciency of the myocardial muscle (JNC, 2003).

Smoking. Cigarette smoking is associated with a number of diseases, including heart disease, chronic obstructive lung disease, and lung cancer. Cigarette smoking can worsen peripheral vascular and coronary artery diseases (JNC, 2003). Inhaled nicotine causes vasoconstriction of peripheral and coronary blood vessels, increasing blood pressure and decreasing blood flow to peripheral vessels. Women who take birth control pills and smoke cigarettes are at increased risk for cardiovascular problems such as thrombophlebitis and pulmonary emboli.

✳ BOX 39-3 FOCUS ON OLDER ADULTS

- The tuberculin skin test is an unreliable indicator of tuberculosis in older clients. They frequently display false-positive or false-negative skin test reactions.
- Older clients are at an increased risk for reactivation of dormant organisms that have been present for decades, as a result of age-related changes in the immune system.
- The standard 5-TU Mantoux test is given and repeated or repeated with the 250-TU strength to create a booster effect.
- If the older client has a positive reaction, a complete history is necessary to determine any risk factors.
- Older adults have more atypical signs and symptoms of coronary artery disease (Meiner & Leuckenotte, 2006).
- The incidence of atrial fibrillation increases with age and is the leading contributing factor for stroke in the older adult (Meiner & Leuckenotte, 2006).
- Mental status changes are often the first signs of respiratory problems and may include forgetfulness and irritability.
- Older adults may not complain of dyspnea until it affects the activities of daily living that are important to them.
- Changes in the older adult's cough mechanism may lead to retention of pulmonary secretions, airway plugging, and atelectasis if cough suppressants are not used with caution.

✳ BOX 39-4 FOCUS ON PRIMARY HEALTH CARE

Positive Lifestyle Practices for Cardiopulmonary Health Promotion

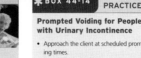

As part of a primary health care focus, it is important to educate young to older adults about the following lifestyle practices that promote cardiopulmonary health:
- Maintain ideal body weight.
- Eat a low-fat, low-salt, calorie-appropriate diet.
- Engage in regular aerobic exercise of 1 hour daily.
- Use a filter mask when exposed to occupational hazards.
- Use stress-reduction techniques.
- Reduce exposure to secondary infections.
- Be smoke free.
- Avoid second-hand smoke and other pollutants.
- Have annual visits with a health care professional.
- Monitor blood pressure.
- Monitor cholesterol and triglyceride levels.
- Get an annual influenza vaccine if at risk for the development of influenza.
- Get a pneumococcal vaccine if appropriate.

Focus on Older Adults boxes prepare you to address the special needs of older adults.

Focus on Primary Health Care boxes draw attention to principles of primary health care and their application.

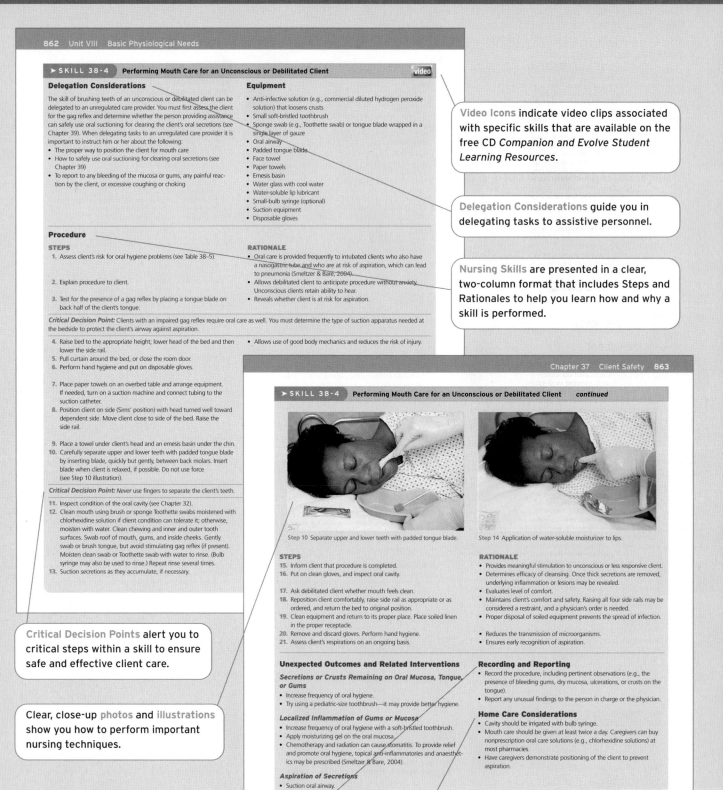

► SKILL 38-4   Performing Mouth Care for an Unconscious or Debilitated Client   video

Delegation Considerations

The skill of brushing teeth of an unconscious or debilitated client can be delegated to an unregulated care provider. You must first assess the client for the gag reflex and determine whether the person providing assistance can safely use oral suctioning for clearing the client's oral secretions (see Chapter 39). When delegating tasks to an unregulated care provider it is important to instruct him or her about the following:

- The proper way to position the client for mouth care
- How to safely use oral suctioning for clearing oral secretions (see Chapter 39)
- To report to any bleeding of the mucosa or gums, any painful reaction by the client, or excessive coughing or choking

Equipment

- Anti-infective solution (e.g., commercial diluted hydrogen peroxide solution) that loosens crusts
- Small soft-bristled toothbrush
- Sponge swab (e.g., Toothette swab) or tongue blade wrapped in a single layer of gauze
- Oral airway
- Padded tongue blade
- Face towel
- Paper towels
- Emesis basin
- Water glass with cool water
- Water-soluble lip lubricant
- Small-bulb syringe (optional)
- Suction equipment
- Disposable gloves

Procedure

STEPS	RATIONALE
1. Assess client's risk for oral hygiene problems (see Table 38–5).	- Oral care is provided frequently to intubated clients who also have a nasogastric tube and who are at risk of aspiration, which can lead to pneumonia (Smeltzer & Bare, 2004).
2. Explain procedure to client.	- Allows debilitated client to anticipate procedure without anxiety. Unconscious clients retain ability to hear.
3. Test for the presence of a gag reflex by placing a tongue blade on back half of the client's tongue.	- Reveals whether client is at risk for aspiration.

Critical Decision Point: Clients with an impaired gag reflex require oral care as well. You must determine the type of suction apparatus needed at the bedside to protect the client's airway against aspiration.

4. Raise bed to the appropriate height; lower head of the bed and then lower the side rail.	- Allows use of good body mechanics and reduces the risk of injury.
5. Pull curtain around the bed, or close the room door.	
6. Perform hand hygiene and put on disposable gloves.	
7. Place paper towels on an overbed table and arrange equipment. If needed, turn on a suction machine and connect tubing to the suction catheter.	
8. Position client on side (Sims' position) with head turned well toward dependent side. Move client close to side of the bed. Raise the side rail.	
9. Place a towel under client's head and an emesis basin under the chin.	
10. Carefully separate upper and lower teeth with padded tongue blade by inserting blade, quickly but gently, between back molars. Insert blade when client is relaxed, if possible. Do not use force (see Step 10 illustration).	

Critical Decision Point: Never use fingers to separate the client's teeth.

11. Inspect condition of the oral cavity (see Chapter 32).
12. Clean mouth using brush or sponge Toothette swabs moistened with chlorhexidine solution if client condition can tolerate it; otherwise, moisten with water. Clean chewing and inner and outer tooth surfaces. Swab roof of mouth, gums, and inside cheeks. Gently swab or brush tongue, but avoid stimulating gag reflex (if present). Moisten clean swab or Toothette swab with water to rinse. (Bulb syringe may also be used to rinse.) Repeat rinse several times.
13. Suction secretions as they accumulate, if necessary.

► SKILL 38-4   Performing Mouth Care for an Unconscious or Debilitated Client   *continued*

Step 10 Separate upper and lower teeth with padded tongue blade.

Step 14 Application of water-soluble moisturizer to lips.

STEPS	RATIONALE
15. Inform client that procedure is completed.	- Provides meaningful stimulation to unconscious or less responsive client.
16. Put on clean gloves, and inspect oral cavity.	- Determines efficacy of cleansing. Once thick secretions are removed, underlying inflammation or lesions may be revealed.
17. Ask debilitated client whether mouth feels clean.	- Evaluates level of comfort.
18. Reposition client comfortably, raise side rail as appropriate or as ordered, and return the bed to original position.	- Maintains client's comfort and safety. Raising all four side rails may be considered a restraint, and a physician's order is needed.
19. Clean equipment and return to its proper place. Place soiled linen in the proper receptacle.	- Proper disposal of soiled equipment prevents the spread of infection.
20. Remove and discard gloves. Perform hand hygiene.	- Reduces the transmission of microorganisms.
21. Assess client's respirations on an ongoing basis.	- Ensures early recognition of aspiration.

Unexpected Outcomes and Related Interventions

Secretions or Crusts Remaining on Oral Mucosa, Tongue, or Gums
- Increase frequency of oral hygiene.
- Try using a pediatric-size toothbrush—it may provide better hygiene.

Localized Inflammation of Gums or Mucosa
- Increase frequency of oral hygiene with a soft-bristled toothbrush.
- Apply moisturizing gel on the oral mucosa.
- Chemotherapy and radiation can cause stomatitis. To provide relief and promote oral hygiene, topical anti-inflammatories and anaesthetics may be prescribed (Smeltzer & Bare, 2004).

Aspiration of Secretions
- Suction oral airway.
- Perform tracheal bronchial suctioning.
- Notify the physician.

Recording and Reporting
- Record the procedure, including pertinent observations (e.g., the presence of bleeding gums, dry mucosa, ulcerations, or crusts on the tongue).
- Report any unusual findings to the person in charge or the physician.

Home Care Considerations
- Cavity should be irrigated with bulb syringe.
- Mouth care should be given at least twice a day. Caregivers can buy nonprescription oral care solutions (e.g., chlorhexidine solutions) at most pharmacies.
- Have caregivers demonstrate positioning of the client to prevent aspiration.

Video Icons indicate video clips associated with specific skills that are available on the free CD *Companion and Evolve Student Learning Resources.*

Delegation Considerations guide you in delegating tasks to assistive personnel.

Nursing Skills are presented in a clear, two-column format that includes Steps and Rationales to help you learn how and why a skill is performed.

Critical Decision Points alert you to critical steps within a skill to ensure safe and effective client care.

Clear, close-up **photos** and **illustrations** show you how to perform important nursing techniques.

Recording and Reporting sections provide guidelines for what to chart and report with each skill.

Home Care Considerations explain how to adapt skills for the home setting.

✻ BOX 30-5   CULTURAL ASPECTS OF CARE

Cultural context shapes the types of environmental stimuli that produce stress. For example, diverse cultures address developmental transitions and life's turning points differently. How a person leaves the parental home, experiences health crises or chronic illness, cares for the family, or becomes disabled or dependent are all culturally bound. Furthermore, how a person appraises stress is also dependent on the person's culture. Coping strategies are also influenced by culture. According to Aldwin (1992), cultures vary in their emotion-focused and problem-focused coping strategies. According to some cultures, emotions should be controlled; according to others, they should be expressed. *Problem-focused coping* refers to controlling or managing stress. In addition, cultures provide different institutions for coping with stress. These include the legal system for conflict resolution, advice givers or support groups, and rituals.

Implications for Practice

- Realize that stressors and coping styles vary with different cultures.
- Use introspection to examine your own perceptions of stress and coping in a cultural context.
- Assess the influence of culture on a client's appraisal of stress.
- Determine the available resources within a client's culture that may facilitate coping.

From Aldwin, C. M. (2000). *Stress, coping and development: An integrative perspective* (pp. 30–22). New York: Guilford Press.

Nursing Process

❖ Assessment

When assessing a client's stress level and coping resources, you must ask the client to share personal and sensitive information. Therefore, you must first establish a trusting nurse–client relationship. By asking open-ended questions, listening carefully, observing the client's nonverbal behaviour, and observing the client's environment, you learn about the client's stress. You use critical thinking skills to synthesize and analyze information (Figure 30–3). Often clients have difficulty expressing what is troubling them until they have the opportunity to talk with someone who has time to listen.

Subjective Findings

When assessing a client's level of stress and coping resources, you arrange a nonthreatening physical environment, without a desk as a barrier, for the interaction (Varcarolis, 2002). You assume the same height as the client, arranging the interview environment so that eye contact can be comfortably maintained or avoided. By placing chairs at a 90-degree angle or side by side, you can reduce the intensity of the interaction (Varcarolis, 2002). You use the interview to determine the client's view of the stress, past successful coping resources, any possible maladaptive coping, and adherence to prescribed medical recommendations, such as medication or diet (Monat & Lazarus, 1991; Table 30–1). If the client is using denial as a coping mechanism, you must be alert to whether he or she is overlooking necessary information. Other clients may state that they feel overwhelmed and unable to cope, but with help, they can reduce their multiple interacting stressors to manageable pieces. As in all interactions with the client, you must respect the confidentiality and sensitivity of the information shared.

safety alert Medical conditions such as sleep apnea and thyroid dysfunction that are common in older adults can initially cause symptoms that mimic stress-related symptoms. For this reason, a thorough physical assessment of an older adult who appears stressed or anxious is necessary to rule out potentially serious medical disorders. In addition, in older adults, signs of stress and crisis must be differentiated from emerging dementia and also from acute confusion, a condition that can be life-threatening.

Objective Findings

You obtain further findings about stress and coping by observing the client's appearance and nonverbal behaviour during the interview, including grooming and hygiene, handshake and gait, body language, speech quality, eye contact, and attitude. Before or at the end of the interview, depending on the client's anxiety level, you take basic vital signs to assess for physiological signs of stress, such as elevated blood pressure, heart rate, or respiratory rate (Figure 30–4).

Client Expectations

It is crucial that you understand the meaning the client attaches to the precipitating event and how stress is affecting the client's life. You must allow the client time to express priorities for coping. For example, if a woman has just been told that a breast mass was identified on a routine mammogram, you must discern what the client wants and needs most from you. Some clients identify an immediate need for information about biopsy or mastectomy; others need guidance and support on how to share the news with family members. In some cases, when nothing can be done to change or improve the situation, allowing the client to use denial as a coping mechanism can be help-

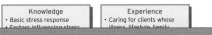

Knowledge	Experience
• Basic stress response	• Caring for clients whose
• Factors influencing stress	illness, lifestyle, family...

Safety Alerts indicate techniques you can use to ensure client and nurse safety.

Cultural Aspects of Care boxes prepare you to care for clients of diverse populations and suggest actions needed to meet different cultural needs and preferences.

▶ BOX 45-9   Procedural Guidelines

Digital Removal of Stool

Delegation Considerations: The digital removal of stool procedure should not be delegated to unregulated care providers.

Equipment

- Bath blanket
- Waterproof pad
- Disposable gloves
- Lubricant
- Towel
- Washcloth
- Soap and water
- Bedpan

Procedure

1. Explain the procedure to the client.
2. Perform hand hygiene. Take baseline vital signs prior to the procedure. Help the client to lie on the left side with knees flexed and back toward you.
3. Drape the trunk and lower extremities with a bath blanket and place a waterproof pad under the buttocks. Keep a bedpan next to the client.
4. Apply disposable gloves and lubricate the index finger of your dominant hand with lubricating jelly.
5. Gently insert the gloved index finger into the rectum and advance the finger slowly along the rectal wall toward the umbilicus.
6. Gently loosen the fecal mass by massaging around it. Work the finger into the hardened mass.
7. Work the feces downward toward the end of the rectum. Remove small pieces at a time and discard into the bedpan.
8. Reassess the client's vital signs and look for signs of fatigue. Stop the procedure if the heart rate drops significantly or if the heart rhythm changes.
9. Continue to remove feces and allow the client to rest at intervals.
10. After completion, wash and dry the buttocks and anal area.
11. Remove the bedpan and dispose of the feces. Remove gloves by turning them inside out, and then discard.
12. Assist the client to the toilet or position the client on a clean bedpan if the urge to defecate develops.
13. Perform hand hygiene. Record results of the removal of the impaction by describing the fecal characteristics.
14. Follow the procedure with enemas or cathartics as ordered by physician.
15. Reassess the client's vital signs and level of comfort.

✻ BOX 45-10   NURSING STORY

Disimpaction Is a Painful Stimulus

The first time I, as a newly hired nursing instructor, took fourth-year students to a clinical experience, we attended a small (8-bed) neurological intensive care unit. One client, a young man in his late teens who was conscious but still confused, was recovering from a motorbike accident. The student who was assigned to this client read the doctor's order for rectal disimpaction (the client's bowels had not moved since the accident five days previously). The student and I discussed in great detail the procedure and came to a disagreement about the highest priority for the client after safety. I said that the student required assistance, but she said no the greater need was for the client's privacy. As I hovered near the curtains, she explained the procedure to the young man, assessed his vital signs, prepared the bedpan, put on her gloves, lubricated her index finger, and drew the curtains ever tighter. She then attempted to insert the gloved, lubricated finger into the rectum. To the young man, this was a startling procedure (although it had been verbally explained to him). I heard a loud yell from the client and the clatter of a bedpan bouncing across the floor, and then a bedraggled nursing cap sailed under the curtains. I rushed behind the curtains to rescue the student from the flailing arms of the strong young man. No harm was done and the student gratefully accepted assistance from the orderly.

Lesson learned: disimpaction is a strong, noxious stimulus and the client's reactions may be unpredictable. In an older adult client, the reaction may even be pathological, such as a cardiovascular response or increased heart rate and blood pressure from sympathetic stimulation. In very ill clients, the crash cart should be present at the bedside because a cardiac arrest could ensue.

As a footnote to the story, this student and I had a several further disagreements that year. Several years later, however, I received a note from this woman, who was now teaching nursing herself. She apologized for her behaviour. She had taught several students who had reminded her of herself when she was a student, she said; and now she wondered how I ever put up with her behaviour.

Procedural Guidelines provide streamlined, step-by-step instructions for performing basic skills.

Nursing Story boxes tell a real-life story concerning one or more topics in the chapter.

▶ TABLE 45-6   Purposes of Nasogastric Intubation

Purpose	Description	Type of Tube
Decompression	Removal of secretions and gaseous substances from the gastrointestinal tract to prevent or relieve abdominal distension	Salem sump, Levin, Miller-Abbott
Feeding (i.e., gavage; see Chapter 43)	Instillation of liquid nutritional supplements or feedings into the stomach for clients unable to swallow fluid	Duo, Dobhoff, Levin
Compression	Internal application of pressure by means of an inflated balloon to prevent internal esophageal or gastrointestinal hemorrhage	Sengstaken-Blakemore
Lavage	Irrigation of the stomach in cases of active bleeding, poisoning, or gastric dilation	Levin, Ewald, Salem sump

The future of nursing in Canada looks promising. Dynamic change and ongoing development of the discipline point to the need for extensive and wide-ranging knowledge as the foundation of good care. The nurses of tomorrow will need to practise outstanding nursing and demonstrate its importance in maintaining and improving the health of Canadians. Nursing practice will be characterized by critical thinking, client advocacy, excellence in clinical decision making, and client teaching within a broad spectrum of health services.

Canadian Fundamentals of Nursing is designed for beginning students in all types of professional nursing programs. The text provides comprehensive coverage of fundamental nursing concepts, skills, and techniques required for safe and competent nursing practice.

The fourth edition of *Canadian Fundamentals of Nursing* has been extensively revised and thoroughly edited for easier reading and understanding. Across its 49 chapters, the text is more concise than in the previous edition. All chapters have been written or revised so that they reflect Canadian standards, traditions, research, and practice. The text is organized to indicate the order in which topics are usually taught. For example, foundational chapters such as "The Development of Nursing in Canada" and "Research as a Basis for Practice" appear in Units 1 and 2.

Canadian Fundamentals of Nursing includes content covering the entire scope of primary, acute, and restorative care. The focus is on the central role of primary health care in all areas of nursing practice. Emphasis is also placed on evidence-informed practice in skills and care plans to foster understanding of how research findings should guide clinical decision making. The book includes concept maps that demonstrate the relationships among nursing assessment, diagnosis, planning, intervention, and evaluation. In the form of Nursing Stories, first-person accounts of issues that have arisen in nursing practice are designed to engage the student's attention and encourage more detailed reading and understanding.

New to this edition is an **Editorial Advisory Board** comprising three prominent Canadian nurses who are leaders in nursing education in Canada. For this task, we chose three accomplished individuals from diverse regions of the country: Dr. Sally Thorne, Director and Professor of the School of Nursing at the University of British Columbia, is well known as a researcher and theoretician in nursing. Her research has focused upon applying conceptual knowledge to nursing practice, critical thinking, nursing theory and the philosophy of nursing science. Dr. Shirley Solberg, Associate Professor, School of Nursing, Memorial University of Newfoundland, researches women's health, health promotion and education, primary care, and cancer care. Dr. Ann Tournageau, Associate Professor, Faculty of Nursing, University of Toronto and Adjunct Scientist, Institute for Clinical Evaluative Studies in Ontario, holds a Career Scientist award from the Ontario Ministry of Health and Long-Term Care. Her research and teaching centre on nursing outcomes, in which she evaluates the contribution of nursing care and nursing work environments to client and organizational outcomes. Moreover, our Editorial Advisory Board consulted with us to ensure that all aspects of the book are current and attuned to the needs of beginning nursing students across the country.

One of the many issues about which we consulted our board was our choice of terminology. For this edition, we have chosen not to use the familiar term "evidence-based practice." We have chosen instead to use **evidence-*informed*** practice because although "evidence-based policy" is used in the literature, it largely relates to one type of evidence only: research. Using the term "evidence-influenced" or "evidence-informed" reflects the need to be context sensitive and to consider use of the best available evidence in dealing with everyday circumstances. A variety of distinct pieces of evidence and sources of knowledge inform policy, such as histories and experience, beliefs, values, competency or skills, legislation, politics and politicians, protocols, and research results.

This textbook is the result of the combined efforts of many talented professionals committed to excellence. Expert contributors from across Canada approached the revision with enthusiasm, and worked hard to ensure that the content is current and reflects the Canadian health care system, Canadian health and social organizations, and uniquely Canadian health care issues. Reviewers scrutinized the chapters and made many helpful suggestions. We appreciate the conscientiousness and enthusiasm of all these dedicated professionals.

Classic Features

- **Comprehensive** coverage and readability of all fundamental nursing content are provided.
- **Full-colour** text is used to enhance visual appeal and instructional value.
- **Primary health care and health promotion** issues are discussed throughout the text.
- **Focus on Primary Health Care** boxes highlight how the principles of primary health care can be applied to the topic of the chapter; the context of each of these boxes pertains uniquely to Canadian health care.
- **Health promotion, acute and tertiary care**, and **restorative care** are covered in order to address today's practice in various settings.
- **Cultural diversity** is presented in Chapter 10, stressed in clinical examples throughout the text, and highlighted in special boxes.
- **Research Highlight** boxes are integrated throughout the text to provide current nursing research studies and explain the implications for daily practice; many of these present Canadian research.
- **Client education** is stressed in boxes that list teaching objectives, strategies, and evaluation for clinical topics throughout the text.
- **Evidence-informed practice** is discussed throughout the text.
- **Evidence-Informed Practice Guidelines** boxes provide examples of recent state-of-the-science guidelines for nursing practice.
- **Gerontological nursing** principles are addressed in Chapter 25, as well as in special **Focus on Older Adults** boxes throughout the text.
- **Health Assessment and Physical Examination** (Chapter 32) provides students with important background in this important area of practice.
- **Diverse clinical settings**, including clinics, long-term-care facilities, and the home, as well as acute care settings, are described.
- **Historical boxes** entitled **"Milestones in Canadian History"** provide information about nursing leaders and critical events in Canadian nursing history.

- **Critical thinking** in clinical chapters is presented through a dimensional **critical thinking model** that visually demonstrates the ongoing assimilation of knowledge, critical thinking attitudes, intellectual and professional standards, and experience in relationship to clinical decision making and the nursing process.
- **Nursing Care Plans** guide students on how to conduct an assessment and analyze the defining characteristics that indicate nursing diagnoses. The plans include Nursing Interventions Classification (NIC) and Nursing Outcomes Classification (NOC) to familiarize students with this important nomenclature. The evaluation sections of the plans show students how to determine the expected outcomes and evaluate the results of care.
- Important nursing skills are presented in a clear, two-column format with a rationale for all steps; whenever possible, rationales are based on the most current research evidence.
- **Unexpected Outcomes and Related Interventions** are highlighted within discussions of nursing skills.
- **Critical pathways** address collaborative care in home and acute care settings.
- **Concept maps** demonstrate the relationship between nursing assessment, diagnosis, planning, intervention, and evaluation.
- **Procedural Guidelines** boxes provide streamlined, step-by-step instructions about how to perform basic skills.
- **Video Icons** indicate video clips associated with specific skills that are available on the free CD-Companion and Evolve Student Learning Resources.
- **End-of-chapter review questions** help students review and evaluate what they have learned. Answers and rationales are provided at the end of the book.
- The annotated **Recommended Web Sites** sections at the end of each chapter direct the student to current Web-based resources, most of which are Canadian.

New Features

- New chapter on **Nursing Informatics and Canadian Nursing Practice** (Chapter 17), written by leading Canadian nursing authorities, helps students to understand the growing dimensions of computerization in nursing practice.
- New chapter on **Caring for the Cancer Survivor** (Chapter 5) helps students support clients and families facing cancer.
- Extensively revised **Community Health Nursing Practice** chapter (Chapter 4) now includes discussions of home care and rural health care.
- **Nursing process content** has been condensed and is presented in Chapters 13, 14, and 15, making key concepts clearer for students.
- **Nursing Story** boxes present first-person accounts of issues in relation to chapter content.
- **References** have been updated throughout to include Canadian research and practice standards, such as the best nursing practice guidelines of Health Canada, Statistics Canada, the Canadian Nurses Association, and the Registered Nurses Association of Ontario. References have been organized by chapter and compiled at the end of the text.
- **Media Resources** boxes detail available electronic resources.
- Free **CD Companion** in each text has been enhanced to include Test-Taking Skills, in addition to Butterfield's Fluids and Electrolytes program, interactive exercises, and a glossary.
- Updated **Practical Nursing in Canada** appendix (Appendix A) provides important information on this nursing role in Canada.

- New **Laboratory Values** appendix (Appendix B) is a concise, up-to-date source of current laboratory values for use in clinical practice.

Ancillaries

For the Student

Free Companion CD-ROM in each text includes Test-Taking Skills and Review Questions, in addition to Butterfield's Fluids and Electrolytes program, interactive learning activities, and an audio glossary.

Evolve Course Web site enables students to access downloadable audio and video clips for on-the-go learning with portable media devices, plus review questions, Mosby's Nursing Skills video clips, audio chapter summaries, a searchable Spanish–English audio glossary, Butterfield's Fluids and Electrolytes Tutorial, test-taking tips, and chapter-specific Web links.

Study Guide and Skills Performance Checklists provide ideal supplements to help students understand and apply the content of the text. Each chapter includes multiple sections:

- Preliminary reading includes a chapter assignment from the text.
- Comprehensive understanding provides a variety of activities to reinforce the topics and main ideas from the text.
- Review questions are multiple-choice, requiring students to provide rationales for their answers. Answers and rationales are provided in the answer key.
- Clinical chapters include critical thinking models that expand the case study from the chapter's care plan; students are asked to develop a step in the model on the basis of the actions of the nurse and client in the scenario. This helps students learn to apply both content learned and the critical thinking synthesis model.
- Skills performance checklists are included so that students can evaluate skill competency.

Clinical Companion is a concise, portable guide that features all of the facts and figures that students need to know in their early clinical experiences.

Virtual Clinical Excursions is a workbook and CD-ROM package that provides a hands-on learning experience in which students care for a variety of clients on a multifloor virtual hospital.

Nursing Skills Online focuses on the skills that are most difficult to teach and those that pose the greatest risk to client safety; this one-of-a-kind, interactive, and evaluative online course engages students in media-rich learning modules with realistic, case-based lessons to help students review and evaluate their competency before performing skills in the clinical setting.

For the Instructor

Integrated lesson plans give you everything you need to deliver effective lectures, engage student learning, and provide application opportunities, including live links to teaching resources and classroom teaching strategies.

Evolve Online Courseware includes secure access to integrated lesson plans, an ExamView computerized test bank, an electronic image collection, PowerPoint slides, and all student online resources.

Mosby's Nursing Video Skills on DVD helps you show your students how to perform nursing skills safely. Version 3.0 includes all-new footage and an exciting, interactive format on basic, intermediate, and advanced DVDs. Sold separately.

Acknowledgements

Developing a nursing text for the Canadian market is an enormous undertaking, and in this fourth Canadian edition, every chapter has been written by expert Canadian nurses. We acknowledge the contributions of each of our Canadian authors, who developed and wrote outstanding material in a short time frame. Their dedication and expertise is evident throughout, and we thank them for the extraordinary effort they put forward to make this book a success.

The Editorial Advisory Board, composed of three experts—Dr. Shirley Solberg, Dr. Sally Thorne, and Dr. Ann Tourangeau—provided outstanding direction for the fourth Canadian edition. In addition, the appointment of section editors was a new feature of this edition. The individuals who served in this capacity, providing support to the authors and editors, were Dr. Barbara Astle, Dr. Sonya Grypma, and Dr. Nicole Letourneau.

Toni Chahley, Developmental Editor, provided excellent leadership and capable organization of all parts of the developmental process and has been extremely supportive of all the authors and editors. We are grateful to her for her skill, hard work, and dedication to the task. We would also like to thank Lise Dupont, Managing Production Editor, Elsevier Canada.

Ann Millar, Publisher, Elsevier Canada, is a visionary leader who was highly involved in the development of the fourth Canadian edition of *Canadian Fundamentals of Nursing*. We thank her for all her efforts; without her, this edition would not have been possible.

Janet C. Ross-Kerr
Marilynn J. Wood

Canadian Contributors

Kaysi Eastlick Kushner, RN, PhD
Associate Professor
University of Alberta
Edmonton, Alberta

Nancy Edgecombe, RN-NP, BN, MN, PhD
Assistant Professor
School of Nursing
Dalhousie University
Halifax, Nova Scotia

Frances Fothergill-Bourbonnais, RN, PhD
Full Professor
School of Nursing, Faculty of Health Sciences
University of Ottawa
Ottawa, Ontario

Jo-Ann E.T. Fox-Threlkeld, RN, BN, MSc, PhD
Professor Emeritus
McMaster University
Hamilton, Ontario

Nancy Goddard, RN, PhD
Nursing Instructor
Red Deer College
Red Deer, Alberta

Kathryn J. Hannah, RN, PhD
President
HECS Inc.
and
Professor (ADJ)
Department of Community Health Science
Faculty of Medicine
University of Calgary
Calgary, Alberta

Giuliana Harvey, RN, MN
Lecturer
University of Toronto
Toronto, Ontario

Kathy Hegadoren, RN, PhD
Professor
University of Alberta
Edmonton, Alberta

Deborah Hobbs, RN, BScN, CIC
Infection Control Practitioner
University of Alberta Hospital
Edmonton, Alberta

Carnett Howell, RN, MN
Clinical Nurse Specialist—Acute Care and
    Chronic Medicine
Mount Sinai Hospital
Toronto, Ontario

Jim Hunter, RN, MSN
Program Head, Year 2
British Columbia Institute of Technology
Burnaby, British Columbia

Kathleen F. Hunter, RN, NP, PhD GNC(C)
Assistant Professor
Faculty of Nursing, University of Alberta
and
Nurse Practitioner
Capital Health Specialized Geriatric Services
Edmonton, Alberta

Darlaine Jantzen, RN, MA, PhD(c)
University of Alberta
Nursing Faculty
Camosun College
Victoria, British Columbia

Willy Kabotoff, RN, BScN, MN
Faculty Lecturer
University of Alberta
Edmonton, Alberta

Anne Katz, RN, PhD
Adjunct Professor
University of Manitoba
Winnipeg, Manitoba

Margaret Ann Kennedy, RN, PhD
President
Kennedy Health Informatics Inc.
Merigomish, Nova Scotia

Rosemary Kohr, RN, PhD, ACNP(cert)
Advanced Practice Nurse
London Health Sciences Centre
and
Assistant Professor
Faculty of Health Sciences
University of Western Ontario
London, Ontario

Francis Loos, RN, MN, CNCC(C)
Clinical Nurse–Post Anesthetic Care Unit
Regina Qu'Appelle Health Region
Regina, Saskatchewan

Jeannie McClennon-Leong, RN, MN, APNP
ADN Instructor
Northeast Wisconsin Technical College
Green Bay, Wisconsin

Jill Milne, RN, PhD
Research Associate, Adjunct Assistant Professor
Faculty of Medicine
University of Calgary
Calgary, Alberta

Anita E. Molzahn, RN, MN, PhD
Professor and Dean
Faculty of Nursing
University of Alberta
Edmonton, Alberta

Judee E. Onyskiw, RN, BScN, MN, PhD
Educator, and Research and Scholarship Advisor
Faculty of Health and Community Studies
MacEwan College
Edmonton, Alberta

Jan Park Dorsay, RN(EC), MN, NP, CON(C)
Advanced Practice Nurse,
Rehabilitation
Hamilton Health Sciences
and
Assistant Clinical Professor
School of Nursing
McMaster University
Hamilton, Ontario

Barb Pesut, RN, PhD
Assistant Professor
School of Nursing
University of British Columbia Okanagan
Kelowna, British Columbia

Pammla Petrucka, RN, PhD
Associate Professor
University of Saskatchewan (Regina Site)
Regina, Saskatchewan

Shelley Raffin Bouchal, RN, PhD
Associate Professor
Faculty of Nursing
University of Calgary
Calgary, Alberta

Linda Reutter, RN, PhD
Professor
Faculty of Nursing
University of Alberta
Edmonton, Alberta

Daria Romaniuk, RN, BN, MN, PhD(c)
Assistant Professor
Daphne Cockwell School of Nursing
Ryerson University
Toronto, Ontario

Donna M. Romyn, RN, PhD
Director and Associate Professor
Centre for Nursing and Health Studies
Athabasca University
Athabasca, Alberta

Cheryl Sams, RN, MSN
Professor
Seneca College
Toronto, Ontario

Brett Sanderson, BScPT
Physiotherapist
Hamilton Health Sciences
Henderson Hospital
Hamilton, Ontario

Carla Shapiro, RN, MN
Instructor II
University of Manitoba
Winnipeg, Manitoba

D. Lynn Skillen, RN, PhD
Professor Emerita
University of Alberta
Edmonton, Alberta

Kathryn A. Smith Higuchi, RN, PhD
Assistant Professor
School of Nursing
University of Ottawa
Ottawa, Ontario

Shirley M. Solberg, RN, PhD
Professor
Memorial University of Newfoundland
St. John's, Newfoundland and Labrador

Tracey C. Stephen, RN, MN
Faculty Lecturer
University of Alberta
Edmonton, Alberta

Sally Thorne, RN, PhD
Professor and Director
University of British Columbia
Vancouver, British Columbia

Jill E. Vihos, RN, BScN, MN, PhD(c)
Faculty Lecturer
University of Alberta
Edmonton, Alberta

Fay F. Warnock, RN, PhD
Michael Smith Foundation for Health Research Scholar
Nurse Scientist, Children's and Women's Health
        Centre of British Columbia
and
Assistant Professor
School of Nursing
University of British Columbia
Vancouver, British Columbia

Kathryn Weaver, RN, PhD
Associate Professor
Faculty of Nursing
University of New Brunswick
Fredericton, New Brunswick

US Contributors

Marjorie Baier, RN, PhD
Associate Professor
School of Nursing
Southern Illinois University
Edwardsville, Illinois

Sylvia K. Baird, RN, BSN, MM
Manager of Nursing Quality
Spectrum Health
Grand Rapids, Michigan

Karen Balakas, RN, PhD, CNE
Associate Professor
Goldfarb School of Nursing at Barnes-Jewish College
St. Louis, Missouri

Lois Bentler-Lampe, RN, MS
Instructor
Saint Francis Medical Center College of Nursing
Peoria, Illinois

Sheryl Buckner, RN-BC, MS, CNE
Academic and Staff Developer and Clinical Instructor
College of Nursing
University of Oklahoma
Oklahoma City, Oklahoma

Jeri Burger, RN, PhD
Assistant Professor
College of Nursing and Health Professions
University of Southern Indiana
Evansville, Indiana

Janice C. Colwell, RN, MS, CWOCN, FAAN
Clinical Nurse Specialist
University of Chicago Hospitals
Chicago, Illinois

Eileen Costantinou, RN, MSN, BC
Consultant
Center for Practice Excellence
Barnes-Jewish Hospital
St. Louis, Missouri

Margaret Ecker, RN, MS
Director, Nursing Quality
Kaiser Permanente Los Angeles Medical Center
Los Angeles, California

Susan J. Fetzer, RN, PA, BSN, MSN, MBA, PhD
Associate Professor
College of Health and Human Services
University of New Hampshire
Durham, New Hampshire

Victoria N. Folse, APRN, BC, LCPC, PhD
Assistant Professor
School of Nursing, Illinois Wesleyan University
Bloomington, Illinois

Steve Kilkus, RN, MSN
Faculty
Edgewood College School of Nursing
Madison, Wisconsin

Judith Ann Kilpatrick, RN, MSN, DNSc
Assistant Professor
Widener University School of Nursing
Chester, Pennsylvania

Lori Klingman, RN, MSN
Faculty
School of Nursing
Ohio Valley General Hospital
McKees Rocks, Pennsylvania

Anahid Kulwicki, RN, DNS, FAAN
Deputy Director
Wayne County Department of Health and Human Services
and
Professor
Oakland University
School of Nursing
Rochester, Michigan

Annette Lueckenotte, RN, MS, BC, GNP, GCNS
Gerontologic Clinical Nurse Specialist
Barnes-Jewish West County Hospital
Creve Coeur, Missouri

Barbara Maxwell, RN, BSN, MS, MSN, CNS
Associate Professor of Nursing
Ulster Department of Nursing
The State University New York
Stone Ridge, New York

Elaine Neel, RN, BSN, MSN
Nursing Instructor
Graham Hospital School of Nursing
Canton, Illinois

Wendy Ostendorf, BSN, MS, EdD
Associate Professor
Neumann College
Aston, Pennsylvania

Patsy Ruchala, RN, DNSc
Director and Professor
Orvis School of Nursing
University of Nevada–Reno
Reno, Nevada

Lynn Schallom, MSN, CCRN, CCNS
Clinical Nurse Specialist
Surgical Critical Care
Barnes-Jewish Hospital
St. Louis, Missouri

Ann Tritak, BS, MS, EdD
Dean of Nursing
School of Nursing
Saint Peter's College
Jersey City, New Jersey

Janis Waite, RN, MSN, EdD
Professor of Nursing
Saint Francis Medical Center College of Nursing
Peoria, Illinois

Jill Weberski, RN, MSN, PCCN, CNS
Instructor
Saint Francis Medical Center College of Nursing
Peoria, Illinois

Mary Ann Wehmer, RN, MSN, CNOR
Nursing Faculty
College of Nursing and Health Professions
University of Southern Indiana
Evansville, Indiana

Joan Wentz, RN, MSN
(Retired) Assistant Professor of Nursing
Goldfarb School of Nursing at Barnes-Jewish College
St. Louis, Missouri

Katherine West, BSN, MSEd, CIC
Infection Control Consultant
Infection Control/Emerging Concepts, Inc.
Manassas, Virginia

Rita Wunderlich, RN, MSN(R), PhD
Chair, Baccalaureate Nursing Program
St. Louis University School of Nursing
St. Louis, Missouri

Valerie Yancey, RN, PhD
Associate Professor
Southern Illinois University
Edwardsville, Illinois

Reviewers

Catherine Aquino-Rusell, BScN, MN, PhD
Associate Professor, Faculty of Nursing
University of New Brunswick
Moncton, New Brunswick

Heidi Matarasso Bakerman, RN, BA, MScN
Nursing Instructor
Vanier College
St. Laurent, Quebec

Lisa Barrett, RN, MN, RPN
Faculty Lecturer, Faculty of Nursing
University of Alberta
Edmonton, Alberta

Kathleen Barrington, RN, MEd
Coordinator, PN Program
Centre for Nursing Studies
St. John's, Newfoundland and Labrador

Maureen Barry, RN, MScN
Senior Lecturer, Lawrence S. Bloomberg Faculty
of Nursing
University of Toronto
Toronto, Ontario

Zoraida DeCastro Beekhoo, RN, MA
Lecturer, Lawrence S. Bloomberg Faculty of Nursing
University of Toronto
Toronto, Ontario

Arleigh Bell, RN, BSN, MN
BSN Faculty
Kwantlen Polytechnic University
Surrey, British Columbia

Christine Boyle, RN, BScN, MA
Faculty
Mount Royal College
Calgary, Alberta

Roni Clubb, RN, BScN, MScN
Faculty, Practical Nursing Program
Saskatchewan Institute of Applied Science and Technology
Regina, Saskatchewan

Mary Jane Comiskey, RN, BScN, BEd
Professor, Nursing
School of Health and Community Services
Lambton College of Applied Arts and Technology
Sarnia, Ontario

Michelle Connell, BScN, MEd
Professor and Coordinator, Collaborative Nursing Degree
Program
Centennial College
Scarborough, Ontario

Donna Cooke, RN, BSN, MN
Faculty, Nursing Education Program
Saskatchewan Institute of Applied Science and Technology
Regina, Saskatchewan

Fiona D'Costa-Box, RN, BA (Hons.), BScN, MScN
Professor, Nursing
School of Health and Community Services
Lambton College of Applied Arts and Technology
Sarnia, Ontario

Julie Duff Cloutier, RN, BScN, MSc
Assistant Professor, School of Nursing
Laurentian University
Sudbury, Ontario

Lynne Esson, RN, BSN
Lecturer, School of Nursing
University of British Columbia
Vancouver, British Columbia

Wendy Fostey, RN, BHScN, MHScN
Professor, Nursing
NEOCNP Collaborative BScN Program
Sault College
Sault Ste. Marie, Ontario

Marla Fraser, RN, BSN
Faculty, Practical Nursing Program
Saskatchewan Institute of Science and Technology
Regina, Saskatchewan

Jacalynne Glover, RN, MN, IBCLC
Faculty, Nursing Education in Southwestern Alberta (NESA)
Lethbridge College
Lethbridge, Alberta

Jackie Halliday, RN, BSN, MN
Instructor, Faculty of Community and Health Studies BSN
Program
Kwantlen Polytechnic University
Surrey, British Columbia

Rae Harwood, RN, BN, MA
Clinical Course Leader, Faculty of Nursing
University of Manitoba
Winnipeg, Manitoba

Vicki Holmes, RN, BScN, MScN
Assistant Professor, School of Nursing
Thompson Rivers University
Kamloops, British Columbia

Kerri L. Honeychurch, RN, BScN, MEd
Coordinator and Professor, School of Health Sciences
Seneca College of Applied Arts and Technology
Toronto, Ontario

Jean Jackson, RN, MEd
Professor, School of Health and Community Services
Durham College
Oshawa, Ontario

Lynda Johnston, RN, BSN, MEd
Program Faculty, BSN Program
Douglas College
Coquitlam, British Columbia

Jo-Ann MacDonald, RN, BScN, MN, PhD(c)
Assistant Professor, Faculty of Nursing
University of Prince Edward Island
Charlottetown, Prince Edward Island

M. Star Mahara, RN, BSN, MSN
Assistant Professor, School of Nursing
Thompson Rivers University
Kamloops, British Columbia

Claire Marshall, RN, CMH, BTSN
Instructor, Practical Nursing Program
Vancouver Island University
Nanaimo, British Columbia

Karey D. McCullough, BScN, MScN, PhD(c)
Assistant Professor, School of Nursing
Nipissing University
North Bay, Ontario

Florence Melchior, RN, PhD
Nursing Instructor, Health Studies
Medicine Hat College
Medicine Hat, Alberta

Barbara Morrison, RN, HBScN, MEd
Professor, Nursing
Confederation College
Thunder Bay, Ontario

Enid Muirhead, RN, BScN, MEd
Clinical Associate
University of British Columbia
Vancouver, British Columbia

Denise Newton-Mathur, RN, BA, MA
Assistant Professor, School of Nursing
Laurentian University
Sudbury, Ontario

Wanda Pierson, BSN, MSN, MA, PhD
Chair, Nursing Department
Langara College
Vancouver, British Columbia

Joanne Profetto-McGrath, RN, BScN, BA Psych, MEd, PhD
Associate Professor, Faculty of Nursing
and
Associate Dean, Executive and Partnership Development
University of Alberta
Edmonton, Alberta

Michael Scarcello, RN, HBScN, MA(N)(c)
Professor, Practical Nursing Program
School of Health and Community Services
Confederation College
Thunder Bay, Ontario

Candide Sloboda, BN, MEd
Faculty Lecturer, Faculty of Nursing
University of Alberta
Edmonton, Alberta

Lynne Thibeault, RN(EC), BScN, MEd, DNP(c)
Professor, Nursing
Confederation College
Thunder Bay, Ontario

Wendy Wagner, RN, BScN, MA, CACE, RYT
Nursing Instructor
Malaspina University-College
Nanaimo, British Columbia

Molly Westland, RN, BScN, MN, CCHN(c)
Program Coordinator, Trent/Fleming School of Nursing
Trent University
Peterborough, Ontario

Lucille Wittstock, RN, MN
Associate Director, Undergraduate Student Affairs
School of Nursing
Dalhousie University
Halifax, Nova Scotia

Pat Woods, BSN, MSN
Student and Curriculum Coordinator, Department of Nursing
Langara College
Vancouver, British Columbia

1

Health and Wellness

Written by Linda Reutter, RN, PhD,

and Kaysi Eastlick Kushner, RN, PhD

media resources

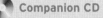 **Web Site**

- Audio Chapter Summaries
- Glossary
- Multiple-Choice Review Questions
- Student Learning Activities
- Weblinks

Companion CD

- Glossary
- Interactive Learning Activities
- Fluids and Electrolytes Tutorial
- Test-Taking Skills

Concepts of health and what determines health have changed significantly since the 1970s. This conceptual change has major implications for Canadian nursing in the twenty-first century because how you perceive health—and what determines it—influences the nature and scope of nursing practice. The importance of health to nursing is reflected in nursing models and frameworks, in which health is one of the four "metaparadigm" concepts along with *person, environment,* and *nursing* (see Chapter 6). In each framework, health concepts are congruent with the assumptions and focus of the model.

Conceptualizations of Health

Discussion about the nature of health revolves around its relationship to *disease, illness,* and *wellness.* Often, debates focus on whether health is defined in negative or positive terms. When health is negatively defined as the absence of disease, health and illness are represented on a continuum, with maximum health at one end and death at the other. When health is positively defined, however, health and illness are viewed as distinct but interrelated concepts. Therefore, a person can have disease, such as a chronic pathological condition, and have healthy characteristics as well.

Many people use the words *illness* and *disease* interchangeably. Others suggest that **disease** is an objective state of ill health, the pathological process of which can be detected by medical science, whereas **illness** is a subjective experience of loss of health (Jensen & Allen, 1993; Labonte, 1993; Naidoo & Wills, 1994). Figure 1–1 shows the relationships among health, illness, and disease.

Definitions of health beyond the absence of disease usually have multidimensional components, including physical, mental, social, and spiritual health (e.g., the widely accepted biopsychosocial conceptualization of health put forward by Engel in 1977). Although some scholars have considered this broad definition of health to be synonymous with wellness (Labonte, 1993; Pender et al., 2006), others have argued that health and wellness are different concepts. That is, others have argued that **health** is an objective process characterized by functional stability, balance, and integrity, whereas **wellness** is a subjective experience (Jensen & Allen, 1993; Orem, 1995).

The word *health* is derived from the Old English word *hoelth,* meaning whole of body. Historically, physical wholeness was important for social acceptance, and people with contagious or disfiguring diseases were often ostracized. Good health was considered natural, whereas disease was considered unnatural. As science progressed, disease was regarded less negatively because it could be countered by scientific medicine. After World War II, the World Health Organization (WHO, 1947) in its constitution defined health as "a state of complete physical, mental and social well-being, and not merely the absence of disease or infirmity." This is still the most commonly cited definition of health.

Classifications of Health Conceptualizations

Pender et al. (2006) classified health in three ways:

- **Health as stability.** Health is defined as the maintenance of physiological, functional, and social norms, and it relates to concepts of adaptation and homeostasis.
- **Health as actualization.** Health is defined as the actualization of human potential. Scholars and researchers who adhere to this definition often use the terms *health* and *wellness* interchangeably.
- **Health as actualization and stability.** Both actualization and stabilization concepts are incorporated in the definition of health as "the

actualization of inherent and acquired human potential through goal-directed behaviour, competent self-care and satisfying relationships with others, while making adjustments as needed to maintain structural integrity and harmony with relevant environments" (Pender et al., 2006, p. 23).

In 1984, the WHO updated its conceptualization of health as follows:

". . . the extent to which an individual or group is able, on the one hand, to realize aspirations and satisfy needs; and, on the other hand, to change or cope with the environment. Health is, therefore, seen as a resource for everyday life, not the objective of living; it is a positive concept emphasizing social and personal resources, as well as physical capacities." (p. 3)

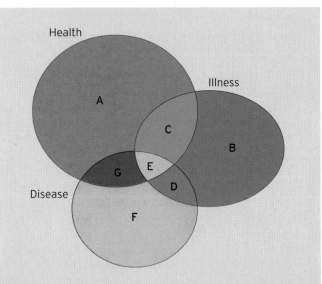

Legend

Circle A represents health or wellness, the clear area being experiences such as feeling vital, enjoying good social relationships, having a sense of purpose in life, and experiencing a connectedness to "community."

Circle B represents experiences of illness, the clear area representing illness that cannot be explained by conventional biomedical concepts and research.

Shaded area C is feeling "so-so," where little is required to tip one into wellness or illness.

Shaded area D is where a diagnosed pathology objectively validates and explains the subjective experience of illness.

Shaded area E represents feeling "so-so," being diagnosed with a pathology, and becoming sick.

Circle F represents diagnosed pathology, the clear area being undiagnosed or silent pathology, such as hypertension, CVD, congenital diseases, or cancers.

Shaded area G represents being diagnosed with a pathology, but still reporting oneself as feeling well or healthy.

Figure 1-1 Health, illness, and disease. **Source:** From Labonte, R. (1993). *Issues in health promotion series. 3. Health promotion and empowerment: Practice frameworks* (p. 18). Toronto, ON: Centre for Health Promotion, University of Toronto, & ParticipACTION.

Rather than viewing health as an ideal state of well-being (as in the 1947 WHO definition), this definition, incorporating both actualization and stability dimensions, suggests that people in a variety of situations—even those with physical disease or nearing death—could be considered healthy.

Labonte (1993) developed a multidimensional conceptualization of health that reflects both actualization and stability perspectives. Aspects include the following qualities:

- Feeling vitalized and full of energy.
- Having satisfying social relationships.
- Having a feeling of control over one's life and living conditions.
- Being able to do things that one enjoys.
- Having a sense of purpose.
- Feeling connected to community.

Using the WHO dimensions of physical, mental, and social well-being, Labonte (1993) categorized these characteristics into a Venn diagram (Figure 1–2). The diagram clearly depicts the concept of holism, whereby health is more than the sum of the component parts in that the interrelationships between and among different components result in different aspects of health.

Nurse scholars use nursing frameworks to conceptualize health in different ways (see Chapter 6). For example, the McGill model concept of health as coping and development is very congruent with the WHO (1984) definition (Gottlieb & Rowat, 1987). Jones and Meleis (1993) articulated health as empowerment: "health is being empowered to define, seek, and find conditions, resources, and processes to be an effective agent in meeting the significant needs perceived by individuals" (p. 12). This conceptualization is congruent with Labonte's (1993) focus and reflects the essence of health promotion, to be discussed later. In a review of the concept of health, Raeburn and Rootman (2007) suggested that in view of current realities of the

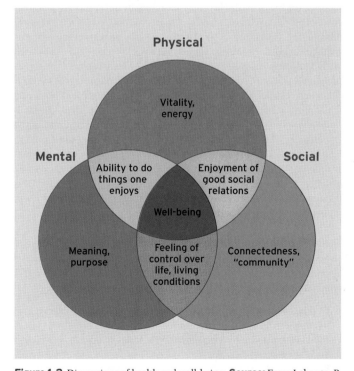

Figure 1-2 Dimensions of health and well-being. **Source:** From Labonte, R. (1993). *Issues in health promotion series. 3. Health promotion and empowerment: Practice frameworks* (p. 20). Toronto, ON: Centre for Health Promotion, University of Toronto, & ParticipACTION.

twenty-first century, a definition of health needs to be positive (not based on pathology or deficit), comprehensive (with a broad set of determinants), particularly attentive to the mental health dimension, and inclusive of quality of life and spirituality.

Historical Approaches to Health in Canada

Definitions of health emerge from different contexts. In modern times, the three major approaches to health have been medical, behavioural, and socioenvironmental (Labonte, 1993). These approaches offer a useful framework for examining the evolution of health orientations in Canada.

Medical Approach

The **medical approach**, which represents a stability orientation to health, dominated Western thinking for most of the twentieth century. It emphasizes that medical intervention restores health. Health problems are defined primarily as **physiological risk factors**—physiologically defined characteristics that are precursors to or risk factors for disease. Examples include hypertension, hypercholesterolemia, genetic predispositions, and obesity. The biopsychosocial view of health (Engel, 1977) includes psychological and social elements; however, in practice, a medical focus on pathology was retained (Antonovsky, 1987). In the medical approach, an adequate health care system is paramount to ensuring that populations remain healthy.

Focusing on treatment of disease was strongly supported after World War II, when new technological and scientific medical advances facilitated the medical approach. In Canada, postwar economic growth increased funding to build new hospitals. National health insurance was created to remove financial barriers to care. Many people believed that scientific medicine could solve most health problems and that accessible and quality health care (or, more correctly, illness care) would improve the health of Canadians. Within this approach, less emphasis was given to health promotion and disease prevention.

Behavioural Approach

By the early 1970s, increasingly large amounts of money were spent on health care, but the health status of the population did not improve proportionately. To better understand what contributed to illness and death, the Minister of Health and Welfare, Marc Lalonde, commissioned a study that resulted in the 1974 report *A New Perspective on the Health of Canadians*. This so-called *Lalonde Report* shifted emphasis from a medical to a **behavioural approach** to health. The report concluded that the traditional medical approach to health care was inadequate and that "further improvements in the environment, reductions in self-imposed risks, and a greater knowledge of human biology" were necessary to improve the health status of Canadians (p. 6). The *Lalonde Report* was the first modern government document in the Western world to acknowledge the inadequacy of a strictly biomedical health care system.

The *Lalonde Report* broadly defined health determinants as *lifestyle, environment, human biology,* and the *organization of health care.* This **health field concept** was widely used, modified, and expanded by other countries, and its release was a turning point in broadening Canadians' attitudes about factors that contribute to health, along with the role of government in promoting health (Health Canada, 1998). Of the four determinants, lifestyle received the most attention, perhaps because lifestyle behaviours contributed to chronic diseases (such as cancer and heart disease) and to injuries—both of which are the leading causes of morbidity and mortality in Canada (Labonte, 1993). In addition, greater understanding of behavioural social psychology revealed factors that motivated individuals to engage in healthy or unhealthy behaviours. In 1978, the Canadian government established the Health Promotion Directorate in the Department of National Health and Welfare, the first official health promotion undertaking of its kind. Its aim was to decrease **behavioural risk factors** such as smoking, substance abuse, lack of exercise, and an unhealthy diet. Public health programs such as Operation Lifestyle and ParticipACTION were developed through this department.

The behavioural approach places responsibility for health on the individual, thereby favouring health promotion strategies such as education and social marketing. Strategies are often based on the assumption that if people know the risk factors for disease, then they will engage in healthy behaviours. Indeed, health-enhancing practices among Canadians increased during this time. With the ParticipACTION initiative, for instance, many people increased their physical activity. Antismoking campaigns led to a substantial decrease in tobacco use.

Socioenvironmental Approach

By the mid-1980s, however, the behavioural approach to health and illness prevention fell into disfavour. Studies showed that lifestyle improvements were made primarily by well-educated, well-employed, and higher income Canadians. The *Lalonde Report* was criticized for deflecting attention from the environment and for how environment and lifestyle were defined. Lifestyle was viewed as being within an individual's control, with health risks as "self-imposed" behaviours. This supported "victim-blaming" and views that health was largely an individual responsibility. Critics suggested that health-related behaviours could not be separated from the social contexts (environments) in which they occurred. For example, living and working conditions were perceived as barriers to engaging in healthy behaviours (Labonte, 1993).

In the **socioenvironmental approach**, health is closely tied to social structures. For example, poverty and unhealthy physical and social environments, such as air pollution, poor water quality, and workplace hazards, are recognized as influencing health directly. Thus, Canadian public health professionals expanded Lalonde's (1974) health field concept to emphasize the social context of health and the relationship between personal health behaviours and social and physical environments (Hancock & Perkins, 1985).

Internationally, more attention was also given to the social context of health. The WHO Regional Conference in Europe produced a discussion paper identifying the social conditions that influence health (WHO, 1984). Just as Canada led the behavioural approach to health with the *Lalonde Report,* it was now instrumental in focusing on social and environmental conditions. In 1986, the First International Conference on Health Promotion was held in Ottawa, sponsored by the WHO, the Canadian Public Health Association (CPHA), and Health and Welfare Canada. It produced a watershed document—the *Ottawa Charter for Health Promotion*—that supported a socioenvironmental approach. This document has since been translated into more than 40 languages.

Ottawa Charter. The *Ottawa Charter for Health Promotion* (WHO, 1986) identified **prerequisites for health** as peace, shelter, education, food, income, a stable ecosystem, sustainable resources, social justice, and equity. These prerequisites clearly go beyond lifestyles or personal health practices to include social, environmental, and political contexts.

They place responsibility for health on society rather than only on individuals. The *Charter's* focus on social justice and equity also incorporated the concept of *empowerment*—a person's ability to define, analyze, and solve problems—as an important goal for health care professionals (Registered Nurses Association of British Columbia, 1994). Indeed, Wallerstein (1992) contended that powerlessness could be the underlying health determinant influencing other risk factors. Consequently, health promotion literature emphasizes the concept of empowerment. The *Ottawa Charter* incorporated the then-new 1984 WHO definition of health (discussed previously), which identified health as having both social and individual dimensions, emphasized its dynamic and positive nature, and viewed it as a fundamental human right (Naidoo & Wills, 1994). The *Charter* outlined five major strategies to promote health: building healthy public policy, creating supportive environments, strengthening community action, developing personal skills, and reorienting health services (detailed later in this chapter).

Achieving Health for All. Concepts from the *Ottawa Charter* were incorporated into another important Canadian document, *Achieving Health for All: A Framework for Health Promotion* (Epp, 1986). This report, developed under the leadership of Jake Epp, Minister of National Health and Welfare from 1984 to 1989, became Canada's blueprint for achieving the WHO goal of "Health for All 2000" (Figure 1–3).

Epp's (1986) report identified three major health challenges: reducing inequities, increasing prevention, and enhancing coping mechanisms. It acknowledged disparities in health, particularly between low- and high-income people, and that living and working conditions were critical determinants of health. It emphasized the need for effective ways to prevent injuries, illnesses, chronic conditions, and disabilities. Enhancing coping was an acknowledgment that the dominant diseases in Canada were chronic conditions that could not be cured. Therefore, the challenge is assisting people to manage and cope with chronic conditions in order to live meaningful and productive lives. The *Epp Report* emphasized society's responsibility for providing supports for people experiencing chronic medical conditions, stress, mental illness, and problems associated with aging, as well as the need for supports for caregivers. The report identified self-care, mutual aid, and healthy environments as ways that these challenges could be addressed, which reflected both personal and social responsibility. Specific strategies to address the challenges included fostering public participation, strengthening community health services, and coordinating healthy public policy.

The *Ottawa Charter* and the *Epp Report* each reflect a socioenvironmental approach in which health is seen as more than just the absence of disease and engaging in healthy behaviours; rather, this approach emphasizes connectedness, self-efficacy, and capacity to engage in meaningful activities (see Figure 1–2).

Risk Factors and Risk Conditions. Labonte (1993) categorized the major determinants of health in a socioenvironmental approach as psychosocial risk factors and socioenvironmental risk conditions:

- **Psychosocial risk factors** are complex psychological experiences resulting from social circumstances that include isolation, lack of social support, limited social networks, low self-esteem, self-blame, and low perceived power.
- **Socioenvironmental risk conditions** are social and environmental living conditions that include poverty, low educational or occupational status, dangerous or stressful work, dangerous physical environments, pollution, discrimination, relative political or economic powerlessness, and inequalities of income or power.

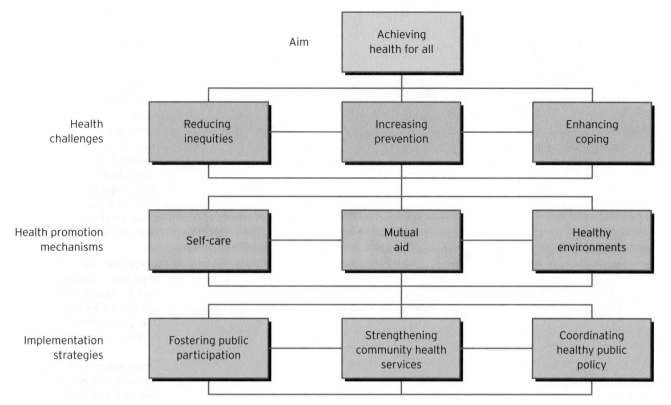

Figure 1-3 Achieving health for all: A framework for health promotion. **Source:** From Epp, J. (1986). *Achieving health for all: A framework for health promotion* (p. 8). Ottawa, ON: Health and Welfare Canada. Reproduced with the permission of the Minister of Public Works and Government Services Canada, 2005.

According to a socioenvironmental approach to health, political, social, and cultural forces affect health and well-being both directly and indirectly through their influence on personal health behaviours. Socioenvironmental risk conditions can contribute to psychosocial risk factors, which can then result in unhealthy behaviours (Figure 1–4). This means that health care professionals should recognize the influence of environment on personal behaviours and that "health-inhibiting" behaviours could be coping strategies for managing the stress created by living and working conditions that decrease access to resources. In other words, "to change behaviour it may be necessary to change more than behaviour" (Wilkinson, 1996, p. 64). For example, in addition to working "downstream" to assist people who are experiencing the negative health effects of socioenvironmental conditions, nurses need to work "upstream" by advocating for policies that ensure affordable housing, financial support to clients with low incomes, and safe, fulfilling work environments.

Strategies for Population Health. In Canada, the determinants of health have been further emphasized through the **population health approach**. This approach, initiated by the Canadian Institute for Advanced Research, was officially endorsed by the federal, provincial, and territorial ministers of health in the report titled *Strategies for Population Health: Investing in the Health of Canadians* (Federal, Provincial, and Territorial Advisory Committee on Population Health [ACPH], 1994). In a population health approach, "the entire range of known individual and collective factors and conditions that determine population health status, and the interactions among them, are taken into account in planning action to improve health" (Health Canada, 1998). The population health approach emphasizes the use of epidemiological data to determine the etiology of health and disease.

The key health determinants identified in the *Strategies for Population Health* report are as follows:

- Income and social status.
- Social support networks.
- Education.
- Employment and working conditions.
- Physical environments.
- Biology and genetic endowment.
- Personal health practices and coping skills.
- Healthy child development.
- Health services.

In 1996, Health Canada added *gender, culture,* and *social environments* to this list. Note that the list includes determinants at the individual level (personal health practices and coping skills; biology and genetic endowment) and at the population level (education, employment, and income distribution).

Jakarta Declaration. The *Jakarta Declaration on Health Promotion into the 21st Century* (WHO, 1997) emerged from the 4th International Conference on Health Promotion, the first to be held in a developing country and to involve the private sector. The *Jakarta Declaration* affirmed the *Ottawa Charter* prerequisites for health; added four other prerequisites (*empowerment of women, social security, respect for human rights,* and *social relations*); and declared poverty to be the greatest threat to health. The Declaration identified the following priorities for action: promoting social responsibility for health in public and private sectors; increasing investments for health in all sectors; consolidating and expanding partnerships for health to all levels of government and the private sector; increasing community capacity and empowering the individual; and securing adequate infrastructure for health promotion.

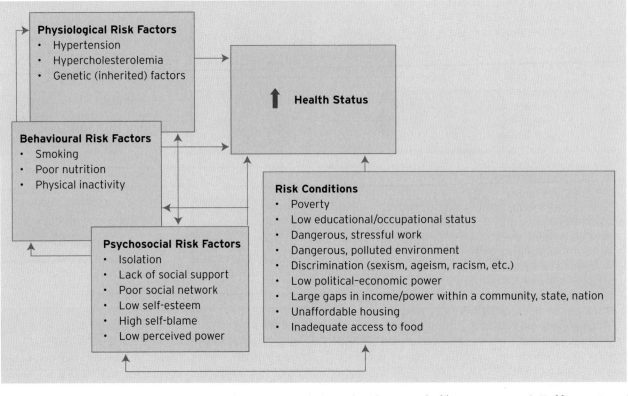

Figure 1-4 Socioenvironmental approach to health. **Source:** From Labonte, R. (1993). *Issues in health promotion series. 3. Health promotion and empowerment: Practice frameworks* (p. 11). Toronto, ON: Centre for Health Promotion, University of Toronto, & ParticipACTION.

Bangkok Charter. The *Bangkok Charter for Health Promotion in a Globalized World* (WHO, 2005) affirmed health as a human right and emphasized mental and spiritual well-being as important elements. It identified critical factors influencing health, such as the increasing inequalities within and between countries, global environmental change, and urbanization. The *Charter* emphasized strong political action and sustained advocacy, empowering communities with adequate resources, and corporate sector commitment to healthy workplaces and ethical business practices.

Toronto Charter. In the early to middle 1990s, Canadian social and health policies resulted in increased social and economic inequalities (Bryant, 2002; Raphael et al., 2004) and health disparities. These concerns culminated in the *Toronto Charter on the Social Determinants of Health,* which identified the following social determinants as particularly important for health: early childhood development, education, employment and working conditions, food security, health care services, housing shortages, income and its equitable distribution, social safety nets, social exclusion, and unemployment and employment security. **Social determinants of health** can be defined as "the *economic and social conditions* that influence the health of individuals, communities, and jurisdictions as a whole . . . [and] determine the extent to which a person possesses the physical, social, and personal resources to identify and achieve personal aspirations, satisfy needs, and cope with the environment" (Raphael, 2004, p. 1; italics ours). This conceptualization of health determinants emphasizes *societal* responsibility for reducing health disparities because it focuses on how a society distributes economic and social resources through its economic and social policies.

Concern about **health disparities** (i.e., differences in health status among different population groups) has been raised worldwide. The WHO Commission on Social Determinants of Health (WHO,

2006) was charged with developing strategies to narrow health disparities through action on the social determinants of health. Nationally, the Health Disparities Task Group (2005), commissioned by the Public Health Agency of Canada (PHAC), identified socioeconomic status, Aboriginal identity, gender, and geographic location as the most important factors related to health disparities. Health disparities are associated with inequitable access (unfair or unjust lack of access) to health determinants, resulting from economic and social policies. You will see how some of these factors play out in the discussion of determinants in the following sections.

Determinants of Health

The following section introduces you to some of the major determinants of health affecting Canadians (Health Canada, 1996). Although each determinant contributes individually to health (enhances or inhibits health), the determinants are also interrelated and influence each other.

Income and Social Status (Income Distribution)

Income and social status is the greatest **determinant of health** (Canadian Institute for Health Information [CIHI], 2004; Raphael et al., 2004). According to Statistics Canada pretax low-income cut-offs in 2004, 16% of Canadians lived in poverty, with much higher rates among single mothers (47%) and unattached individuals younger than 65 years (38%) (National Council of Welfare, 2007) and among Aboriginal peoples (34%), Canadians of colour (28%), people with disabilities (23%), and recent urban immigrants (43%) (Canadian Council on Social Development, 2007).

Poverty exerts its effect on health through lack of material resources that support health, through higher levels of psychosocial stress, and through health-threatening behaviours to cope with limited resources and stress (Raphael, 2004). Low-income Canadians are more likely to die early and to suffer from most diseases, regardless of age, sex, race, culture, or place of residence. It is estimated that 23% of Canadians' premature loss of life can be accounted for by income differences (Raphael, 2004). People with lower incomes are more likely to have chronic health problems, particularly cardiovascular disease and type II diabetes (Raphael et al., 2003; Raphael & Farrell, 2002; Wilkins et al., 2002); lower self-esteem, lower sense of mastery and coherence; and higher levels of depression (Federal, Provincial, and Territorial ACPH, 1999).

Low birth weight, an important marker for subsequent poor child and adult health, has a 43% higher incidence in poor neighbourhoods than in higher income neighbourhoods (Wilkins et al., 2002). Children living in poverty are more likely to have chronic diseases such as asthma, to visit emergency rooms, and to die from injuries (Canadian Institute on Children's Health, 2000) and are at greater risk for cognitive difficulties, delayed vocabulary development, and behavioural problems (CIHI, 2004).

With each step up the economic ladder, Canadians' health status improves. This suggests that ill health is related to more than absolute material deprivation. Social deprivation may also influence health, perhaps through its effects on personal control and uncertainty (Wilkinson & Marmot, 1998).

Income inequality (i.e., the increasing gap between the rich and the poor [Dunn, 2002; Phipps, 2003]), also influences population health, and some academics have suggested that it is the greatest threat to the well-being of Western societies (Kawachi & Kennedy, 1997). Countries with economic inequality have higher levels of poverty, fewer public services, weaker social safety nets (Raphael, 2004), and lower overall health and life expectancies (Dunn, 2002; Wilkinson, 1996).

Social Support Networks

Social support affects health, health behaviours, and health care utilization (Carpiano, 2007; Stewart, 2000) through practical, emotional, informational, and affirmational support (House, 1981). Indeed, some experts believe that relationships may be as important to health as established risk factors such as obesity, smoking, and high blood pressure (Federal, Provincial, and Territorial ACPH, 1999). A strong body of research links social support with positive health outcomes (Berkman, 1995; Carpiano, 2007; Cohen, 1992; Tomaka et al., 2006).

In general, Canadians have reported high levels of support (Federal, Provincial, and Territorial ACPH, 1999). Four of five Canadians reported they had someone to confide in, whom they could count on in a crisis or for advice, and who made them feel loved and cared for. Nevertheless, men, single parents, and lower income Canadians generally reported less support than did their respective counterparts. Support from families and friends and from informal and formal groups can provide practical aid during times of crisis and emotional support in times of distress and change. Social support can decrease stress (Kosteniuk & Dickinson, 2003). Social support also assists coping and behavioural changes and can help individuals solve problems and maintain a sense of mastery and control over their lives. A survey of young parents in Alberta identified spouses, family, and friends as major sources of support in encouraging healthy behaviours (exercise, diet) by providing emotional, affirmational, and practical support, including child care and financial assistance (Reutter et al., 2001). In another study, a support intervention helped mothers of very preterm infants gain confidence in their parenting skills and understand their infants' medical conditions (Preyde, 2007).

Education and Literacy

Education and literacy are important influences on health status because they affect many other health determinants. Literacy can influence health both directly (e.g., medication use, safety practices) and indirectly through use of services, lifestyles, income, work environments, and stress levels. For example, people with low literacy skills are more likely to be unemployed, earn minimum wages in unskilled jobs, and make less use of preventive services (Rootman & Ronson, 2005). Education increases job opportunities and income security, which provide knowledge and skills to solve problems and gain a sense of control (PHAC, 2004). People with higher education levels tend to smoke less, be more physically active, and have access to healthier foods and physical environments (Federal, Provincial, and Territorial ACPH, 1999).

Employment and Working Conditions

Employment and working conditions significantly affect physical, mental, and social health. Paid work provides financial resources, a sense of identity and purpose, social contacts, and opportunities for personal growth (CPHA, 1996a). Unemployed people have reduced life expectancy and experience significantly more health problems than do employed people (Bartley et al., 1999).

Working conditions themselves can support health or pose health hazards. Healthy workplaces include job and employment security, safe physical conditions, reasonable work pace, low stress, opportunities for self-expression and individual development, participation, and work–life balance (Jackson, 2004). Temporary employees, part-time workers, and people working in low-wage jobs have high levels of job insecurity and frequent periods of unemployment. Often such jobs do not provide benefits or pensions, which can lead to uncertainty and stress (Menendez et al., 2007; Tompa et al., 2007). In 2000, more than one in four Canadian workers believed that their place of work was not healthy (Canadian Policy Research Networks, 2008). One third of Canadian workers in 2003 reported high stress at work, with even higher rates (45%) for health care workers (Wilkins, 2007). Indeed, the concern regarding negative workplace conditions in the health sector is considerable; nurses have had the highest or second-highest rates of absenteeism of all workers in Canada since the early 1990s (Villeneuve & MacDonald, 2006). Workplace stress is linked to increased risk of physical injuries, high blood pressure, cardiovascular disease, depression, and increases in tobacco and alcohol use (Jackson, 2004). In 2003, almost 10% of Canadian workers in trades, transport, and equipment operation sustained on-the-job injuries, which is more than four times the rate among workers in the "white-collar" sector (Wilkins & Mackenzie, 2007).

Physical Environments

Housing, indoor air quality, and community planning are important determinants of health. Contaminants in air, water, food, and soil also adversely affect health, sometimes contributing to cancer, birth defects, respiratory illness, and gastrointestinal ailments. Children from low-income families, who often live in substandard housing and in neighbourhoods near highways and industrial areas, are particularly likely to be exposed to these contaminants (Federal, Provincial, and Territorial ACPH, 1999). Asthma, which is characterized by high sensitivity to airborne contaminants, is the most common chronic respiratory disease among children, accounting for 25% of all school absenteeism (Canadian Council on Social Development, 2006); children in poverty are particularly vulnerable to this disease (Lethbridge & Phipps, 2005).

Involuntary exposure to tobacco smoke (second-hand smoke) has received considerable attention in Canada. Children exposed to tobacco smoke are at increased risk for sudden infant death syndrome

(SIDS), acute respiratory infections, ear problems, and reduced lung development, and exposure of adults to second-hand smoke can lead to coronary heart disease and lung cancer (US Department of Health and Human Services, 2006). Municipalities throughout Canada have incorporated smoking bans in public places, which has reduced exposure to second-hand smoke. In 2005, 23% of nonsmokers reported regular exposure in at least one venue (public place, home, or vehicles), and children were at highest risk for exposure (Shields, 2007).

Another important aspect of the environment is affordable and adequate housing. Homelessness in Canada is increasing, in part because of reduced government funding of social housing and lack of affordable rental accommodation (Bryant, 2004; Khandor & Mason, 2007). The number of working poor homeless is also on the rise, particularly in areas experiencing economic boom, such as Alberta. Homeless populations are at greater risk for a variety of health problems, including mental illness, substance abuse, suicide, tuberculosis, injuries and assaults, chronic medical conditions (e.g., respiratory and musculoskeletal), and poor oral and dental health, and for early death (Frankish et al., 2005; Khandor & Mason, 2007). Whereas inadequate housing can affect health directly, lack of affordable housing can also *indirectly* affect health through its influence on other determinants (Bryant, 2004). Spending a disproportionate amount of income on rent, for example, reduces the amount of money that families can spend on food, clothing, recreation, and health care.

The determinant of physical environment also includes the effects of climate change on the health of populations and the planet itself. The Canadian Nurses Association and Canadian Medical Association (2005) developed position statements on ecosystem health and environmentally responsible activity in the health sector. The need for sustainable ecosystems, included as a prerequisite for health in the *Ottawa Charter,* is becoming more critical.

Biological and Genetic Endowment

Heredity is strongly influenced by social and physical environments, and considerable effort has been expended to prevent congenital defects through monitoring and improved preconception and prenatal care (Federal, Provincial, and Territorial ACPH, 1999). This effort has led to substantial decreases in anomalies at birth.

Age is also a strong determinant of health. Many older people develop chronic diseases, although disability can be reduced with healthy aging (Healthy Aging and Wellness Working Group, 2006). Indeed, 70% of older people in Canada report good overall health, including good functional health and independence in activities of daily living (Shields & Martel, 2006). Nurses need to consider how much of the decline associated with aging is related to biological aging versus other determinants such as socioeconomic status, social support, and individual health practices.

Individual Health Practices and Coping Skills

Effective coping skills help people face challenges without resorting to risk behaviours such as substance abuse. Many so-called risk behaviours may, in fact, be coping strategies for stress and strain caused by living circumstances. For example, considerable evidence reveals that low-income women use smoking as a coping strategy (Stewart et al., 2004). Three risk behaviours with major detrimental health consequences are physical inactivity, poor nutrition, and tobacco use.

Physical inactivity is a major risk factor for some types of cancer, diabetes, cardiovascular disease, osteoporosis, obesity, hypertension, depression, stress, and anxiety. In 2004, just over half (52%) of Canadians aged 12 and older were at least moderately active during their leisure time (equivalent to walking at least 30 to 60 minutes a day). Those who were active were more likely to rate their health as excellent or very good and to report lower levels of stress and were less likely to be overweight, obese, or hypertensive (Gilmour, 2007).

Poor nutrition, particularly overconsumption of fats, sugars, and salt, is linked to such diseases as some cancers, cardiovascular diseases, type 2 diabetes, hypertension, osteoarthritis, and gallbladder disease and to functional limitations and disabilities (Tjepkema, 2006). Obesity is now considered a major public health problem. The 2004 Canadian Community Health Survey (CCHS) revealed that 23% of adult Canadians were obese (body mass index [BMI] of 30 or more) and 36% were overweight (Shields 2006); as BMI increased, so did the likelihood of reporting high blood pressure, diabetes, and heart disease. About 26% of children (aged 2–17 years) were overweight or obese (Shields, 2006). The 2004 CCHS (Nutrition section) revealed that 70% of children aged 4–8 years ate fewer than the minimum five servings of vegetables and fruit daily. Moreover, 25% of Canadians overall (and one third of teenagers aged 14–18) had eaten at fast-food outlets the previous day (Garriguet, 2007), which feature foods high in fats and salt. Several factors influence food consumption patterns, including household income, food advertising, and availability of nutritious choices. Food insecurity (the limited or uncertain availability of nutritious foods) is a growing problem in Canada. In 2004, more than 40% of households with low or lower middle incomes reported food insecurity (Ledrou & Gervais, 2005); those receiving social assistance were particularly vulnerable. Food insecurity is significantly associated with multiple chronic conditions, obesity, distress, and depression (Che & Chen, 2001; Tarasuk, 2004).

Tobacco use remains the leading preventable cause of death, disease, and disability (Makamowski Illing & Kaiserman, 2004). Smoking is linked to many diseases, such as cancer, cardiovascular disease, and respiratory illnesses, and it reduces the health of smokers in general (US Department of Health and Human Services, 2004). The smoking rate in Canada in 2007 was 19% (Health Canada, 2008). People most likely to smoke are men and women in their 40s, those living in poverty (Physicians for a Smoke-free Canada, 2005), and Aboriginal people (Health Canada, 2007) People with mental illness are twice as likely as the general population to smoke tobacco and to smoke more heavily (Lasser et al., 2000).

Clearly, many factors influence individual health behaviours (e.g., income, education, gender, culture, and social support). Resources to develop and maintain health-enhancing behaviours need to include not only health education but also social policies such as income security and anti-smoking legislation to make healthy choices the "easy" choices.

Healthy Child Development

All determinants influence child development, but healthy child development is a separate determinant because of its importance to lifelong health. Increasing evidence reveals that events during conception and through the age of 6 years influence children's health for the rest of their lives (CIHI, 2004). Three conditions for healthy child development are adequate and equitable income, effective parents and families, and supportive community environments (CIHI, 2004; Stroick & Jenson, 1999).

From conception to birth, two significant health risks are low birth weight and maternal tobacco, alcohol, and drug use (Steinhauer, 1998). Low birth weight contributes to perinatal illness and death; is associated with higher rates of long-term health problems, including cerebral palsy and learning difficulties, and with more frequent hospitalizations (Canadian Institute on Children's Health, 2000); and is related to development of chronic diseases in adulthood, especially heart disease and type II diabetes (Raphael et al., 2003; Raphael & Farrell, 2002). From birth through the toddler years, family environment is important, particularly establishing attachment to a primary caregiver during the first two years of life (Steinhauer, 1998). Throughout the toddler, preschool, and school-aged years, meeting a child's development needs is crucial. Family conflict, violence, and poverty threaten healthy child development. Schools in which students feel secure, respected, challenged, and cared for help ensure that children succeed academically. Community support is also important (Steinhauer, 1998).

Quality early childhood education and care are particularly important in early child development, so much so that they have been singled out by some researchers as a combined social determinant of health (Friendly, 2004). High-quality programs promote cognitive development and social competence and support parents in education and employment. Canada has acknowledged the importance of early childhood intervention through its Early Childhood Development Initiative (Health Council of Canada, 2006); however, Canada lacks a national child care program.

Health Services

Approximately 25% of a population's health status is attributed to the quality of health care services (Saskatchewan Public Health Association, 1994). Quality, accessible acute-care treatment, long-term care, home care, and preventive services are therefore important. More funding is given to acute-care services than to health promotion and disease prevention, and yet the latter services contribute even more to population health. Prenatal care, well-child and immunization clinics, education services about healthy lifestyles, and services that maintain older adults' health and independence are important examples of preventive and primary health care services (discussed further in Chapters 2 and 4) that Canadians should continue to develop. Canada's national health insurance scheme is considered a hallmark of society. Principles of the *Canada Health Act*—universality, portability, accessibility, comprehensiveness, and public administration—apply to the provision of medically insured services. Increasingly, the trends in health care service provision are from institutionalized care to community-based care, toward decision making that is based on the best available evidence, and toward more regional administration. In Canada, considerable monies have been invested in initiatives that incorporate principles of primary health care; however, the progress in this regard has been relatively slow.

Gender

Gender is "the array of society-determined roles, personality traits, attitudes, behaviours, values, relative power, and influence that society ascribes to the two sexes on a differential basis" (PHAC, 2004). Many health issues are a function of gender-based social roles, and gender can influence health status, behaviours, and care (Spitzer, 2005). In Canada, men are more likely than women to die prematurely, largely as a result of heart disease, unintentional fatal injuries, cancer, and suicide. Women, however, are more likely to suffer from depression, stress (often resulting from efforts to balance work and family life), chronic conditions such as arthritis and allergies, and injuries and death from family violence (Federal, Provincial, and Territorial ACPH, 1999). Moreover, gender influences men's and women's experience of sex-specific health concerns (e.g., pregnancy, prostate cancer, presentation of cardiovascular signs and symptoms), exposure to potential risk conditions (e.g., caregiving demands as traditionally women's responsibility), and interactions with health care professionals (e.g., gender stereotypes, medicalization of health experience) (Pederson & Raphael, 2006).

Culture

Cultural and ethnic factors influence people's interactions with a health care system, their participation in prevention and health promotion programs, their access to health information, their health-related lifestyle choices, and their understanding of health and illness (Health Canada, 1996). Cultural factors also influence whether and how determinants are met (see Chapter 10). For example, among immigrants and refugees, unmet expectations and challenges to successful social integration negatively impact individual health (Simich et al., 2003, 2005). Language differences can lead to isolation and decreased social support networks. Prejudice can cause individuals to be denied opportunities for education, employment, and access to housing (Health Canada, 1996). First Nations people are much more likely to suffer ill health; however, it is important to acknowledge the intersection of culture with other health determinants such as social support and income.

Social Environments

Social environments are defined as "the array of values and norms of a society [that] influence in varying ways the health and well-being of populations. In addition, social stability, recognition of diversity, safety, good working relationships, and cohesive communities provide a supportive society that reduces or avoids many potential risks to good health" (PHAC, 2004). The social environment is clearly related to other factors and expands on the social support determinant by incorporating broader community characteristics, norms, and values. Healthy social environments include freedom from discrimination and prejudice—particularly for people marginalized by income, age, gender, activity limitations, ethnicity, and sexual orientation. The determinant of social environment is also evident in the *Jakarta Declaration's* prerequisites of human rights, social security, and social relations (WHO, 1997). These prerequisities relate to social exclusion——the process by which people are denied opportunities to participate in many aspects of cultural, economic, social, and political life (Galabuzi, 2004). People most likely to be excluded are poor citizens, Aboriginal people, New Canadians, and members of racialized or nonwhite groups. Social exclusion limits people's access to the resources that support health and their participation in community life (Stewart et al., 2008).

Another important aspect of the social environment is the absence of violence, both in the home and in the community. In 2004, 7% of Canadians aged 15 years and older had experienced spousal violence in the previous 5 years; Aboriginal people were at a three-fold greater risk, and women were more likely to suffer from serious types of violence. Children accounted for 21% of cases of physical assault and 61% of cases of sexual assault, and close to 40% of elderly women suffered some kind of assault from family members (Canadian Centre for Justice Statistics, 2005). The health effects of family violence are devastating, for those experiencing or exposed to violence and for the perpetrators, and include psychological, physical, behavioural, academic, sexual, interpersonal, self-perceptual, or spiritual consequences, which may appear immediately or over time (Department of Justice Canada, 2008).

Violence is also experienced in other venues, particularly schools and workplaces. More than one third (36%) of Canadian students in grades 6–10 reported being victims of bullying. Victimized children are at risk for anxiety, depression, loss of self-esteem, and somatic complaints; perpetrators are also at risk for long-term problems such as antisocial behaviour and substance use (Craig & Edge, 2008). Health care workers, including nurses, have experienced violence perpetrated by clients, family members, and coworkers (Duncan et al., 2001).

Strategies to Influence Health Determinants

Health Promotion and Disease Prevention

The understanding that health is qualitatively different from disease has led to a differentiation of the concepts of health promotion and disease prevention, although they are interrelated. Pender et al. (2006) differentiated between health promotion and disease prevention as follows: **health promotion** is "directed toward increasing the level of well-being and self-actualization" (p. 37); **disease prevention** (particularly primary prevention) is "action to avoid illness/disease" (p. 36). On the other hand, other researchers consider health promotion as one aspect of primary prevention (Leavell & Clark, 1965; Neuman, 1995) and not necessarily disease specific (Leavell & Clark, 1965). In contrast, the *Ottawa Charter* views health promotion as the overarching concept, defined as "the process of enabling people to increase control over, and improve, their health" (WHO, 1986). The following more comprehensive definition was offered by Nutbeam (1998):

> *"Health promotion represents a comprehensive social and political process, it not only embraces actions directed at strengthening the skills and capabilities of individuals, but also action directed towards changing social, environmental and economic conditions so as to alleviate their impact on public and individual health. Health promotion is the process of enabling people to increase control over the determinants of health and thereby improve their health. Participation is essential to sustain health promotion action."* (p. 351)

Three levels of disease prevention correspond to the natural history of disease:

- *Primary prevention* activities protect against a disease before signs and symptoms occur (prepathogenesis stage of disease). Examples include immunization (to prevent infectious diseases) and reduction of risk factors (such as inactivity, smoking, and exposure to air pollution).
- *Secondary prevention* activities promote early detection of disease once pathogenesis has occurred, so that prompt treatment can be initiated to halt disease and limit disability. Examples include preventive screening for cancer (e.g., mammography, testicular self-examination); blood pressure screening to detect hypertension; and blood glucose screening to detect diabetes.
- *Tertiary prevention* activities are initiated in the convalescence stage of disease and are directed toward minimizing residual disability and helping people to live productively with limitations. An example is a cardiac rehabilitation program after a myocardial infarction.

Nursing strategies guided by a prevention framework focus on assessment and alleviation of risk factors for disease. On the other hand, health promotion may be viewed more broadly than disease prevention (Laffrey & Craig, 2000) inasmuch as it emphasizes enhancing personal competencies and capacities and is committed to empowerment and community-based health planning (Robertson, 1998). Health promotion strategies, therefore, are often political because they emphasize addressing structural and systemic inequities and have a strong philosophy of social justice. Health promotion is guided by the following principles (CPHA, 1996b):

- Health promotion addresses health issues in context.
- Health promotion supports a holistic approach.
- Health promotion requires a long-term perspective.
- Health promotion is multisectoral.
- Health promotion draws on knowledge from social, economic, political, environmental, medical, and nursing sciences, as well as from first-hand experiences.

Health Promotion Strategies

The *Ottawa Charter* identified five broad strategies to enhance health. The following is a brief introduction to each of these **health promotion strategies**.

1. Build Healthy Public Policy. Advocating healthy public policies is a priority strategy for health promotion in Canada. Indeed, some academics have suggested that this strategy is the foundation of all others because policies shape how money, power, and material resources are distributed to society (CPHA, 1996b). Advocating healthy public policy is a collaborative effort to identify the most important areas in which policy can make a difference. As a nurse, you might work with others to develop policy options, encourage public dialogue, persuade decision makers to adopt the healthiest option, and follow up to make sure the policy is implemented (CPHA,

---

BOX 1-1   NURSING STORY

Cathy Crowe: Advocating Healthy Public Policy

Cathy Crowe is a Toronto street nurse who has advocated for policies related to a variety of social determinants. Her work as an outreach street nurse in Toronto since the 1980s exemplifies nursing's role not only in attending to immediate health needs of people who are homeless but also advocating for policies that will provide more adequate and affordable housing to alleviate the root causes of these health problems. Ms. Crowe cofounded the Toronto Disaster Relief Committee (TDRC) in 1998, which declared homelessness a national disaster in Canada. The Committee advocated a "1% solution," calling on the federal, provincial, and territorial governments to allocate an additional 1% of their budget to fully fund a national affordable housing program. The efforts of the TDRC increased awareness, both in large cities in Canada and at the United Nations, of Canada's housing problem. This awareness led to the appointment of a federal minister responsible for homelessness and federal emergency relief monies (e.g., for shelter beds, food banks, programs for homeless youth). Although monies were also made available to provide housing, the goal of a fully funded national housing strategy has not yet been realized, and homelessness continues to increase across Canada.

Ms. Crowe has fostered numerous coalitions and advocacy initiatives, working with homeless people and other organizations. The TDRC was involved in fighting the evictions of Toronto's Tent City in 2002 and succeeded in eventually securing housing for many residents. Ms. Crowe is currently on the Board of Directors of a nonprofit organization that is building affordable housing in Toronto. To raise awareness about children who are homeless, she is currently producing a film set in several Canadian cities. As part of this initiative, a children's forum on homelessness was organized to provide children the opportunity to voice their concerns to the United Nations Special Rapporteur on Adequate Housing when he visited Canada. Ms. Crowe has also written a book, *Dying for a Home,* co-authored with activists who are homeless themselves.

Ms. Crowe has received numerous awards for her advocacy work. She sees advocacy as a critical nursing role and responsibility. You are encouraged to view her many speeches and activities on the TDRC Web site at http://www.tdrc.net or at http://tdrc.net/index.php?page=cathy-crowe.

1996b). Cathy Crowe, a Toronto "street nurse," is an excellent example of a nurse who advocates for healthy public policy: she works to reduce homelessness (Box 1–1).

The CPHA recommends that more emphasis be placed on policies that create healthy living conditions and enable people who are least powerful to express their concerns. This priority is also reflected in the *Toronto Charter on the Social Determinants of Health,* discussed earlier, which focuses specifically on determinants that have policy implications. Because the determinants of health are broad, healthy public policy necessarily extends beyond traditional health agencies and government health departments to other sectors such as agriculture, education, transportation, labour, social services, energy, and housing. Therefore, policymakers in all government sectors and organizations should ensure that their policies have positive health consequences.

Increasingly, policy advocacy is incorporated into nursing role statements (e.g., Community Health Nurses Association of Canada, 2003; International Council of Nurses, 2001) and nursing education curricula (Rains & Barton-Kriese, 2001; Reutter & Duncan, 2002; Reutter & Williamson, 2000). You should think about what policies have contributed to health problems, what policies would help alleviate the problem, and how you can champion public policies. For example, how do current welfare incomes, which are lower than poverty "lines" (low-income cut-offs), influence recipients' abilities to obtain adequate food and shelter and participate meaningfully in Canadian society? Cohen and Reutter (2007) outlined several ways that nurses can engage in policy advocacy in relation to child and family poverty.

2. Create Supportive Environments.

The *Ottawa Charter* (WHO, 1986) states that "the overall guiding principle . . . is the need to encourage reciprocal maintenance, to take care of each other, our communities and our natural environment" (p. 2). This strategy helps ensure that physical environments are healthy and safe and that living and working conditions are stimulating and satisfying. Creating supportive environments also means protecting the natural environment and conserving natural resources (WHO, 1986).

An excellent example of an initiative that helps create supportive environments is the Comprehensive School Health Initiative, which focuses on improving school environments by providing health instruction, social support, support services, and positive physical environments (Mitchell & Laforet-Fliesser, 2003). Other examples of supportive environments include flexible workplace policies and quality child care programs that support early child development and parental employment.

3. Strengthen Community Action.

Strengthening communities is a requisite for successful health promotion and for community health nursing practices in Canada (Community Health Nurses Association of Canada, 2003; CPHA, 1996b). In this strategy, often referred to as *community development,* communities identify issues and work together to make changes that will enhance health. In a community development approach, health professionals help community groups identify important issues and organize and implement plans and strategies to resolve these issues, often partnering with other community organizations (see Chapter 4). Public participation in all phases of community programming is key to community development (Labonte, 1993).

4. Develop Personal Skills.

This strategy, which is probably most familiar to nurses, helps clients develop personal skills, enhance coping strategies, and gain control over their health and environments so that they can make healthy lifestyle choices. Personal skills development includes health education, but it also emphasizes adequate support and resources. Some examples of interventions to enhance personal skills include early intervention programs for children, home visiting by public health nurses, and parenting classes. School health education focusing on developing interpersonal skills and health practices is another example.

5. Reorient Health Services.

Health system reform has two objectives: to shift emphasis from treating disease to improving health and to make the health care system more efficient and effective (CPHA, 1996b). A proactive approach to health requires improved access to primary health care services, increased community development, improved community-based care services, increased family-based care, and public participation. In Canada, there is considerable emphasis on developing the primary health care model, which nursing associations have advocated for many years (Reutter & Ogilvie, in press).

Population Health Promotion Model: Putting It All Together

This chapter has presented two major approaches to health: health promotion and population health. Hamilton and Bhatti (1996) integrated these two concepts into one model that shows their relationship to each other (Figure 1–5). Aimed at developing actions to improve health, the model explores four major questions: "On *what* can we take action?"; "*How* can we take action?"; "With *whom* can we act?"; and "*Why* take action?" (Saskatchewan Health, Population Health Branch, 2002).

The document *Strategies for Population Health* (Federal, Provincial, and Territorial ACPH, 1994) indicates health determinants actions that could be taken (the "what"). The *Ottawa Charter* provides a comprehensive set of five strategies to enhance health (the "how"). Together, these documents suggest that to enhance population health, action must be taken on a variety of levels (the "who"). Clearly, nurses must direct these strategies toward individuals and families, communities, individual sectors of society (such as health or environmental sectors), and society as a whole. For example, to promote the health of lower income clients, you can help them access resources and supports that will enhance their personal skills. Community programs such as school lunch programs, recreational activities, collective kitchens, and support groups can be provided. You can lobby government sectors responsible for housing and employment to implement healthy public policies pertaining to affordable housing, job creation, child care, income security, and financially accessible health services. On a societal level, nurses can raise awareness about the negative effects of poverty on health and well-being and can advocate for policies that will decrease poverty. The population health promotion model shows how evidence-informed decision making is a foundation to ensure that policies and programs focus on the right issues, take effective action, and produce successful results (Hamilton & Bhatti, 1996), the "why" of action (Saskatchewan Health, Population Health Branch, 2002). Evidence is informed by research, experiential learning, and evaluation of programs, policies, and projects. Values and assumptions that are the foundation of the model include the following:

- Stakeholders representing the various determinants must collaborate to address health determinants.
- Society is responsible for its members' health status.
- Health status is a result of people's health practices and their social and physical environments.

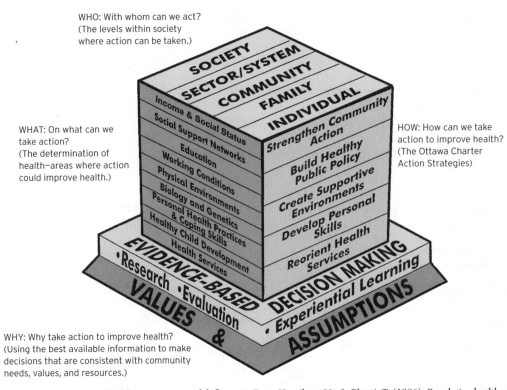

WHO: With whom can we act?
(The levels within society where action can be taken.)

WHAT: On what can we take action?
(The determination of health—areas where action could improve health.)

HOW: How can we take action to improve health?
(The Ottawa Charter Action Strategies)

WHY: Why take action to improve health?
(Using the best available information to make decisions that are consistent with community needs, values, and resources.)

Figure 1-5 Population health promotion model. **Source:** From Hamilton, N., & Bhatti, T. (1996). *Population health promotion: An integrated model of population health and health promotion.* Ottawa, ON: Health Promotion Development Division, Health Canada. Copyright 1996 © by Minister of Public Works and Government Services Canada.

- Opportunities for healthy living are based on social justice, equity, and relationships of mutual trust and caring, rather than on power and status.
- Health care, health protection, and disease prevention complement health promotion.
- Active participation in policies and programs is essential.

Summary

This chapter has introduced you to different ways of viewing health and health determinants, including the historical development of these concepts within the Canadian context. The content of the chapter challenges you to approach health situations broadly by identifying the myriad determinants that influence health. An increased understanding of health determinants should enable you to provide more sensitive care at the individual level and to consider strategies at the community and policy levels that will address the root causes of health situations.

✳ KEY CONCEPTS

- Health conceptualizations and determinants influence the nature and scope of professional practice.
- Definitions of health can be classified in several ways; recent definitions reflect a multidimensional perspective and a positive orientation.
- Three recent approaches to health are medical, behavioural, and socioenvironmental.
- Behavioural approaches focus primarily on health practices.

- Socioenvironmental approaches emphasize psychosocial factors and socioenvironmental conditions.
- Health determinants are interrelated.
- Canada is a leader in ever-changing views of health and health determinants.
- Health promotion differs from disease prevention.
- Three levels of disease prevention are primary (protection against disease), secondary (activities that promote early detection), and tertiary (activities directed toward minimizing disability from disease and helping clients learn to live productively with their limitations).
- The *Ottawa Charter* identifies five major categories of health promotion strategies: building healthy public policies; creating supportive environments; strengthening community action; developing personal skills; and reorienting health care services.

✳ CRITICAL THINKING EXERCISES

1. Describe your current level of health. What criteria did you use? Which definition of health discussed in this chapter best matches your understanding of health? Consider another definition of health discussed in this chapter. Does your current level of health change on the basis of this definition? How might your nursing practice differ depending on which conceptualization of health you choose to guide your practice? How might your definition of health change as you experience different life transitions (e.g., aging, parenthood)?

2. What do you consider to be the three most important health problems facing Canadians today? What are the major determinants of these problems? Which health promotion strategies would you consider the most appropriate to address them?

3. Imagine you are a community health nurse working in an area where many low-income women smoke. In a socioenvironmental approach to health, what questions would you need to address to decrease smoking behaviour in your area? How would your approach differ if you were using a behavioural approach to health?

✳ REVIEW QUESTIONS

1. The *Lalonde Report* is significant in that it was the first to emphasize
   1. A behavioural approach to health
   2. A medical approach to health
   3. A socioenvironmental approach to health
   4. Physiological risk factors

2. The "watershed" document that marked the shift from a lifestyle to a socioenvironmental approach to health was the
   1. *Lalonde Report*
   2. National Forum on Health (1997)
   3. *Toronto Charter*
   4. *Ottawa Charter*

3. From a socioenvironmental perspective, the major determinants of health are
   1. Psychosocial risk factors and socioenvironmental risk conditions
   2. Physiological risk factors and behavioural risk factors
   3. Behavioural and psychosocial risk factors
   4. Behavioural and socioenvironmental risk factors

4. The main reason that intersectoral collaboration is a necessary strategy to reach the goal of "Health for All" is
   1. The determinants of health are broad
   2. Intersectoral collaboration is cost-effective
   3. Intersectoral collaboration encourages problem solving at a local level
   4. Intersectoral collaboration is less likely to result in conflict

5. Providing immunizations against measles is an example of
   1. Health promotion
   2. Primary prevention
   3. Secondary prevention
   4. Tertiary prevention

6. Which one of the following statements does *not* accurately characterize health promotion?
   1. Health promotion addresses health issues within the context of the social, economic, and political environment.
   2. Health promotion emphasizes empowerment.
   3. Health promotion strategies focus primarily on helping people develop healthy behaviours.
   4. Health promotion is political.

7. The belief that health is primarily an individual responsibility is most congruent with the _____ approach to health.
   1. Medical
   2. Behavioural
   3. Socioenvironmental
   4. Public health

8. All of the following statements accurately describe the Population Health Promotion Model *except*
   1. The model suggests that action can address the full range of health determinants
   2. The model incorporates the health promotion strategies of the *Ottawa Charter*
   3. The model focuses primarily on interventions at the societal level
   4. The model attempts to integrate population health and health promotion concepts

9. Which of the following is the most influential health determinant?
   1. Personal health practices
   2. Income and social status
   3. Health care services
   4. Physical environment

10. Health promotion activities are aimed at
    1. Providing protection against disease
    2. Increasing the level of well-being
    3. Avoiding injury or illness
    4. Teaching clients to learn to live with their limitations

✳ RECOMMENDED WEB SITES

Canadian Institute for Health Information (CIHI): http://secure.cihi.ca/cihiweb/dispPage.jsp?cw_page=home_e
The CIHI is a not-for-profit Canadian organization working to improve the health of Canadians and the health care system. One of its goals is to generate public awareness about factors affecting good health. This Web site offers current information and numerous links to government health reports.

Public Health Agency of Canada: http://www.phac-aspc.gc.ca
The Web site of the Public Health Agency of Canada provides excellent information on many aspects of public health, including the population health approach and the determinants of health.

Population Health: Determinants of Health: http://www.phac-aspc.gc.ca/ph-sp/determinants/determinants-eng.php#income
This Web page also provides links to health promotion research and documents.

World Health Organization publications: http://www.who.int/pub/en/
This Web site provides links to the publications of the World Health Organization, including the *World Health Report*.

WHO Commission on Social Determinants of Health: http://www.who.int/social_determinants/en/
This Web page provides many excellent papers pertaining to several determinants of health and provides a global perspective.

2

The Canadian Health Care System

Written by Pammla Petrucka, RN, BSc, BScN, MN, PhD

objectives

Mastery of content in this chapter will enable you to:

- Define the key terms.
- Discuss the evolution of Canada's social safety net and Medicare program.
- Identify and define the principles of the *Canada Health Act* and significant legislations related to the Canadian health care system.
- Discuss principal factors influencing health care reform and the current health care system.
- Discuss clients' rights to health care.
- Discuss multiple roles of nurses and challenges faced by them in different health care settings.
- Describe five levels of health care and the types of services aligned with each.
- Identify various settings and models of care delivery in the Canadian health care system.
- Identify initiatives related to enhancing the quality of the Canadian health care system.

media resources

evolve Web Site

- Audio Chapter Summaries
- Glossary
- Multiple-Choice Review Questions
- Student Learning Activities
- Weblinks

Companion CD

- Glossary
- Interactive Learning Activities
- Fluids and Electrolytes Tutorial
- Test-Taking Skills

Nurses are an essential part of the Canadian health care system, constituting the largest employment group within the health care system and recognized as invaluable to the health of Canadians. Nursing services are necessary for virtually every client seeking care of any type. In 2006, there were 252,948 registered nurses (77.8% of the regulated nursing workforce), 67,300 (20.7%) licensed practical nurses, and 5051 (1.6%) registered psychiatric nurses, which reflected an overall increase of 1.3% in the 2005 numbers (Canadian Institute for Health Information [CIHI], 2007a, 2007b, 2007c; see Box 2–1). Since the late 1990s, the size of the Canadian nursing workforce has remained relatively stable, despite a 9.1% increase in the general population, which means a decrease in the number of nurses per capita (CIHI, 2004a, 2004b). *Building the Future* (2005) was the first national study endorsed by stakeholder groups to outline a long-term strategy for ensuring adequate nursing human resources in Canada. The nursing workforce is challenged by the aging of its workers, a high retirement rate, and a lack of full-time positions.

Nursing is an integral part of the health care system, and so you must understand the system and the issues that affect how care is provided to clients. As a practicing nurse, you must appreciate the complexities of a health care system faced with rising costs, human resource challenges, and lack of availability of quality services. Financial pressures have forced hospitals and other institutions to shift priorities and to control costs by cutting the workforce and support services. Nursing professionals can help restructure delivery systems and achieve excellence in health care. The role of nurses in client advocacy is crucial for ensuring that everyone's health care needs are served. The success of health care depends on the participation of nurses to create systems that deliver quality, cost-effective care. Nurses must lead the way, advocating, reinforcing, and retaining its values for safe, quality, and **evidence-informed** client care.

> **BOX 2-1**   **Facts About Nursing in Canada, 2007**

- Of all registered nurses, 33% were degree-prepared; 13.9% had a baccalaureate degree when they entered practice.
- Nearly half (46.3%) of post-2000 registered nurses entered practice with a baccalaureate degree.
- Of the registered nurse workforce, 7.7% were foreign graduates; 1.8% of licensed practical nurses were foreign graduates.
- Of all registered nurses, 63.2% practiced in the hospital sector; 11.1%, in **long-term care;** 13.8%, in community and **home care;** and 11.9%, in other settings.
- Of all licensed practical nurses, 45.2% practiced in hospitals and 39.3% in long-term care.
- Of all registered nurses, 94.5% were female and 5.5% were male; of licensed practical nurses, 93.0% were female and 7% were male.
- Average age of registered nurses was 45; that of licensed practical nurses was 44.1; and that of registered psychiatric nurses was 47.2.
- Of all registered nurses, 20.8% were aged 55 years or older; 8.0% were aged 60 years or older; and 1.9% were aged 65 years or older. There were more Canadian registered nurses aged 55–59 than there were aged 25–29.
- More than 50% of the registered nurses had graduated more than 20 years earlier.
- Of all licensed practical nurses, 35.9% were aged 50 years or older.

Sources: Canadian Institute for Health Information (CIHI). (2007a). *Workforce trends of licensed practical nurses in Canada, 2006*. Ottawa, ON: Author; CIHI. (2007b). *Workforce trends of registered nurses in Canada, 2006*. Ottawa, ON: Author; and CIHI. (2007c). *Workforce trends of registered psychiatric nurses in Canada, 2006*. Ottawa, ON: Author.

Evolution of the Canadian Health Care System

Despite significant changes since the 1960s, a network of national provincial, and territorial social programs, referred to as the **social safety net**, is still needed to protect the most vulnerable members of Canadian society. Most programs are targeted to specific populations (e.g., elderly persons, children), but a few are universally accessible to all Canadians. For example, provincial social assistance programs provide income support to clients who are unemployed for a long time, and the federal Employment Insurance program provides income support for those with short-term interruption of employment. A key component of Canada's social safety net for citizens is the provision of hospital and medical insurance, known as **Medicare**, which is funded by general taxation.

Although often referred to as a "national" program, Medicare is, in fact, an interlocking set of 10 provincial and three territorial insurance schemes that provide "free" access to medically necessary hospital and physician services to all citizens, landed immigrants, and permanent residents (Health Canada, 2006a). Medicare is a source of significant national pride as a Canadian commitment to the well-being of its citizens, as well as a source of national debate regarding its costs, effectiveness, and sustainability. Few issues are as important and controversial to Canadians as health care.

Early Health Care in Canada

Europeans who came to Canada in the fifteenth century brought infectious diseases that flourished under conditions of poor sanitation. Settlements enacted public health laws to control the spread of diseases. For years, government care was limited to essential services (i.e., care of insane persons and epidemics). Permanent boards of health did not exist; families, churches, and local communities were expected to be self-reliant in handling all other medical and social problems. The first Canadian nurses were nuns from religious orders, such as the legendary Marguerite d'Youville (see Box 2–2).

Canada became a self-governing colony with the passage of the *British North America Act* (also known as the *Constitution Act*) in 1867 which united three colonies into the original four provinces of

---

> **BOX 2-2**   **Moments in Canadian Nursing History***

Throughout Canada's history, nurses have been meeting the health care needs of individuals, families, and communities. As nurses encountered changing practice environments, such as World Wars or the Great Depression in the 1930s, they transformed their practices and skills to meet the new situations. During English–French hostilities from 1756 to 1760, the Grey Nuns cared for sick and wounded soldiers, including British prisoners of war. This order was known for its excellent hospitals, offering care regardless of race, colour, creed, or financial status. By the middle of the twentieth century, nursing transformed from a predominately spiritual vocation to a secular profession (Mansell, 2004). Most nurses worked in hospitals and communities but were also present in nursing and health care organizations such as the Red Cross, the Victorian Order of Nurses, military or navy service, tuberculosis sanatoria, professional nursing associations, and nursing unions. Although "the practice of nursing is perceived as an integral part of health care services in Canada" (Mansell, 2004, p. 204), the struggle for professionalism and recognition has not been an easy one.

*Section Contributor: S. L. Bassendowski, RN, EdD

Ontario, Quebec, Nova Scotia, and New Brunswick. This Act accorded certain powers to the national (federal) government and certain powers to the provincial governments. Responsibility for health, education, and social services was accorded to the provinces; the federal government retained jurisdiction for parts of these public policies (Storch, 2006). For example, health care for Canada's Aboriginal peoples and pharmaceutical safety remain federal responsibilities, but regulation of hospitals is a provincial jurisdiction.

As Canada's population grew and became more urban and industrial, crowded living conditions, poor housing, and sanitation led to more disease. Provinces enacted public health acts to establish local boards of health to hire medical health officers and sanitation inspectors. The nurses working directly in the community and with the poor were the first public health nurses.

By 1920, health and social programs had expanded, and **voluntary agencies** formed; the latter included the Children's Aid Society (formed in 1891), the Red Cross (in 1896), the Victorian Order of Nurses (in 1897), and the Canadian Mental Health Association (in 1918). Municipalities organized services for the poor and established hospitals. Clients who could not pay depended on charity (Figure 2–1). Fraternal societies (e.g., Knights of Columbus) and unions created trusts that members could access when ill, injured at work, or unemployed. Such programs were precursors of modern employment insurance.

As urbanization continued, rural communities had difficulty attracting and paying physicians. The federal *Municipality Act* of 1916 gave communities the power to levy taxes to pay for physicians. The Great Depression during the 1930s dramatically affected the health care system. Many families could not pay their medical bills, and hospital stays caused financial ruin. As needs increased, it became apparent that many provinces did not have the tax base to fund these services and to ensure that they were similar in scope across the country.

These hardships inspired the Canadian provincial governments to create a prepaid medical and hospitalization insurance plan. In 1947, Premier Tommy Douglas of Saskatchewan introduced a public, universal hospital insurance plan. This program became the basis of the first major federal initiative to expand hospital insurance across the country with the passage of the *Hospital Insurance and Diagnostic*

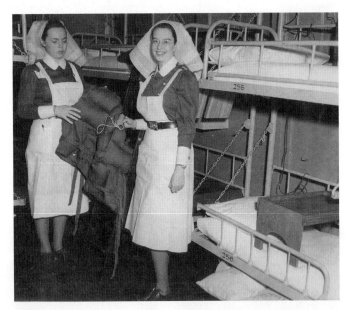

Figure 2-1 Military nurses. **Source:** Photo courtesy of WJR Bateman.

Services Act (HIDSA) in 1956. For provinces that agreed to set up universal hospital insurance, *HIDSA* provided federal funds to cover approximately half of service cost. By 1961, all provinces and territories were in agreement to provide coverage for **inpatient** hospital care.

The next step was to ensure medical services outside hospitals. Again, Saskatchewan took the lead. Because the federal government now covered half of the cost of hospital insurance in the province, Saskatchewan could now afford to provide medical insurance, and in 1962, the *Medical Care Insurance Act* was passed. The legislation was opposed by the province's physicians, who went on a 23-day strike. They eventually reached a compromise with the government in which the physicians' autonomy to practice as they wished was preserved in exchange for agreeing to a single-payer insurance system to fund their services.

In 1964, the Royal Commission on Health Services was appointed to study the provision of hospital and medical care to all Canadians and concluded that "strong federal government leadership and financial support for medical care" was needed (Wilson, 1995). The *Hall Commission Report,* named after lead commissioner, Justice Emmett Hall, called for the expansion of the Saskatchewan model across the country on a cost-shared basis similar to that of *HIDSA* (Royal Commission on Health Services, 1964, 1965).

On the basis of these recommendations, the federal government passed the *Medical Care Act* in 1966. Federal grants were awarded on a cost-sharing basis with the provinces if programs provided universal, comprehensive, portable, and publicly administered coverage of hospital and physician services. The federal, provincial, and territorial governments agreed to share health care expenses equally. By 1972, all provincial and territorial insurance plans had extended their coverage to include medical services provided outside hospitals. Thus began modern Medicare, inasmuch as all Canadians now had free access to hospital and medical care, regardless of personal wealth.

Although programs prospered, cost sharing did not last. In 1977, the Canadian government enacted the *Federal Provincial Fiscal Arrangements and Established Programs Financing Act* to replace cost sharing with block transfers of funds and a complicated formula of transferring tax points from the federal government to the provinces and territories. These block transfers resulted in decreased federal contributions. To make up this shortfall, some provinces allowed the so-called extra billing of clients by hospitals and provider groups over the amount that the universal insurance program covered. These charges were seen by Medicare's defenders as a threat to the universality of Canada's medical insurance scheme and as a violation of the principle that care should be accessible on the basis of need and not on the ability to pay.

The federal government's response was to enact the *Canada Health Act* in 1984, which amalgamated the previous acts of *HIDSA* and *Medical Care Act* and effectively banned extra billing and user fees. The *Canada Health Act* added the principle of **accessibility** to the principles of **public administration, comprehensiveness, universality,** and **portability** (see Table 2–1). These principles apply to all **insured residents** (i.e., eligible residents) of a province or territory but exclude members of the Canadian Forces, Royal Canadian Mounted Police (RCMP), veterans, and inmates of federal penitentiaries. First Nations and Inuit health services receive special consideration, which is discussed later in this chapter. Under previous acts, access to services was through physician gatekeepers. Revisions to the *Canada Health Act* allowed multiple points of access and insurance for care providers other than physicians. Although opposition to the *Canada Health Act* arose, all provinces and territories were following its principles by 1987 (Health Canada, 1992). According to the *Canada Health Act,* the primary objective of Canadian health care policy is ". . . to protect, promote and restore the physical and mental well

> **TABLE 2-1**   **Principles of the Canada Health Act of 1984**

Public administration	A public authority administers and operates the plan on a nonprofit basis; it is responsible to the provincial and territorial governments for decision making on benefit levels and services and is subject to financial audits.
Comprehensiveness	The plan covers all medically necessary hospital and physician services and, as the province or territory permits, services of other health care practitioners. The palette of services publicly funded for each province and territory varies, which is controversial and under review (e.g., Commission on the Future of Health Care in Canada [Romanow, 2002]; Ontario Health Services Restructuring Commission, 2000).
Universality	Insured residents are entitled to health care services provided by the plan on uniform terms and conditions. Universality negates discrimination based on race, gender, income, ethnicity, or religion (Health Canada, 2006b; Romanow, 2002).
Portability	Insured residents can access health care services in another province or territory without cost or penalty. Personal coverage must be maintained when an insured person moves or travels within Canada or travels outside of Canada.
Accessibility	Insured residents have reasonable access to medically necessary hospital and physician services, regardless of income, age, health status, gender, or geographical location. Additional charges for insured services are not permitted, and *essential* health care services must be available to all Canadians on the basis of need (Romanow, 2002).

Adapted from Health Canada. (2007c). *Canada Health Act: Introduction.* Retrieved March 31, 2008, from http://www.hc-sc.gc.ca/hcs-sss/pubs/cha-lcs/2006-cha-lcs-ar-ra/intro-eng.php

being of residents of Canada and to facilitate reasonable access to health services without financial or other barriers"(Health Canada, 2007a).

The *Canada Health Act* is a major piece of legislation that influences the delivery of health care services across Canada. A wide array of other legislation (see Table 2–2) at the federal level influences health and health services for the people of Canada in areas such as tobacco use, environmental health, and health research.

Aboriginal Health Care

Another major source of legislation is the *Indian Act* of 1985, which identifies the federal government's role in providing health care services to First Nations and Inuit people (Department of Justice Canada, 2003). First Nations and Inuit Health (FNIH), a part of Health

Canada, and Indian and Northern Affairs Canada (INAC) share responsibility for ensuring that health care services are provided to Canada's First Nations and Inuit people (Health Canada, 2006a; INAC, 2004). Treaties with so-called Indian bands in Canada were signed before Confederation with the British government and after Confederation with the government of Canada (Natural Resources Canada, 2003). These treaties outlined agreements regarding land, services, and relationships; some (such as Treaty 6) included a provision for health care services to be provided by the government to the First Nations communities, often referred to as the "medicine chest" clause (INAC, 2004). These treaties have enabled direct delivery of services to First Nations and Inuit peoples, regardless of where they live in Canada, including **primary health care (PHC)** and emergency services on remote and isolated reserves where provincial or territorial

> **TABLE 2-2**   **Relevant Health-Related Legislation***

Legislation and Date Passed	Purpose
Canadian Environmental Protection Act, 1999	Regulates pollution prevention; environmental protection and human health contribute to sustainable development
Canadian Institutes of Health Research Act, 2000	Strategizes and funds health-related research
Controlled Drugs and Substances Act, 1996	Controls certain drugs, their precursors, and related substances
Emergency Preparedness Act, 1988	Develops and implements civil emergency plans by facilitating and coordinating among government institutions and with provincial and territorial governments, foreign governments, and international organizations
Food and Drugs Act, 1985	Regulates food, drugs, cosmetics, and therapeutic devices
Quarantine Act, 1985	Controls introduction and spread of infectious or contagious diseases
Tobacco Act, 1997	Regulates manufacture, sale, labelling, and promotion of tobacco products

*Section contributor: T. McIntosh, PhD.

services are not readily available; community-based health programs both on reserves and in Inuit communities; and noninsured health benefits programs (e.g., pharmaceuticals, dental, vision, and medical transportation). All three levels of government (federal, provincial and territorial, and Aboriginal) are working together to improve and integrate health service delivery (Health Canada, 2006a). Aboriginal self-governance has been enabled through the "inherent right of self-government" under Section 35 of the *Canadian Constitution Act* of 1982. As self-governance models emerge, health care, as part of the palette of services and programs within Aboriginal jurisdiction, will challenge health care professionals to be "responsive to their particular political, economic, legal, historical, cultural, and social circumstances" (INAC, 2008).

The Organization and Governance of Health Care

Under the Canadian constitution, administration and delivery of health care services are primarily provincial or territorial responsibilities. The federal government has a role in health care financing, enforcement of the *Canada Health Act,* delivery of services to previously described targeted groups, and setting national agendas such as those relating to public health and safety, pharmaceuticals, and biomedical and health services research.

Federal Jurisdiction
The federal government accomplishes the following tasks:

- Sets and administers national principles for the health care system through the *Canada Health Act.*
- Assists in financing of provincial and territorial health care services through transfer payments (i.e., transferring tax money to share cost of health care services) on the basis of adherence to the *Canada Health Act* principles.
- Delivers health services for targeted groups, including First Nations and Inuit people, military veterans, federal inmates, and the RCMP.
- Provides national policy and programming to promote health and prevent disease, such as healthy environment and consumer safety programs and public health programs.

Provincial and Territorial Jurisdiction
Each provincial and territorial government accomplishes the following tasks:

- Develops and administers its own health care insurance plan.
- Manages, finances, and plans insurable health care services and delivery, in alignment with *Canada Health Act* principles (see Table 2–1).
- Determines organization and location of hospitals or long-term care facilities; the mix of health care professionals employed in hospitals or health care facilities; and the amount of money dedicated to health care services.
- Reimburses physician and hospital expenses; provides some **rehabilitation** and long-term care services, usually on the basis of copayments with individual users.

Each provincial and territorial plan is unique, and what is covered and by how much varies across the country. For example, coverage for drugs taken outside of hospitals, ambulance services, and home care varies widely by province and territory. Marchildon (2006) reviewed what is and is not covered by each province and territory. To offset costs for services not covered by provincial or territorial insurance, Canadians can buy private health insurance or participate in employer-offered individual or group insurance plans.

Professional Jurisdiction
Most health professions (i.e., medicine, nursing, pharmacology) in Canada are self-regulated, which means they determine standards, competencies, codes of ethics, and disciplinary actions for their respective members. Some professions are regulated through governments (e.g., emergency medical technicians in British Columbia, Manitoba, Ontario, and Saskatchewan) or other regulatory mechanisms (e.g., osteopathic physicians in Alberta and British Columbia). In some cases, so-called omnibus legislations regulate several professions simultaneously (e.g., *Alberta's Health Disciplines Act* of 2000).

Health Care Spending

"Canadians pay, directly or indirectly, for every aspect of our health care system through a combination of taxes, payments to government, private insurance premiums, and direct out-of-pocket fees of varying types and amounts" (Romanow, 2002, p. 24). In a 2005 Commonwealth Fund International Health Policy Survey, Schoen et al. (2005) found that Canadians are dissatisfied with their health care system; 78% asserted that fundamental change or a complete overhaul was needed. This dissatisfaction exists despite steady growth in health care costs since the late 1950s—faster on average than the economy as a whole.

In 2006, Canada spent an estimated $148 billion on health services, more than three times what was spent in 1975, adjusted for inflation (CIHI, 2006). Overall, in Canada, about $4548 per person was spent on health care in 2006, in comparison with $3572 in 2002 (CIHI, 2006). In addition, the average Canadian household expended $1870 (Statistics Canada, 2008) for health care, an amount up 6% from that of the previous year. Furthermore, per capita spending is higher for children and older adults than for younger adults. Although older adults constitute 12.6% of the population, they account for approximately 50% of hospital costs (CIHI, 2004b). In 2006, health care spending as a share of Canada's gross domestic product was 10.3% (CIHI, 2006), in comparison with 16% in the United States (National Coalition on Health Care, 2008) or 9.4% in Sweden (Vårdguiden, 2007). In 2006, hospital and health care institutions (30%), retail drug sales (17%) and physician services (13%) accounted for more than half of health care spending. In 2005, this translated to hospital expenditures of $40.35 billion, drug expenditures of $23.34 billion, and physician services expenditures of $18.34 billion, in contrast to $8.46 billion for public health services and $15.21 billion for other health care professionals' services. Despite these significant expenditures, Canada ranks 8th of 17 industrialized countries in the Organization for Economic Cooperation and Development (Conference Board of Canada, 2007) on a series of indicators such as life expectancy, perceived health status, disease specific mortality rates, and lifestyle behaviours (e.g., smoking, obesity).

Trends and Reforms in Canada's Health Care System

Since the 1980s, rapid and significant changes in health care delivery, technology, and public expectations have challenged the Canadian federal, provincial, and territorial governments to reconstruct a health care system that balances current and future political, legal, economic, and social realities (Petrucka, 2005). In most provinces, restructuring has become entrusted to **regional health authorities**, which are led by appointed or elected community representatives and whose mandates, roles, and responsibilities are guided by provincial legislations (Lewis & Kouri, 2004). Regionalization was intended to streamline health services, to reduce fragmentation, to respond to local needs, to improve public participation, and to address the continuum of health care services from disease prevention and health promotion to curative, supportive, restorative, and **palliative** treatments (Lewis & Kouri, 2004). Although these principles were initially attractive and promising, the process has not lived up to its potential; instead, it has become primarily a fiscal exercise rather than a philosophical or health-motivated reform (Petrucka, 2005).

According to Armstrong (1999), health reform *concerns primarily continuity and integration, quality and accountability, and disease prevention and health promotion. Framed within the determinants of health literature, the reforms are intended to deliver better quality and more appropriate care at lower cost, primarily by adopting managerial strategies from the business sector.* Numerous federally and provincially sponsored reports have made recommendations for reforming the health care system. Two influential national reports on Canada's health care system include the *Kirby Report* (Kirby, 2002) and the report of the Romanow Commission (Romanow, 2002; see Box 2–3).

Many experts claim that Canadians' current rate of health care expenditures is unsustainable. As discussed previously, health care spending has continued to grow exponentially, and some academics have predicted that by 2020, it will near $250 billion (Conference Board of Canada, 2007). Because health care costs are rising faster than government revenues, some Canadian citizens and decision makers believe that spending on health care will eventually crowd out spending on other programs in the social safety net and will consume 100% of all monies (MacKinnon, 2004). If health care spending absorbs all available monies, the future of education programs, social services, transportation safety, and environmental protection—all of which have a profound impact on health—will be uncertain.

The Canadian Nurses Association (CNA) is a strong proponent of a health care system that continues to respect the principles of the *Canada Health Act* and acknowledges the advancement of nursing as a primary access point to health care (see CNA, 2005; Smadu, 2006).

Role of Nurses in Health Care Policy

Nurses play a key role in health care policy, both as leaders at the political and community level and in their everyday work lives. Individually and collectively, nurses are integral to policy development (Falk-Raphael, 2005; Hart, 2004). For most of the years since the late 1950s, the position of a senior or chief nurse has existed at the federal government level, and many provincial governments employ nurses in similar positions. These nurses bring the nursing perspectives to health policy decisions, present government perspectives to nurses and clients, and articulate the potential impact of policy decisions to politicians and other stakeholders. Referring to a broader level, Villeneuve and MacDonald (2006) stated that all nurses can be at the forefront of the coming changes, setting the agenda to create a health care system that truly serves and reflects the priorities of Canadians. Falk-Rafael (2005) stated that "nurses . . . are ideally situated and morally obligated to include political advocacy and efforts to influence health public policy in their practice" (p. 212). Health care across the country needs a coordinated, integrated approach by nurses if they are to inform policy decisions and help shape the country's health care systems (Villeneuve & MacDonald, 2006).

> **BOX 2-3**   **Influential Health Care Reports**

The Romanow Commission

Romanow (2002) concluded that Medicare is sustainable and must be preserved because it represents Canadians' core values. His top priority was to modernize the *Canada Health Act* through appropriate funding and to initiate the following changes:

- Create a new diagnostic service fund
- Build information technology infrastructure
- Improve access (e.g., in rural and remote areas and for Aboriginal peoples)
- Ensure and measure quality
- Improve and expand PHC
- Strengthen and expand home care
- Offer catastrophic drug coverage
- Create a National Health Council responsible for indicators, benchmarks, and performance measures

Romanow (2002) did not attach a specific cost to any of his recommendations, but he did stress accountability for funding and services provided.

The *Kirby Report*

Kirby (2002) concluded that the current Medicare system is not sustainable. He advocated stronger private sector involvement in health care delivery. Although Kirby did not address the core values or recommend changes to the *Canada Health Act,* he clarified the impact of spiraling health care costs on other social programs. Kirby recommended the following priorities:

- Shift funding for hospitals to a service-based model
- Grant more responsibility to regional health authorities for delivering publicly insured health services, contracting out these services, or both
- Reform PHC
- Offer a health care guarantee to Canadians (e.g., time limits for wait times; if the wait time is exceeded, the government pays for care provided elsewhere)

Like Romanow (2002), Kirby (2002) emphasized accountability for services and funding. Instead of a National Health Council (as recommended by Romanow), he suggested an appointed council with limited advisory functions.

Based on Romanow, R. J. (2002). *Building on values: The future of health care in Canada—Final report.* Ottawa, ON: Commission on the Future of Health Care in Canada; and Kirby, M. J. L. (2002). *The health of Canadians—The federal role. Vol. 6: Recommendations for reform.* Ottawa ON: Standing Senate Committee on Social Affairs, Science and Technology, retrieved August 8, 2008, from http://www.parl.gc.ca/37/2/parlbus/commbus/senate/com-e/soci-e/rep-e/repoct02vol6-e.htm

---

Right to Health Care

The consensus in Canada is that everyone has a right to health care. Upon entering the health care system, a person becomes a client with certain rights. In general, consumers have a right to determine what kind of health care should be available to them. However, the *Canadian Charter of Rights and Freedoms* of 1982 does not explicitly include health care as a right; therefore, federal and provincial legislation must prove legal entitlement. (Only Quebec has health care rights in its legislation.) The *Canada Health Act* influences rights by setting conditions for federal funding, giving insured persons the right to have health care costs covered, but the right to health care itself is not guaranteed in the Act.

Rights Within the Health Care System

Sutherland and Fulton (1992) articulated a number of rights that Canadian health care workers expect: namely, the right to reasonable working conditions, including safety and absence of discrimination. The Commission on the Future of Health Care in Canada called for the adoption of a health covenant that would specify the rights, obligations, and expectations of governments, citizens, and health care professionals (Romanow, 2002), but, to date, governments have shown little interest in ratifying this kind of arrangement. Although, in practice, no statutory requirement exists in Canada to include client advocacy (or other stakeholder) groups in the policymaking process, a number of national groups (e.g., Canadian Cancer Society, Canadian Diabetes Association), as well as disease-specific client groups, are involved. These groups often share information, endorse, report on, or criticize health care policy decisions (Health Consumer Powerhouse AB & Frontier Centre for Public Policy, 2008).

Primary Health Care

PHC is a foundation of Canada's health care system, providing entry point of contact into the health care system, as well as the vehicle for **continuity of care** (Health Council of Canada, 2008). Rooted in a 1974 document by then–Minister of Health and Welfare Marc Lalonde, who advocated a broad strategy, PHC involves addressing nonmedical determinants of health in order to improve the health of citizens (Health Canada, 2006a). The report outlined the connection between health status and the social determinants of health, including employment, poverty, lifestyle, environment, and genetic endowment. Other documents, such as the Alma-Ata declaration on PHC (World Health Organization [WHO], 1978) and the *Ottawa Charter for Health Promotion* (Lalonde, 1986), built the framework that has informed population health and **health promotion** approaches globally. The WHO has continued its focus on population health, and Canadian federal, provincial, and territorial health departments have established units or branches that focus on and fund programs and services to promote this approach.

According to the CNA, PHC is a philosophy and a model for improving health that supports essential health care services (promotive, preventive, curative, rehabilitative, and supportive), with a strong emphasis on the principles of health promotion and disease prevention. Most definitions of PHC recognize the importance of placing stronger emphasis on the determinants of health and strategies to advance individual and population health (Health Council of Canada, 2008). PHC is cited as the key to health care reform and sustainability. In June 2002, Romanow stated, "PHC is the single most important basis from which to renew the health care system" (CNA, 2003).

PHC, as an integrated approach, refers to health and a related spectrum of services external to the traditional health care system. These services represent health in its broadest sense, such as income, housing, education, and environment (Health Canada, 2006b). The PHC model (see Figure 2–2) focuses on collaboration among health professionals, community members, and others working in multiple sectors, emphasizing health promotion, development of health policies, and prevention of diseases for all individuals. According to the National Primary Health Care Awareness Strategy [NPHCAS] (2006a), PHC accomplishes the following:

- Prevents people from becoming ill or injured.
- Enables clients to manage chronic conditions.

- Optimizes use of health care professional expertise.
- Enables health care workers to treat acute and episodic illness.
- Coordinates for efficiency and access.
- Enables individuals to participate fully in their health care.
- Recognizes factors external to the health care system that affect individual and community health.

Throughout this book, "Focus on Primary Health Care" boxes highlight the vital role that nurses play in providing PHC. Box 2–4 links health care situations to PHC principles.

Barriers to Primary Health Care

The meaning of PHC has caused confusion among health care consumers and even health care professionals. The distinction between PHC and **primary care (PC)** is difficult to understand. Access to PC is a key element of PHC, but it is only one component. PC focuses on personal health services, whereas PHC extends beyond PC to include health education, proper nutrition, maternal and child health care, family planning, immunizations, and control of locally endemic diseases. This broader concept of PHC proposed for Canada relates to the continuum of care by interprofessional teams of providers working with the client as the driver (Annapolis Valley Health, 2007).

Challenging the adoption of PHC is an underlying concern that "Many Canadians see the health system as an 'illness care' system that will be there when they need it" (CNA, 2003). Some experts fear that if monies are dedicated to PHC priorities and implementation, benefits will be limited, at least in the near term. PHC is a sensible approach to health care that is cost-effective and benefits people most in need. It offers vulnerable people the chance for a healthy life. For example, by attending a community health program on infant and child care, parents learn the importance of recognizing signs and symptoms of urinary tract infection (UTI) in children and the importance of seeking medical treatment if they suspect their child has a UTI. With this knowledge, parents may prevent long-term serious complications of untreated UTIs, such as kidney damage and distress, as well as reduce health care costs.

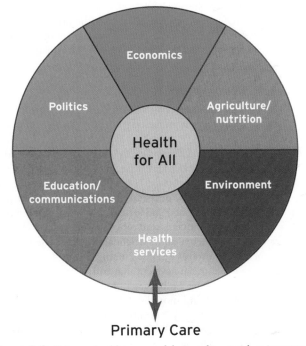

Figure 2-2 Primary health care model: A multisectoral or intersectoral approach. **Source:** From Shoultz, J., & Hatcher, P. A. (1997). Looking beyond primary health care: An approach to community-based action. *Nursing Outlook, 45*(1), 24. © 1996 by P. Hatcher, J. Shoulz, and W. Patrick.

The Canadian Health Services Research Foundation (2005) stated that clients seeking interdisciplinary care "in addition to their PC physicians fare at least as well as those receiving care from their doctors alone, and many studies find significant improvements." Despite this finding, some professionals do not support a PHC model, which requires interdisciplinary collaboration and flexible boundaries between health care professions. Smadu (2005) stated that many health care professionals are socialized to believe—and act as if—they alone must have all the answers and provide all the direction for their clients. In response, Health Canada (2007b) introduced the Interprofessional Education for Collaborative Patient-Centred Practice strategy, which provided interprofessional education opportunities across Canada aimed at improving socialization, decision making, respect, understanding, and competencies related to enhancing collaborative practice. This program strives to highlight changes in the way health care professionals are educated with the knowledge and skills to work interprofessionally and to be responsive in achieving health care change.

✳ BOX 2-4   FOCUS ON PRIMARY HEALTH CARE

The Four Pillars of Primary Health Care*

A number of models for PHC have been described. The NPHCAS (2006b) described four pillars of PHC as follows: teams, access, information, and healthy living.

Teams

PHC requires a team of health care providers working together to improve continuity of care, reduce duplication, and ensure access to appropriate health care professionals (Mang, 2005). Of importance is that clients are at the centre of the team and are empowered to make decisions about their own care (Smadu, 2005).

West Winds Primary Health Centre (WWPHC) in Saskatoon is a **PHC centre** addressing the health care needs of men, pregnant and nonpregnant women, adolescents, children, new immigrants, First Nations and Métis peoples, and older adults. WWPHC functions as a partnership with the University of Saskatchewan and the Saskatoon Health Region to deliver PHC in a community setting. WWPHC offers outstanding research and program evaluation opportunities for students in the health sciences, including medicine. Transdisciplinary, intersectoral collaboration is evolving at WWPHC, providing a full range of services that include but are not limited to health promotion, chronic disease prevention and management, the Healthy Mother Healthy Baby program, maternal mental health, the Food for Thought program, mental health and addiction services, diabetes education, public health services, and dental clinics. Staff includes physicians, nutritionists, clinical health psychologists, clinic nurses, nurse practitioners, occupational therapists, physical therapists, speech-language pathologists, pharmacists, social workers, public health nurses, and clinical researchers. A community participation working group and a collaborative practice resource group provide direction and support development of evidence-informed programs.

Access

PHC is rooted in ensuring that Canadians have greater access to the appropriate services when and where they are needed. According to Mang (2005), PHC recognizes the need for advice, information, and care outside of office hours. PHC improves access in three ways: It provides faster entry into the health care system, maximizes scopes of practice for all health professionals, and reduces demands for heath care by making clients healthier (Rachlis, 2005).

In urban settings, teams of nurses, physicians, social workers, counsellors, nutritionists, and other professionals bring PHC to the streets. They seek out the vulnerable groups—people who are in poor health (often with addictions, human immunodeficiency virus [HIV] infection or acquired immunodeficiency syndrome [AIDS], and hepatitis C), homeless, and malnourished and who lack support—to assess and monitor the health status and provide care "in place." Nurses on "PHC street teams" care for individuals who are in need, as well as for the needs of entire communities. For example, one nurse visits a 17-year-old prostitute who is 8 months pregnant, is addicted to crack, and lives within a boxcar community. The nurse also runs a community program called "Having Healthy Babies" for young, vulnerable women, which is located at a centre near the train tracks, to increase accessibility.

Information

PHC is about sharing and increasing access to information between health care professionals and Canadians who use the health care system or seek health care advice (NPHCAS, 2006b). Tools (e.g., electronic health records; diagnostic equipment) and skills (e.g., telehealth) are needed to facilitate quality, access, and coordination of information. An appropriate technology is the telephone triage systems now used successfully in many provinces and territories. Individuals dial a toll-free number and are immediately connected to a qualified nurse who can answer their health questions. This technology has addressed access to health care, especially in rural and remote areas. For example, nurses in the New Brunswick program have responded to the questions and concerns of almost 75% of callers.

Canada Health Infoway (Infoway) is a federally funded, independent, not-for-profit organization with representation from 14 federal, provincial, and territorial health ministries. Infoway fosters and accelerates development and adoption of electronic health information systems with compatible standards and communications technologies on a pan-Canadian basis. The vision is of a high-quality, sustainable, and effective infostructure that provides Canadians and health care professionals with timely, appropriate, and secure access to the appropriate information when and where they enter into the health care system. This infostructure further empowers clients by providing a cumulative personal health history that provides health care professionals with accurate health information (Alvarez, 2005).

Healthy Living

PHC, with its wellness focus, embraces strategies of prevention, management of chronic illness, and self-care. It recognizes that factors outside the health care system (e.g., social, economic, environmental) influence individual and community health. At the individual level, healthy living means making positive choices; at a broader level, it addresses factors that influence people's health and their ability to make healthy choices (Harvey, 2005).

A case in point is the story of a public health nurse in southern Ontario who was running a program that educated low-income mothers about nutrition, child development, and community action. The women shared their ideas about how to meet their family's nutritional requirements on tight budgets. They were alarmed to learn that a national bakery was closing its local day-old–bread outlet. The nurse coached the women to call a local newspaper reporter, who, in turn, contacted the bakery's president, and persuaded the owner to keep the outlet open. The nurse's health promotion activities resulted in a decision that benefited the community.

---

*Section contributor: V. R. Ramsden, RN, PhD.

Source: Canadian Nurses Association. (2003). Primary health care—The time has come. *Nursing Now, 16,* 1–4.

Future of Primary Health Care

In a restructured health care system that emphasizes PHC, programs necessarily will cross sectors. For example, trauma programs will have health promotion activities (road safety education), preventive programming (helmet legislation), **secondary** and **tertiary care** (emergency transportation), and rehabilitation (head injury–related recovery programs). Programs will cover multiple sites, may be defined by a particular disease or population group (e.g., children), and will comprise multiple disciplines and sectors of society (e.g., health care, education, justice systems). Nursing will have a significant role in every aspect of a PHC-integrated program.

Because of its integrated approach, PHC may hold the key to Canada's looming health care crisis. If Canadians stay healthier because more money is spent on PHC, they will need less medical care, and the proportion of money going to medical care will decline. If health care, education, social services, and the voluntary sector have integrated programs, competition among the various sectors for government monies may decline. This integration requires each sector to think beyond its own boundaries (see Box 2–5). If the PHC agenda in Canada is to progress, a number of resources and strategies are considered necessary, including the following (Health Canada, 2006b):

- An adequate supply of health care human resources.
- A team approach focused on client needs, to ensure that the greatest number of appropriate providers work collectively to optimize outcomes.
- Information technology (i.e., electronic health records).
- Governance and funding models that support team-based care.
- Links to public health.
- A culture of accountability, performance measurement, and quality improvement.

Settings for Health Care Delivery

Although health care organization and delivery varies across Canada, three types of delivery agencies are comparable: institutional agencies, formal community agencies, and voluntary and private sector agencies.

Institutional Sector

The institutional agencies include hospitals, long-term care facilities, psychiatric facilities, and **rehabilitation centres**. All offer health care services to inpatients (clients who stay at an institution for diagnosis, treatment, or rehabilitation). Most offer services to **outpatients** (clients who visit an institution for these services).

BOX 2-5   CASE STUDY

Primary Health Care

During a community meeting in a core area of a small city, parents, educators, health care professionals, and volunteers agreed to pilot an integrated program to prevent obesity in children. Social services and volunteers run a breakfast program. Fruits and vegetables for twice-daily snacks are donated by a local grocery store. Nutritionists and kinesiologists educate the teachers to integrate nutrition and physical fitness into the curriculum. Schools commit to having students and teachers participate in activities for at least 15 minutes every day and establish rules for school lunches (e.g., no soda pop). Nurse practitioners arrange visits with the parents of children identified as being overweight or at risk. If only 10% of the children in the program develop a healthier lifestyle, future savings to the health care system will pay for program costs.

Hospitals. Hospitals have traditionally been considered major health care agencies, most specializing in **acute care** services. Hospital services may include emergency and diagnostic, inpatient, surgical intervention, intensive care, outpatient, and rehabilitation services. The numbers of hospitals, hospital beds, and admissions in Canada have decreased significantly since the 1990s; the results are a higher proportion of clients with more acute needs and rapid turnover of clients in hospitals, in turn creating more intense, specialized, and increased workloads for health care providers (CIHI, 2007a, 2007b, 2007c). Hospitals strive to provide the highest quality of care possible and to facilitate early client discharge safely to the home, community, or a facility that can adequately manage remaining health care needs. Acute care is health care delivered for a short time (usually days to weeks, typically less than 3 months) in which an immediate health problem is diagnosed, treated, or both.

Hospitals are distinguished by their size (e.g., community hospitals), service provision (e.g., cancer care hospitals), and connection to academic institutions (e.g., university health science centres), as well as by public or private status. Public hospitals are financed and operated by a government agency at the local, provincial, or national level and constitute the largest group of health employers in Canada. Private hospitals are owned and operated by groups such as churches, corporations, and charitable organizations. Military hospitals, although limited in Canada, provide medical services to members of the military and their families. Veterans' hospitals provide residential, extended care, and rehabilitation to aging, injured, and disabled military veterans.

Roles and functions of hospitals and hospital-based health care professionals have rapidly evolved in this era of health care reform. Hospital nurses use critical thinking skills (see Chapter 12), apply the nursing process (see Chapter 13), coordinate and delegate care elements (see Chapter 11), and stress client teaching and postdischarge self-care (see Chapter 21). A trend is currently emerging toward evidence-informed practice when client interventions are determined. Nurses participate in discharge planning as a critical interdisciplinary coordination strategy in the continuity of care for clients, ensuring the smooth and safe transitions of clients between levels of care and the community. Many hospital nurses specialize as clinical nurse specialists, for example, in caring for clients with specific needs (e.g., palliative) or specific diseases (e.g., cardiovascular). Other hospital roles include nurse manager, infection control coordinator, clinical educator, and clinical nurse researcher.

Long-Term Care Facilities. A long-term care (extended care) facility provides accommodations and 24-hour intermediate and custodial care (e.g., nursing, rehabilitation, dietary, recreational, social, and spiritual services) for residents of any age with chronic or debilitating illnesses or disabilities. Most residents are frail, older adults with multiple health issues (see Chapter 25). Some are younger adults with severe, chronic health conditions (see Chapter 24). A long-term care facility functions as the resident's temporary or permanent home; therefore, the surroundings should be as homelike as possible. The philosophy of care is to provide a planned, systematic, and interdisciplinary approach that helps residents reach and maintain their highest level of function. Long-term care facilities are not part of the insured services bundle within the *Canada Health Act*, although many provincial and territorial plans do provide some coverage. In these settings, nurses plan and coordinate resident care, manage chronic illnesses, and conduct rehabilitation programs. Nursing roles involving education (see Chapter 21), communication (see Chapter 18), and family-related interventions (see Chapter 20) are prevalent in this setting.

Psychiatric Facilities. Located in hospitals, independent outpatient clinics, or mental health clinics, psychiatric facilities offer inpatient and outpatient services. Mental health is often seen as one of the "orphan children of Medicare," never being fully integrated into the health care system (Romanow, 2002). Nurses in these facilities collaborate with doctors, psychologists, social workers, and therapists to make plans that enable a client to return to the community. At discharge from inpatient facilities, clients are usually referred for follow-up through community-based agencies. Nurses working in these settings are especially skillful in communication skills (see Chapter 18) and client safety (see Chapter 37).

Rehabilitation Centres. A rehabilitation centre is a residential institution that provides therapy and restorative training, the goal being to decrease clients' dependence on care. Many centres offer programs that teach the client, the client's family, or both to achieve maximum function after a stroke, head or spinal cord injury, or other impairment. Drug rehabilitation centres help clients withdraw from drug dependence and return to the community. Nurses in rehabilitation centres collaborate closely with physical and occupational therapists, psychologists, and social workers. They work with clients experiencing stress and adaptation (see Chapter 30) and those who are at risk of challenges to mobility (see Chapter 46) and to safety (see Chapter 37).

Community Sector

Community services are directed at primary and secondary care, described later in this chapter, and should be accessible to clients in locations where they live, work, play, and engage. The focus in the community sector is on empowerment and community development opportunities that effect change at the broadest social level (Health Canada, 2006c). Community health nurses oversee and participate in outreach programs that provide services and locate clients who might not seek care at traditional health care centres. Community health care agencies include physicians' offices, clinics, community health centres, home health care agencies, and crisis intervention centres. Nurses practicing in the community sector are involved in community-based nursing (see Chapter 4) and caring throughout the lifespan (see Unit V).

Public Health. Public health is committed to ensuring conditions and circumstances in which people can be healthy through appropriate screening, assessment, development, monitoring, and support (i.e., public policy). Whether it concerns environmental, biological, or disease issues, public health differs from many clinical practice settings in its focus on entire populations rather than on individual clients.

Activities related to pandemic planning, severe acute respiratory syndrome (SARS), West Nile virus, and global surveillance have put public health into the forefront (refer to the *Canadian Pandemic Influenza Plan for the Health Sector* [Public Health Agency of Canada, 2006]) in terms of protection and promotion efforts. Public health nurses work closely with a range of health care professionals, including medical health officers, environmental and public health inspectors, psychologists, nutritionists, and therapists. Nurses are the primary professionals in public health clinics offering well-baby clinics, school health programs, sexually transmitted infections surveillance, and screening programs, as well as health promotion (e.g., tobacco reduction) and disease prevention programs. For example, during an outbreak of a communicable disease such as meningitis, the public health care system mobilizes to detect cases early and prevent transmission, often through mass vaccination, communication, and public education.

Physician Offices. Physician offices offer PC and tend to focus on the diagnosis and treatment of specific illnesses rather than on health promotion. The majority of physicians function as private contractors within the publicly funded health care system, working on a fee-for-service basis. In this setting, nurses record vital signs, prepare clients for examination, and collaborate with physicians to conduct physical examinations, document histories, offer health education, and recommend therapies.

Community Health Centres (CHCs) and Clinics. Staff at these centres plan, manage, and deliver comprehensive services to designated geographic areas or specific at-risk populations. CHCs typically offer a variety of health and social services, including family medicine, social work, counselling, health promotion, and community development programs. CHCs are cost-effective, reduce hospitalization, and function interprofessionally (Yalnizyan & Macdonald, 2005). Increasingly, nurse practitioners and nurses are managing CHCs, with the intention of enabling clients to assume more responsibility for their health. Nurse practitioners have become CHC team members focused on prevention and supportive services rather than on family practitioner–driven curative and rehabilitative care.

Assisted Living. Assisted living facilities are community-based residential facilities where adults live and receive a range of support services, including personalized assistance in achieving a level of independence. Personal assistance services are "designed to promote maximum dignity and independence," including meal preparation, personal hygiene practice, mobility, and socialization. These facilities usually have a combination of professional and nonprofessional staff available on a round-the-clock basis.

Home Care. Canadian health care is shifting from an institution-based system to one in which community care is playing a greater role (see Chapter 4). Home care is the provision of health care services and equipment to clients and families in their homes and is offered in all jurisdictions in Canada. Home care is not included in the *Canada Health Act* as a medically necessary service, and so the range of public funding varies significantly among jurisdictions (Health Canada, 2006a). All provinces and territories fund assessment and case management, nursing care, and support services for eligible clients. Clients may pay for extra professional or support services through insurance programs or pay-for-service arrangements. The federal government delivers home care services to First Nations people on reserves and Inuit people in designated communities, to members of the armed forces and the RCMP, to federal inmates, and to eligible veterans.

Home care involves primarily nursing care but also includes other professional and nonprofessional services, such as physiotherapy; social work; nutrition counselling; and occupational, respiratory, and speech therapy. Support services are nonmedical services and include personal care, assistance with activities of daily living, and assistance with home management.

Home care was created to provide individualized care for people after hospital discharge but has increasingly included clients in a range of ages from very young to very old; those with mental, physical or developmental challenges; and those needing recovery to end-stage care. A cost-effective alternative to institutional care, home care assists clients in maintaining health and independence longer (Hollander & Chappell, 2001). Nurses working in home care have experience with all levels of care occurring within the home setting (see "Levels of Care" section), as well as complex caseloads. Home care nurses must respond to issues of cultural diversity (see Chapter 10), family nursing (see Chapter 20), and client safety (see Chapter 37).

Adult Day Care Centres. Adult day care centres are associated with a hospital or long-term care facility or exist as independent centres. Frequently, rather than hospitalization, continuous health care services are needed for specific clients (e.g., those with dementia, those needing physical rehabilitation or counselling, or those with chemical dependency). These centres enable family members to participate in providing care, while maintaining employment and other activities (Meiner & Lueckenotte, 2006). Nurses in adult day care centres provide continuity between the care delivered at home and care delivered in the centre. For instance, nurses administer treatments, encourage clients to adhere to prescribed medication regimens (see Chapter 34), link clients with community resources (see Chapter 4), and provide counselling services (see Chapter 20).

Community and Voluntary Agencies. National, provincial, and regional voluntary agencies (e.g., the Heart and Stroke Foundation of Canada; Canadian Diabetes Association) meet specific needs. Most voluntary agencies offer programs to educate about, prevent, and detect specific conditions, rather than treat them. Voluntary agencies depend on the help of professional volunteers (e.g., Victorian Order of Nurses) and lay volunteers (e.g., Meals on Wheels); financial support for training physicians and nurses is often derived from fundraising and donations.

Occupational Health. More than 2000 members of the Canadian Occupational Health Nurses Association (2008) deliver integrated occupational health and safety services to individual and communities of workers. Nurses certified in occupational health have met specific eligibility requirements, have passed a written examination, and have met a national standard of competency. Occupational health nurses often work with physiotherapists, occupational therapists, and psychologists for large corporations in broad-based programs that encompass the range of promotion, maintenance, and restoration of health and prevention of illness and injury.

Hospice and Palliative Care. A hospice is a family-centred care system that enables a person to live in comfort, with independence and dignity, while living with a life-threatening illness. Hospice care is palliative, not curative (see Chapter 29). Its multidisciplinary approach involving physicians, nurses, social workers, pharmacists, and pastoral care staff is crucial. Hospice nurses work in hospitals, free-standing structures called *hospices,* or the client's home, caring for the client and family during the terminal phase of illness and at the time of death. They may offer continued services in the form of bereavement counselling to the family after the client's death.

Parish Nursing. Parish nursing is becoming more popular as faith-based communities promote and maintain members' health. According to the Canadian Association for Parish Nursing Ministry [CAPNM] (2007), a parish nurse is a registered nurse with specialized knowledge who is called to ministry and affirmed by a faith-based community to promote health, healing, and wholeness. Currently, more than 200 members of the CAPNM promote the integration of faith and health through advocacy, counselling, education, and linkages to health and intersectoral services (Caiger, 2006; CAPNM, 2007).

Levels of Care

Five **levels of health care** exist: promotive, preventive, curative (diagnosis and treatment), rehabilitative, and supportive (including home care, long-term care, and palliative care) (CNA, 2003; WHO, 1978).

Level 1: Health Promotion

The first level of health care, health promotion, focuses on "the process of enabling people to increase control over, and to improve their health" (Health Canada, 2006b). Examples of this process include the provision of wellness services, antismoking education, promotion of self-esteem in children and adolescents, and advocacy for healthy public policy.

Health promotion takes place in many settings. For example, community clinics offer prenatal nutrition classes that promote the health of the woman, fetus, and infant. The *Ottawa Charter for Health Promotion* (Lalonde, 1986) lists five action strategies for health promotion: building healthy public policy, creating supportive environments, strengthening community action, developing personal skills, and reorienting health care services. The *Ottawa Charter for Health Promotion* details how health care professionals can enable clients to make decisions that affect their health. Furthermore, it states that the foundation of health promotion consists of "the fundamental conditions and resources for health [which] are peace, shelter, education, food, income, a stable ecosystem, sustainable resources, social justice, and equity" (see Chapter 1).

Level 2: Disease and Injury Prevention

The second level of health care delivery includes illness prevention services to help clients, families, and communities reduce risk factors for disease and injury (see Chapter 4). Prevention strategies include clinical actions (screening, immunizing), behavioural aspects (lifestyle change, support groups), and environmental actions (societal pressure for a healthy environment)(see Chapter 1).

Level 3: Diagnosis and Treatment

Diagnosis and treatment, which are the services most often used, focus on recognizing and treating clients' existing health problems. Within this level of care, three sublevels exist: primary, secondary, and tertiary care. These typically refer to health care activities aimed at individuals, rather than at families or communities.

- PC is the first contact of a client with the health care system that leads to a decision regarding a course of action to resolve any actual or potential health problem. PC providers include physicians and nurse practitioners in practice settings such as physicians' offices, nurse-managed clinics, schools, and occupational settings. The focus is on early detection and routine care, with emphasis on education to prevent recurrences. (Recall and note the difference from PHC.)
- Secondary care, which occurs usually in hospital or home settings, involves provision of a specialized medical service by a physician specialist or a hospital on referral from a PC practitioner. Secondary care deals with clients seeking definitive diagnosis or requiring further diagnostic review.
- Tertiary care is specialized and highly technical care in diagnosing and treating complicated or unusual health problems. Clients requiring tertiary care have an extensive, often complicated pathological condition. Tertiary care occurs in regional, teaching, university, or specialized hospitals that house sophisticated diagnostic equipment and perform complex therapeutic procedures.

Level 4: Rehabilitation

Rehabilitation is the restoration of a person to his or her fullest physical, mental, social, and vocational functioning possible (Clemen-Stone et al., 2002). Clients require rehabilitation after a physical or mental illness, injury, or chemical addiction. Initially, rehabilitation may focus on preventing complications from the illness or injury. As a condition stabilizes, rehabilitation is necessary until clients return to their previous level of function or reach a new level of function limited by their illness or disease. The goal is to assist a client in regaining maximal functional status, thereby enhancing quality of life while promoting independence and self-care.

Rehabilitation nurses work closely with physiotherapy, occupational and speech therapy, and social services. Ideally, rehabilitation begins the moment a client enters a health care setting for treatment. For example, some orthopedic programs have clients undergo physiotherapy exercises before major joint repair so as to enhance their recovery (see Chapter 36). Nurses have a key role in the continuity of care aspects of rehabilitation, which occurs in many health care settings, including institutions, outpatient settings, and the community.

Level 5: Supportive Care

Clients of all ages with illnesses or disabilities that are chronic (i.e., are long-term) or progressive (i.e., worsen over time) may require supportive care. **Supportive care** consists of health, personal, and social services provided over a prolonged period to people who are disabled, who do not function independently, or who have a terminal disease. The need for supportive care is evolving. People are living longer; chronic conditions are becoming more common; and care settings (i.e., institutional, community, and home) are becoming more diverse.

Palliative care is a component of supportive care. Palliative care is services for people living with progressive, life-threatening illnesses or conditions. *Palliate* means to soothe or relieve. The goal of palliative care is to meet the physical, emotional, social, and spiritual needs of the client and family. Palliative care can be provided in hospitals, hospices, or homes.

Respite care is another component of supportive care that provides short-term relief or time off for family caregivers. Adult day care is one form of respite care. However, respite care can be provided within the home by health care professionals and trained volunteers.

Challenges to the Health Care System

Canada's health care system is faced with many issues and challenges, which can be categorized either as cost accelerators or as costs associated with trying to provide equal care and access to care for all.

Cost Accelerators

Technologies. New technologies, such as new-generation antibiotics, diagnostic imaging equipment, and specialized beds, have become integral in the treatment of diseases and disabilities. The effectiveness of these technical advances have contributed to reductions in mortality and morbidity rates; however, costs have increased with these innovations.

The overarching term **e-health** is used to describe the application of information and communications technologies in the health care sector (see Chapter 17). As part of this strategy, there is an emphasis on developing a national health infostructure to support direct care, telehealth, and the maintenance of electronic health records. For nurses, the area of **nursing informatics** is an emerging area of practice that "integrates nursing science, computer science, and information science to manage and communicate data, information, and knowledge in nursing practice. Nursing informatics facilitates the integration of data, information, and knowledge to support clients, nurses, and other providers in their decision-making in all roles and settings" (Canadian Nursing Informatics Association, 2008).

Demographics. As the population ages, chronic and age-related diseases are increasing in frequency, largely because older people are more likely to become ill and disabled. They require more treatment and drugs, which results in higher costs to the health care system. According to a Statistics Canada (2007) report titled *Canada's Population by Age and Sex*, "nationally, 13.4 per cent of Canada's population was comprised of seniors aged 65 and over, up from 12.7 per cent in 2002 . . . . This number should increase for another 20 years, when people born during the peak of the baby-boom generation reach retirement age. At that time, more than half a million will turn 65 each year" (Corbella, 2008).

Another demographic that has resulted in higher health care costs is maternal age, the average of which has risen steadily since the mid-1980s.

Consumer Involvement. Canadians are better informed than ever about their health care options and demand **high-quality care** for their tax dollars. For example, clients might ask a physician to order an expensive diagnostic test such as magnetic resonance imaging (MRI), whereas previously they would have been satisfied with an X-ray film.

There is a growing presence of and demand for **self-care**, which Health Canada (2006d) described as one of the pillars of health care and health care reform. According to the CNA (2002) and Health Canada (2006d), self-care is a range of activities (e.g., information exchange, decision making, networking) undertaken to improve health with the involvement of informal and family caregivers.

Equality and Quality

The Canadian health care system strives to provide equal care and access to care for all.

Income Status. Income assistance programs for older adults and social assistance recipients cover some health care expenses not covered by Medicare, such as optometric, dental, and pharmaceutical care. However, Canadians with low wages may experience poorer access and, consequently, poorer health status. Lower income Canadians visit dentists less often than do middle- or upper income Canadians and are less likely to seek preventive eye care.

Cultural Competence. Canada is a country of diversity; regardless of the health status and needs of Aboriginal peoples or of newcomers, it is apparent that the health care system and its providers are challenged to be responsive and respectful (see Chapter 10). As discussed earlier, the federal government has a key role in the provision of health care services to First Nations and Inuit people. Since 1986, a movement to transfer responsibility and control for health services to First Nations and Inuit governance has emerged (Health Canada, 2003). The shift in the health structures and PHC seem to hold the promise of aligning with Aboriginal peoples' beliefs, especially in terms of holism and integration.

Immigration has shaped Canada's population historically and currently. Between 2001 and 2006, newcomers represented two thirds of the population growth, with significant influxes in urban centres and neighbouring municipalities (Chui et al., 2007). Linguistic and cultural diversity is immense, more than 70% of newcomers having reported a mother tongue other than English or French (mostly Chinese) (Chui et al., 2007). Variations in the health status of the newcomers are based on their reasons for immigration, place or circumstances of origin, and social supports (Wayland, 2006). Issues of income, psychological well-being, and ethnic support are identified as important aspects of adjustment and risk reduction (Wayland, 2006).

Evidence-Informed Practice. Nursing practice is constantly evolving, and nurses must remain responsive to new developments, innovations, and information. **Evidence-informed practice** has become the gold standard in clinical decision making that is informed by *both* best available research evidence and clinical considerations (e.g., experience and client preferences) (Melnyk & Fineout-Overholt, 2005).

Evidence-informed practice resources are available on CNA's portal called NurseONE/INF-Fusion (http://www.nurseone.ca/). NurseONE is a personalized, interactive web-based resource providing a gateway for nurses and nursing students to resources to enhance client care, manage their careers, pursue life-long learning opportunities, and connect to colleagues (Bassendowski et al., 2008).

Quality and Client Safety. According to the International Society for Quality in Health Care (ISQua, 2007), quality practice and performance improvement underpin the work of the health care team across the continuum of care. Quality and safety in health care involve health facilities and providers, clinicians, and other professionals, providing the right care for the right people at the right first time and in the right amount (ISQua, 2007). The ISQua reported that consumers consistently rank quality and safety of their care high among their concerns.

According to Baker and Norton (2004), approximately 70,000 preventable adverse events occur annually in Canadian hospitals, which translated to between 9000 and 24,000 deaths in 2000. One per nine clients contracts an infection while in hospital, and the same number experiences a medication-related error (Baker et al., 2004). The Canadian Patient Safety Institute (2005) is charged with providing leadership in building and advancing a safer health care system.

Quality Workplaces. According to Law et al. (2007), the health of health care workers and healthy workplaces is a critical aspect of health care sustainability and a target for investment in the Canadian health care system. Health care has the most diverse range of work environments, which further challenges addressing quality issues and potentially affects recruitment and retention.

Privatization of Services. Governments are struggling to maintain the principle of universality against the benefits and challenges of privatization. At present, not all health care services are available and accessible to all Canadians. For example, some infertility treatments and laser eye surgical procedures are performed in private offices and are available to only to clients who can pay for them. Discussions continue about what constitutes "medically necessary services" and what core services should be available and accessible to everyone. Many experts contend that Medicare can be saved only by privatizing more parts of the health care system.

Health Care Human Resources. According to Chui et al. (2007), in 2006, more than 1 million people (about 6% of the total workforce) in Canada worked directly in health-related occupations. Despite these numbers, accessibility to health care services is compromised by shortages of physicians, nurses, and other health care professionals. According to Health Canada (2007b), health and human resources planning must occur within the context of the broader health care system and must recognize the systemic challenges of wait times, client safety, and bed closures.

Aboriginal peoples are significantly under-represented in health care roles. In response, Health Canada established a five-year initiative, known as the Aboriginal Health Human Resources Initiative (AHHRI), which focuses on increasing representation of Aboriginal peoples in health care and retention of health care providers who work with Aboriginal peoples.

Nursing's Future in the Emerging Health Care System

This chapter has included an extensive discussion about restructuring and challenges within the Canadian health care system. In response to this context, nursing roles continue to evolve and diversify. In the future, nurses will increasingly be regarded as critical stakeholders, partners, and providers within the emerging health care system. Nurses will continue to draw on their historical legacy, forge ahead, and use evidence to inform their pursuit of excellence and quality in care, while advocating and innovating for the benefit of their clients.

✳ KEY CONCEPTS

- Medicare is a key component of Canada's social safety net.
- Government plays a major role in the Canadian health care system by funding national health insurance and by setting health care policy according to the principles of the *Canada Health Act*.
- The *Canada Health Act* forbids extra billing and user fees and stresses the principles of public administration, comprehensiveness, universality, portability, and accessibility.
- Health care services are provided in institutional and community settings, across all age groups, and for individual, family, group, community, and population clients.
- The five levels of health care are as follows: promotive, preventive, curative, rehabilitative, and supportive.
- Escalating costs are driving health care reform efforts, challenging health care institutions to deliver quality care more efficiently.
- Issues of equality, access, and continuity of care challenge the health care system.
- To achieve continuity of care when a client is discharged from a hospital, the staff nurse must anticipate and identify the client's continuing needs and then work with all members of the multidisciplinary team to develop a plan that transfers the client's care from the hospital to another environment.
- The rise of PHC and home care is a result of reforms to the health care system.
- Successful health promotion and disease prevention programs, such as those found in community health centres, schools, and community clinics, are designed to help clients acquire healthier lifestyles and achieve a decent standard of living.
- Home care is one of the fastest growing components of the health care system partly because clients are sent home from hospital sooner than they used to be.
- Demographic, geographical, and technological realities affect the functioning of the Canadian health care system.
- The existence of sufficient and qualified health human resources is a key challenge to the Canadian health care system.
- Enhancing the health of Aboriginal peoples in Canada is a significant challenge to society and to the health care system.
- Nurses must continually seek out information and evidence to remain responsive to providing quality and safe client care.

✳ CRITICAL THINKING EXERCISES

1. Debate the following issues in relation to the future of the Canadian health care system: escalating costs, privatization, continuity of care, accessibility.

2. Consider and describe how the national economy, changes in the population, and technology have changed the Canadian health care system. Identify what implications these changes have for nursing practice.

3. Consider Mr. W., a 68-year-old widower with no immediate family supports, who is scheduled to have major surgery to replace the joint in his hip. He is generally in good health otherwise and lives in a seniors-only apartment complex in the centre of town. After surgery, he will need extensive therapy in order to walk normally again. Describe the type of health care services and client safety issues that might become involved in his care.

✳ REVIEW QUESTIONS

1. Canada contributes 10.3% of its gross domestic product to health care. Which one of the following countries contributes a greater percentage to its health care system?
   1. United Kingdom
   2. United States
   3. Japan
   4. Sweden

2. Which of the following people are insured under the *Canada Health Act*?
   1. Aboriginal peoples
   2. RCMP members
   3. Members of military services
   4. Persons in transit between provinces

3. Public health focuses on
   1. Treatment
   2. Promotion
   3. Intervention
   4. Institutionalization

4. The *Canada Health Act* embraces the following five principles:
   1. Public administration, comprehensiveness, universality, portability, accessibility
   2. Social justice, equity, acceptability, efficiency, effectiveness
   3. Accountability, equality, economy, collaboration, coordination
   4. Insured health services, compensation for providers, hospital services, community care, and prescription drugs

5. An adult day care centre is an example of
   1. A home care organization
   2. An institutional agency
   3. A community agency
   4. An ambulatory care centre

6. What are the five levels of health care services?
   1. Promotive, preventive, curative, rehabilitative, supportive
   2. Prevention, protection, diagnosis, treatment, palliative care
   3. Promotion, prevention, treatment, PHC, diagnosis
   4. Assessment, diagnosis, planning, implementation, evaluation

7. The largest share of health expenditures in Canada goes to
   1. Physicians
   2. Home care
   3. Prescription drugs
   4. Hospitals

8. Which is *not* a cause of Canada's increasing health care costs?
   1. Workplace injuries
   2. Aging of the population
   3. New technologies and drugs
   4. Chronic and new diseases

9. A nurse organizes a blood pressure screening program. This is an example of
   1. Health promotion
   2. Disease prevention
   3. Continuing care
   4. Rehabilitation

10. The provision of specialized medical services by a physician specialist or a hospital is known as
   1. PC
   2. PHC
   3. Secondary care
   4. Tertiary care

✳ RECOMMENDED WEB SITES

Canadian Health Services Research Foundation: Research Theme: Primary Health Care: http://www.chsrf.ca/research_themes/ph_e.php
This site addresses initiatives of the Foundation that relate to PHC reform and research.

Canadian Institute of Health Information: http://www.cihi.ca
This is a not-for-profit organization seeking to improve the health care system and the health of Canadians by providing health information.

Canadian Public Health Association: http://www.cpha.ca
This is a national, not-for-profit association seeking excellence in public health nationally and internationally.

Commission on the Future of Health Care in Canada: http://www.hc-sc.gc.ca/hcs-sss/hhr-rhs/strateg/romanow-eng.php
This site provides an overview of the Romanow Commission and access to the full report.

Health Canada: http://www.hc-sc.gc.ca
This Web site provides links to information about the Canadian health care system, including a link to the *Canada Health Act* (http://www.hc-sc.gc.ca/hcs-sss/medi-assur/cha-lcs/index-eng.php), legislation, federal reports, and related publications.

Canadian Patient Safety Institute: http://www.patientsafetyinstitute.ca
This Institute was established in 2003 to build and advance a safer health care system for Canadians. This site reports on activities in leadership role across health sectors and health care systems, highlights promising practices, and raises awareness with stakeholders and the public about client safety.

Health Quality Council (Saskatchewan): http://www.hqc.sk.ca
The Saskatchewan Health Quality Council was established in 2002 through provincial legislation to improve health care in Saskatchewan by encouraging the use of best evidence.

Health Council of Canada: http://www.healthcouncilcanada.ca/en/
This council fosters accountability and transparency by assessing progress in improving quality, effectiveness, and sustainability of the health care system. The Web site reports monitoring and facilitates informed discussion regarding barriers and facilitators to health care renewal and the well-being of Canadians.

3

The Development of Nursing in Canada

Written by Janet C. Ross-Kerr, RN, BScN, MS, PhD

media resources

evolve Web Site

- Audio Chapter Summaries
- Glossary
- Multiple-Choice Review Questions
- Student Learning Activities
- Weblinks

Companion CD

- Glossary
- Interactive Learning Activities
- Fluids and Electrolytes Tutorial
- Test-Taking Skills

Over the centuries, the goals of nursing have been to help people maintain their health and to provide comfort and care to the sick. Modern nursing is a professional discipline with a unique body of knowledge applied to the needs of individuals and families. The foundations of professional practice emerge from historical and philosophical traditions in nursing and health care, social policy and practice, and ongoing research in nursing. It is interesting to explore the origins of nursing because they have contributed to modern nursing. The evolution of nursing has brought the profession to a challenging and exciting time in its history. There are tremendous opportunities to improve the health and quality of life of clients and communities with advances in professional knowledge and practice.

The philosophical and theoretical basis of the profession provides the necessary foundation for practice (see Chapter 6). Henderson's (1966) famous definition of nursing was adopted by the **International Council of Nurses (ICN)** in 1973 and continues to be the primary description of the role of the nurse:

> "The unique function of the nurse is to assist the individual, sick or well, in the performance of those activities contributing to health [and] its recovery, or to a peaceful death that the client would perform unaided if he had the necessary strength, will, or knowledge. And to do this in such a way as to help the client gain independence as rapidly as possible." (p. 15)

As a profession, nursing is committed to public service. The practice of nursing requires specialized knowledge that must be acquired and carries a high degree of responsibility. Nursing has practical and theoretical components, is motivated by altruism, and is based on ethical standards. The profession evolves as society, health care, and social policies change. This chapter traces the roots of the nursing profession over many centuries to its establishment and development in Canada. Although there has been a dramatic increase in the nature and extent of knowledge and skills required for nursing, the professional mandate has remained relatively constant over time and continues to be an inspiring force for the profession. The transformation of the profession to the modern era is highlighted.

Highlights of World Nursing History

Nursing's historical roots are deep and honourable and can be traced over many centuries. In the sixteenth century B.C., the ancient Egyptians recognized the importance of preventing illness and maintaining health. They understood that a good diet was important in maintaining health, and consumed a reasonably well-balanced diet of fruits, vegetables, fish, milk, legumes, seeds, and oil. Priest-physicians ministered to the people, using herbs to relieve pain and a variety of treatments for illness that were based on spiritual or mythological beliefs about its causation. The Papyrus Ebers and the Edwin Smith Papyrus, came to light in Thebes (now Luxor) in 1862 and document the Egyptians' knowledge of disease and treatment. These ancient manuscripts have helped modern scholars understand how they dealt with health and illness as far back as 3300–1500 B.C.

The theories of health and illness of the ancient Egyptians provided a framework for the development of medicine in ancient Greece. Although the early Greeks believed in the spiritual causes of disease, Hippocrates (circa 460–370 B.C.) was the first to make observations of patients and develop treatments on the basis of symptoms. He founded a school of medicine on the island of Cos and wrote numerous books on disease. Hippocrates is considered the father of scientific medicine and Western medical ethics; he developed methods of treating disease

and establishing ethical principles upon which practice was based. Through his influence, medicine developed into a science. Galen (circa A.D. 130–203), another Greek physician-scientist, made important contributions to the field of physiology through research on animals and also wrote a number of books, eventually moving to Rome and becoming physician to the gladiators. Knowledge acquired through Galen and other Greek physicians had a significant influence on the Romans.

The Romans recognized the importance of fresh water and hygiene for public health. As their cities grew and the water supply became inadequate, Roman engineers developed aqueducts in Rome between 312 B.C. and 226 A.D. to carry fresh water from distant springs. They also developed public baths and constructed public toilets and sewers, which greatly improved the health of the population.

The ancient Hebrews believed in a spiritual basis of illness and that following the Ten Commandments promoted health. They also recognized the importance of nutrition and developed dietary laws that protected the public by prescribing what foods could or could not be eaten together, or eaten at all, as well as guidelines for safely eating the meat of slaughtered animals. Nurses cared for the sick in the home and community and served as midwives during childbirth.

During the early Christian period, with the emphasis of Christianity on love for others, nursing became a caring service undertaken by women. The Benedictine Order originated with St. Benedict of Nursia in A.D. 529 and is the oldest of the Catholic nursing orders. Fabiola, a well-to-do Christian woman in Rome, offered respite to ill and fatigued pilgrims travelling to the Holy Land. Later, during the twelfth and thirteenth centuries, hospitals were built to provide care for the sick. The Knights Hospitallers of the Order of St. John of Jerusalem emerged from the Benedictine nursing tradition to become one of a number of religious orders formed during the Crusades (eleventh to thirteenth centuries) that were committed to caring for and defending pilgrims. Hospices were constructed for pilgrims. When the Protestant Reformation took hold in Europe after the Crusades, monasteries were disbanded, and the hospitals and other institutions where monks and nuns cared for the sick and weary were closed. When new hospitals were built, untrained and unsuitable individuals were responsible for nursing patients. Conditions deteriorated as lack of sanitation prevailed and disease spread rapidly.

During the seventeenth century, conditions began to improve and there was greater emphasis on nursing. St. Vincent de Paul founded the Sisters of Charity in 1633 to care for the sick, poor, and orphaned. Because this order was noncloistered (the first such order), the nuns were able to go into the community to care for people. For the most part, women who entered convents to become nurses came from the upper classes and were well educated. In Germany, Pastor Theodore Fliedner established his now rather famous Institute of Deaconesses at Kaiserwerth in 1836 to prepare women to serve as nurses.

Nineteenth Century and Florence Nightingale

The movement to improve standards of nursing care in the mid-nineteenth century was spearheaded by Florence Nightingale, who is considered the founder of modern nursing. Brought up in a wealthy family, Nightingale railed against the customs of her time that did not allow middle- and upper class women to work outside the home: "Why have women passion, intellect, moral activity—these three—and a place in society where no one of the three can be exercised?" (Nightingale, 1872/1979). She was well educated and, against the wishes of her family, sought to prepare herself for nursing in 1850 by travelling to Kaiserwerth, Germany, where she worked with the German deaconesses under Pastor Fliedner. She later worked in

France with nuns in the French nursing orders. Then, in 1853, she accepted the post of superintendent at Harley Street Hospital in London and developed the nursing services there. When reports reached London of the appalling conditions for British wounded soldiers, Nightingale was asked to organize a group of nurses to go to the Crimea in 1854.

Nightingale and her staff of nurses made every possible attempt to care for the wounded and make them comfortable in ways that would foster their recovery. These women were able to achieve dramatic reductions in morbidity and mortality rates, saving the lives of thousands of wounded British soldiers by applying principles of cleanliness and comfort to nursing care. Accounts of Nightingale's work were distributed to the British press by a reporter covering the war. She achieved worldwide fame because of her success in reducing morbidity and mortality through exemplary nursing care. Nightingale helped to elevate the status of nursing so that it became accepted as a suitable field of work for women outside the home. At the same time, remarkable advances in health care and the expansion in the number and importance of hospitals created a need for nurses, and the nursing profession became one of the most significant avenues of work for women in the nineteenth century. Nursing thus became an instrument of women's emancipation against the prevailing middle-class restrictions on women working outside the home.

After her remarkable service during the Crimean War, Nightingale was plagued by continuing ill health. She became an advocate for the health of people, reform of the health care system of the British army, and educational preparation for nursing. She made her views known through her voluminous writings and lobbied members of parliament and acquaintances to support and act on her views. She drew her conclusions from health data that she collected and analyzed. She thus became known as the first health statistician. Nightingale is the subject of a large, ongoing scholarly writing project spearheaded by McDonald (2008) that incorporates the most significant analyses of her work to date.

Early History of Nursing in Canada

The roots of nursing and health care in North America may be found in the values and ideals of the European settlers in New France. At a time when knowledge of disease was primitive, technology was virtually nonexistent, and a few herbal remedies were the only medicines available, the practice of nursing developed as an integral part of the emerging health care system. Nursing care was often the sole weapon in fighting infectious disease. Its importance is underscored in accounts of the devastating epidemics of smallpox, diphtheria, cholera, and other infectious diseases that continually ravaged the population (Paul & Ross-Kerr, in press).

A long-established indigenous society existed in North America before the arrival of the first settlers. At the time of the first sustained contact with European people, the estimated number of indigenous people in North America was about 500,000, although this is acknowledged as probably a conservative number (Royal Commission on Aboriginal Peoples, 1996). The Aboriginal peoples also had health care knowledge of their own, including the use of herbal remedies.

The First Nurses and Hospitals in New France

In 1608, Samuel de Champlain selected Quebec as the site for a colony of settlers to support the growing fur trade. For the next two decades, the first colonists in New France provided their own health care. The first laywoman to provide nursing care in New France was Marie Rollet Hébert. She and her husband, Louis Hébert, who was a surgeon-apothecary, emigrated with their three children at the request of Champlain in 1617. Mme Hébert became the first woman to emigrate to the new world from France and cared for Native people and settlers alike. Her husband's apothecary and agricultural skills helped prevent starvation and mitigate illness (Brown, 2002). Although she was a layperson, Madame Hébert extended care to Aboriginal people and settlers who were ill, just as she would for ill family members, the latter being a customary role for women at the time.

The first nurses to tend the sick in a type of health care centre were male attendants at a "sick bay" established at the French garrison in Port Royal in Acadia in 1629 (Gibbon & Mathewson, 1947). The Jesuit priests, who were missionary immigrants to New France, also served as nurses. They found that in order to carry out their mission to convert the Aboriginal people to Christianity, they had to minister to the sick. Many religious orders and laypersons came to New France voluntarily to assist the Jesuits. Most of the women who came to New France were motivated by Christian ideals of educating Native children and caring for the sick. Although small in number, these women led the young colony's efforts in health care and teaching. They proved remarkably resilient as they battled smallpox epidemics and tended to people injured in the Iroquois wars.

The first nursing mission was established in 1639 at Sillery, outside the citadel of Quebec, by three Augustinian nuns who were Hospitalières de la Miséricorde de Jésus. As a result of the Iroquois wars, the nuns abandoned this mission in 1644 and opened another mission inside the citadel, where they nursed French settlers. This mission later became known as Hôtel-Dieu, Quebec's first hospital. In 1641, Jeanne Mance came to New France to found a hospital in the yet unsettled region of Ville Marie (later Montreal); Mance and her fellow travellers were not warmly received. Their intentions to care for the sick were viewed with suspicion by the settlers. When she arrived at Ville Marie in 1642, Mance was the only person with health care knowledge in the new settlement. She was a leader in the community and became an inspiration for later generations of nurses (Box 3–1).

A Canadian order of nuns, the Sisters of Charity of Montreal, formed in 1737 by Marguerite d'Youville (see Chapter 2), became the first visiting nurses in Canada. They began as a small group of women who pooled their possessions to form a refuge for the poor and needy (Gibbon & Mathewson, 1947). Because some colonists doubted their charitable intentions, the women were called "les soeurs grises," a derogatory term meaning both "the grey nuns" and "the tipsy nuns." However, the goodness of their intentions was clear, and they were respected for their work. They proudly referred to themselves as the "Grey Nuns" from then on, and were given a charter to take over the General Hospital of Montreal. To meet their hospital expenses, these resourceful women made military garments and tents, started a brewery and a tobacco plant, and operated a freight and cartage business (Paul & Ross-Kerr, in press).

Nursing During the British Regime

During the war between the British and the French in 1756, the Grey Nuns designated a ward of the General Hospital of Montreal for the care of English soldiers, thus caring for soldiers on both sides of the conflict. The status of nursing and the quality of care provided at this time differed markedly between Canada and Great Britain. Nursing in Britain had fallen into disrepute after Henry VIII's renunciation of the Catholic Church. The nursing orders of nuns, which had previously provided the nursing services in the large London hospitals, were replaced by women of questionable morals and little knowledge. However, nursing remained strong in early Canada because of the influence of France, where nursing was performed at a highter standard.

➤ **BOX 3-1**   **Milestones in Canadian Nursing History**

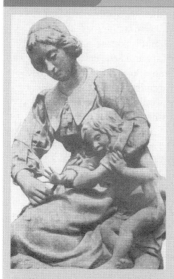

Jeanne Mance, 1606-1673

Jeanne Mance was born in a wealthy family in Langres, France, in 1606. She was the daughter of a wealthy legal advisor to the court of the King of France and decided early to devote her life to God. She learned about New France from a cousin, a Recollet priest who had served there. She gained nursing knowledge and skills in Langres, where an epidemic of plague occurred and many people were wounded in the Thirty Years' War. Supported by a wealthy widow who wanted to finance a hospital at Ville Marie, Jeanne Mance sailed to New France with Paul de Chomédey, Sieur de Maisonneuve, and his band of 40. Maisonneuve's mission was to establish a settlement at Ville Marie, but arriving in Quebec after a 2-month voyage, the settlers learned that the governor was suspicious of their mission, and he tried to dissuade them from it.

They decided that it was too late in the summer to try to build the colony, and so they remained in Quebec, involving themselves in the community. Mance spent time learning about nursing and health care in New France from the Augustinian nuns in their hospital.

In the spring, the settlers set out for Ville Marie in three boats and immediately began building houses and the Hôtel-Dieu. The next year, during an attack by the Iroquois, several settlers were killed, and others were taken hostage. The remaining settlers managed to finish the hospital and build a stockade around their colony. However, the attacks increased, and Mance was kept busy caring for both wounded settlers and Aboriginal people. By 1649, the settlers' funds were low, and the colony was close to having to disband. Mance sailed to Paris, where she raised money and recruited settlers. Over the next few years, relations with the Iroquois continued to be poor. A guard was placed at the hospital and Mance slept within the fort. In 1650, the Iroquois killed 30 of 70 settlers.

Maisonneuve went to France in 1651 to gain further support and did not return for 2 years. This period was difficult, but Mance held the colony together during his absence. After a truce reached between the French and the Iroquois in 1654, Mance was able to move back to the Hôtel-Dieu. In 1657, Mance fell on the ice, and fractured her right arm in two places, and dislocated her wrist, and she experienced continuing disability. She decided to make another trip to France to ask the order of nuns at La Flèche to come and help her in the hospital. While in Paris during prayer at the Seminary of Saint Sulpice, she discovered she could move her arm without pain, and it healed miraculously. She made her last trip to France in 1663, again to solicit funding for the colony because it was, again, close to bankruptcy. En route back, she contracted typhus and nearly died. She was shocked to find upon her return that Maisonneuve had been replaced as governor. In declining health, Mance was less able to help at the hospital. She died peacefully in her sleep in 1673.

As well as founding and managing the Hôtel-Dieu, Mance assisted Maisonneuve in running the colony as confidant, advisor, and accountant. She is hailed as a founder of the city of Montreal. Today, the Canadian Nurses Association (CNA) awards its highest honour in the name of this courageous pioneer.

Infectious diseases carried by immigrants and travellers spread rapidly in the British colonies. The increasing populace and continuing epidemics created a need for more health care facilities. In areas not served by the French-Canadian nursing orders, institutions were established with standards similar to those in Britain at the time (CNA, 1968). Laywomen offered their services and organized groups to provide proper care, but because they lacked knowledge and skill, these efforts were largely unsuccessful. The established French-Canadian orders expanded their services, and new English-speaking orders were founded to help the sick and the poor.

Opening of the West and the Grey Nuns

In 1844, four Grey Nuns embarked on a perilous canoe journey from Montreal to St. Boniface, Manitoba, where their mission was to care for the sick. Soon after their arrival, a series of epidemics began. The nuns visited the sick at home, where they cared for people with measles, dysentery, and smallpox and treated them with medicines and local herbs.

In 1859, another group of Grey Nuns travelled from Montreal by rail through the United States and then North to St. Boniface. After resting for a time, they set off by ox cart over rough terrain to arrive in what is now Alberta to establish their first mission in Lac Ste. Anne, where they visited clients in their homes and cared for them in the convent. Arriving before most of the settlers, the sisters established systems of health care to care for the sick. Demand from the populace was such that they later built a separate hospital building. Later, they established small missions in what is now northern Saskatchewan and the Northwest Territories to provide health care in Native settlements. In 1895, they were asked to construct a hospital in Edmonton (the General Hospital) because settlement was burgeoning there.

Nursing Education in Canada

In 1860, Florence Nightingale established a financially independent school of nursing in association with St. Thomas's Hospital in London, England. Interest in the new school was high. Soon hospital training schools for nurses were established throughout Europe and North America.

Unfortunately, the educational model of the Nightingale school was missing from the new hospital schools. This was largely because the new schools had no financing and required students to provide nursing service to the hospital in return for their education and living expenses, which enabled hospitals to provide nursing services at minimal cost. The race to establish hospitals in the early 1890s was undoubtedly spurred on by the financial benefits of establishing associated schools of nursing. The early hospitals were challenged financially because they did not charge poor clients. Services thus had to be of high enough quality to attract paying clients, and a training school attached to a hospital ensured a higher standard of care than one without a school (Young, 1994).

The First Canadian Nursing Schools

The first hospital diploma school in Canada, the St. Catharines Training School, opened in 1874 at the St. Catharines General and Marine Hospital. Admission standards were "plain English education, good character, and Christian motives" (*St. Catharines Annual Report*, cited by Healey, 1990). At that time, nursing was still considered an undesirable vocation for a refined lady in Canada, the only acceptable profession being teaching (Healey, 1990). Students learned chemistry, sanitary science, physiology, anatomy, and hygiene. They were taught to observe patients for changes in temperature, skin condition, pulse, respirations, and functions of organs and to report "faithfully" to the attending physician (Healey, 1990).

The School for Nurses at the Toronto General Hospital was established in 1881; Mary Agnes Snively was appointed superintendent in 1884 (Box 3–2). Although work and living conditions were poor, Miss Snively worked hard to improve the program. In 1896, she introduced a 3-year course with 84 hours of practical nursing and 119 hours of instruction by the medical staff (Gibbon & Mathewson, 1947).

In Montreal, after several unsuccessful attempts, The School for Nurses at the Montreal General Hospital was established in 1890 under the direction of Nora Livingston. Conditions were deplorable,

but Livingston quickly made improvements. The popularity of the school increased rapidly. Livingston reported 169 applications in the first year, from which 80 students were accepted (Gibbon & Mathewson, 1947).

The move to establish hospital schools of nursing swept the country. The Winnipeg General Hospital initiated the first Training School for Nurses in 1887 in western Canada. A measure of its success was that 134 of its graduates served as nurses in World War I (Gibbon & Mathewson, 1947). By 1890, hospitals in Fredericton, Saint John, Halifax, and Charlottetown had opened schools. Vancouver General Hospital began a school in 1891, and in Alberta, a school was opened in Medicine Hat in 1894. By 1930, there were approximately 330 schools of nursing in Canada (CNA, 1968; Box 3–3).

The Impact of Nursing Organizations on Nursing Education

At the same time that hospital training schools for nurses were being established, nurses began to advocate for improved educational standards and passage of legislation for their profession. Women's associations were instrumental in the public health care crusade in Canada and in the rise of nursing organizations. The National Council of Women under the presidency of Lady Ishbel Aberdeen, wife of the governor general of Canada, approved the formation of the Victorian Order of Nurses (VON) in 1898. Lady Aberdeen had conceived the idea of establishing the VON after she discovered the plight of women in Western Canada who had to give birth in remote locations with no assistance. The formation of the VON signified a professional standard of education for Canadian nurses that recognized the need not only for altruism and compassion but also for nursing knowledge.

Nurses from around the world were beginning to form organizations, inspired by the leadership of women such as Ethel Gordon Bedford Fenwick. Editor of the *British Journal of Nursing,* she attended the 1893 Congress of Charities, Corrections, and Philanthropy in Chicago, where she spoke of British struggles to achieve registration for nurses. Her North American colleagues had similar concerns. After the Congress, they formed the American Society of Superintendents of Training Schools for Nurses of the United States and Canada, later to become the National League for Nursing Education, whose goal was to raise standards of nursing education. Soon afterward in 1896, the Nurses' Associated Alumnae of the United States and Canada was formed, becoming the American Nurses Association in 1911. A major goal was to secure legislation to differentiate between trained and untrained nurses (CNA, 1968).

In 1899, Bedford Fenwick founded the ICN, with Britain, Germany, and the United States as member organizations. Nations without national nursing organizations could not become members. As mentioned previously, although Canada did not yet have a national nursing organization, Mary Agnes Snively, Superintendent of Nurses at Toronto General Hospital, was elected the first honourary treasurer of the ICN in 1899 (CNA, 1968).

The Origins of the Canadian Nurses Association and Provincial Nursing Associations.
The Canadian Society of Superintendents of Training Schools for Nurses was formed in 1907. The next year, the Provisional Society of the Canadian National Association of Trained Nurses (CNATN) was formed. Mary Agnes Snively served as founding president of both organizations (CNA, 1968). Membership in this new national organization was through affiliated societies in the provinces. At the ICN meeting in 1909, Canada became a full-fledged member of the organization. Later, the CNATN streamlined its organization when registration of nurses was established through legislation in each province. Its name was

---

> **BOX 3-2** | **Milestones in Canadian Nursing History**

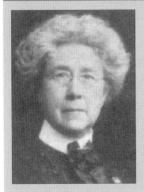

Mary Agnes Snively, 1847–1933

Born in St. Catharines, Ontario, Mary Agnes Snively was a teacher before she was a nurse. Upon graduation from the school of nursing at Bellevue Hospital, New York, in 1894, she was appointed Lady Superintendent of Nurses at Toronto General Hospital and director of the school of nursing. The school, founded along with the hospital 3 years earlier, was in a state of disorganization. Students provided most of the nursing care at Toronto General Hospital at little cost to the hospital. Snively found no organized plan for classes or clinical experience, nor was there a residence (students were housed in various locations in the hospital). Written records of nursing care, medical orders, and client histories were also lacking. Recruiting desirable applicants was difficult because students in the school faced so many hardships that parents were reluctant to allow their daughters to seek admission.

Snively rectified all these deficiencies. A residence was soon built; she developed a curriculum plan, including nursing theory and practice; and she lengthened the education period to 3 years. By the end of her tenure in 1910, the Toronto General Hospital school was thriving as the largest school of nursing in Canada with hundreds of graduates, a full complement of students, and many more seeking admission. All parental skepticism had been overcome, and Toronto General Hospital served as a model for others across the country.

Snively achieved acclaim for her organizational work. She helped found the first nurses' alumnae association in Canada at Toronto General Hospital in 1894. She also attended the historic 1899 founding meeting of the ICN in London, England and was elected first honorary treasurer of the ICN, even though Canada did not have the necessary national nursing association to become an ICN member at the time. In 1907, Snively established the Canadian Society of Superintendents of Training Schools of Nursing, and, recognizing that an organization that would include all nurses would be needed for Canada to become a member of the ICN, she was the driving force behind the 1908 founding of the Provisional Organization of the Canadian National Association of Trained Nurses (later the CNA), becoming its first president. She shepherded the entry of the fledgling Canadian organization to membership in the ICN and served later as ICN vice president.

Sources: Gibbon, J. M., & Mathewson, M. S. (1947). *Three centuries of Canadian nursing.* Toronto, ON: Macmillan; and Riegler, N. (1997). *Jean I. Gunn, nursing leader.* Markham, ON: Associated Medical Services with Fitzhenry and Whiteside.

> ### BOX 3-3   Milestones in Canadian Nursing History

Jean I. Gunn, 1882-1941

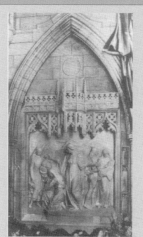

Born in 1882 in Belleville, Ontario, Jean I. Gunn completed teacher training studies at Albert College in Belleville; her father was not in favour of her pursuing a career in nursing. Assisted by her mother, she went to New York to visit her sister and investigate nursing schools there. She then enrolled in the School of Nursing at Presbyterian Hospital, New York, graduating in 1905. After experience at her alma mater and in community nursing, Gunn was appointed superintendent of nurses at the Toronto General Hospital in 1913. In this position, she was also responsible for the school of nursing.

Gunn recruited outstanding nursing administrators to assist her and became involved in provincial, national, and international health care and nursing organizations. She was a tireless worker and served with many organizations. Gunn was very supportive of the Toronto General Hospital alumnae association that in 1904 helped establish the Graduate Nurses' Association of Ontario (later the Registered Nurses Association of Ontario) and pressed for legislation for the registration of nurses. She became secretary of the Canadian National Association of Trained Nurses in 1914 and president in 1917. She served on the executive of the National Council of Women and became very involved in the Canadian Red Cross Society, in which she chaired a committee on surgical dressings during World War II. In this role, she oversaw production of millions of dressings by female civilian volunteers.

Nurses were in short supply during this time. With most men in the armed forces, many industrial jobs were now open to women and at wages far surpassing those of nurses. In 1917, Gunn pressed for the establishment of a permanent cadre of trained nurses for national service. She continued to work for the registration of nurses, which came to fruition in Ontario in 1922.

Gunn advocated for nursing and nurses on many fronts. She castigated hospital boards for reviewing costs of hospital services while ignoring the savings that accrued from educating a nurse. She was passionately interested in improving standards of nursing education. She decried the exploitation of nurses in schools of nursing and worked with other nursing leaders to establish the Weir study of nursing and nursing education, jointly sponsored by the CNA and the Canadian Medical Association. The 1932 Weir report confirmed the deficiencies that she and other nursing leaders had publicized for so long, and she campaigned for the implementation of its recommendations.

Gunn also envisioned university degree programs in nursing and in 1914 arranged for the Department of Social Service at the University of Toronto to give lectures to third-year Toronto General Hospital students. In 1917, a course in chemistry taught by university instructors was implemented. The following year, field experience in public health nursing was introduced, and Gunn organized centralized lectures among Toronto schools of nursing held at the University of Toronto.

Gunn is perhaps best remembered for her work toward the Nurses' War Memorial, which recognized the service of military nurses during World War I. She lobbied politicians and other health care organizations extensively and raised money from 10,000 nurses and their organizations from all over Canada. The result was a bas-relief sculpture in white Carrara marble that was unveiled in 1924 in a prominent position in the Centre Block of the Parliament Buildings, located in the Hall of Honour, separating the House of Commons from the Senate. In 1932, Gunn was responsible for having the crest of the CNA added to the sculpture.

In recognition of her outstanding service to nursing and health care throughout her life, Gunn received a number of honours in her final years, including a King's Jubilee Medal in 1935 and a Doctor of Laws degree from the University of Toronto in 1938. Jean Gunn was a leader among leaders in nursing and an individual who was able to inspire nurses to contribute to the common good.

Source: Riegler, N. (1997). *Jean I. Gunn, nursing leader*. Markham, ON: Associated Medical Services with Fitzhenry and Whiteside.

changed to the *Canadian Nurses Association* in 1924, and it became a federation of provincial associations in 1930.

The struggle for women's rights helped nurses to secure laws to regulate their profession. Nurses formed provincial nurses' associations and sought legislation that would set educational standards and improve nursing care. The first province to gain legislation was Nova Scotia, where a voluntary registration act was passed in 1910. It also allowed nongraduate nurses to register. Initial acts passed in other provinces contained more restrictive standards. Admission criteria and curricula were set for nursing schools, as were rules governing the registration and discipline of practising nurses.

All provinces and two territories eventually secured mandatory registration, requiring that all practising nurses register with the regulatory body approved by the provincial nursing act (Canadian Institute for Health Information, 2006). The distinguishing feature of mandatory rather than permissive legislation is a statute containing a definition of the scope of nursing practice, as well as protecting the use of the title of *registered nurse*. Permissive legislation only protects the title of *registered nurse* (Wood, in press). Licensure laws are designed to protect the public against unqualified and incompetent practitioners.

The First University Programs

The devastating consequences of World War I and the influenza pandemic of 1918 led to support for public health programs and new patterns of health care delivery. Community health care was promoted, and nurses were seen as central participants who needed university-level education. To this end, the Canadian Red Cross Society awarded grants to a number of Canadian universities to develop postgraduate courses in public health nursing: University of Toronto, McGill University, University of British Columbia, University of Alberta, Dalhousie University, and University of Western Ontario (Canadian Red Cross Society, 1962).

The first Canadian undergraduate nursing degree program was established at the University of British Columbia in 1919, with Ethel Johns as director. The operating costs of the new department were to be borne by the hospital, an incentive for the university to support the program. The program was nonintegrated—that is, "the university assumed no responsibility for the two or three years of nursing preparation in a hospital school of nursing" (Bonin, 1976, p. 7).

Several new 5-year, nonintegrated degree programs began at Canadian universities in the 1920s and 1930s: the University of

Western Ontario, the University of Alberta, l'Institut Marguerite d'Youville, the University of Ottawa, and St. Francis Xavier University. The religious order associated with the University of Ottawa launched what was essentially a hospital diploma program in 1933.

From the Depression to the Post-World War II Years

When nursing schools were established, women's education was a low priority. Nursing students were exploited in the hospital-based programs: in effect, subsidizing hospital operations. Nursing leaders fought to improve education at nursing schools and limit service, developing a standard curriculum that they urged schools to use. To eliminate weak programs, they encouraged the closure of hospital schools with insufficient beds. In 1932, the Weir report confirmed what nurses already knew about nursing schools: The conditions were deplorable, the health of students was in jeopardy, and education was secondary to hospital service (Weir, 1932).

The Great Depression "brought unemployment and hardship to nurses" (Allemang, 1974, p. 172). Clients could no longer afford to employ private-duty nurses, which had been the most promising area of employment for graduate nurses (Gunn, 1933). During the Depression, Canadian universities faced reduced revenues, staff layoffs, and difficult working conditions. The Depression was especially hard on McGill University, which depended on funds from private sources. During the Depression, raising private funds became next to impossible. Leaders of McGill's nursing school had fought unsuccessfully for years for a degree program. Once the university's finances began to deteriorate, the Board of Governors threatened to close the school altogether. The school's director, Bertha Harmer, gave up her salary, the faculty bought books for the library, and nursing alumnae groups all over the country raised funds to ensure the survival of the McGill nursing school (Tunis, 1966).

During World War II, health education became a priority as doctors and nurses were needed to care for military personnel, as well as civilians. Nurses who held critical positions as administrators, supervisors, teachers, and public health nurses were recruited for military service and left their positions. A shortage of nurses soon developed.

During and after the war, a new interest in nursing education led to increased external university funding, more scholarships and bursaries from private foundations, the growth of existing schools, and the founding of new programs. Programs were initiated at Queen's and McMaster Universities in 1941, followed by the University of Manitoba in 1943, Mount Saint Vincent University in 1947, and Dalhousie University in 1949. At McGill, new funds flowed in, and in 1944, supporters of the school were rewarded with a 5-year nonintegrated degree program.

Most nonintegrated programs offered a 2- to 3-year apprenticeship-based hospital diploma program sandwiched between 2 years of university study. The nonintegrated degree pattern with its stepladder approach to nursing education was well established, and the hospital programs on which this approach depended had been entrenched for many years. However, the new interest in nursing education led to exciting innovations.

In 1942, the University of Toronto introduced an integrated basic degree program. Under the leadership of Edith Kathleen Russell (see Chapter 4), courses in arts and sciences were taught concurrently with nursing courses to enhance student development. Also, university instructors supervised student clinical practice in the health care agencies. Four years after the introduction of the University of Toronto basic degree program, a second basic degree program was developed at McMaster University under Gladys Sharpe's direction.

Expansion in the 1950s and 1960s

In the 1960s, existing nursing degree programs expanded, and new programs emerged in other universities. The first master's degree program in nursing was established at the University of Western Ontario in 1959, followed in the 1960s and 1970s by similar programs in universities across the country. In 1962, the Canadian Nurses Foundation was established as an entity separate from the CNA, to provide scholarships, bursaries, and fellowships for graduate study in nursing.

Nursing schools' financial dependence left them at the mercy of hospital administrators. "The lack of nursing instructors and of other graduate nurses on patient care units meant that there were few role models for students for observation, questions and general discussion. In most cases senior students were left in charge of teaching junior students, and this with very limited supervision" (Paul, 1998, pp. 133–134). Many authorities have suggested that this was not a true apprenticeship model because it lacked the "master craftsman" to guide the students (Chapman, 1969).

Nursing leaders called for better faculty preparation, more integrated programs, and more university-based opportunities for students, such as student placements and increased enrolments. The movement to separate nursing education programs from the authority of hospitals began in earnest. Studies of nursing education identified persistent problems. Helen K. Mussallem found that hours on duty for students in hospital schools of nursing were too long, nursing instructors were too few, and the instructors were not qualified (CNA, 1965). In a 1965 survey, 65% of hospital schools reported that clinical assignments were based on the service needs of the patient care units, not on the students' educational needs (CNA, 1965).

Universities resisted introducing basic integrated degree programs because of the costs associated with the low student–teacher ratios required for clinical nursing. It was cheaper for them to let hospitals finance clinical education, but this meant that universities granted degrees for work over which they had no control. In 1964, the Royal Commission on Health Services castigated universities for this practice. By the late 1960s, the basic integrated degree program modeled on the program at the University of Toronto finally became the prototype for the establishment of integrated programs in nursing in universities across the nation.

From the 1970s to 2000

In 1975, the Alberta Task Force on Nursing Education proposed a postion on entry to practice, a radical proposal at the time, that recommended that all new nursing graduates be qualified at the baccalaureate level by 1995. Provincial governments gradually accepted the proposal and increased the capacity of degree-granting nursing education programs to accommodate all students studying nursing at the undergraduate level (CNA, 1991). Most provincial and regulatory bodies have now made the baccalaureate degree a requirement for the practice of nursing (CNA & Canadian Association of Schools of Nursing, 2004).

Throughout the 1970s and 1980s, university faculties and schools of nursing developed research resources so that they could offer graduate programs first at the master's level and then at the doctoral level. The first doctoral nursing program was established at the University of Alberta Faculty of Nursing on January 1, 1991, and others quickly followed.

The CNA has developed a position statement on promoting nursing history (CNA, 2008d), noting that learning from the lessons of history is "critical to advancing the profession in the interests of the Canadian public." This statement outlined the responsibilities of nurses across the whole gamut of roles and settings to promote nursing history.

Nursing Education Today

With continuing expansion of health care knowledge and technology, beginning practitioners require a broad educational foundation. New curricula and collaborative baccalaureate programs across the country attest to the profession's commitment to maintaining high standards of health care and responding to society's changing health care needs. The Internet, computerized learning programs, shared faculty through teleconferencing, and weekend and evening courses provide practising nurses with many options to complete degrees. The CNA's nursing portal, NurseOne, has made database information available to nurses across the country. Some universities have innovative programs at the baccalaureate level, including accelerated programs in which candidates hold baccalaureate degree in other fields. Baccalaureate programs, master's degree programs, and some courses in doctoral programs are also offered through distance education.

Standards for nursing education are monitored by each province to ensure that educational programs are of appropriate quality and respond to changes in health care. As professionals, nurses must acquire, maintain, and continuously enhance the knowledge, skills, attitudes, and judgment necessary to meet client needs in an evolving health care system. The responsibility for educational support for competent nursing practice is shared among individual nurses, professional nursing organizations, educational institutions, and governments (Wood, in press).

The need for nurses with graduate degrees is rising, along with the need for research. A master's degree in nursing is necessary for nurses seeking positions as clinical nurse specialists, nurse practitioners, nurse administrators, or nurse educators. Most master's programs in Canada now offer a concentration in advanced nursing practice for clinical nurse specialists and nurse practititioners. This provides advanced preparation in nursing science, theory, and practice, with emphasis on evidence-based clinical practice. Nurses with doctorates can undertake research that advances knowledge and evidence-based practice in clinical settings (see Chapter 7). This research enhances the quality of nursing care and improves Canadians' health outcomes. Today, there are 30 master's programs and 12 doctoral programs in nursing in Canada.

Continuing and In-Service Education

Nurses need to continually update their skills and knowledge to practise in a constantly changing health care environment. **Continuing education** includes formal, organized, and educational programs offered by provincial associations and educational and health care institutions. In addition, health care agencies and institutions offer **in-service education** programs, designed to increase the knowledge, skills, and competencies of nurses and other health care professionals employed by the institution. A growing number of professional associations are developing continuing competence programs in which nurses must provide evidence that they are taking steps to update their knowledge and skills.

Professional Roles and Responsibilities

Contemporary nursing requires that the nurse possess knowledge and skills for a variety of professional roles and responsibilities. In the past, the principal role of nurses was to provide care and treatment, as well as comfort. This role has grown to include increased emphasis on health promotion and on concern for clients and families. The role of the nurse in primary health care (see Chapter 1) is an evolving and important one because nurses are involved with assisting clients and families to learn as much as possible about their health and health care in order to ensure health and well-being. Nurses also help clients make the transition from home to the health care agency, or vice versa, as seamless as possible.

As advanced knowledge and technology are being rapidly incorporated into care, nursing roles have also been evolving. Thus, nursing offers expanded roles and a broad range of career opportunities (Figure 3–1). Examples of career roles include those as nurse educators, managers or **administrators**, **researchers**, quality improvement nurses, consultants, and even business owners. Many nurses are employed in the areas of education and administration.

Since the late 1980s, there have been significant developments in the expansion of nursing roles, specifically in advanced nursing practice. *Advanced nursing practice* is an umbrella term that refers to two advanced nursing roles in Canada: namely, the clinical nurse specialist and the nurse practitioner. The CNA (2008c) developed a national framework intended to guide the development of advanced nursing practice in Canada in which it defined core competencies in five areas: clinical nursing, research, leadership, collaboration, and change agency. It also stipulated a graduate degree in nursing as the minimum educational requirement and recommended that regulation of practice be part of the current scope of nursing practice and regulation.

The **clinical nurse specialist** role is one that involves a high level of nursing practice in a specialized area such as oncology or gerontology, and this role has been integrated into health care. The difference between the roles of nurse practitioners and clinical nurse specialists is an important one. **Nurse practitioners** provide mainly primary care, whereas clinical nurse specialists function in a more consultative way as expert clinicians and educators. Although nurse practitioners have

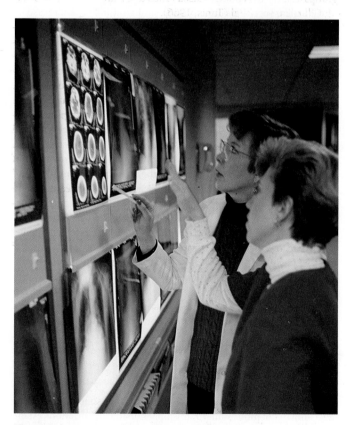

Figure 3-1 Nurse specialists consult on a difficult case.

been practising in Ontario since the 1970s, this was the culmination of a movement that began a decade previously. Furthermore, legislation to govern their practice in primary health care settings has more recently been developed as part of existing legislation in all jurisdictions (MacDonald et al, 2005). Although there is variation from one jurisdiction to another, the nurse practitioner may prescribe medications with certain exclusions and treat health problems within the scope of nursing practice. Developments in the educational programs for and licensing of nurse practitioners have been taking place at a rapid pace and have greatly extended the scope of practice for this group of nurses. There have been discussion and some controversy about advanced practice roles that could be developed in Canada, including roles such as nurse anesthetist and nurse midwife (Schreiber & MacDonald, 2008).

Gender and Diversity in Nursing

Nursing is a profession in transition from one that has been predominantly female in character to one that is gender balanced. Traditional societal values that negate nurturing roles for men have been changing. However, even though the number of men employed in nursing in Canada has increased, the current proportion of male nurses represents only 5.6% of the total nurse population, a slight increase over the 4.7% it represented in 2000 (CNA, 2006). This is remarkable at a time when the proportion of women in traditionally male-dominated professions has increased at a phenomenal rate. O'Lynn and Tranbarger (2006) pointed to communication problems, reverse discriminatory practices, and gender-based barriers for male students in nursing. However, although many factors have deterred men from pursuing careers in nursing, some of the negative influences are slowly beginning to change.

Canadian society has also become multicultural. The increase in racial, ethnic, and cultural diversity has meant that individuals of different races, ethnic descent, and cultural backgrounds are present in every major population and occupational group. The benefit to Canada of this new diversity is inestimable and provides a far richer background for local, national, and international relationships. Some groups have historically been underrepresented in certain professions, including nursing, in comparison with their representation in the population. Recognition of the contributions of different ethnic and cultural groups, including Aboriginal groups, to the cultural mosaic in Canadian society has been slow in coming.

Villeneuve (2002–2003) decried the fact that the majority of nurses in Canada remain white and female, a situation that is common in the health care professions. Gates (2007) found that the greater the perceived increased difference in status between a staff nurse and others in the setting, the weaker was the nurse's intent to remain on the job. There has been pressure for the profession to enhance and improve programs in order to encourage nurses with minority cultural and racial backgrounds to enter programs and remain committed to their choices. The development of shared value systems, along with defined strategies to enhance recruitment, retention, and management, has been seen as crucial for retaining staff (Gates, 2007).

Professional Nursing Organizations

A **professional organization** deals with issues of concern to people practising in the profession. Professional nursing organizations establish educational and practice standards for nurses, carry out the regulatory functions of registration and licensure, and discipline members who do not meet the standards. Most of these organizations have continuing competence programs to ensure that their members maintain competence through continuing education. The terms *registration* and *licensure* have different meanings, although they are often used interchangeably. *Registration* refers to the listing of a member in good standing on the membership roster of an organization, whereas *licensure* refers to the exclusive right to practise a profession, granted by a government body to a member in good standing. In most provinces and territories (except Ontario), governments entrust administration of the legislation to the professional nursing association.

Nursing associations at the provincial or territorial level are organizations that serve as official representatives of the nursing profession and interact with provincial or territorial government officials on issues concerning the health of the populace and the roles of nurses. In most provinces, these organizations perform the regulatory functions of registration and professional conduct. Professional organizations are concerned with standards of practice and education. They present education programs, publish journals or newsletters, and work to increase public understanding of nursing and nursing outcomes on the health of individuals, families, and communities. They also collaborate with other health care professions on matters of mutual interest. Some professional organizations and special interest groups focus on specific areas such as critical care, nursing administration, or research. Examples include the Canadian Gerontological Nursing Association, the Canadian Association of Neuroscience Nurses, and the Aboriginal Nurses Association of Canada. These organizations seek to improve the standards of practice, to expand nursing roles, and to foster the welfare of nurses within the specialty areas. In some provinces or territories, "colleges" of registered nurses have been established through new legislation to replace existing nursing legislation. Although the primary mandates in these "colleges" are registration, professional conduct, and standards of practice and education, the degree of involvement in professional association matters varies. For example, in British Columbia (personal communication, Laurel Brunke, May 22, 2008) and Ontario, the respective "colleges" are concerned solely with matters pertaining to registration, professional conduct, and standards of education and practice. However, in other jurisdictions, such as Alberta (personal communication, Kim Campbell, June 11, 2008), Manitoba, and Nova Scotia, the "college" assumes regulatory functions in addition to those of a professional association speaking for and representing nurses on issues and concerns of the profession.

Nurses form a large and very powerful group and have made important contributions to public health through the leadership provided by their professional organizations. The CNA works at the national level for the improvement of health standards and the availability of health care services for all people, fosters high standards of nursing, stimulates and promotes the professional development of nurses, and advances their economic and general welfare. As the national voice of professional nurses, the CNA represents nurses across the country to the federal government and national organizations (Box 3–4). It regularly presents briefs to the House of Commons on areas such as taxation, poverty, health care, unemployment insurance, employment opportunities, part-time work, economic and social affairs, science and technology, and federal and provincial fiscal arrangements, including funding for health care. The CNA also collaborates with other national nursing and health organizations on issues related to practice, education, and research, and it holds regular meetings and discussions with government officials to ensure that the federal government is aware of CNA positions on health care and policy issues.

The CNA also gives individual nurses a collective means to influence health care policy at the national level. For example, in February 2000, after extensive lobbying by the CNA, the federal government

> **BOX 3-4** **Canadian Nurses Association: Vision and Mission Statement**

CNA is the national professional voice of registered nurses, supporting them in their practice and advocating for public health policy and a quality, publicly funded, not-for-profit health care system.

In pursuit of its vision and mission, CNA (2008e) has established the following goals:

- Advancing the discipline of nursing in the interest of the public.
- Advocating public policy that incorporates the principles of primary health care (access; interdisciplinary practice; patient and community involvement; health promotion, including determinants of health and appropriate technology, roles, or models) and respects the principles, conditions, and spirit of the *Canada Health Act*.
- Advancing the regulation of registered nurses in the interest of the public.
- Working in collaboration with nurses, other health care providers, health care system stakeholders, and the public to achieve and sustain quality practice environments and positive client outcomes.
- Advancing international health care policy and development in Canada and abroad to support global health care and equity.
- Promoting awareness of the nursing profession so that the roles and expertise of registered nurses are understood, respected, and optimized within the health care system.

Adapted from Canadian Nurses Association. (2008). *Vision and mission statement*. Ottawa, ON: Author.

committed $2.5 billion to the Canada Health and Social Transfer, earmarking a substantial portion of that amount for nursing. After the 2004 federal election, the CNA lobbied federally for its *Common Vision for the Canadian Health System* on health care in order to develop an agreement with the provinces to ensure "an adequate supply of health providers, pan-Canadian benchmarks and real targets for timely access to care, the expansion of the continuum of care and sufficient, on-going and predictable federal long-term funding" (*Media Statement*, 2004).

Unions

Nursing unions represent nurses in job-related negotiations with their employers. The primary interest of the unions is the economic welfare of the nurses they represent, but bargaining covers a broad area, including benefits, working conditions, and responsibilities.

A movement to establish a national voice for unionized nurses began in the early 1960s, when nurses pressed their professional associations to become involved in collective bargaining for them. Thus, professional organizations initially were responsible for collective bargaining. However, the 1973 Supreme Court decision in the appeal of the Saskatchewan case *Service Employees International Union [SEIU] v. Nipiwan District Staff Nurses Association* (in which the Staff Nurses Association was a unit of the Saskatchewan Registered Nurses Association) led to the separation of professional associations across the country (SEIU Local 333, 1973). The Staff Nurses Association had applied to be certified as a bargaining unit, but certification was denied on the basis of the potential conflict of interest in determining salaries of registered nurses because the Staff Nurses Association's Board of Directors could include nurse managers. Within a decade, every province had both a separate nursing association and a union. Some nursing unions represent both registered nurses and registered practical nurses (licensed practical nurses).

In 1981, the National Federation of Nurses' Unions was formed to represent the interests of nurses in both watchdog and lobbying activities. This organization became the Canadian Confederation of Nurses' Unions (CCNU) and by 2004 all provinces except Quebec were members. Nursing unions have lobbied for professional responsibility clauses in union contracts and are the representatives of nurses in particular provinces or territories when new contracts are negotiated. The CCNU has been active in raising the issues for nurses concerning current and projected nursing shortages and in arguing the case for public health care.

Standards of Nursing Practice

As a self-regulating profession, nursing sets its own standards of practice, which serve as objective guidelines for nurses to provide and evaluate care. Standards are based on research and clinical evidence and help assure clients that they are receiving high-quality care. Quality assurance programs incorporate measures to ensure high standards of practice. Because health is a provincial responsibility, each professional nursing organization is responsible for developing its own standards of nursing practice. In Table 3–1, the nursing practice standards developed for the province of Ontario by the College of Nurses of Ontario (2002) are presented as an example.

Ethical Standards of Practice

Ethical standards that guide practice are fundamental to all professions. Normally, these standards are expressed as "codes" of ethics; they emerged as a result of the Nuremberg Code, developed in 1947 from the post–World War II war crimes investigation of experimentation on human beings. The first **code of ethics** for nursing was developed by the ICN in 1953. The CNA adopted the ICN code the next year and in 1980 developed its first code of ethics. The *Code of Ethics for Registered Nurses* was most recently updated (CNA, 2008b). The Code of Ethics provides nurses with direction for ethical decision making and practice in everyday situations. Because nursing in Canada is a provincial responsibility, each province and territory is responsible for its code of ethics. Therefore, each provincial statute regulating nursing incorporates a code of ethics. Many provinces use the CNA Code of Ethics in their statutes (see Chapter 8).

Registration and Licensure

Because constitutional responsibility for education and health falls under the purview of the provinces and territories, each has a nursing practice act to regulate the licensure and practice of nursing. The scope of nursing practice is defined within the legislation in each province and territory. Provincial and territorial nursing practice acts are revised regularly to reflect changes in nursing practice. In all provinces except Ontario and Quebec, provincial and territorial nursing associations assume responsibility for defining and monitoring standards. In addition, nurses working in hospitals and other health care agencies also practice according to hospital or agency policies. These policies are more detailed and are specific to the nature of the care provided in the the particular health setting. In most jurisdictions, to be eligible for registration, students must complete a prescribed course of study from a nursing program approved by the body legislatively responsible for the regulation of nursing. The legislation governing nursing in all Canadian jurisdictions has been amended since the 1990s to allow for licensing of nurse practitioners (CNA, 2004).

Certification

With the development of highly specialized knowledge in a variety of discrete areas of nursing, there arose a need to ensure that clients received care from nurses who had developed the necessary knowledge and skills to work in particular specialized areas. The CNA

> **TABLE 3-1**   **Standards of Professional Practice**

The following are broad descriptions of the expectations of nurses and apply to all nurses in every area of practice. Although written by the College of Nurses of Ontario for nurses in Ontario, the general themes are relevant for nurses across the country.

Accountability

Each nurse is accountable to the public and responsible for ensuring that her/his practice and conduct meets legislative requirements and the standards of the profession.

Nurses are responsible for their actions and the consequences of those actions. Part of this accountability includes conducting themselves in ways that promote respect for the profession. Nurses are not accountable for the decisions or actions of other care providers when there was no way of knowing about those actions.

Continuing Competence

Each nurse maintains and continually improves her/his competence by participating in the College of Nurses of Ontario's Quality Assurance (QA) Program.

Competence is the nurse's ability to use her / his knowledge, skill, judgment, attitudes, values and beliefs to perform in a given role, situation and practice setting. Continuing competence ensures the nurse is able to perform in a changing health environment. Continuing competence also contributes to quality nursing practice and increases the public's confidence in the nursing profession.

Participation in the College's QA Program assists nurses to engage in activities that promote or foster lifelong learning. The program helps nurses to maintain and improve their competence and is a professional requirement.

Ethics

Each nurse understands, upholds, and promotes the values and beliefs described in the College's ethics practice standard.

Ethical nursing care means promoting the values of client well-being, respecting client choice, assuring privacy and confidentiality, respecting sanctity and quality of life, maintaining commitments, respecting truthfulness, and ensuring fairness in the use of resources. It also includes acting with integrity, honesty, and professionalism in all dealings with the client and other health team members.

Knowledge

Each nurse possesses, through basic education and continuing learning, knowledge relevant to her/his professional practice.

RNs and RPNs study from the same body of nursing knowledge. RPNs study for a shorter period of time, resulting in a more focused or basic foundation of knowledge in clinical practice, decision making, critical thinking, research, and leadership. RNs study for a longer period of time for a greater breadth and depth of knowledge in clinical practice, decision making, critical thinking, research utilization, leadership, health care delivery systems, and resource management. All nurses add to their basic education and foundational knowledge throughout their careers by pursuing ongoing learning.

Knowledge Application

Each nurse continually improves the application of professional knowledge.

The quality of professional nursing practice reflects nurses' application of knowledge. Nurses apply knowledge to practice using nursing frameworks, theories and/or processes. This includes the performance of clinical skills because the technical and cognitive aspects of care are closely related and cannot be separated.

Leadership

Nurses demonstrate [their] leadership by providing, facilitating and promoting the best possible care/service to the public.

Leadership requires self-knowledge (understanding one's beliefs and values and being aware of how one's behaviour affects others), respect, trust, integrity, shared vision, learning, participation, good communication techniques, and the ability to be a change facilitator. The leadership expectation is not limited to nurses in formal leadership positions. All nurses, regardless of their positions, have opportunities for leadership.

Relationships

Each nurse establishes and maintains respectful, collaborative, therapeutic, and professional relationships.

Relationships include therapeutic nurse–client relationships and professional relationships with colleagues, health team members and employers.

Therapeutic Nurse-Client Relationships

The client's needs are the focus of the relationship, which is based on trust, respect, intimacy, and the appropriate use of power. Nurses demonstrate empathy and caring in all relationships with clients, families, and significant others. It is the responsibility of the nurse to establish and maintain the therapeutic relationship.

Professional Relationships

Professional relationships are based on trust and respect, and result in improved client care.

Adapted from College of Nurses of Ontario. (2002). *Professional Standards, Revised 2002.* Toronto, ON: Author. For links to indicators of each standard, see http://www.cno.org/docs/prac/41006_ProfStds.pdf

passed a resolution at its convention in 1980 to explore the feasibility of developing certification examinations in major nursing specialties. As a first step, the CNA Testing Service developed a certification examination for the Canadian Council of Occcupational Health Nurses. The CNA then developed policies for a voluntary certification program, and the Canadian Association of Neuroscience Nurses became the first to sponsor such a program in conjunction with the CNA. As of 2008, the CNA, along with national nursing specialty organizations, offered certification in 18 specialties: cardiovascular care, community health care, critical care, critical care–pediatrics, emergency care, gastroenterology, gerontology, hospice palliative care, nephrology, neuroscience, occupational health care, oncology, orthopedics, perinatal care, perioperative care, psychiatric or mental health care, rehabilitation, and enterostomal therapy (CNA, 2008a). The CNA certification program has been highly successful, inasmuch as it has provided a means of recognizing the specialized knowledge and skills necessary in a great number of areas of practice. It is likely that even more specialty groups will apply to be part of the certification program in the future.

Conclusion

Organized nursing has been a part of the social setting in Canada since the early days of the European settlement at Quebec, a period of more than three and a half centuries. The first nurses who came to found hospitals and to provide care for Aboriginal people and settlers were motivated by altruism and serve as excellent role models for nurses today. Altruism, a hallmark of any profession, remains an important characteristic of the nursing profession despite vast difference between the health care settings of the early days and those of today.

A fundamental and guiding principle of the French-Canadian hospitals that survived largely intact into the twentieth century was that care was available to all people regardless of their background, status in life, or ability to pay. This continues to be a principle for which nurses, through their professional organizations, have argued for determinedly in national debates on the nature and continuing direction of Canada's national health care insurance program. In the presence of pressure to reshape Medicare, nurses have continued to strongly resist calls for privatization of more aspects of the health system. They have also repeatedly called for all health care professionals to be remunerated on a salary or contract basis (Ross-Kerr, in press).

Multidisciplinary teams are an integral component of the health care organization in the community. However, nurses are the primary health care professionals both in home care and in community health settings. Thus, expanded and enhanced educational systems for nurses that incorporate knowledge and skills for community health and home care nursing are essential to meet the health needs of the populace today.

Nursing today requires a vast range of knowledge and skills, and thus educational programs to prepare nurses for the health systems of today and the future are demanding. Nurses have unlimited opportunities for fulfilling careers in a vast array of general and specialty areas. Numerous educational opportunities are open to nurses throughout their careers to enhance knowledge and skills and to move into new areas if desired. In nursing practice, nurses carry more responsibility than ever before. Nurse educators have challenging opportunities in practice, education, and research. Nursing scientists are leaders in health research, and the results of their investigations have changed health practices around the world.

The transformation of the nursing profession and of the educational programs that support it since the nineteenth century has been truly remarkable. Despite monumental obstacles, nurses have demonstrated the value of their service, the integrity of their goals, the quality of their educational programs, and the strength of their commitment. Although developments through the twenty-first century are as yet unknown, it is certain that the nursing profession will continue to evolve in the interest of providing a high quality of nursing care to the populace.

✳ KEY CONCEPTS

- Nursing has responded to the health care needs of society, influenced over time by economic, social, and cultural factors.
- Nursing in Canada is rooted in the traditions of good nursing that developed in New France.
- Florence Nightingale revolutionized nursing as an acceptable profession for women as lay nurses in the late 1800s and early 1900s.
- The development of a system of nursing education in Canada emerged from the early nursing sisterhoods and from schools of nursing associated with hospitals.
- Baccalaureate entry to practice is almost fully implemented in Canada.
- Basic nursing education is acquired in college, collaborative college-university, or university programs.
- Nurses have a variety of career opportunities and roles, including those of clinical nurse, clinical nurse specialist, nurse practitioner, educator, administrator, and researcher.
- The ranks of the profession are moving toward gender balance and a racial, ethnic, and cultural mix that reflects the Canadian population.
- Professional nursing organizations establish standards of education and practice for nurses, perform the regulatory functions of registration and professional conduct, deal with issues of concern to nurses and specialist groups within the nursing profession, and empower nurses to influence health care policy and practice.
- Nursing sets its own standards of practice—from scientific research and the work of nurse clinical experts—to ensure high-quality care.

✳ CRITICAL THINKING EXERCISES

1. Explain the importance of Florence Nightingale's work to establish nursing as a profession.

2. Identify some of the enduring values that have emerged from the history of nursing in Canada.

3. Observe various levels of nursing practice, such as a staff nurse, nurse practitioner, and nurse educator. Identify similarities and differences in their roles and educational preparation.

4. Outline some career objectives for yourself after completing your nursing program. Think about what you want to do as a professional nurse, and then outline strategies for achieving these goals.

✳ REVIEW QUESTIONS

1. The founder of modern nursing is
    1. Hippocrates
    2. Florence Nightingale
    3. Jeanne Mance
    4. Mary Agnes Snively

2. The founder of the Sisters of Charity of Montreal, which later became known as the Grey Nuns, is
   1. Marie Rollet Hébert
   2. St. Vincent de Paul
   3. Marguerite d'Youville
   4. Lady Ishbel Aberdeen

3. The first doctoral nursing program in Canada was established in
   1. 1890
   2. 1933
   3. 1975
   4. 1991

4. Nurse practitioners in Canada
   1. Work in university health settings
   2. Are able to function independently
   3. Are licensed under nursing legislation in jurisdictions
   4. Function as unit directors in health agencies

5. Nursing has a code of ethics that professional registered nurses follow, which
   1. Defines the principles of nursing care
   2. Ensures identical care to all clients
   3. Protects the client from harm
   4. Improves self-health care

6. Which of the following is *not* a function of a professional nursing organization?
   1. Regulating registration and professional conduct
   2. Monitoring unregulated care providers
   3. Collaborating with other health care organizations on matters of mutual interest
   4. Establishing standards of education and professional practice

7. The practice of nursing is regulated by
   1. The CNA
   2. Nursing practice acts
   3. Best practice guidelines
   4. Hospital administrators

8. Some of the professional standards outlined by the College of Nurses of Ontario include
   1. Accountability, ethics, leadership
   2. Administering medications, personal hygiene and grooming
   3. Care of vulnerable populations
   4. Care of people in financial crises

9. Except for Ontario and Quebec, minimum standards for nursing education are set by
   1. The nursing school
   2. The provincial or territorial nursing association
   3. The Canadian Nurses Association
   4. The Canadian Nurses Federation

10. A role of a nursing union is to
    1. Devise ethical standards to guide practice
    2. Set the standards of practice for nursing
    3. Represent nurses in bargaining for new contracts
    4. Carry out registration and licensure

✳ RECOMMENDED WEB SITES

Canadian Association for the History of Nursing (CAHN): http://www.cahn-achn.ca/
An affiliate group of the CNA, the CAHN offers information about Canadian nursing history and promotes historical research.

Canadian nursing organizations: http://www.canadianrn.com/directory/assoc.htm
This site offers a list of current Canadian nursing organizations, including contact information.

4

Community Health Nursing Practice

Written by Kaysi Eastlick Kushner, RN, PhD

media resources

evolve Web Site
- Audio Chapter Summaries
- Glossary
- Multiple-Choice Review Questions
- Student Learning Activities
- Weblinks

Companion CD
- Glossary
- Interactive Learning Activities
- Fluids and Electrolytes Tutorial
- Test-Taking Skills

Today's health care climate is rapidly changing in response to economic pressures, technological and medical advances, and client participation in health care. As a result, many clients are receiving care in the community rather than in hospital. There is a growing need to deliver health care where people live, work, and learn through a community health nursing practice model (Community Health Nurses Association of Canada [CHNAC], 2003). Community health nursing care focuses on health promotion, disease prevention, and restorative and palliative care. The goals of community health nursing are to keep individuals healthy, encourage client participation and choice in care, promote health-enhancing social environments, and provide in-home care for ill or disabled clients.

Promoting individual and community health has always been key to the holistic practice of nursing. In the 1730s, the Grey Nuns were established as Canada's first community nursing order. More than a century later, in England, Florence Nightingale articulated a nursing philosophy grounded in knowledge of environmental conditions. By the end of the century, the Victorian Order of Nurses was providing in-home nursing, often in outpost and remote regions. After World War I, community nursing responsibilities "extended to screening programs to detect disease at early stages, to helping to maintain a healthy environment, and to providing nursing care" (Ross-Kerr, 1996, p. 11).

Canadians such as Kate Brighty Colley (Box 4–1) and Edith Kathleen Russell (Box 4–2) pioneered community health nursing and public health nursing in Canada. Today, nursing is leading the way in assessing, implementing, and evaluating all types of public and community-based health services needed by clients. Community health nursing is essential for improving the health of the general public.

Promoting the Health of Populations and Community Groups

Nurses practising in the community face many challenges in promoting the health of populations and community groups. A **population** is a collection of individuals who have in common one or more personal or environmental characteristics (Maurer & Smith, 2005). Examples of populations include Canadians inclusively and, more specifically, high-risk infants, older adults, or a cultural group such as Aboriginal peoples. A healthy population is composed of healthy individuals, and the health status of individuals is considered an overall aggregate that reflects an average or general health status. To determine a population's health status, individual characteristics (such as occurrence of illness, disability, and death; lifespan; education; and living conditions) are considered. A **community** is a group of people who share a geographic (locational) dimension and a social (relational) dimension (Edwards & Moyer, 2000; Laverack, 2004). The social dimension—which comprises individual relationships, interactions among groups, and shared characteristics among members—distinguishes a community from a population. Examples of communities include geographic groupings (e.g., neighbourhoods) and shared interest groups (e.g., women's health networks). A healthy community consists of healthy individuals engaged in collective relationships that create a supportive living environment. Both individual and community characteristics are used to determine community health status. Key characteristics of a healthy community include a collective capacity to solve problems; adequate living conditions; a safe environment; and sustainable resources such as employment, health care, and educational facilities.

Community Health Nursing Practice

The scope of **community health nursing practice** includes population health promotion, protection, maintenance, and restoration; community, family, and individual health promotion; and individual rehabilitation or palliative care. Community health nursing promotes

> ### ➤ BOX 4-1   Milestones in Canadian Nursing History

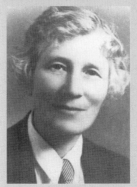

Kate Brighty Colley, 1883-1985

Born in England in 1883, Kate Brighty immigrated with her parents to Nova Scotia at the age of 3 years. She graduated from the Royal Alexandra Hospital School of Nursing in Edmonton in 1917, after which she enlisted with the Canadian Army Medical Corps in Calgary.

After completing a course in public health nursing at the University of Alberta in 1919, Brighty was one of the first nurses to be appointed to the staff of the new Alberta Department of Public Health. Soon afterward, the Alberta Department of Agriculture engaged her to teach home nursing, bedside care, and hygiene in Grande Prairie.

In the same year, Brighty was appointed matron of the second municipal hospital in Alberta, the Mission Hospital at Onoway. Because there were no physicians in the region, she and her two employees staffed the hospital and visited rural patients on horseback. In 1923, she returned to the Department of Public Health to establish a district nursing centre at Buck Lake near Pendryl, southwest of Edmonton—an area that had no roads at the time—and then another centre, farther north at Wanham, near the Peace River. Here she travelled by cutter to assist women in labour and those who were ill.

In 1925, Brighty took a postgraduate course in public health nursing at Columbia University, New York. Upon her return to Alberta in 1928, she was appointed director of the Department of Public Health Nursing. Her responsibilities were expanded a year later to include the post of inspector of hospitals.

In her new post, Brighty established a number of new district nursing centres. As a former district nurse, she understood the problems these nurses faced, and she travelled widely to visit staff. She expanded the health education program and gave talks on the radio on health, hygiene, nutrition, and child welfare. These broadcasts were important to residents of remote areas, where little formal health care was available.

Brighty was active in the Alberta Association of Registered Nurses (AARN) and, in 1936, was elected president of the organization. She wrote the first history of nursing in Alberta, the *AARN Blue Book* (Brighty, 1942).

After 24 years of service to the Department of Public Health Nursing, she retired in 1943 to Vancouver Island, where she contributed regularly to the *Halifax Chronicle, Atlantic Monthly,* and other magazines. She married W. H. Colley after her retirement, and in 1970, she published *While Rivers Flow: Stories of Early Alberta,* experiences and short stories based on her public health nursing practice.

Sources: Brighty, K. (1942). *Collection of facts for a history of nursing in Alberta: 1864–1942.* Edmonton, AB: Alberta Association of Registered Nurses; and Brighty Colley, K. (1970). *While rivers flow: Stories of early Alberta.* Saskatoon, SK: The Western Producer; and Stewart, I. (1979). *These were our yesterdays: A history of district nursing in Alberta.* Altona, MB: Friesen Printers.

and protects the health of individuals, families, groups, communities, and populations (CHNAC, 2003). It involves coordinating care and planning services, programs, and policies by collaborating with individuals, caregivers, families, other disciplines, communities, and governments (CHNAC, 2003). It combines knowledge of nursing theory, social sciences, and public health sciences.

Community health nursing includes public health nursing, home health (community-based) nursing, and community mental health nursing, as well as a variety of other specialities such as street health, telehealth, and parish nursing (CHNAC, 2003; see also Stamler & Yiu, 2008, and Stanhope et al., 2008, for in-depth descriptions of community health nursing roles in Canada). Occupational health nursing has emerged as a distinctive specialized practice, although it is arguably within the inclusive focus of community health nursing. The community health nursing focus is broader than that of public health nursing, emphasizing both the community's health and direct care to subpopulations within that community. By focusing on subpopulations, the community health nurse cares for the whole community and considers the individual to be one member of a group. The practice focus of various specialties within community health nursing can be compared to the shifting perspective of a camera lens: For example, home health nurses "zoom in" to focus on individual clients, then enlarge their view (wide angle) to consider family and community, whereas public health nurses more often shift from a "wide-angle" view of populations to a "close-up" view of specific vulnerable groups or families (CHNAC, 2003).

Regardless of specific role, function, or setting, community health nursing practice is guided by values and beliefs in caring, multiple ways of knowing, individual–community partnerships, primary health care, and empowerment (CHNAC, 2003). **Primary health care** focuses on education, rehabilitation, support services, health promotion, and disease prevention. It involves multidisciplinary teams and collaboration with other sectors, as well as with secondary and tertiary care facilities (see Chapter 2). Primary health care principles guide community health nurses to use empowerment-based models of community practice (Chalmers & Bramadat, 1996; CHNAC, 2003). **Empowerment** may be most simply described as a means by which people, individually and collectively in organizations and communities, exercise their ability to effect change to enhance control, quality of life, and social justice (CHNAC, 2003). Empowerment is both an outcome and a process by which that outcome is achieved. Empowerment exists in dynamic power relations among people, which from a health promotion perspective are expressed as "power-with" rather than "power-over" relations (Labonte, 1993). Although empowerment is commonly conceptualized as a process continuum from personal to small group to community organzation to partnership to social and political action (Laverack, 2004), Labonte's holosphere (Venn diagram) better depicts the interrelated and nonlinear dynamic of these empowering processes in practice. Criticisms that empowerment is often misinterpreted as increasing individual responsibility but overlooking power and control (Cooke, 2002) highlight the importance of action to ensure that adequate resources are available for individuals and for groups and communities collectively. Such action would be grounded in ethical commitment to inclusion, diversity, participation, social justice, advocacy, and interdependence as a complementary foundation to the Canadian Nurses Association (CNA) Code of Ethics intended to guide all nursing practice (Racher, 2007).

Empowerment-based skills of client advocacy, communication, and the design of new systems in cooperation with existing systems help make community health nursing practice effective. Figure 4–1 depicts the Canadian Community Health Nursing Practice Model. The model shows how community health nursing care encompasses action aimed at illness care; prevention of illness, disease, or injury;

and health promotion. These actions complement one another, even as their underlying aims, approaches to care, and perceptions of clients differ.

Community health nursing practice requires a distinct set of skills and knowledge. Expert community health nurses understand the needs of a population or community through experiences with individuals, families, and groups. They think critically in applying a wide range of knowledge to find the best approaches for partnering with their clients. In 2006, the CNA introduced a certification process for nurses in community health nursing (CNA, 2006). Certification confirms practitioner competence in the specialty, recognizes nurses who meet the national standards of the specialty, and, most important, promotes excellence in nursing care for the Canadian population (see CNA, 2006, and CHNAC, 2003, for details about standards and certification procedures).

Public Health Nursing

Public health nursing merges knowledge from the public health sciences with professional nursing theories to safeguard and improve the health of populations in the community (Canadian Public Health Association, 1990; CHNAC, 2003). To understand public health

---

> **BOX 4-2**   **Milestones in Canadian Nursing History**

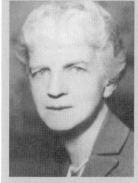

Edith Kathleen Russell, 1886–1964

Edith Kathleen Russell was born in Windsor, Nova Scotia, in 1886. She entered the Toronto General Hospital School of Nursing in 1915 and, after graduating, worked with the Department of Public Health in Toronto. In 1920, the Department of Public Health Nursing at the University of Toronto was established, and Russell was appointed its first director.

Russell recognized the great need for improved nursing education. At the time, the norm was an apprenticeship system in hospital schools, in which students, rather than graduate nurses, fulfilled nursing tasks. The primary focus of the hospital school system was not education but hospital service; the incentive was mainly financial. Although public health nursing was her department's original focus, Russell turned her attention to hospital nursing. She gained the support of the University of Toronto and the Rockefeller Foundation for an experiment in basic nursing education and obtained a grant of more than $250,000. This was at the height of the Great Depression, when other university schools were fighting for their very existence.

Russell's diploma program, begun in 1933, prepared nurses for hospital and public health nursing. In 1942, her program evolved into an integrated basic degree program controlled by the university, in which clinical practice was obtained at affiliated hospitals under supervision of university instructors. This program was the first of its kind in Canada and was hailed throughout the world as an important new system of nursing education. Today, hospital-based schools of nursing have largely given way to schools in the general educational system, either in community colleges or in universities, and most provinces are adopting the degree as the basic credential for nursing practice. Edith Kathleen Russell is widely recognized as the architect of the integrated degree nursing program.

Source: Carpenter, H. (1982). *A divine discontent: Edith Kathleen Russell, reforming educator.* Toronto, ON: University of Toronto Faculty of Nursing.
Photo: Reproduced by permission of Helen M. Carpenter (BS, MPH, EdD).

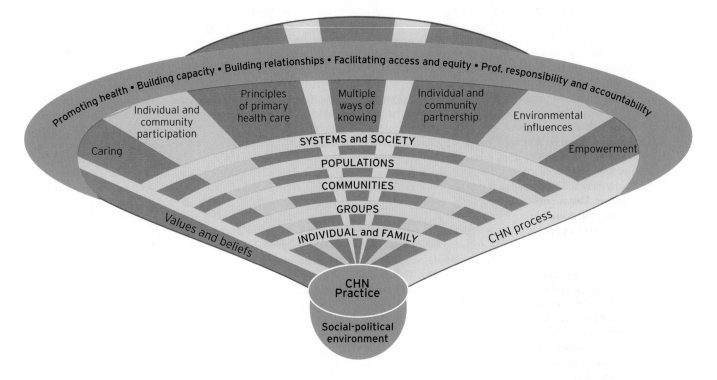

Figure 4-1 The Canadian community health nursing practice model. The model illustrates the dynamic nature of community health nursing (CHN) practice, embracing the present and projecting into the future. The values and beliefs (*green* or *shaded*) ground practice in the present and yet guide the evolution of community health nursing practice over time. The community health nursing process (*pink* or *unshaded*) provides the vehicle through which community health nurses work with people, and supports practice that exemplifies the standards of community health nursing. The standards of practice revolve around both the values and beliefs and the nursing process, and the energies of community health nursing are always being focused on improving the health of the people in the community and facilitating change in systems or society in support of health. Community health nursing practice occurs not in isolation but rather within an environmental context, such as policies within nurses' workplace and the legislative framework applicable to their work. **Source:** Adapted from Community Health Nurses Association of Canada. (2008). *Canadian community health nursing standards of practice.* Retrieved September 10, 2008, from http://www.chnac.ca/images/downloads/standards/chn_standards_of_practice_mar08_english.pdf

nursing, it is necessary to know how public health works. The emphasis in **public health** is on the health of the entire population. Historically, government-funded agencies have supported public health programs that improve food and water safety and provide adequate sewage disposal. Public health policy has largely been responsible for the dramatic gain in life expectancy for North Americans during the past century (McKay, 2008; Shah, 2003). The goal of public health is to achieve a healthy environment for everyone. **Public health principles** of disease prevention, health promotion and protection, and healthy public policy (Canadian Public Health Association, 2008) can be applied to individuals, families, groups, or communities. Public health practice calls for competencies (i.e., knowledge, skills, attitudes) that cross the boundaries of specific disciplines and are independent of programs and roles (Public Health Agency of Canada, 2007). These competencies include "population health assessment, surveillance, disease and injury prevention, health promotion, and health protection" (Public Health Agency of Canada, 2007, p. 1).

A public health focus requires understanding the needs of a population. Focus may be narrowed to vulnerable populations, such as low-income families or recent immigrants. Public health professionals must understand factors influencing the health promotion and health maintenance of groups, trends and patterns influencing the occurrence of disease or risks within populations, environmental factors contributing to health and illness, and political processes used to influence public policy (see Chapter 1, "Determinants of Health" section).

As discussed in Chapter 1, **population health** emerged in Canada in the 1990s as an approach to public health care. The overall goals of a population health approach are to maintain and improve the health of the entire population and to eliminate health disparities (Health Canada, 1998). The population health promotion approach (Hamilton & Bhatti, 1996) provides a framework for thinking about health and for taking action to improve the health of populations. Action is directed primarily at community levels. Strategies address the determinants of health in order to improve population health and reduce risks (see Chapter 1). Most health determinants involve other sectors of society such as education, agriculture, business, and government. Multisectoral collaboration between the health sector and other sectors is essential in a population health approach. This approach further broadens the scope of nursing practice in the community. Population-based public health programs focus on disease prevention, health protection, and health promotion, which provide the foundation for health care services at all levels (see Chapter 2).

Public health nurses perceive value in their distinctive practice, which enables them to see "the big picture" as a result of their "broad health knowledge base, in-depth understanding of the community and community resources, and . . . appreciation of individual–family–community inter-relationships" (Reutter & Ford, 1996, p. 8). By using public health principles, the nurse is better able to understand the environments in which clients live, the factors that influence client health, and the types of interventions supportive of client health. Figure 4–2 illustrates a framework for public health programs that provides a means of organizing program development in public health practice (Edwards & Moyer, 2000).

Successful public health nursing practice involves empowerment-based strategies initiated by building relationships with the community and being responsive to changes within it (Canadian Public Health Association, 1990; CHNAC, 2003; Diekemper et al., 1999). For example, when increasing numbers of grandparents are caring for their grandchildren in a particular community, nurses can collaborate with local schools and agencies to create a program that might include opportunity for peer support and education about available resources. The public health nurse is responsive by being active in the community; knowing its members, needs, and resources; and working collaboratively to establish health promotion and disease prevention programs. This means developing and maintaining relationships with other professional systems and individuals and encouraging them to respond to a population's needs.

Home Health Nursing

Home health nursing, also known as **community-based nursing,** involves acute, chronic, and palliative care of individuals and their families that enhances their capacity for self-care and promotes autonomy in decision making (Ayers et al., 1999; CHNAC, 2003). Nursing takes place in community settings such as the home, a long-term care facility, or a clinic. The nurse's competence is based on critical thinking and decision making at the level of the individual client: assessing health status, selecting nursing interventions, and evaluating care outcomes. Because they provide care where clients live, work, and play, home health nurses need to be individual- and family-oriented

and also need to appreciate a community's values (CHNAC, 2003; Zotti et al., 1996).

Components of home health nursing practice include self-care as a client and family responsibility; preventive care; care within the community context; continuity of care between home and health system services; and collaborative client care among health practitioners (CHNAC, 2003; Hunt & Zurek, 1997). Nurses use their clinical expertise to provide direct care (e.g., a case manager monitors clients recovering from stroke and provides rehabilitation services). Nursing supports and improves clients' quality of life. Illness is seen as one aspect of clients' everyday lives. Nursing tends to be problem focused, addressing client needs for primary, secondary, and tertiary prevention (CHNAC, 2003; Hunt, 1998).

A strong theoretical foundation for home health nursing is provided by the human ecological model, which conceptualizes human systems as open and interactive with the environment (Chalmers et al., 1998). In an ecological model, the individual is viewed within the larger systems of family, social network, community, and society, which can be depicted as four concentric circles: the innermost circle of the client and the immediate family, the second circle of people and settings that have frequent contact with the client and family, the third circle of the local community and its values and policies, and the outermost circle of larger social systems such as business and government (Ayers et al., 1999). A home health nurse must understand the interaction of all systems while caring for clients and families in their home environment. Nurses typically become involved in the domain of the first three circles. For example, as a home health nurse, you work closely with a client in whom diabetes

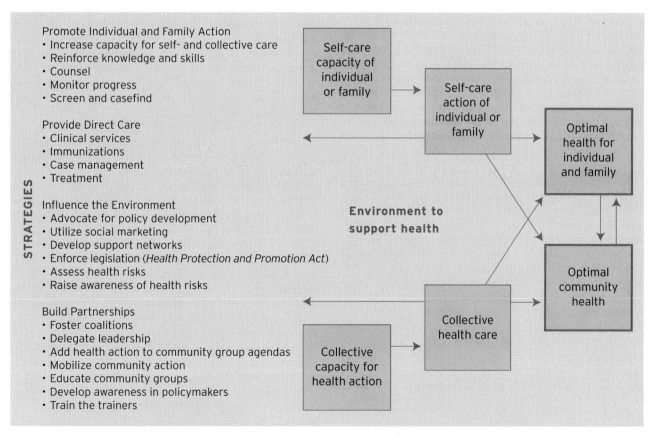

Figure 4-2 Framework for public health programs. **Source:** From N. Edwards et al. (1995). *Building and sustaining collective health action: A framework for community health practitioners.* Ottawa, ON: Community Health Research Unit, Pub. No. DP95-1, as cited by Edwards, N. C., & Moyer, A. (2000). Community needs and capacity assessment: Critical component of program planning. In M. J. Stewart (Ed.): *Community nursing: Promoting Canadians' health* (2nd ed., pp. 433), Toronto, ON: W. B. Saunders.

was recently diagnosed and with the family to establish a care plan. You use your observations of the client's lifestyle when considering an exercise schedule and meal routines. Knowing community resources (e.g., shops with glucose-monitoring supplies and local diabetes support groups) enables you to provide comprehensive support.

Home health nursing is family-centred care (Ayers et al., 1999; CHNAC, 2003). This care requires knowledge of family theory (see Chapter 20), cultural diversity (see Chapter 10), communication (see Chapter 18), and group dynamics. Empowerment-based strategies guide you to work in partnership with clients and families to support them and help them participate in their health care decisions (Toofany, 2007). The client and family are partners with you in planning, decision making, implementation, and evaluation of health care approaches.

The Changing Focus of Community Health Nursing Practice

Community health nursing practice has changed since the 1960s in response to social, economic, and political influences. Changes were documented by Chalmers et al. (1998), who interviewed community health nurse educators, administrators, and staff nurses who worked in public health agencies, home health services, and community health centres in Manitoba. The nurses noted shifts in practice focus from universal programs to programs directed to high-risk or vulnerable groups, from generalized to specialized practice, and from delivery of traditional public health services to more community-based acute care. These shifts have resulted in increasing demands placed on community health nurses, who are faced with more complex care situations. In 2005, Meagher-Stewart et al. reported the practice challenges articulated by public health nurses and nurse administrators in Nova Scotia (Box 4–3). The trends identified by Chalmers et al. remain relevant because they reflect continuing shifts and related challenges in community health nursing practice a decade after they were publicized.

Although many changes are consistent with the principles of primary health care and health promotion, there is concern that some changes put universal accessibility of public health nursing services at risk (Meagher-Stewart et al., 2005; Reutter & Ford, 1998). This concern also has emerged in home health practice, in which a policy agenda of increasing medicalization "stands in contrast to the principles of primary health care, and potentially leads to further marginalization of the most vulnerable" (Duncan & Reutter, 2006, p. 242). Home health care case managers expressed concern about limits on their practice arising from a conflict between professional discourse that guides practice and economic discourses that drive organizational priorities (Ceci, 2006).

Vulnerable Populations

Community health nurses care for clients from diverse cultures and backgrounds and with various health conditions. However, because of changes in the health care delivery system, high-risk groups have become the nurses' principal clients.

Vulnerable populations of clients are those who are likely to develop health problems as a result of excessive risks, who experience barriers when trying to access health care services, or who are dependent on others for care. Vulnerability can be understood in relation to the determinants of health, particularly social determinants that compromise socioeconomic status, literacy, and social inclusion (see Chapter 1). People living in poverty, homeless people, people in precarious circumstances (such as women in abusive interpersonal relationships), people with chronic conditions and disabilities, and people who engage in stigmatizing risk behaviours (including substance abuse and unsafe sexual practices), as well as Aboriginal peoples and new immigrants and refugees, are examples of vulnerable populations (Beiser & Stewart, 2005). Vulnerable individuals and their families often belong to more than one of these groups and may live in communities that can be characterized as vulnerable. Frequently, vulnerable clients come from a variety of cultures, have beliefs and values different from the mainstream culture, face language barriers, and have few sources of social support (Chalmers et al., 1998). Their special needs contribute to the challenges that community nurses face in caring for increasingly complex acute and chronic health conditions.

To provide competent care to vulnerable populations, nurses in community health care practice must be comfortable with diversity. Culture, ethnicity, ability, economic status, gender, and sexual orientation are all aspects of diversity in Canadian society. Sensitivity to diversity requires more than tolerance of difference, which implies that the dominant culture is the reference point. Rather, community health nursing practice that is sensitive to diversity embraces diversity as valuable to individual and social well-being. Chapter 10 addresses factors influencing individual differences within cultural groups and the nurse's role in providing culturally sensitive, competent, and safe care. To be culturally competent and safe, you must be more than just sensitive to a client's cultural uniqueness. You must be able to appraise and understand clients' cultural beliefs, values, and practices in order to work with them to determine their needs and the interventions most likely to improve their health. You cannot judge or evaluate a client's beliefs and values about health in terms of your own culture. Communication and caring practices are crucial for understanding clients' perceptions of their problems and for planning effective, culturally competent, and safe health care. You need to be aware of cultural and ethnic determinants of health, differing beliefs about health and medicine among ethnic communities, and barriers to accessing care that affect members of ethnic minorities.

Vulnerable populations typically experience poorer health outcomes than do people with ready access to resources and health care services (Beiser & Stewart, 2005). Higher morbidity and mortality

---

▶ BOX 4-3   Challenges to Community Health Nursing Practice

- Pulled between documenting work and valued practice with clients
- Torn between prescribed programs and community partnership activities
- "Never enough time," especially for higher needs
- Increased task orientation, specialization, and working in silos
- Lack of evaluation of program effectiveness
- Increasing inequity of programs to rural, seniors, and low income populations
- Feeling stretched related to shortage of nursing and administrative support staff
- Staying current on health information
- Loss of connection and visibility with the community

From Meagher-Stewart, D., Aston, M., Edwards, N., Smith, D., Young, L., Woodford, E., et al. (2005). *The study of public health nurses in primary health care. Fostering citizen participation and collaborative practice: Tapping the wisdom and voices of public health nurses in Nova Scotia. Research Report* (p. 6). Halifax, NS: Dalhousie University. Retrieved August 12, 2008, from http://preventionresearch.dal.ca/pdf/PHN_study_Nov25.pdf

rates characterize members of ethnically and racially diverse minority groups (Barr et al., 2002; Hwang, 2000). Members of vulnerable groups frequently experience cumulative risk factors or combinations of risk conditions that make them more sensitive to the adverse effects of individual risk factors that others might overcome (Rew et al., 2001). Community health nurses must assess clients from vulnerable populations by considering multiple risk factors and the clients' ability to deal with stressors. Box 4–4 summarizes guidelines for assessing clients from vulnerable population groups.

Poor and Homeless People. People who live in poverty are more likely to live in hazardous environments, work at high-risk jobs, eat less nutritious foods, and experience multiple stressors. They face practical problems such as limited access to transportation, limited quality child care to support employment, and limited medication or dental coverage from supplementary health benefits. Low-income status is prevalent among lone-parent families, unattached older adults (mostly women), and Aboriginal families (Canadian Population Health Initiative, 2004). Homeless people have even fewer resources than do low-income people. Their vulnerability lies in their social condition, lifestyle, and environment, which diminish their ability to maintain or improve their health or access health care. Homeless people live on the streets or in temporary accommodation such as shelters and boarding houses. They may distrust health and social services as bureaucratic and judgmental, using them only when their health has deteriorated (Thibaudeau & Denoncourt, 2000). Chronic health problems worsen because of barriers to supportive self-care and medical care. Homeless people have a high incidence of mental illness and substance abuse. Nurses can help low-income and homeless people identify their capacities and resources, their eligibility for assistance, and interventions to help improve their health. For example, Cathy Crowe's work as a street nurse in Toronto includes direct care such as "dressing a wound under a highway overpass," "treating frostbite," and "providing intravenous rehydration to patients in shelters during a Nowalk virus outbreak," as well as advocacy such as "constantly seeking donations like Gatorade to counter dehydration" and "documenting police-inflicted injuries" (Crowe, 2007, p. 6).

People in Precarious Circumstances. Women are at greater risk for problems related to low income, violence, and the stressors associated with unpaid caregiving. Such risks are further complicated for some by geographically isolated settings that challenge women's resilience in maintaining their health (Leipert & Reutter, 2005). Community health nurses's work is guided by their recognition of the need to listen to, respect, and communicate with women in their communities (Leipert, 1999).

Physical, emotional, and sexual abuse, as well as neglect, are major public health problems, particularly affecting older adults, women, and children (Canadian Public Health Association, 1994; Sebastian, 2006). Abuse occurs in many settings, including the home, workplace, school, health care facility, and public areas, and is most often committed by an acquaintance of the victim (Canadian Public Health Association, 1994). When dealing with clients at risk for or who may have suffered abuse, you must provide protection for them. Interviews with clients should occur in private when the individual suspected of being the perpetrator is not present. Clients who have been abused often fear retribution if they discuss their problems with a health care professional. Most regions have reporting agencies or hotlines for notification when an individual has been identified as being at risk, and you can work with clients to reflect on concerns, identify acceptable alternatives, and make decisions about their situation.

Unintentional injuries, unemployment, depression, and suicide are a concern among youth, particularly young men and those in Aboriginal communities. "Community health nurses who are

> ### ➤ BOX 4-4 Guidelines for Assessing Members of Vulnerable Population Groups

Setting the Stage

- Create a comfortable, nonthreatening environment.
- Learn as much as you can about the culture of the clients you work with, so that you will understand traditions and values that influence their health care practices.
- Provide culturally competent assessment by understanding the meaning of language and nonverbal behaviour in the client's culture.
- Be sensitive to the fact that the individual or family may have priorities, such as financial or legal problems, that are more important to them than traditional health concerns. Within your scope as a nurse, you may need to help them deal with these priority concerns before you can address specific health concerns.
- Collaborate with others as appropriate; connect your client with someone who can help.

Nursing History of an Individual or a Family

- You may have only one opportunity to work with a vulnerable person or family. Try to document a history that provides essential information you need to help on that day. Organize what you need to ask, and be prepared to explain why the information is necessary.
- Use a modified comprehensive assessment form to focus on the special needs of the vulnerable group. Be flexible. With some clients, it is impractical and unethical to ask all questions on the form. If you expect to see the client again, ask less urgent questions at the next visit.
- Include questions about social support, economic status, resources for health care, developmental issues, current health problems, medication, and how the person or family manages health status. Your goal is to obtain information that will enable you to provide family-centred care.
- Determine whether the individual has any condition that compromises his or her immune status, such as human immunodeficiency virus (HIV) infection or acquired immunodeficiency syndrome (AIDS), or is receiving therapy that would result in immunodeficiency, such as cancer chemotherapy.

Physical Examination or Home Assessment

- Complete as thorough a physical examination (on an individual) or home assessment as you can. Collect only information you can use to work with the individual or family.
- Be alert for indications of mental or physical abuse, substance use, or differences from normal physical examination findings.
- Observe a family's living environment. Does the family have running water, functioning plumbing, electricity, and access to a telephone? Is perishable food left on tables and countertops? Are surfaces reasonably clean? Is paint peeling on the walls and ceilings? Are room ventilation and temperature adequate? Is the home next to a busy highway, exposing the family to high noise levels and automobile exhaust?

Adapted from Sebastian, J. G. (2006). Vulnerability and vulnerable populations: An overview. In M. Stanhope & J. Lancaster (Eds.), *Foundations of nursing in the community: Community-oriented practice* (pp. 403–417). St. Louis, MO: Mosby.

concerned with adolescent health promotion must consider the broad range of factors that affect adolescent health decisions and behaviours. Individual, family and environmental factors must be considered, together with many structural and societal factors" (Gillis, 2000, p. 257).

People with Chronic Conditions and Disabilities.

"Chronic conditions are impairments in function, development, or disease states that are irreversible or have a cumulative effect" (Ogden Burke et al., 2000, p. 211). There are physical and emotional aspects of living with chronic conditions. Societal trends toward greater family mobility, maternal employment, smaller families, and female-headed lone-parent low-income families are challenges for families caring for children with chronic conditions (Ogden Burke et al., 2000). Older adults experience more chronic conditions as they age (Health Canada, 1999). The shift in health care service delivery from institutional to community-based care places demands on families, particularly women, to provide caregiving in the community. You need to work with individuals, families, and communities to promote adequate support for family caregivers and access to resources and services.

For a client with a severe mental illness, multiple health and socioeconomic problems must be explored. Many such clients are homeless or marginally housed. Others are unable to work or provide self-care. They require medication therapy, counselling, housing, and vocational assistance. No longer hospitalized in long-term psychiatric institutions, clients with mental illness are offered resources within their community. However, many communities face continuing difficulties in the establishment of comprehensive, coordinated, and accessible community-based service networks (Health Canada, 2002; Shah, 2003). Many clients who lack functional skills are left with fewer and more fragmented services. An increasing number of young mentally ill people have only episodic hospital care.

Collaboration among community resources is key to helping mentally ill people obtain health care. For example, the interdisciplinary Psychiatric Outreach Team of the Royal Ottawa Hospital provides mobile services to shelters and drop-in centres to initiate mental health care, assist in linking clients to community resources, and provide education and assistance in connecting with mental health and addiction treatment (Farrell et al., 2005).

With the increasing population of older adults, there is a corresponding increase in the number of clients with chronic disease and a greater demand for health care (Craig, 2000). You must view health promotion from a broad perspective, by understanding what health means to older adults and ways they can maintain their own health. Among individuals who feel empowered to control their own health, the incidence of disability from chronic disease is lower (Baas et al., 2002). You can help improve the quality of life for older adults.

People Who Engage in Stigmatizing Risk Behaviours.

Potentially stigmatizing risk behaviours include substance abuse and unsafe sexual practices. The social determinants of health provide a holistic perspective to address social and structural conditions that influence behaviour and to challenge the "unprecedented reliance on interventions that focus on addressing what is wrong with the individual" (Shoveller & Johnson, 2006, p. 56). *Substance abuse* is a general term for the use of illegal drugs and the abuse of alcohol and prescribed medications such as antianxiety agents and narcotic analgesics. Clients who abuse substances also frequently have health and socioeconomic problems. A substantial proportion of adult HIV and AIDS cases have been attributed to injection drug use (Geduld & Gatali, 2003). Substance abuse, particularly alcohol abuse, remains a serious problem among Canadian adolescents (Gillis, 2000). Socioeconomic problems often result from financial strain, employment loss, and family breakdown. The incidences of

---

✳ BOX 4-5   RESEARCH HIGHLIGHT

AIDS Prevention Street Nurse Program

Research Focus

The AIDS Prevention Street Nurse Program in Vancouver provides outreach services for preventing HIV and sexually transmitted infection in vulnerable, high-risk clients (Hilton, Thompson, & Moore-Dempsey, 2000; Hilton, Thompson, Moore-Dempsey, & Hutchinson, 2000, 2001). The program was awarded the Provincial Health Officer's Award of Excellence in 2007 and acknowledged as symbolizing best nursing practices and organizational commitment. Community health nurses with the program use harm reduction and health promotion approaches in their work. Harm reduction includes needle exchange for injection drug use, education to promote safer drug use and sexual behaviour, and support to clients in addiction treatment programs. Nurses go where the clients are: clinics, drop-in centres, detoxification centres, jails, door-to-door in hotels, or on the street.

Research Abstract

The purpose of the program evaluation study was to describe the nurses' work and its impact on clients, the challenges that nurses faced, and the program fit with other services (Hilton, Thompson, Moore-Dempsey, & Hutchinson, 2001). Program nurses were interviewed, as were clients of the program, including youths living on the streets, sex trade workers, and injection drug users. Challenges facing nurses include building trust with clients, providing needed care or resources, and involving other health care professionals. Clients reported gaining knowledge, feeling better about themselves,

being supported, and changing their behaviours to help themselves and others (Hilton, Thompson, Moore-Dempsey, & Hutchinson, 2000, 2001).

Evidence-Informed Practice

- Key strategies for reaching vulnerable populations include working with clients "at their location, on their own terms, and according to their own agenda" (Hilton, Thompson, Moore-Dempsey, & Hutchinson, 2001, p. 274) and encouraging and facilitating client participation and choice.
- Client empowerment can be promoted through nurses' nonjudgmental care, trust, and respect.
- Educating marginalized clients about health promotion and harm prevention increases their self-concept and encourages them to change their behaviour.

References: Hilton, A. B., Thompson, R., & Moore-Dempsey. L. (2000). Evaluation of the AIDS prevention street nurse program: One step at a time. *Canadian Journal of Nursing Research, 32*(1), 17–38; Hilton, A. B., Thompson, R., Moore-Dempsey, L., & Hutchinson, K. (2001). Urban outpost nursing: The nature of the nurses' work in the AIDS prevention street nurse program. *Public Health Nursing, 18*(4), 273–280; and Thompson, R., Hilton, A. B., Moore-Dempsey, L., & Hutchinson, K. (2000). AIDS prevention on the streets: Vancouver nurses are taking AIDS prevention to the streets. *Canadian Nurse, 96*(8), 24–28.

unsafe sexual practices and multiple risk-taking behaviours remain high among young people, particularly young men (Health Canada, 1999). Unsafe sex creates serious health and social risks, including the risks of unplanned pregnancy and acquiring sexually transmitted infections (e.g., HIV infection and AIDS). Unplanned adolescent pregnancy poses risks for both mothers and infants, including pregnancy complications (DiCenso & Van Dover, 2000), low income, low academic achievement, unemployment, violence (Gillis, 2000), and stigma (Fulford & Ford-Gilboe, 2004). You can partner with clients to assess the circumstances that contribute to substance use, unsafe sexual practices, and other high-risk behaviours and identify strategies to address the often multiple and interrelated concerns. For example, Steenbeek (2004) identified strategies such as peer leader training and self-advocacy skill development within an empowering health promotion framework to prevent sexually transmitted infections among Aboriginal youth. The AIDS Prevention Street Nurse Program (Box 4–5) and the Nursing Story (Box 4–6) illustrate **harm reduction,** an important but controversial approach to health promotion, that is based on user input and demand, compassionate pragmatism, and commitment to offer alternatives to reduce risk behaviour consequences, to accept alternatives to abstinence, and to reduce barriers to treatment by providing user-friendly access (Hilton, Thompson, Moore-Dempsey, & Janzen, 2001; Pauly et al., 2007; Shah, 2003).

Competencies, Roles, and Activities in Community Health Nursing

Nurses in community health practice must have a broad base of knowledge and skills in order to work with clients to meet their health care needs and develop community relationships. Primary health care and health promotion approaches help nurses recognize the interplay between individual experience and social conditions, the value of diversity, and the importance of building capacity to promote health-enhancing change. In community health nursing practice, "nurses are responsible for the maintenance of professional nursing standards and of public health standards by being accountable for the quality of their own practice, striving for excellence, ensuring that their knowledge is current and taking advantage of opportunities for life long learning" (Canadian Public Health Association, 1990, p. 5). Cradduck (2000) concluded that the "legacy of community health nursing is its multidimensional role, community orientation, and advocacy" (p. 367). The CHNAC (2003) identified five standards of practice for community health nurses: promoting health, building individual and community capacity, building relationships, facilitating access and equity, and demonstrating professional responsibility and accountability. These standards reflect the nursing process "of assessment, planning, intervention, and evaluation. Community health nurses enhance this process through individual or community participation in each component multiple ways of knowing awareness of the influence of the broader environment on the individual or community that is the focus of their care (e.g., the community will be affected by provincial or territorial policies, its own economic status and the actions of its individual citizens) (CHNAC, 2008, p. 9). A summary of key roles and practice dimensions identified by the Canadian Public Health Association (1990) and that remain relevant to current community health nursing practice is presented in the following sections.

Communicator. Communication skills support all other activities in community health nursing practice. Skill as an effective communicator is closely related to the leadership, enabling, and advocacy skills of the facilitator. As communicators, you may use negotiation and mediation to foster collaboration.

Facilitator. To facilitate is to promote. Community health nurses work within a participatory process to identify issues, develop goals for change, and implement strategies for action and evaluation of results. Leadership, enabling, and advocacy skills are key to these activities. Leadership focuses on supporting processes that build capacity among participants, rather than on directing or controlling decision making. Enabling encourages client participation and experiential learning. Advocacy fosters equity and accessibility of care, especially among vulnerable populations.

Collaborator. Collaboration is a way of working together that is characterized by recognition of interdependence, collective responsibility, and negotiated equity in relationships (Gray, 1989; Labonte, 1993). Collaboration involves more than linking or networking with others. Community health nurses participate in a collective process

BOX 4-6   NURSING STORY

Harm Reduction Nursing

Harm reduction initiatives, such as needle exchange programs now available in most Canadian provinces, exemplify community nursing practice guided by primary health care, health promotion, empowerment, and ethical principles. The leadership, creativity, and dedication of nurses have contributed significantly to the development of these initiatives. For example, Wood et al. (2003) successfully advocated for the establishment of a supervised injection site for injection drug users as part of the Day Program services provided by the Dr. Peter Centre in Vancouver's Downtown Eastside. Collaborating with local HIV and AIDS network members, researchers, and street nurses (see Box 4–4), they developed policies, procedures, and protocols to deliver harm reduction services to a highly vulnerable population in which stigmatizing risk behaviours were compounded by homelessness, precarious life circumstances, and chronic conditions and disabilities. In addition to the supervised injection site, nurses provide sterile drug injection supplies through a needle exchange program, teach about safe sex, offer condoms, talk with sex trade workers about safer ways of dealing with johns, counsel on addiction, support methadone maintenance regimens, and help when individuals are ready to enter detoxification programs or rehabilitation (Griffiths, 2002, p. 12). Serving the same population, Insite, North America's first dedicated legal supervised drug injection site, opened in 2003 and provides health care, counseling, education, and support from a multidisciplinary team that includes nurses. Since 1989, nurses with the Streetworks initiative in Edmonton have worked from several fixed daytime sites and from a mobile van for evening outreach to offer harm reduction strategies in partnership with agencies serving the inner city community. Nurses' work in these initiatives illustrates many of the role dimensions needed for community health practice, including activities as communicator, facilitator, collaborator, coordinator, educator, care or service provider, community developer, policy formulator, and researcher. "Using professional practice to create change, the passion and leadership of a few nurses are resulting in an innovative approach. If such an approach were adopted across Canada, the number of human lives and health care dollars saved would be monumental" (Wood et al., 2003, p. 24). You are encouraged to reflect on these nursing roles and activities by reading more about these and similar programs in communities across the country.

Web Sites
Dr. Peter Centre http://www.drpeter.org/
Insite http://www.vch.ca/sis/
StreetWorks http://www.streetworks.ca/pro/index.html

as a collaborator with clients, community members, agencies, and sectors. This process is supported by developing honest relationships and mutual respect, recognizing many forms of expertise, valuing diversity, and being organized and committed.

Coordinator. The coordinator's role has long been associated with nursing practice. Community health nurses work with clients and diverse agencies to coordinate or organize activities, resources, access, and care to promote client health. Coordinator activities complement activities as educator, direct care or service provider, community developer, and social marketer.

Consultant. As consultants, community health nurses rely on a broad knowledge base to provide information and to support participation in health activities. As a nurse, you involve not only clients but also community members, health care professionals, professionals from other disciplines, members of other sectors, policymakers, and government officials. You respond to inquiries about and make referrals to community resources. By developing collaborative relationships, you support client access to these resources.

Educator. Competence in client education with individuals and groups requires a broad knowledge base, as well as communication and learning process theory. Nurses provide information to support community, family, and individual decision making. You may participate in formal education sessions, such as prenatal classes, or in informal sessions, such as discussions with families during home visits. Clients need information to make decisions about health issues, but this is not enough to produce behavioural change. You support clients in applying information to their everyday lives.

Direct Care or Service Provider. Community health nurses act as direct care or service providers when they work with clients to promote and protect health and to prevent injury and illness. In many communities, home visiting remains integral to community health nursing practice, as do services such as health assessment and immunization clinics. Care may involve treating illness, monitoring risk conditions, educating or guiding informed decision making, and supporting client self-care.

Community Developer. As a community developer, community health nurses must support community participation. Participation encourages open identification of issues, shared decision making, egalitarian relationships, and collective ownership of action (Labonte, 1993). Participation and empowerment are closely linked.

Social Marketer. Social marketing is an approach to social change related to health behaviours in which marketing and change theory are used to design and manage programs (Kotler & Roberto, 1989). Interdisciplinary and intersectoral collaboration provides a broad base of expertise. Community health nurses may act as social marketers to promote public awareness of issues and available programs and to build support for social action initiatives.

Policy Formulator. Activities as a policy formulator include identifying the need for policy and program development; participating in program development, implementation, and evaluation; and helping establish policies to support their practice. Community health nurses can support the collective voice of their professional associations (e.g., CNA, CHNAC) to advocate for health-enhancing public policy.

Researcher. Research is used to generate information, identify issues, determine directions for action, consider strategies to promote change, and evaluate results. Community health nurses need to review research and apply knowledge to practice. They also engage in research projects as participants or investigators to support evidence-informed practice.

Community Assessment

As a community health nurse, you need to assess the community—the environment in which people live and work. Without an understanding of that environment, any effort to promote health and to support change is unlikely to succeed, whether you work with an individual, a family, a group, or a community as client.

The community can be seen as having three components: the locale or structure, the social systems, and the people. A complete assessment involves studying each component to understand the health status of the people and the health determinants that influence their health as a basis on which to identify needs for health policy, health program development, and service provision (see Chapter 1; for detailed descriptions of community assessment strategies, see also community health nursing textbooks such as Stamler & Yiu, 2008; Stanhope et al., 2008; and Vollman et al., 2008). To assess the locale or structure, you might travel around the community and observe the physical environment, the location of services, and the places where residents congregate (completing a windshield or walking survey). Information about social systems, such as schools, health care facilities, recreation, transportation, and government, may be acquired by visiting various sites and learning about their services (observing activities, interviewing key informants). Community statistics from a local library or health department can help assess a population's demographics and health status (reviewing population data). Discussion with community members is also helpful (interviewing key informants, holding focus groups) to identify priority issues within the community. It is essential to identify community resources and capacities, as well as issues and problems (Edwards & Moyer, 2000).

Recall the determinants of health as you consider the following scenario. As a community health nurse, you wish to familiarize yourself with the local area to help you begin to identify potential health concerns and available resources that will guide your work with the community. Your windshield and walking surveys reveal an older, high-density neighbourhood where pawn shops and bars outnumber grocery stores, schools, and community recreation facilities. You observe a culturally diverse population, including young families and older people, who interact with each other at community events sponsored by faith-based groups and social agencies. Your observations are reinforced in discussions as you develop relationships with community leaders and with health and social agency staff, whose perspectives are supported by census tract data and regional health statistics. Neighbourhood Watch members, however, alert you to tensions related to high unemployment, language barriers to services, and youth crime, particularly break-ins and vandalism. Once you have a good understanding of the community, you may then perform individual or family client assessment against that background. For example, consider assessment of an older couple's safety. Are windows in their apartment secure and intact? Is lighting along walkways and entryways operational? Do they feel comfortable calling on their neighbours for assistance if necessary? Are health and social services easy to reach when needed? How safe do they feel in the neighbourhood? No individual or family assessment should occur in isolation from the environment and conditions of the community setting. A collaborative approach to community assessment grounded in an empowerment process helps you establish working relationships, identify shared concerns, recognize collective capacities, and develop effective strategies to enhance health.

Promoting Clients' Health

The challenge for nurses in community health practice is how to promote and protect the health of clients, whether within the context of their community or with the community as the focus. You may bring together the resources necessary to improve the continuity of client care. In collaboration with clients, health care and social service professionals, and other community members, you coordinate health care services, locate appropriate social services, and develop innovative approaches to address clients' health issues.

Perhaps the key to being an effective community health nurse is the ability to understand clients' everyday lives. The foundation for this understanding is the establishment of strong, caring relationships with clients (see Chapters 18 and 19) that support empowerment as an active growth process rooted in cultural, religious, and personal belief systems (Falk-Rafael, 2001). The quasi-insider status of nurses in a community often enables them to identify local patterns and needs that can be addressed through programs, policies, and advocacy (SmithBattle et al., 2004) that are responsive, supportive, and effective. This is difficult because the time that nurses have to spend with clients continues to decline. However, the expert nurse is able to advise, counsel, and teach after being accepted into the client's family or the community and by understanding what makes clients unique. The day-to-day activities of family and community life and the cultural, economic, and political environment influence how you adapt nursing interventions. The time of day an individual client goes to work, the availability of the spouse and client's parents to provide child care, and the family values that shape views about health are just a few examples of the many factors you must consider in community health practice. Once you acquire an understanding of a client's life, interventions designed to promote health and prevent disease can be introduced. Similarly, understanding the relationships, activities, and concerns of client groups and communities is central to health promotion practice.

Community health nursing practice is influenced by trends that focus attention on consumer participation, aggregates and communities, independent and interdependent practice, health promotion (Stewart & Leipert, 2000), population health, and health and social system reform that emphasizes service delivery in the community. A continuing challenge articulated by Stewart and Leipert is "to translate all these trends into the everyday practice of community health nurses in Canada" (p. 609) in ways that respect and promote collective empowerment, as well as individual and family empowerment, to enhance health in everyday life.

✳ KEY CONCEPTS

- A successful community health nursing practice involves building relationships with the community members and being responsive to changes within the community.
- The principles of public health nursing practice aim at assisting individuals in acquiring a healthy environment in which to live.
- The public health nurse cares for the community as a whole and considers the individual or family to be one member of a population or potential group at risk.
- The home health nurse's competence is based on decision making at the level of the individual client.
- Within an ecological model of home health nursing, the individual is viewed within the larger systems of family, social network, community, and society.

- Vulnerable individuals and their families often belong to more than one vulnerable group.
- The special needs of vulnerable populations contribute to the challenges that nurses face in caring for these clients' increasingly complex acute and chronic health conditions.
- Exacerbations of chronic health problems are common among homeless people because they have few resources.
- An important principle in dealing with clients at risk for or who may have suffered abuse is protection of the client.
- Clients who engage in risk behaviours such as substance abuse may respond to a harm reduction approach.
- In community health practice, it is important to understand what health means to clients and the steps they can take to maintain their own health.
- A community health nurse must be competent in fulfilling a multidimensional role, including activities as communicator, facilitator, collaborator, coordinator, consultant, educator, care or service provider, community developer, social marketer, policy formulator, and researcher.
- Assessment of a community includes assessing population health status and relevant determinants of health in relation to three elements: locale or structure, the social systems, and the people.
- An important consideration in becoming an effective community health nurse is to strive to understand clients' lives.

✳ CRITICAL THINKING EXERCISES

1. You are working with the family of a severely disabled child and learn that no respite services to provide parental support, and only limited educational resources, are available in your community. What activities or roles of the community health nurse would be important to establish a special-education day care service, operated by volunteer educators?

2. Mr. Crowder is a 42-year-old man with diabetes mellitus and visual impairment. Your assessment reveals that he is homeless and spends nights in a local shelter. He is not able to buy medications or ensure adequate diet to control his blood glucose. What factors might you consider to support Mr. Crowder's self-care?

3. Conduct a community assessment of an area that you have visited infrequently. Observe the community locale by driving or walking through the more populated area. Look for the following services: hospital, clinic, pharmacy, grocery store, schools, park or playground, and police and fire departments.

✳ REVIEW QUESTIONS

1. The overall goals of a population health approach are to
   1. Maintain and improve the population's health and eliminate health disparities
   2. Gather information on incidence rates of certain diseases and social problems
   3. Assess the health care needs of individuals, families, or communities
   4. Develop and implement public health policies and improve access to acute care

2. Public health nursing merges knowledge from professional nursing theories and the
   1. Population sciences
   2. Public health sciences
   3. Environmental sciences
   4. Social sciences

3. Home health nursing involves acute, chronic, and palliative care of clients and families to enhance their capacity for
   1. Nursing care that promotes autonomy in decision making
   2. Improving their health care and self-care
   3. Self-care and autonomy in decision making
   4. Learning about their illnesses

4. Vulnerable populations are more likely to develop health problems as a result of
   1. Acute diseases, homelessness, and poverty
   2. Lack of transportation, dependence on others for care, and lack of initiative
   3. Poverty, lack of education, and mental illness
   4. Excess risks, barriers to health care services, and dependence on others for care

5. Which is *not* an aspect of competent care of vulnerable populations?
   1. Providing culturally appropriate care
   2. Creating a comfortable, nonthreatening environment
   3. Assessing living conditions
   4. Offering financial or legal advice

6. Major public health problems affecting older adults, women, and children are
   1. Prescribed medication abuse, poverty, sexual abuse
   2. Physical, emotional, and sexual abuse, as well as neglect
   3. Acute illnesses, neglect, substance abuse
   4. Financial strain, poverty, physical abuse

7. A successful community health nursing practice requires
   1. A graduate degree in health education or health promotion
   2. Building relationships with and responding to changes in the community
   3. Taking a passive role to allow the community to initiate change
   4. Subspecialty education in public health sciences

8. Teaching classes about infant care, cancer screening, and home safety adaptations for older people are examples of a nurse in the role of
   1. Consultant
   2. Collaborator
   3. Educator
   4. Facilitator

9. A community health nurse who is directing a client to community resources is an example of a nurse in the role of a
   1. Consultant
   2. Collaborator
   3. Coordinator
   4. Researcher

10. A community includes the following three elements, each of which must be assessed:
    1. Locale or structure, social systems, and people
    2. People, neighbourhoods, and social systems
    3. Health care systems, geographic boundaries, and people
    4. Environment, families, and social systems

✳ RECOMMENDED WEB SITES

Canadian Public Health Association: http://www.cpha.ca
The Canadian Public Health Association (CPHA) is a national, independent, not-for-profit, voluntary association representing public health care in Canada.

Community Health Nurses Association of Canada: http://www.chnac.ca/
The CHNAC is a national-level organization. It provides standards and information on community health nursing.

Fact Sheet: The Primary Health Care Approach: http://cna-aiic.ca/ CNA/documents/pdf/publications/FS02_Primary_Health_Care_ Approach_June_2000_e.pdf
This Canadian Nurses Association publication defines and describes primary health care in Canada.

Public Health Agency of Canada: Health Promotion: http://www.phac-aspc.gc.ca/hp-ps/index-eng.php
This federal Web site provides links to many useful health promotion resources and guides that will aid health professionals and community leaders.

Victorian Order of Nurses: http://www.von.ca/
The Victorian Order of Nurses (VON) is Canada's leading charitable organization addressing community health and social needs.

5

Caring for the Cancer Survivor

Original chapter by Patricia A. Potter, RN, MSN, PhD, GMAC, FAAN

Canadian content written by Willy Kabotoff, RN, BScN, MN

objectives

Mastery of content in this chapter will enable you to:

- Define the key terms listed.
- Discuss the concept of cancer survivorship.
- Describe the influence of cancer survivorship on clients' quality of life.
- Discuss the effects cancer has on the family.
- Explain the nursing implications related to cancer survivorship.
- Discuss the essential components of survivorship care.

key terms

Biological response modifiers (biotherapy), p. 54
Cancer-related fatigue, p. 55
Cancer survivor, p. 54
Chemotherapy, p. 54
Hormone therapy, p. 54
Lumpectomy, p. 56

Mastectomy, p. 56
Neuropathy, p. 55
Oncology, p. 61
Paresthesias, p. 55
Post-traumatic stress disorder (PTSD), p. 56
Radiation therapy, p. 54

media resources

evolve Web Site
- Audio Chapter Summaries
- Glossary
- Multiple-Choice Review Questions
- Student Learning Activities
- Weblinks

Companion CD
- Glossary
- Interactive Learning Activities
- Fluids and Electrolytes Tutorial
- Test-Taking Skills

Cancer survivors have not been recognized for the extent and nature of the health problems that they experience. Cancer has been diagnosed in approximately 833,100 Canadians at some time during the previous 15 years (Canadian Cancer Society [CCS], 2007). The number of survivors will continue to grow because more than 159,000 new cases of cancer are diagnosed each year (CCS, 2007). Cancer survivors' health care problems have largely been ignored or misunderstood because of the belief that for those who receive treatment, survive, and are given a "clean bill of health," their health problems are over. Such is not the case; different trajectories or courses for cancer survival exist (Box 5–1). With the advances made in diagnosis and treatment, more clients are becoming long-term survivors of cancer, whereas others with cancers such as lymphoma control the disease with ongoing or periodic treatment. The major forms of cancer therapy—**surgery, chemotherapy, hormone therapy, biological response modifiers (biotherapy),** and **radiation therapy**—often create unwanted, long-term effects on tissues and organ systems that impair a person's health and quality of life in small and large ways (Institute of Medicine [IOM] & National Research Council [NRC], 2006). A diagnosis of cancer presents many physical, emotional, and spiritual challenges to clients, families, and other loved ones. Although many individuals who survive cancer continue to live productive and rewarding lives, these challenges may persist beyond the physical recovery of the cancer itself. A large number of Canadians living with the effects of cancer require repeated active treatment, as well as extensive use of rehabilitation and supportive care resources. This increased demand and the complexity of survivors' health care needs must be considered in the planning and development of interdisciplinary health care services (CCS, 2007).

Yabroff et al. (2004) offered one definition of a **cancer survivor:** "An individual is considered a cancer survivor from the time of diagnosis, through the balance of his or her life." Family members and friends should also be considered survivors, because they experience the effects that cancer has on their loved ones. Cancer truly is a life-changing event. One phase of cancer care is often neglected: the period following first diagnosis and initial treatment and before the development of a recurrence of the initial cancer or death (IOM & NRC, 2006). In this phase of their disease, survivors do not have consistent health care follow-up. Frequent contact with a cancer care professional often

stops suddenly, and survivors' unique psychosocial needs often go unnoticed or untreated. Despite the incredible advances made in cancer care, many long-term survivors suffer unnecessarily and die as a result of delayed cancer diagnoses or treatment-related chronic disease.

As a nurse, you have the responsibility for better understanding the needs of cancer survivors and for providing the most current evidence-informed approaches to managing late and long-term effects of cancer and cancer treatment. As many as 75% of survivors have serious health deficits, both physical and psychological, that are related to their treatment (Aziz & Rowland, 2003). Disparities in health care among ethnic groups are related to a complex interplay of economic, social, and cultural factors, with poverty being a key factor (IOM & NRC, 2006). Being able to provide comprehensive care to a cancer survivor begins with recognizing the effects of cancer and its treatment and learning about the survivor's own meaning of health.

The Effects of Cancer on Quality of Life

As people live longer after diagnosis and treatment for cancer, it becomes important to understand the types of distress that many survivors experience and how it affects their quality of life (Figure 5–1). Cancer survivors have poorer health outcomes than do similar individuals without cancer (Box 5–2). Cancer survivors report struggles to find a balance in their lives and a sense of wholeness and life purpose (Ferrell, 2006). Quality of life in cancer survivorship means having a balance between the experience of increased dependence while seeking both independence and interdependence. Of course, exceptions exist with regard to the level of distress that survivors face. For some, cancer becomes an experience that provides self-reflection and an enhanced sense of what life is about. Regardless of each survivor's journey with cancer, having cancer affects each person's physical, social, psychological, and spiritual well-being.

> **BOX 5-1**　**The Phases of Cancer Survival**

- **Acute survival:** Starts with the diagnosis of cancer. Diagnostic and therapeutic efforts dominate. Fear and anxiety are constant elements of this phase.
- **Extended survival:** Period during which a client's disease goes into remission or the basic, rigorous course of treatment has ended and a phase of watchful waiting begins. Client undergoes periodic examinations, intermittent therapy, or both. The fear of recurrence is common. This is usually a period of physical limitations. Diminished strength, fatigue, pain, nausea, reduced tolerance for exercise, or hair loss often occurs in the acute phase, but clients now have to deal with the effects of cancer at home, in the community, and in the workplace.
- **Permanent survival:** This phase is roughly equated with "cure," but the experience permanently affects the survivor. Problems with employment and insurance are common. The long-term secondary effects of cancer treatment on health represent an area in which permanent survivors are at risk.

Adapted from Mullan, F. (1985). Seasons of survival: Reflections of a physician with cancer. *New England Journal of Medicine, 313*(4), 270; and Hewitt, M., Greenfield, S., & Stovall, E. (Eds.). (2006). *From cancer client to cancer survivor: Lost in transition.* Washington, DC: National Academies Press.

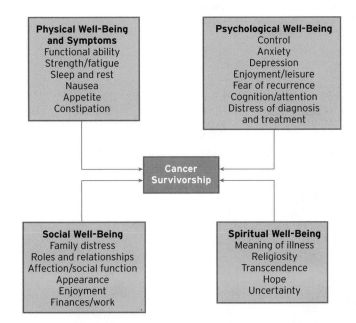

Figure 5-1 Dimensions of quality of life affected by cancer. **Source:** From Ferrell, B. (2006). *Introduction to cancer survivorship strategies for success: Survivorship education for quality cancer care.* Pasadena, CA: City of Hope National Medical Center.

✳ BOX 5-2   EVIDENCE-INFORMED PRACTICE
GUIDELINE

The Burden of Illness for Cancer Survivors

Evidence Summary

Yabroff et al. (2004) wanted to learn about the burden of illness among cancer survivors. The researchers studied more than 1800 cancer survivors, as well as individuals without cancer (the control group) who were matched with cancer survivors by age, sex, and educational attainment. The researchers examined several measures of burden or stress, including a person's sense of utility (feeling useful), a perception of overall health, and days lost from work. The results of the study showed that cancer survivors had poorer outcomes than did matched control subjects across all measures: lower sense of utility, higher levels of lost productivity, and more likelihood of reporting their health as fair or poor.

Application to Nursing Practice

As a nurse, you must learn to assess the many ways in which cancer affects the lives of clients who are survivors. Because cancer causes long-term effects, it is important for you to spend time assessing clients' symptoms, the effects of symptoms on lifestyle and self-care ability, the effects on client relationships, the clients' ability to remain productive and successful in their jobs, their economic security, and their physical well-being. When you attempt any intervention that requires the client to be motivated and involved, it is important to understand the client's self-perceptions.

Source: Yabroff, K. R., Lawrence, W. F., Clauser, S., Davis, W. W., & Brown, M. L. (2004). Burden of illness in cancer survivors: Findings from a population-based national sample. *Journal of the National Cancer Institute, 96*(17), 1322.

Physical Well-Being and Symptoms

Cancer survivors are at increased risk for developing a subsequent cancer (either a recurrence of the cancer for which they were treated or a secondary cancer) and for a wide range of treatment-related problems (IOM & NRC, 2006). The risk for developing a secondary cancer increases as a result of cancer treatment, genetic or other susceptibility, or an interaction between treatment and susceptibility. The risk for treatment-related problems is associated with the complexity of the cancer itself (e.g., type of tumour and stage of disease); the type, variety, and intensity of treatments used; and the age and underlying health status of the client.

The following description (Leigh, 2006) offers an example of how a cancer survivor's physical health problems can be so complex and burdensome.

Susan was an Army nurse, who learned 7 months after discharge from the Army that she had Hodgkin's disease. Hodgkin's is a malignancy of lymphoid tissue. Susan received an aggressive course of treatment, including surgery, 6 months of chemotherapy, and 3 months of total lymph node irradiation. It took many months for her bone marrow to heal and blood values to return to normal. After a few years she had bilateral mastectomies for treatment-related breast cancer. She also received 3 years of immunotherapy for cancer in situ (tumour not metastasized) of the bladder. She continues to experience many noncancer conditions: premature menopause, early osteoporosis, hypothyroidism, lung fibrosis, and atrophy of neck and upper chest muscles. (Leigh, 2006)

Such a story is not unusual among survivors; it highlights the long disease course that many cancer survivors face. Numerous tissues and body systems are impaired as a result of cancer and its treatment (Table 5–1). Late effects of chemotherapy include osteoporosis, congestive heart failure, diabetes, amenorrhea in affected women, sterility in affected men and women, gastrointestinal motility problems, abnormal liver function, impaired immune function, **paresthesias**, hearing loss, and problems with thinking and memory (IOM & NRC, 2006). The cancer itself or its treatment often induces pain and **neuropathy** (Polomano and Farrar, 2006). **Cancer-related fatigue** and associated sleep disturbances are the most frequent and disturbing complaints of people with cancer (Barton-Burke, 2006). Certain conditions resolve over time, but irreversible tissue damage causes conditions to progress and persist indefinitely. Health care professionals do not always recognize these conditions as delayed problems. In many cases, conditions such as osteoporosis, hearing loss, or change in memory are instead considered to be age related. The problem for many survivors is that these conditions go undiagnosed and are never treated.

Cognitive changes are characterized by a set of physical symptoms very common in survivors that develop from the disease, treatment, the complications of treatment, underlying medical conditions, and psychological responses to the diagnosis of cancer (Nail, 2006). Cognitive changes can occur during all phases of the cancer experience, from small deficits in information processing to acute delirium. Often the cognitive impairments that survivors experience are not evident to someone else but are apparent to the person experiencing them, especially in relation to work performance with high cognitive demands (Anderson-Hanley et al., 2003). For example, clients report attention problems, loss of memory, and difficulty in recognizing and solving problems. Studies have revealed that systemic cancer treatment, including chemotherapy or biotherapy, has a generalized, subtle effect on cognitive function. In addition, systemic treatment causes both short-term and persistent cognitive impairment in a variety of cognitive domains. Researchers do not yet understand the effects of specific cognitive changes on survivors' daily lives (Nail, 2006).

The estimates for 2008 indicate that about 69% of new cancer cases will occur in Canadians over the age of 60 (CCS, 2007). The most common cancers in this age group are those of the prostate, lung, and colon. Often, health care professionals wrongly attribute the symptoms of cancer or those from the side effects of treatment to aging. This can lead to late diagnosis or a failure to provide aggressive and effective treatment of symptoms.

Cancer is a chronic disease because of the serious consequences and the persistent nature of some of its late effects (IOM & NRC, 2006). The effects that clients suffer are diverse. For example, a 46-year-old woman with early-stage melanoma on the right arm may undergo successful surgery, and the only effect is an inconspicuous scar. In contrast, Susan, the Canadian Forces nurse diagnosed with Hodgkin's disease, underwent intensive chemotherapy followed by an extended course of radiation. She faced serious and substantial long-term health problems from her treatment. The type of conditions that develop and the length of time the conditions persist vary significantly.

Numerous factors contribute to survivors' not receiving timely and appropriate treatment for the effects of their disease or treatment. Survivors are often reluctant to report symptoms because of a fear of being perceived as ungrateful for being disease-free or a fear of cancer recurrence (Polomano and Farrar, 2006). Survivors are not always aware that painful conditions or syndromes are common and frequently believe that pain relief is not possible (see Chapter 42) (Box 5–3). Health care professionals have limited awareness of the prevalence and incidence of pain and other symptoms among survivors, and education in symptom management is frequently limited. In the case of pain management, health care professionals often do not

> **TABLE 5-1**   Examples of Late Effects of Surgery Among Adult Cancer Survivors

Procedure	Late Effect
Any procedure	Pain, psychosocial distress, impaired wound healing
Surgery involving brain or spinal cord	Impaired cognitive function; motor and sensory alterations; alterations in vision, swallowing, language, and bowel and bladder control
Head and neck surgery	Difficulties with communication, swallowing, and breathing
Abdominal surgery	Intestinal obstruction, hernia, altered bowel function
Lung resection	Difficulty breathing, fatigue, generalized weakness
Prostatectomy	Urinary incontinence, sexual dysfunction, poor body image

Modified from Institute of Medicine and National Research Council. (2006). *From cancer client to cancer survivor: Lost in transition* (M. Hewitt, S. Greenfield, & E. Stovall, Eds.). Washington, DC: National Academies Press.

acknowledge the potential for chronic pain after curative cancer therapies or fail to inform clients about potential long-term consequences of cancer treatment (Polomano and Farrar, 2006). Few health care settings track the health-related quality of life and symptoms of clients over time. Thus, limited evidence exists about the long-term patterns of symptoms most commonly associated with certain forms of cancer and its treatment

Research on breast cancer is extensive. Women with a history of breast cancer constitute the largest group of cancer survivors (IOM & NRC, 2006). After their primary treatment for breast cancer, women generally report decreased physical functioning but good emotional functioning, especially those who undergo **mastectomy** or receive chemotherapy (Ganz, 2004). Symptoms that persist one year after either **lumpectomy** or mastectomy to treat early-stage breast cancer often include numbness in the chest wall or axilla, tightness and a pulling sensation in the arm or axilla, fatigue, difficulty sleeping, and hot flashes (Shimozuma et al., 1999). By two to three years after surgery, breast cancer survivors report a quality of life more favourable

> **BOX 5-3**   Examples of Chronic Pain Syndromes Associated With Cancer Treatments

Postoperative Pain Syndromes

Postmastectomy syndrome
Post–radical neck dissection pain
Postamputation pain
Fistula formation

Postradiation Pain Syndromes

Myelopathy
Enteritis or proctitis
Lymphedema
Brachial or lumbosacral plexopathy

Postchemotherapy Pain Syndromes

Peripheral neuropathy
Avascular necrosis of femur or humerus

Modified from Polomano, R. C., & Farrar, J. T. (2006). Pain and neuropathy in cancer survivors. *American Journal of Nursing, 106*(Suppl. 3), 39.

than that reported by clients with other common medical conditions (Ganz et al., 1996). However, the same breast cancer survivors reported problems with sexual function, body image, and physical function after three years.

Psychological Well-Being

The physical effects of cancer and its treatment sometimes cause serious psychological distress (see Chapter 30). In the context of cancer, distress is defined as a multifactorial unpleasant emotional experience of a psychological, social, and or spiritual nature (see Chapter 28) that interferes with the ability to cope effectively with cancer, its symptoms, and its treatment (Wilkes, 2003). Survivors' feelings of distress range along a continuum from sadness to disabling depression (Vachon, 2006). The long-term presence of fatigue and sleep disturbances, for example, is often associated with anxiety and depression in many cancer survivors (Barton-Burke, 2006). Research has revealed an association between depression and decreased cancer survivorship. A study conducted by Brown et al. (2003) suggested that a cancer diagnosis and its effects predispose people to distress, which if maintained over time will enhance disease progression.

Another common psychological problem for survivors is **posttraumatic stress disorder (PTSD)**. PTSD is a psychiatric disorder characterized by an acute emotional response to a traumatic event or situation. Cancer survivors experience symptoms of PTSD (e.g., grief, nightmares, panic attacks, or fear) at a rate of 4% to 19%, as a result of their diagnosis, treatment, or a past traumatic episode (Kwekkeboom & Seng, 2002). Being female, being younger, being less educated, having a lower income, and having less social and emotional support increase the risk for PTSD. Results of studies of clients with PTSD suggest that the stress response of the hypothalamus–pituitary–adrenal system is abnormal (see Chapter 30). The same response—negative feedback inhibition of cortisol production, which results in alterations in cortisol level—also occurs in cancer (Yehuda, 2003).

The disabling effects of chronic cancer symptoms disrupt family and personal relationships, impair individuals' work performance, and often isolate survivors from normal social activities. Such changes in lifestyle create serious implications for a survivor's psychological well-being. When cancer changes a client's body image or alters sexual function, the survivor frequently experiences significant anxiety and depression with regard to interpersonal relationships. In the case of breast cancer survivors, studies have revealed that poorer self-ratings of quality of life are associated with poor body image, poor coping strategies, and a lack of social support (IOM & NRC, 2006).

The risk of a cancer survivor's having psychological problems is high because of a complex set of factors. Anderson (1993) developed a model for predicting the psychological well-being in women with gynecological cancer (Figure 5–2). The model has applications for other client groups as well. How well a survivor adapts to the cancer experience depends on predisposing factors (e.g., age, gender, race, income, prior psychiatric disorder, marital status, coping style, and social support), the client's current psychological status, and the presence of disruptive signs and symptoms. In a client who has few disruptive signs and symptoms and in which the cancer is less extensive, the risk of poor psychological well-being is low. In contrast, in a client who has numerous disruptive signs and symptoms, an advanced stage of cancer, and other health problems, the risk of psychological distress is high.

Certain factors help ease the psychological stress associated with having cancer. A survivor's appraisal of the cancer experience makes a difference. A survivor who sees cancer as a challenging experience and a controllable threat will have less stress (Jacobsen, 2006). Clients who use problem-oriented, active, and emotionally expressive coping processes also manage stress well (see Chapter 30). Survivors who have social and emotional support systems and maintain open communication with their treatment professionals are also likely to experience less psychological distress (Jacobsen, 2006).

Social Well-Being

Cancer affects all age groups (Figure 5–3). The developmental effects of cancer are perhaps best seen in the social impact that occurs across the lifespan. For adolescents and young adults, cancer seriously alters a young person's social skills, sexual development, body image, and the ability to think about and plan for the future (see Chapter 23). Cancer interrupts their lives, causing young survivors either to feel out of touch with the interests of their peers or to perceive those interests as superficial (Blum, 2006). In addition, because cancer makes them feel different, young survivors, out of fear of rejection, have difficulty dating and developing new relationships. The course of cancer or its treatment often causes young adults to delay leaving their parents. The natural separation that occurs when young adults finish school and look to start their careers is postponed or stopped. Often a young adult with cancer feels ill equipped to take on the real world.

Adults aged 30 to 59 who have cancer experience significant changes in their families. Once a member of the family receives a diagnosis of cancer, every family member's role, plans, and abilities change (Blum, 2006). The healthy spouse often takes on added job responsibilities to provide additional income for the family. A spouse, sibling, grandparent, or child often has to assume caregiving responsibilities for the client with cancer. The marriages of clients who experience changes in sexuality, intimacy, and fertility are affected; too often, this results in divorce. A history of cancer significantly affects employment opportunities and the ability of a survivor to obtain and retain health and life insurance (IOM & NRC, 2006). Often a survivor experiences health-related work limitations (Box 5–4) that necessitate a reduced work schedule or a complete change in employment. However, most cancer survivors who worked before the diagnosis return to work after the treatment (Spelten et al., 2002). The problem is that employers and supervisors often assume that persons with cancer are not able to perform job responsibilities as well as they did before the diagnosis; thus, job discrimination against cancer survivors is common. Cancer survivors report problems in the workplace,

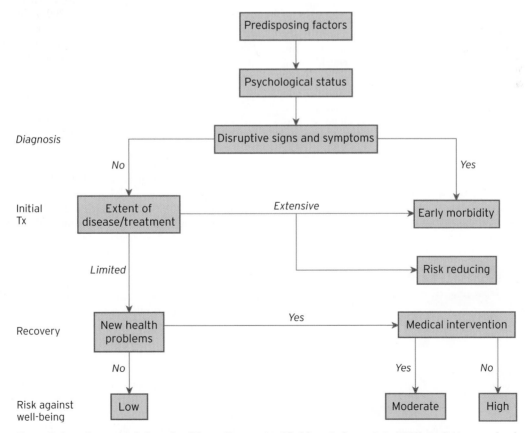

Figure 5-2 Predicting psychological well-being. **Source:** Modified from Anderson, B. L. (1993). Predicting sexual and psychologic morbidity and improving the quality of life for women with gynecologic cancer. *Cancer, 71*(Suppl. 4), 1678.

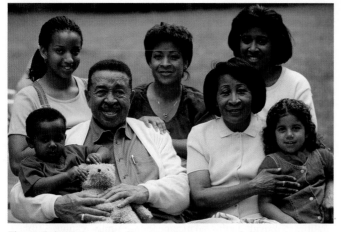

Figure 5-3 Photo of a family, representing young and old.

including dismissal, failure to hire, demotion, and denial of promotion. Many survivors also experience "job lock": A survivor will stay in an undesirable job or in one that has become difficult to perform in order not to lose insurance benefits.

The economic burden of cancer is enormous. If a survivor's illness affects his or her ability to work, the individual and family accrue less income. Also, there is usually an increase in high out-of-pocket expenses for prescription drugs, medical devices, and supplies (CCS, 2005). Some expenses may not be covered by provincial or private health insurance plans. Older adults face numerous social concerns as a result of cancer. The disease often causes clients to retire prematurely.

Many older adults have a fixed income. The older cancer survivors can see their retirement pensions erode away quickly. The survivors often have to use their income for basic expenses and cancer care costs, which limits opportunities for any social activities. Older adults who have moved to retirement residences in other provinces may find themselves isolated from the social support of family, which is especially important once cancer is diagnosed. Older adults also face a high level of disability as a result of cancer and cancer treatment. Older adults with cancer report a higher incidence of limitations in activities of daily living than do older adults without cancer (IOM & NRC, 2006). As a result, many older cancer survivors require ongoing caregiving support from either family members or professional caregivers.

Spiritual Well-Being

The experience of cancer challenges a person's spiritual well-being (see Chapter 28). Key features of spiritual well-being include a harmonious interconnectedness, creative energy, and a faith in a higher power or life force (Brown-Saltzman, 2006). Cancer and its treatment create

physical and psychological changes that cause survivors to ask the question "Why me?" and to wonder whether perhaps the disease is some form of punishment. Survivors often experience a level of spiritual distress, a disruption in a person's spirit or life principle. Survivors most at risk for spiritual distress are those with energy-consuming anxiety, an inability to forgive, low self-esteem, maturational losses, and mental illness (Brown-Saltzman, 2006). Additional risk factors include poor relationships and situational losses (see Chapter 29).

Relationships, whether with a higher power, nature, family, or community, are crucial for cancer survivors. Cancer threatens relationships because it makes it difficult for survivors to maintain a connection and a sense of belonging with what is important to them. Cancer may isolate survivors from meaningful interaction and support, which then threatens their ability to maintain hope. The long courses of treatment, the reoccurrence of cancer, and the lingering side effects of treatment all create uncertainty for survivors.

Cancer and Families

A survivor's family takes different forms: the traditional nuclear family, the extended family, single-parent family, close friends, and the blended family (see Chapter 20). Once cancer affects a member of the family, it affects all other members as well. It is usually a member of the family who becomes the client's caregiver. Family caregiving is a stressful experience, depending on the relationship between client and caregiver and on the nature and extent of the client's disease. Many caregivers who are 30 to 50 years old must care for their own immediate family in addition to a parent with cancer. The demands are many, from providing ongoing encouragement and support and assisting with household chores to providing hands-on physical care (e.g., bathing, assisting with toileting, or changing a dressing) when cancer is advanced. Caregiving also involves the psychological demands of communicating, problem solving, and decision making; social demands of remaining active in the community and work; and economic demands of meeting financial obligations.

Family Distress

Relationships between cancer survivors and family members become difficult to maintain because family members often do not know, do not understand, or report not having the skills or confidence to support the family's reactions to cancer. Changes in family roles and the burden on family caregivers negatively affect the quality of life and well-being of caregivers and cancer survivors (Stetz and Brown, 2004; Strang and Koop, 2003). Mellon et al. (2006) interviewed cancer survivors and their family caregivers and found that one of the strongest predictors for cancer survivors' quality of life were family stressors and social support. In the Mellon et al. study, family caregivers reported a quality of life lower than that of their family members. The researchers also noted that ongoing concerns and problems facing survivors and their family are important determinants of adjustment and quality of life. Families generally find themselves ill prepared to deal with cancer. Cancer survivorship has not yet become a distinct phase of cancer care; thus, professional caregivers often fail to inform and educate clients and their families about what to expect during the cancer experience. Professional caregivers do not usually address the psychosocial needs of cancer clients and their families.

For couples in which a woman experiences the acute phase of breast cancer treatment, the couple often functions in a survival mode, during which competing demands from their jobs or other family members distract the couple from attending to each other's needs, thoughts, and feelings (Lewis, 2006). Many such couples struggle with interpersonal problem solving, because they do not have the commu-

► BOX 5-4	Limitations Imposed by Cancer and Its Treatment as Reported by Survivors	
Physical tasks	18%	
Lift heavy loads	26%	
Stoop, kneel, crouch	14%	
Concentrate for long periods	12%	
Analyze data	11%	
Keep pace with others	22%	
Learn new things	14%	

Adapted from Bradley, C. J., & Bednarek, H. L. (2002). Employment patterns of long-term cancer survivors. *Psycho-Oncology, 11,* 188.

nication or problem-solving skills to understand one another's views, concerns, or fears. Less is known about what happens to family relationships in long-term survivorship. Lewis (2006) suggested two possible outcomes: benefit-finding behaviour (identifying positive aspects in the cancer experience) and heightened interpersonal tension.

Families struggle to maintain core functions when one of their members is a cancer survivor. Core family functions include maintaining an emotionally and physically safe environment, interpreting and reducing the threat of stressful events (including the cancer) for family members, and nurturing and supporting the development of individual family members (Lewis, 2006). In child-rearing families, this means providing attentive parenting for children and providing information and support to children when their sense of well-being is threatened.

When a member of the family has cancer, these core functions become threatened. Women with cancer who were mothers of young and adolescent children reported the inability to be the parent they wanted to be during the treatment phase of the disease (Zahlis & Lewis, 1998). Spouses often do not know what to do to support the survivor, and they struggle with how to help. In the end, family functions become fragmented, and family members develop an uncertainty about their roles.

Implications for Nursing

Cancer survivorship creates many implications for nursing. As a professional nurse, you must play a leadership role in helping survivors plan for optimal lifelong health. Much needs to be done in conducting nursing research to find appropriate interventions for the effects of cancer and its treatment. Nurses are in a strong position to take the lead in improving public health care efforts to manage the long-term consequences of cancer. Improvement is also necessary in the education of nurses and survivors about the phenomenon of survivorship. As a nursing student, you too can make a difference. This section addresses approaches to incorporate cancer survivorship into your nursing practice.

Survivor Assessment

Knowing that there are many cancer survivors in the health care system, you can consider how to assess clients who report a history of cancer. It is important that assessment of cancer survivors' needs is a standard part of your practice. While you are documenting a health nursing history (see Chapter 32), explore with your clients their history of cancer, including the diagnosis and type of treatment they either are undergoing or have received in the past. You must be aware that some clients do not always report that they have had cancer. So, when a client tells you he or she has had surgery, ask whether it was cancer related. When a client reveals a history of chemotherapy, radiation, biotherapy, or hormone therapy, you need to refer to resources to help you understand how those therapies typically affect clients in both the short and long term. Once you do so, extend your assessment to determine whether these treatment effects exist for your client. Remember that you need to consider not only the effects of the cancer and its treatment but also how it will affect any other medical condition. For example, if a client also has heart disease, how will the fatigue related to chemotherapy affect this individual?

From a client's own story, you can achieve an understanding of the cancer experience. By asking a general question about the client's being a cancer survivor, you can encourage the client to reveal his or her story. For example, you might ask, "Having cancer is a journey for many. How does the disease most affect you right now?" or "What is the biggest problem that you are experiencing from cancer?" This type of question helps you focus on the area that is most important to the client. Communicate to clients your interest in their situation. Show a caring approach so that clients know that you hear their story (see Chapter 19). You might further ask, "What can I do to help you at this point?"

Symptom management is an ongoing problem for many cancer survivors. If cancer is their primary diagnosis, it will be natural for you will explore any presenting symptoms. Be sure to learn specifically how any symptoms are affecting the client. For example, is pain also causing fatigue, or is a neuropathy causing the client to walk with an abnormal gait? If cancer is secondary, then important symptoms must not go unrecognized. Ask the client, "Since your diagnosis and treatment of cancer, what physical changes or symptoms have you had?" and "Tell me how these changes affect you now." Depending on the symptoms that a client identifies, you will explore each one in order to gain a complete understanding of the client's health status (Table 5–2). Remember that some clients are reluctant to report or discuss their symptoms. Be patient, and once you identify a symptom, explore the extent to which the symptom is currently affecting the client.

Because you know that cancer affects a client's quality of life in many ways, be sure to explore the client's psychological, social, and spiritual needs and resources. Sometimes you will not be able to conduct a thorough assessment when you document an initial health

▶ TABLE 5-2	Assessment Questions for Cancer Survivors
Category	**Examples of Questions**
Symptoms	• Have you had any pain or discomfort in the area where you had surgery or radiation; discomfort, pain, or unusual sensations in your hands or feet; weakness in your legs or arms; or problems moving around? • Do you experience fatigue, sleeplessness, or shortness of breath? If so, please describe them. • Sometimes people feel as if they are starting to have problems after chemotherapy, such as paying attention, remembering things, or finding words. Have you noticed any changes like these?
Psychosocial problems	• How distressed are you feeling at this point on a scale of 0 to 10, with 10 being the worst distress that you could imagine? • How do you think your family is dealing with your cancer? • What do you see in your family members' responses to your cancer that is a concern for you?
Sexuality problems	• If you have had sexual changes, what strategies have you tried to make things better? Have these strategies worked? • Would you be open to a health care professional who knows how to help you? • Since your cancer diagnosis, do you see yourself differently as a person?

nursing history. If this is the case, incorporate your assessment into your ongoing client care. Observe your client's interactions with family members and friends. When you are administering care to clients, talk about their daily lives and determine the extent to which cancer has changed their lifestyle.

One area that is often difficult for nurses to assess well is a client's sexuality. Sexuality is more than simply the physical ability to perform a sex act or conceive a child. It also includes a person's body image, sexual response (e.g., interest and satisfaction), and sexual roles and relationships (see Chapter 27). Surgery for many cancers is disfiguring, and chemotherapy and radiation often alter a client's sexual response. Cancer therapies have the potential to cause fatigue, apathy, nausea, vomiting, malaise, and sleep disturbances, all of which interfere with a client's libido (Pelusi, 2006).

It is important to realize that cancer often does influence the client's sexuality. This realization helps you develop a comfort level in acknowledging with clients that sexual changes are common at any age level. Ask a client, "Since your diagnosis and treatment of cancer, has your ability or interest in sexual activity changed? If so, how?" Clients will appreciate your sensitivity and interest in their well-being. When clients begin to discuss their sexual problems, you need to know the expert resources in your institution (e.g., psychologist or social worker) available for client referral.

Client Education

It is nurses' responsibility to educate survivors and their families about the consequences of cancer and cancer treatment. This means that when you care for a cancer survivor, you need to understand the nature of the client's particular disease and know the effects of each therapy that a client receives and the short- and long-term consequences. You play a key role in preparing a cancer survivor with the knowledge and resources needed for ongoing self-management. Lorig (2003) defined the purpose of self-management education as the provision of skills for clients to live an active and meaningful life with chronic disease. In designing education that promotes self-management in caregiving, plan activities on the basis of the caregiver's and cancer survivor's perceived disease-related problems, and assist them with problem solving and gaining the self-efficacy or confidence to deal with these problems. Client education helps survivors assume more healthy lifestyle behaviours that will then give them control of some aspects of their health and improve outcomes from cancer and chronic illness.

When caring for clients with an initial diagnosis of cancer, reinforce their health care professional's explanations of the risks related to their cancer and treatment, what they need to self-monitor (e.g., appetite, weight, and effects of fatigue and sleeplessness), and what to discuss with health care professionals in the future. If clients learn about the potential for adverse treatment effects such as pain, neuropathy, or cognitive change, they are more likely to report their symptoms. Survivors need to learn how to manage problems related to persistent symptoms. For example, survivors with neuropathy need to learn how to protect their hands and feet, prevent falls, and avoid accidental burns.

Because survivors are at increased risk for developing a secondary cancer, a chronic illness, or both, it is important for them to learn about lifestyle behaviours that will improve the quality of their lives. Health promotion education is timely after an initial cancer diagnosis, when many survivors become motivated to change their behaviour (Satia et al., 2004). Many survivors become interested in learning more about dietary supplements and nutritional complementary therapies to manage disease symptoms (IOM & NRC, 2006). Scientific evidence reveals several health promotion areas of interest to cancer

survivors: smoking cessation, physical activity, diet and nutrition (see Chapter 43), and the use of complementary and alternative medicine (see Chapter 35). You can explore with clients useful strategies to promote their health. For example, behavioural interventions for increasing physical activity among cancer survivors have yielded positive and consistent effects on vigor, cardiorespiratory fitness, quality of life, fatigue, and depression (Holtzman et al., 2004).

Providing Resources

Numerous organizations and agencies provide resources to cancer survivors. The problem is that many survivors do not receive timely and appropriate referral to these resources. As a nurse, you will find that many people (e.g., friends, neighbours, and family members) ask for your advice about health care before they actually become clients. It is important to know that cancer-related hospital and ambulatory care are not standardized. For example, when a client with cancer is hospitalized, the availability of ancillary services for long-term care varies by care setting.

A designated cancer centre offers the most comprehensive and up-to-date clinical care. National Cancer Institute–designated centres also conduct important clinical trials to investigate the most up-to-date cancer therapies. Many clients benefit when they have the opportunity to participate in these trials. Your role is to tell clients about the different resources available so that clients are able to make informed choices.

A number of cancer-related community support services are available to survivors through voluntary organizations. Most offer their services at no cost. Many supportive services offer call centres and Internet-based information and discussion boards, in addition to direct service delivery (IOM & NRC, 2006). Health care professionals are not consistent in referring clients to these valuable services. In addition, although community-based services help most survivors, gaps exist in service provision for assistance with transportation, home care, child care, and financial assistance. Become knowledgeable about the services within your community. Several national agencies exist; these include the Canadian Cancer Society, National Cancer Institute of Canada, and the Public Health Agency of Canada.

Components of Survivorship Care

Once a cancer client's primary treatment ends, health care professionals must develop an organized plan for survivorship care. This does not always occur, however, because of inadequacies in the health care system, including a failure of any one health care professional to assume responsibility for coordinating care, fragmentation of care between specialists and general practitioners, and a lack of guidance about how survivors can improve their health outcomes (IOM & NRC, 2006). Clients with cancer often do not receive noncancer care (e.g., care for diabetes or heart conditions) when the cancer diagnosis shifts attention away from care that is routine but necessary. Follow-up of cancer care is also poor, even though recommended guidelines exist. For example, some women with a history of breast cancer do not undergo annual mammography, and some clients with colorectal cancer do not undergo regular colorectal examinations. The IOM and NRC (2006) made recommendations for four essential components of survivorship care: (1) prevention and detection of new cancers and recurrent cancer; (2) surveillance for cancer spread, cancer recurrence, or secondary cancers; (3) intervention for consequences of cancer and its treatment (e.g., medical problems, symptoms, and psychological distress); and (4) coordination between specialists and primary care professionals.

Survivorship Care Plan

Just as health care professionals must improve cancer survivorship care, a strategy for survivors' ongoing clinical care is also needed. The IOM and NRC (2006) recommended the provision of a "survivorship care plan" that should be written by the principal health care professional who coordinates the client's **oncology** treatment. Ideally, you would review a survivorship care plan with a client when he or she is formally discharged from a treatment program. The plan would become a guide for any future cancer-related care. Health care professionals would use the plan as a guide for client education. Survivors would use the plan to raise questions with physicians to prompt appropriate care during follow-up visits. Box 5–5 highlights the components of a survivorship care plan.

Few health care agencies provide survivorship care plans. Those that do are usually children's hospitals. Thus, nurses and other health care professionals need to become more vigilant in recognizing cancer survivors and attempting to link them with the support and resources they require. You can make a difference in considering the long-term issues that cancer survivors face after the time of diagnosis and in contributing to solutions to manage or relieve cancer-associated health problems. A strong multidisciplinary approach that includes nurses, oncology specialists, dietitians, social workers, pastoral care, and rehabilitation professionals is necessary. Together, a multidisciplinary team can provide a plan of care that addresses treatment-related problems and future health risks and offers a wellness focus to give clients a sense of hope as they enter their survivor experience.

> ► **BOX 5-5** **Survivorship Care Plan**

Upon discharge from cancer treatment, every client and his or her primary health care professional should receive a record of all care received and a follow-up plan incorporating available evidence-informed standards of care.

Care Summary

- Diagnostic tests performed and their results
- Tumour characteristics (e.g., site, stage, and grade)
- Dates when treatment started and stopped
- Type of therapy (surgery, chemotherapy, radiotherapy, transplant, hormonal therapy, or gene therapy) provided, including the specific agents used
- Psychosocial, nutritional, and other supportive services provided
- Full contact information about the treating institutions and key health care professionals
- Identification of a key point of contact and coordinator of care

Follow-Up Plan

- Likely course of recovery
- Description of recommended cancer screening and other periodic testing and examinations
- Information about possible late and long-term effects of treatment and the symptoms of such effects
- Information about possible signs of recurrence and secondary tumours
- Information about the possible effects of cancer on the marital or partner relationship, on sexual functioning, on work, and on parenting
- Information about the potential insurance-related, employment-related, and financial consequences of cancer and, as necessary, referral for counseling, legal aid, and financial assistance
- Specific recommendations for healthy behaviours
- Information about genetic counselling and testing as appropriate
- Information about known effective chemoprevention strategies for secondary prevention
- Referrals to specific follow-up health care professionals
- A listing of cancer-related resources and information

Adapted from President's Cancer Panel. (2004). *Living beyond cancer: Finding a new balance.* Bethesda, MD: National Cancer Institute; and Hewitt, M., Greenfield, S., & Stovall, E. (Eds.). (2006). *From cancer client to cancer survivor: Lost in transition.* Washington, DC: National Academies Press.

---

* KEY CONCEPTS

- The health care system has largely ignored or misunderstood cancer survivors' health care problems.
- The definition of *cancer survivor* includes family members, friends, and caregivers who are also affected by survivorship.
- The majority of cancer survivors have serious health deficits that are related to their treatments.
- Evidence reveals that cancer survivors have poorer health outcomes than do similar individuals without cancer.
- Survivors are often reluctant to report symptoms because of a fear of being perceived as ungrateful for being disease free or a fear of cancer recurrence.
- How well a survivor adapts to the cancer experience psychologically depends on predisposing factors, the person's current psychological status, the extent of the disease, and the presence of disruptive signs and symptoms.
- The developmental effects of cancer have a social impact that occurs across the lifespan.
- Relationships between cancer survivors and family members become difficult to maintain because family members often do not know, do not understand, or report not having the skills or confidence to support the family's reactions to cancer.
- As a nursing student, you should incorporate cancer survivorship care into your nursing practice through client assessment, education, and referral of clients to available resources.
- Because survivors are at an increased risk for developing a secondary cancer, chronic illness, or both, it is important to educate them about lifestyle behaviours that will improve the quality of their lives.
- Once a cancer client's primary treatment ends, health care professionals should develop an organized plan for survivorship care.
- A client's principal health care professional should write a survivorship care plan that coordinates the client's oncology treatment.
- Ideally, you would review a survivorship care plan with a client when he or she is formally discharged from a treatment program, and it would become a guide for any future cancer-related care.

* CRITICAL THINKING EXERCISES

1. Do you have a friend or family member who has cancer and is willing to talk about it? If so, ask the individual to tell you what the experience has been like and what he or she would recommend to help nurses provide better care for survivors.

2. Ms. Ritter is a 32-year-old woman who visits the medical outpatient clinic for her final course of chemotherapy to treat breast cancer. She is married and has one child, a daughter, who is six years old. She and her husband have hoped to have another child in the near future but now wonder whether that will be possible. She has shared with the nursing staff her concerns about the future and how cancer will affect her and her family. Her

case manager talks with her about a survivorship care plan before discharge from the clinic. Identify two follow-up care plan components that would be important when considering Ms. Ritter's role as a wife and parent.

3 Ms. Ritter tells her nurse, "This chemotherapy has made me feel so tired, and there are many nights I cannot sleep very well. I am looking forward to this going away." What is an appropriate response the nurse might give Ms. Ritter?

✳ REVIEW QUESTIONS

1. Cancer survivors are at risk for treatment-related problems. Which of the clients listed below has the greatest risk for developing such a problem?
   1. An 80-year-old woman undergoing surgery for removal of a basal cell carcinoma on the face
   2. A 71-year-old man receiving chemotherapy and radiation for an advanced-stage lymphoma
   3. A 26-year-old man receiving chemotherapy for testicular cancer that is localized to the testicle
   4. A 48-year-old woman receiving radiation for Hodgkin's disease that involves lymph nodes extending above and below the diaphragm

2. The nurse reviews the medical record of a new client admitted to her nursing unit. She notices in the history that the client had a history of bladder cancer three years ago. Which of the following factors should she consider when conducting an assessment of this client? (Select all that apply.)
   1. The number and type of cancer therapies given to the client
   2. The presence of other medical conditions affecting the client
   3. Use of an approach that encourages the client to tell his or her story
   4. The readiness of cancer survivors to report the symptoms they are experiencing
   5. Assessment of sexuality as to whether the client can perform a sexual act

3. A nurse working in a medicine clinic knows it is important to recognize cancer survivors who are most at risk for post-treatment symptoms. Which of the following clients is probably at greatest risk for post-treatment symptoms?
   1. A 50-year-old mother in whom breast cancer was diagnosed at a late stage
   2. A 20-year-old male college student diagnosed with leukemia whose father had lung cancer
   3. A 32-year-old Cantonese woman with cervical cancer who does not have children and who does have supplemental health insurance.
   4. A 72-year-old First Nations retired Army captain who underwent surgical removal of his colon for cancer and who is now also receiving radiation

4. A 41-year-old man who underwent a craniotomy for the removal of a brain tumour two years ago comes to the clinic for his six-month follow-up visit. In planning your assessment, you anticipate that the client may possibly experience which of the following late effects of surgery? (Select all that apply.)
   1. Intestinal obstruction
   2. Difficulty breathing
   3. Blurred vision
   4. Poor attention span

5. In order to successfully assess whether a client is experiencing cognitive changes as a result of cancer treatment or complications of treatment, which of the following questions is probably be most relevant?
   1. "Can you describe for me your medication schedule?"
   2. "How distressed are you feeling right now, on a scale of 0 to 10?"
   3. "When did you first notice symptoms from your chemotherapy?"
   4. "What differences do you notice in your ability to get work done at your office?"

✳ RECOMMENDED WEB SITES

BC Cancer Agency: http://www.bccancer.bc.ca
This provincial Web site offers resources to the patient, the public, and the health care professional. Resources range from recommended books and pamphlets to online information regarding screening programs to detailed information about specific treatment protocols.

Canadian Breast Cancer Network: http://www.cbcn.ca
This organization is a survivor-directed national network of organizations and individuals. The site provides resources for all Canadians affected by breast cancer and those at risk. Topics include the use of alcohol, issues of beauty and personal care, best practices, and lymphedema.

Canadian Cancer Society: http://www.cancer.ca
This Web site contains French and English content for people affected by cancer (clients, families, and the general public). It presents up-to-date information about cancer prevention, research, and support services, as well as positions and perspectives on cancer-related issues such as tobacco and marijuana use, and occupational exposures.

The Wellness Community: http://www.wellness-community.org
This US site offers virtual as well as actual connections to other cancer survivors and caregivers. It also offers educational resources that range from those supplying general cancer information to those providing very diagnosis-specific information.

6

Theoretical Foundations of Nursing Practice

Written by Sally Thorne, RN, PhD, FCAHS

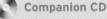

Although certain nursing tasks can be mastered by most people trained to perform them, the hallmark of nursing practice is its unique body of knowledge, as well as the set of principles that guide the systematic application of this knowledge in an expanding array of contexts. **Nursing theory** aims to make sense of knowledge about nursing to enable nurses to use it in a professional and accountable manner (Beckstrand, 1978).

A **theory** is a purposeful set of **assumptions** or **propositions** that identify the relationships between **concepts**. Theories are useful because they provide a systematic view for explaining, predicting, and prescribing phenomena. A nursing theory tends to be not explicitly propositional but rather a **conceptualization** of nursing for the purpose of describing, explaining, predicting, or prescribing care (Meleis, 2007). Theories constitute one aspect of disciplinary knowledge and create vital linkages to how inquiry is approached (Fawcett et al., 2001). Nursing theories provide nurses with a perspective from which to view client situations, a way to organize data, and a method of analyzing and interpreting information to bring about coherent and informed nursing practice.

Early Nursing Practice and the Emergence of Theory

Nursing practices have been documented throughout history (Yura & Walsh, 1973). However, modern nursing practice, in which the knowledge and practice of nursing are formalized into a professional context, is often attributed to the work of Florence Nightingale, a visionary leader in Victorian England who created systems for nursing education and practice (see Chapter 3). Contemporary scholars now consider Nightingale's work as an early theoretical and conceptual **model for nursing**. Her descriptive theory provided nurses with a way to think about nursing practice in a frame of reference that focuses on clients and the environment.

Since Nightingale's era, the status of nursing practice has parallelled that of the authority of women in society. After World War II, major developments in science and technology had a powerful influence on health care, including nursing practice. **Nursing science** came into its own. No longer simply applying the knowledge of other disciplines, nurses now began to acquire a unique body of knowledge about the practice of nursing.

Since the 1960s, scientific knowledge has burgeoned across disciplines. In particular, knowledge about nursing has drawn from and contributed to developments in health sciences, basic physical sciences, social and biobehavioural sciences, social theory, ethical theory, and the **philosophy of science**. Each of these sources has relevance for the interpretation of nursing care and the synthesis of relevant facts and theories for application to practice.

Major developments in nursing theory occurred in the late 1960s (Meleis, 2007). The health care system was expanding and changing, influenced by scientific discoveries and technological applications. Disease intervention became more sophisticated and scientifically driven. The focus of society shifted from simply attending to sick and injured people toward the larger problem of curing and eradicating disease, which expanded physicians' influence over the structure of health care. For the first time, nurses realized the urgency of articulating exactly how their role differed from those of other health care professionals (Chinn & Kramer, 2004; Engebretson, 1997; Fawcett, 2005; Newman, 1972).

The drive for early theorizing about the practice of nursing was led by nursing educators, who noted that traditional ways of preparing professional nurses were rapidly becoming outdated. Until the late 1960s, a nursing apprenticeship model, augmented by lectures offered by physicians, had seemed sufficient. Around this time, nursing educational leaders became inspired to theorize about nursing in order to structure and define what a curriculum oriented to nursing knowledge might contain (Dean, 1995; Orem & Parker, 1964; Torres, 1974). This meant grappling with large theoretical and philosophical questions, such as the following:

- What are the focus and scope of nursing?
- How is nursing unique and different from other health care professions?
- What should be the appropriate disciplinary knowledge for professional nursing practice?

To answer these questions, early theorists developed **conceptual frameworks**, in which they organized core nursing concepts and proposed relationships among these concepts. These conceptual frameworks were "mental maps" whose purpose was to make sense of the information and decisional processes that nurses needed to apply knowledge to nursing practice (Ellis, 1968; Johnson, 1974; McKay, 1969; Wald & Leonard, 1964). Expressing knowledge about nursing in scientific language created a context in which nursing science gained stature and flourished (Cull-Wilby & Peppin, 1987; Jones, 1997). However, these nursing theories were not the kind of scientific theories that could be proved or disproved with empirical evidence (Levine, 1995); rather, they represented ideas about how nurses might organize knowledge, as well as the processes by which they would apply it to unique practice situations. Table 6–1 defines some of the basic terms that are used in theorizing about scientific issues.

Nursing Process

Early nursing theorists sought to organize the knowledge about the practice of nursing that nurses draw upon to direct their approach to clinical encounters. However, theorists generally lacked ways of systematically explaining how nurses work with knowledge in new situations (Field, 1987). An important early step in the application of knowledge to nursing practice was Orlando's (1961) development of a problem-solving approach that came to be known as the **nursing process** (Yura & Walsh, 1973). This process originally involved four steps: assessment, planning, intervention, and evaluation, whereby each step represented a distinct way in which general nursing knowledge could be applied to unique and individual nurse–client situations (Carnevali & Thomas, 1993; Henderson, 1966; Meleis, 2007; Torres, 1986):

- Assessment phase: Nurses would gather information, including biological, sociocultural, environmental, spiritual, and psychological data, to create an understanding of the client's unique health or illness experience. Organizing the data would enable the nurses to interpret major issues and concerns (Barnum, 1998) and produce a **nursing diagnosis**: the nurses's perspective on the appropriate focus for the client (Durand & Prince, 1966).
- Planning phase: Nurses would prioritize the issues raised during assessment in relation to the nursing diagnoses, identify which issues could be supported or assisted by nursing intervention, and create a plan of care.
- Intervention phase: The plan of care would be carried out.
- Evaluation phases: The plan's success or failure would be judged both against the plan itself and against the client's overall health status; that is, it would be determined whether the intended outcomes had been achieved or whether the nursing intervention strategies required revision. The nursing process was intended as

> **TABLE 6-1**   **The Terminology of Scientific Theorizing**

Term	Description	Example
Concept	A mental formulation of objects or events, representing the basic way in which ideas are organized and communicated.	Anxiety
Conceptualization	The process of formulating concepts.	Framing behavioural patterns as anxiety related
Operational definition	A description of concepts, articulated in such a way that they can be applied to decision making in practice. It links concepts with other concepts and with theories, and it often includes the essential properties and distinguishing features of a concept.	Differentiation and measurement of state and trait anxiety
Theory	A purposeful set of assumptions or propositions about concepts; shows relationships between concepts and thereby provides a systematic view of phenomena so that they may be explained predicted, or prescribed.	Social determinants of health
Assumption	A description of concepts or connection of two concepts that are accepted as factual or true; includes "taken for granted" ideas about the nature and purpose of concepts, as well as the structure of theory.	"Nursing exists to serve a social mandate"
Proposition	A declarative assertion.	"Clients who receive appropriate nursing care have better health outcomes"
Phenomenon	An aspect of reality that can be consciously sensed or experienced (Meleis, 2007); nursing concepts and theories represent the theoretical approach to making sense of aspects of reality of concern to nursing.	Pain
Theoretical model	Mental representation of how things work. For example, an architect's plan for a house is not the house itself but rather the set of information necessary to understand how all of the building elements will be brought together to create that particular house.	Biopsychosocial model of health
Conceptual framework	The theoretical structure that links concepts together for a specific purpose. When its purpose is to show how something works, it can also be described as a *theoretical model*. Nursing conceptual frameworks link major nursing concepts and phenomena to direct nursing decisions (e.g., what to assess, how to make sense of data, what to plan, how to enact a plan, and how to evaluate whether the plan has had the intended outcome). Conceptual frameworks are also often referred to as *nursing models* or *nursing theories* (Meleis, 2007).	Orem's (1971) self-care model for nursing

a sequence within which thoughtful interpretation always preceded action, and the effects of action were always evaluated in relation to the original situation.

The nursing process was widely accepted by nurses because it was a logical way to describe basic problem-solving processes in which knowledge was used effectively to guide nursing decisions (Henderson, 1982). Nurses quickly adopted the nursing process because it represented a continuous, rapid cycling of information through each of the phases. Although it was useful for organizing and applying knowledge to clinical practice (Meleis, 2007), some later theorists began to challenge the nursing process as being too linear and rigid for nursing's purposes (Varcoe, 1996).

In current practice, terms such as *clinical judgement* are used to refer to reasoning processes that rely on *critical thinking* and multiple ways of knowing; clinical judgement implies the systematic use of the nursing process to invoke the complex intuitive and conscious thinking strategies that are part of all clinical decision making in nursing (Alfaro-LeFevre, 2004; Benner & Tanner, 1987; Tanner, 1993).

Conceptual Frameworks

The conceptual framework builders of the late 1960s and after are usually referred to as the *nursing theorists*. All were fascinated with how effective nurses systematically organize general knowledge about nursing in order to understand an individual client's situation and determine which of many available strategies would work best to restore health and ameliorate or prevent disease (Orem & Parker, 1964). This reasoning process was different from linear, cause-and-effect reasoning, and it was what the nursing theorists understood to be the hallmark of excellence in nursing practice (Barnum, 1998; Meleis, 2007). Indeed, when effective nurses made intelligent clinical decisions, it was often difficult to determine the precise dynamics that explained how those nurses applied that knowledge (Benner et al., 1996).

The building of nursing models was an attempt to theorize how all nurses might be taught to organize and synthesize knowledge about nursing so that they would develop advanced clinical reasoning skills (Raudonis & Acton, 1997). Theorists who developed these frameworks and models sought to depict theoretical structures that would enable a nurse to grasp all aspects of a clinical situation within the larger context of available options for nursing care. Table 6–2 describes four types of theory: **grand theory**, **middle-range theory**, **descriptive theory**, and **prescriptive theory**.

Metaparadigm Concepts

Each conceptual framework was an attempt to define nursing by creating a theoretical definition for the substance and structure of the key bodies of knowledge that would be needed to understand clinical situations (Figure 6–1). This collective body of knowledge was called the **metaparadigm concepts** and included the concepts of person, environment, health care, and nursing care (Fawcett, 1992).

Client and Person

By the 1960s, professional leaders recognized that nurses did much more than simply care for hospitalized clients. Because of this, nursing theorists started to use the term *client*, rather than *patient*, to refer to the person at the centre of any nursing process. The term signified a range of health states, including both sickness and wellness, and a more interactive relationship between the nurse and the persons to whom care was directed. At the same time, nurses were becoming aware of their potential to deliver care beyond the individual—that is, to families, groups, and communities. Although theories to articulate the role of

nursing care in families and communities also began to arise around this time, most early conceptual models focused on the individual.

To help nurses systematically organize and make sense of the vast amount of information that might be relevant to any particular client, most early models clearly defined the concept of the person. Theorists variously understood a person as a system of interacting parts, a system of competing human needs, or an entity with biological, psychological, social, and spiritual dimensions. Each framework drew attention to multiple aspects of human experience so that the nurse could understand each instance of wellness and illness for its uniqueness within the context of that individual's body, feelings, and situation. Each model depicted a way of thinking about a whole individual, with the aim of helping nurses understand how the implications of any action or intervention could be systematically individualized toward the benefit of all facets of that individual.

Environment

Each conceptual framework reflected an understanding that the person is part of and interacts with a complex environmental system. This environment may involve the person's family and social ties, the community, the health care system, as well as the geopolitical issues that affect health. The early conceptual frameworks helped shape nurses' increasing appreciation of how to work within a larger context of every experience of wellness and illness. In so doing, these frameworks led to a future in which nurses would spearhead advances in social and health care policy, health promotion, and community development.

Health

Because the practice of nursing has a social mandate to improve the health of both the individual and society, the early theorists struggled to articulate a goal for nursing. They defined health as much more than simply the absence of disease or injury but rather as an ideal state of optimal health or total well-being toward which all individuals could strive (see Chapter 1). This definition reflected a vision of

➤ TABLE 6-2	Types of Theory
Type of Theory	**Description**
Grand theory	Global, conceptual framework that provides insight into abstract phenomena, such as human behaviour or nursing science. Grand theories are broad in scope and therefore require further application through research before the ideas they contain can be fully tested (Chinn & Kramer, 2004). They are intended not to provide guidance for specific nursing interventions but rather to provide the structural framework for broad, abstract ideas about nursing. They are sometimes called **paradigms** because they represent distinct world views about those phenomena and provide the structural framework within which narrower-range theories can be developed and tested.
Middle-range theory	Encompasses a more limited scope and is less abstract. Middle-range theories address specific phenomena or concepts and reflect practice (administration, clinical, or teaching). The phenoma or concepts tend to cross different nursing fields and reflect a variety of nursing care situations.
Descriptive theory	Describes phenomena (e.g., responding to illness through patterns of coping), speculates on why phenomena occur, and describes the consequences of phenomena. Descriptive theories have the ability to explain, relate, and in some situations predict phenomena of concern to nursing (Meleis, 2007). Descriptive nursing theories are designed not to direct specific nursing activities but rather to help explain client assessments and possibly guide future nursing research.
Prescriptive theory	Addresses nursing interventions and helps predict the consequences of a specific intervention. A prescriptive nursing theory should designate the prescription (i.e., nursing interventions), the conditions under which the prescription should occur, and the consequences (Meleis, 2007). Prescriptive theories are action oriented, which tests the validity and predictability of a nursing intervention. These theories guide nursing research to develop and test specific nursing interventions (Fawcett, 2005).

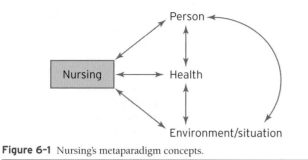

Figure 6-1 Nursing's metaparadigm concepts.

nursing care that applied to both the individual and society and to all clients, sick or well. It recognized that persons with chronic disease could strive for better health and that overall health could be compromised by psychosocial or spiritual challenges, even among the most physically fit individuals. Although perfect health was not always achievable, this conceptualization guided nurses to help all clients reach outcomes that were productive and satisfying.

Nursing

Each early conceptual framework included a unique definition of nursing that linked a view of the client with an understanding of the person's environment, life, and health goals. Built on a distinct subset of knowledge, each conceptual framework presented a coherent and complete belief system about nursing practice, although each did so in different terms and with a different alignment of ideas. Because most nursing scholars of the era assumed that one model would eventually become dominant (Meleis, 2007), competition among the frameworks occurred. Over time, the application of the frameworks in practice became more rigid and codified. The focus, originally on guiding nurses to think systematically, had shifted to using language in particular ways and filling out assessment forms correctly. Many experienced nurses began to conclude that these frameworks actually inhibited their systematic thinking, and much debate ensued with regard to the utility of the models.

Philosophy of Nursing Science

When nursing theorists began developing their frameworks and models, nurses understood the process of building a knowledge base as a matter of science and discovery. In that context, theories were considered logical propositions that could be rigorously tested for their capacity to answer (or not answer) the hypothetical questions posed by a discipline. However, while creating frameworks for the complex reasoning in nursing practice, these early theorists were applying traditional scientific ways of understanding how knowledge works without fully appreciating the limitations of science, especially in relation to complex problems. As thinkers in all disciplines began to move beyond their traditional boundaries, other possibilities for the development of knowledge about the practice of nursing began to emerge.

Scientific Revolutions

Thomas S. Kuhn, a philosopher of science, created a way of thinking about science and knowledge that expanded thought in many disciplines. First published in 1962, his book, *The Structure of Scientific Revolutions,* became popular in the 1970s and 1980s as scholars began to realize the potential of its ideas to support new thinking about how knowledge is built. Kuhn challenged the traditional notion of science as a logical progression of discoveries, arguing that major scientific developments occurred only when scientists thought about problems in radically new ways. These ways of thinking departed

from the traditional to such an extent that an entirely different world view, or "paradigm shift," developed. According to Kuhn, scientific advances happen when people think creatively and look beyond established norms. Such creative thinking could stimulate new undersandings of problems that were once considered irresolvable (e.g., quantum physics introduced the idea that the behaviour of very small particles could explain atomic behaviour in ways that defied explanation through conventional Newtonian physics). This new way of thinking about the philosophy of science led nurses to consider their theoretical frameworks as more than theoretical propositions about logical relationships among concepts, but as actual world views, or *paradigms,* that might help them grasp the complexities of nursing (Fry, 1995).

Complexity Science

A second major shift in scientific thinking occurred with the introduction of chaos theory (Gleick, 1987). Originating from observations in physics that predictable patterns existed among factors that could not be predicted scientifically, this theory created a new way of approaching complex situations. In rejecting the simple cause-and-effect relationships used in traditional science, chaos theory led to what has been termed *complexity science.* In this kind of science, dynamic and interactive phenomena are reduced to the smallest properties that can be observed within their natural context so that their interactions can be interpreted with as little interference as possible from prior assumptions. For example, chaos theory explains how, in sensitive weather systems, minor variations in initial conditions (e.g., barometric pressure) might explain large-scale physical patterns over time (e.g., hurricanes). These ideas created a new language to apply to scientific thinking. Because experiences of health and illness are difficult to understand out of their individual context, chaos theory offered a new way to approach nursing science (Coppa, 1993; Ray, 1998).

Ways of Knowing in Nursing Practice

As ideas shifted, nursing theorists also realized that science was just one of several forms of knowledge necessary for their practice discipline. In 1978, Carper published an influential paper in which she used the expression **ways of knowing** to refer to patterns of knowledge application in nursing practice. Carper articulated a critical role in nursing practice not only for empirical science but also for ethical, personal, and esthetic knowledge. Later theorists added sociopolitical knowledge (White, 1995) and critical thinking (see Chapter 12) to the list of central ways of knowing that are essential to the highest quality of clinical nursing. These ideas contributed to discussions emerging in other social and life sciences around *how* nurses know what they know (Chinn & Kramer, 2004; Kikuchi & Simmons, 1999).

Paradigm Debates Within Nursing

With the new philosophical approach to scientific knowledge, nurses struggled with how to define their work as both an art and a science and as both applied and practical (Donaldson, 1995; Johnson, 1991; Rodgers, 1991; Sarter, 1990). Ideas about the theoretical foundations of nursing practice shifted. Some scholars began to question conceptual models as a valid form of theorizing (Holden, 1990). The frustration resulting from overly formal and rigid approches to applying many of these models led to a period of what has been called *model bashing* (Engebretson, 1997). However, the question confronting the early theorists remained as follows: How does a nurse organize and make sense of all available knowledge and apply it intelligently to the challenges that arise in an individual clinical case?

In this context, many nurse scholars began to appreciate the original theories as being better understood as philosophical statements rather than scientific prescriptions. However, one group of theorists, considering some of the original theories to be overly simplistic and insufficiently holistic, began to categorize various nursing models as reflective of entirely different paradigms of thinking (Parse, 1987). That group of theorists depicted the majority of nursing's models and frameworks as old-fashioned and outdated and, coining the collective term *totality paradigm frameworks,* contended that these models reduced an understanding of the human person to fragmented parts out of context. These theorists identified a contrasting set of conceptual frameworks as radically different by virtue of being both holistic and philosophically sophisticated, and they termed these theories *simultaneity paradigm frameworks* (Parse, 1987). Advocates of simultaneity theories continue to depict the diverse universe of theorizing about nursing as reflecting these two mutually exclusive groupings, positioning one set of conceptual frameworks as philosophically and morally superior to what they understand the other to represent (Cody, 1995; Nagle & Mitchell, 1991; Newman, 1992).

Nursing Diagnosis

Another discussion about nursing theory centred on nursing diagnosis. The scholars who devised conceptual frameworks focused on models to assess and interpret data about individual client situations. However, the conceptual frameworks were less explicit about how to plan, implement, and evaluate nursing care. To fill this gap, nursing diagnosis emerged as an additional phase in that process. It became a discrete focus of theorizing about nursing care.

In the 1970s, scholars noted a need for precise language to categorize and document nursing diagnoses into a taxonomy (Warren & Hoskins, 1990). This resulted in the formation of the North American Nursing Diagnoses Association (NANDA) (see Chapter 14), which held a series of consensus conferences to establish a list of the common client problems addressed by practicing nurses. The nursing diagnosis movement led to considerable general debate on the merits of NANDA's fixed list of nursing diagnoses versus the theoretically infinite options for nursing care intended by the conceptual models (Fitzpatrick, 1990; Roy, 1982). Although it is recognized as practical rather than theoretical (Fitzpatrick, 1990), NANDA's list has become a popular device for organizing nursing care because it enables efficient categorization into electronic databases and the subsequent standardization of nursing care plans (Warren & Hoskins, 1990). Despite its popularity with health care administrators, NANDA's list is recognized by many nurses as a system that relies entirely upon an agreement about what constitutes average wellness and illness experiences. It can therefore create worrisome barriers to the individualized care of clients (Lee et al., 2006).

Reflections on Conceptualizing Nursing

The scientific and philosophical aspects of today's nursing practice is built on the foundation of early nursing theories about nursing. The history of "nursing theory" is the story of an enlightened attempt to articulate excellent clinical reasoning in nursing care. How effective nurses actually use knowledge within the complexity of their clinical reasoning is, however, still undetermined. In this context, theorizing about nursing is perhaps best understood as an extended philosophical struggle to understand how highly skilled nurses actually think. Instead of arguing the advantages of one nursing theory over another, nursing scholars of today appreciate the creativity of their predecessors within the constrained conceptual contexts in which they were expected to operate.

Major Theoretical Models

Some of the major theoretical models are summarized briefly in Table 6–3; the similarities and differences among them are illustrated. Note, however, that because many nursing theorists based their models on complex combinations of theories from many disciplines, the categorization used here is somewhat oversimplistic. It may be helpful to view the conceptual frameworks in terms of larger theories on which they have drawn, such as adaptation theory, systems theory, or human needs theory.

Practice-Based Theories

All conceptual models of nursing are designed to guide and shape practice. Although their theoretical inspiration is derived directly from the practice setting, many conceptual models do not capture all of what might be influencing that practice, such as societal and demographic changes, current health care belief models, and therapeutic strategies, as well as the political struggles inherent to health care delivery. The early practice theories, therefore, reflect the issues that were shaping the role and context of nursing during those specific timeframes.

Florence Nightingale. Whereas most later theorists drew on social and psychological theories, Nightingale was directly inspired by nursing practice. Writing *Notes on Nursing* in 1859, she described conditions necessary to promote health and healing. Her observations during the Crimean War led to the first set of principles for nursing practice, acknowledging the particular importance of the environment, including clean living areas, fresh air, and the presence of light. The role of nursing care included ensuring that wounded soldiers were warm, comfortable, and adequately fed. Torres (1986) noted that Nightingale demonstrated how to think about clients and their environment. By shifting the focus from disease processes toward an environment conducive to healing, Nightingale's conceptualization clearly differentiated the role of nursing from that of medicine.

The McGill Model. Dr. Moyra Allen (Box 6–1) conceived the McGill model, and she and her colleagues developed it (Gottlieb & Rowat, 1987). Systematically studying actual nursing situations, Allen and her colleagues created a way of thinking about nursing that focused on promoting health. They recognized that many clients' health concerns were best approached through changes in lifestyle. The McGill scholars focused on the individual in the context of the family and, like Nightingale, viewed nursing as complementary to medicine. The main features of the McGill model were "a focus on health rather than illness and treatment, on all family members rather than the patient alone, on family goals rather than on the nurse's, and on family strengths rather than their deficits" (Gottlieb & Feeley, 1999, p. 194). Over time, the model has been further developed to demonstrate its application within a range of clinical contexts and settings (e.g., Feeley & Gerez-Lirette, 1992; Feeley & Gottlieb, 1998).

➤ TABLE 6-3	Milestones in the Development of Nursing Theory
1859	Florence Nightingale's *Notes on Nursing: What It Is and What It Is Not* was published (updated version published 1946)
1952	*Nursing Research* (the first peer-reviewed scientific journal about nursing care) was established
1952	Hildegard Peplau's text on *Interpersonal Relations in Nursing* was published
1955	Virginia Henderson's definition of nursing was first published in the 5th edition of Harmer and Henderson's (1955) basic nursing text
1961	Ida Orlando introduced the nursing process
1970	Martha Rogers' model was first published
1970	Callista Roy's model was first published
1971	Dorothea Orem's model was first published
1976	The North American Nursing Diagnosis Association (NANDA) list of nursing diagnoses was first published
1976	The University of British Columbia model of nursing practice was first published (Campbell et al., 1976)
1978	Barbara Carper's paper on fundamental patterns of knowing in nursing practice was published
1979	Evelyn Adam's model was first published (English version published 1981)
1981	Rosemarie Parse's model was first published
1987	The McGill model of nursing was first published (Gottlieb & Rowat, 1987)

Needs Theories

Many early theorists organized their thinking by conceptualizing the client as representing a collection of needs. This reflected a common orientation to studying the nature of people, popularized in the 1960s, in which needs, drives, and competencies were thought to hold potential for explaining human behaviour. Of these theories, Maslow's (1954) hierarchy of needs was one of the best known and most influential. The idea that complex human behaviour can be best explained as a response to the competing demands of various basic needs is featured prominently in many nursing models.

Virginia Henderson. Henderson (Harmer & Henderson, 1955) conceptualized the client as a compilation of 14 basic human needs: to breathe, eat and drink, eliminate waste products, move and maintain posture, rest and sleep, dress and undress, maintain body temperature, be clean, avoid danger, communicate, worship, work, play, and learn. Viewing the client in this way clearly defined the nurse's role. Accordingly, Henderson defined nursing practice as assisting the individual, sick or well, in the performance of activities that contribute to health, recovery, or a peaceful death. Henderson's model has remained popular in practice because its language is familiar and easily comprehensible and because it explains how a person's biological, psychological, social, and spiritual components combine to influence the way illness is experienced and health can be regained.

Dorothea Orem. Orem's (1971) self-care theory, the origins of which lay in Henderson's work, was used widely in both nursing practice and research. Orem's theory addressed the ways in which people are responsible for meeting the following universal self-care requisites:

- Maintaining sufficient intake of air, water, and food.
- Maintaining a balance between activity and rest and between solitude and interaction.
- Providing for elimination processes.
- Preventing hazards to life, functioning, and well-being.
- Promoting functioning and growth in social groups in accordance with human potential.

➤ BOX 6-1	Milestones in Canadian Nursing History

Moyra Allen, 1921-1996

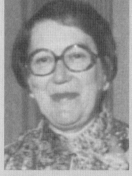

A creative and independent thinker, Moyra Allen was one of the first Canadian nurses to earn a doctoral degree. She lobbied for collective bargaining rights for nurses and was the founding president of the United Nurses of Montreal. She was also the founder of *Nursing Papers*, later renamed the *Canadian Journal of Nursing Research*.

Dr. Allen was a founding member of the World Health Organization committee that developed the criteria for accreditation of nursing schools. She designed an evaluation model for nursing schools and evaluated schools in South America, India, and Ghana. She joined the faculty of the School of Nursing at McGill in 1954 and became professor emeritus in 1985 on her retirement.

In demonstrating her model of nursing, now known as the McGill model, Dr. Allen established The Health Workshop in 1977, a community health facility, in which she put into practice a developmental concept of health and nursing as a prototype of primary health care. The workshop, viewed as complementary to existing services, was staffed with nurses, a community development officer, and a health librarian. The workshop's purpose was to demonstrate the validity of a local health resource managed by nurses that focused on long-term family health. It proved to be an innovative means of improving the health status of families coping with illness and other problems.

Dr. Allen received numerous awards, including the Jeanne Mance Award, which recognizes major contributions to the health of Canadians. In 1987, she became a member of the Order of Canada for her outstanding contributions to Canadian nursing.

Drawing on both human need and developmental theory, Orem's theory focused on the individual's role in maintaining health. This theory emerged at a time when the passive role of the client was being questioned and the health care system was beginning to shift away from full responsibility for people's health. With increased understanding of illness patterns, Orem acknowledged the effects of multiple lifestyle factors such as smoking, diet, and exercise, reminding nurses that clients can look after their own health and that they must learn to care for themselves within their families and communities. Thus, the role of the nurse, according to Orem, was to act temporarily for the client until the client could resume a more independent role in self-care.

Interactionist Theories

Interactionist theories focused on the relationships between nurses and their clients. These theories defined more clearly the specific human communicative and behavioural patterns by which practitioners met their clients' needs. As the theorists reframed definitions of the nursing profession, they drew from the work of psychologists and psychoanalysts such as Harry Stack Sullivan, Abraham Maslow, and Sigmund Freud.

Hildegard Peplau. Peplau, a psychiatric specialist, defined the core of nursing care as the interpersonal relationship between the nurse and the client. Building upon the ideas of psychoanalyst Harry Stack Sullivan, Peplau depicted the practice of nursing as an interactive and therapeutic relationship. Peplau felt that such relationships allowed nurses to challenge the practice of long-term stays in large inpatient psychiatric hospitals and to envision supporting clients to achieve independent living. "The kind of person each nurse becomes makes a substantial difference in what each patient will learn as he is nursed through his experience with illness" (Peplau, 1952, p. vii). According to Peplau, a nurse was "an investigator, prober, interpreter, and reporter, using the rich data she extracts from the patient concerning his life. She develops insights, his and hers, into the meaning of a patient's behaviour and helps the patient recognize and change patterns that obstruct achievement of his goals" (Barnum, 1994, p. 217). An early advocate of an orderly and systematic approach to care, Peplau created a way of thinking about nursing care that directed nurses toward preventing illness and maintaining health.

Joyce Travelbee. Writing in the late 1960s and early 1970s, Travelbee also viewed nursing care as an interpersonal process. In contrast to Peplau's more psychoanalytic orientation, Travelbee drew on a form of thinking known as *existential philosophy* to guide her theorizing. Travelbee (1971) viewed the "client" as including not only the individual but also the client's family and community, and she articulated the role of the nurse as assisting clients to "prevent or cope with the experience of illness and suffering and, if necessary, to find meaning in these experiences" (p. 7). Travelbee emphasized that nurses must recognize the humanity of their clients, suggesting that even the term *patient* should be regarded as a stereotypical categorization. Recognizing the reciprocity of human interaction, Travelbee focused attention on the communication that occurs between nurses and their clients as an important vehicle for finding meaning in illness.

Evelyn Adam. Influenced by Dorothy Johnson, as well as by earlier interactionist theorists (George, 1995), Canadian theorist Evelyn Adam (1979, 1991) articulated the essence of nursing as a helping process. From her perspective, the nurse played a complementary–supplementary role in supporting the client's strength, knowledge, and will. Adam's model drew on Henderson's framework of basic human needs and extended it into a model that would explain not only how nurses conceptualized the client but also how they applied that knowledge in the context of a helping relationship characterized by empathy, caring, and mutual respect.

Systems Theories

In the 1970s and 1980s, as conceptual models of nursing became more sophisticated and structured, several theorists drew on general systems theory (von Bertalanffy, 1968) for guidance in conceptualizing the complexity of human health. The main appeal of systems theory was that it accounted for the whole of an entity (the system) and its component parts (subsystems), as well as the interactions between the parts and the whole. In this way, systems theory allowed theorists to expand the conceptualization of nursing practice through both structure and process, whereby the individual was viewed as an open system in constant interaction with his or her environment. Being outside the system, the nurse became one of the many forces to have an effect on that system. Using this perspective, nurses were encouraged to appreciate the interactions of a system with its component parts and with its environment. Systems approaches helped nurses recognize that intervention in any one part of a system would produce consequent reactions in other parts, as well as in the system as a whole. Regardless of how each theorist depicted the nature of the system, these general principles common to all living systems were featured in each of the nursing systems models.

Dorothy Johnson. Johnson's theoretical work was popularized in the early 1960s through class notes and speeches, but it remained unpublished until much later (Grubbs, 1980; Johnson, 1980). In her nursing model, Johnson identified the individual as a behavioural system with seven subsystems, each of which has a goal, a set of behaviours, and a choice. The notion of goals of the subsystems was based on the drives that were considered universal and applicable to all clients. However, the meanings attributed to each goal and the set of behaviours for achieving goals were seen as highly individual and unique to each client. Together with the choices made by the client in relation to meeting his or her behavioural system goals, each subsystem also had a function that could be considered analogous to the physiological function of a biological system (Meleis, 2007).

The University of British Columbia Model. The behavioural systems model developed at the University of British Columbia (UBC) School of Nursing was inspired by Johnson's model and developed by a committee led by Margaret Campbell that included several of Johnson's former students. Broadening the view of human experience on the basis of behavioural drives, the UBC model depicted the behavioural system as being composed of nine basic human needs, each of which is shaped by the psychological and sociocultural environment in which it is expressed (Campbell et al., 1976). Whereas needs were considered universal and therefore fundamental to human experience, the specific goals toward which needs-related human behaviour were directed and the strategies for achieving those goals were recognized as unique to individuals and their particular physiological, psychological, or social circumstances (Thorne et al., 1993). Thus, the UBC model provided a structure by which general knowledge about human health and illness could be combined with particular knowledge about each individual client. In accordance with the tenets of general systems theory, the goal of nursing practice was balance of the behavioural system. The nurse's role was to foster, protect, sustain, and teach (Campbell, 1987) and thereby bring about not only system balance but also stability and optimal health.

Betty Neuman. Neuman's approach to theorizing about nursing differed from that of other systems theorists in that it did not rely on concepts concerning needs and drives, nor did it break the system into any component parts. Neuman understood the person to be a physiological, psychological, sociocultural, developmental, and spiritual being (Meleis, 2007) and oriented the attention of the nurse to the client system in a health care–oriented and holistic manner (Neuman, 1982). Neuman considered the client system to have innate factors consistent with being human, as well as unique factors that characterized each individual person. According to Neuman, each client had a unique set of response patterns determined and regulated by a core structure. Neuman believed that because the person was vulnerable to environmental stressors, the role of the nurse ought to focus on actual and potential stressors. In this way, Neuman's model focused on prevention.

Sister Callista Roy. In contrast to most other systems theorists, Roy considered the client not as behavioural system but rather as an adaptive one. She viewed the person as a biopsychosocial being in constant interaction with a changing environment (Roy, 1984). Her model depicted four modes of adaptation: physiological needs, self-concept, role function, and interdependence (Roy, 1974). She saw the person as an adaptive system with two major internal processes by which to adapt: the cognator and the regulator subsystems (Roy & Andrews, 1999). Roy used these mechanisms to describe and explain the interconnectedness of all aspects of human adaptation and to conceptualize the role of the nurse in managing the stimuli that influence that adaptation (Meleis, 2007).

Simultaneity Theories

The theorists who identified their work as belonging to the simultaneity paradigm considered their theories to be radically different from the practice, needs, interactionist, and systems theories. Although simultaneity theories were first articulated long before the paradigm debate arose and before the terms *simultaneity* and *totality* were used to categorize the various theories, the language of simultaneity has become prominent in distinguishing this group of nursing theories from others. A characteristic feature of these theories is what Rogers (1970) called the *unitary human being*. Previous theorists had sought to identify aspects of the individual that could represent an abstract conceptualization of the whole but also provided an understanding of the person and his or her problems, needs, or goals. In contrast, the simultaneity theorists viewed the individual as an entirely irreducible whole, inherently and "holographically" connected with the universal environment (Parse, 2004). Thus, these theories represented a distinct way of articulating an understanding of the client of nursing and of nursing's role in relation to that client.

Martha Rogers. Martha Rogers's (1970) model was revolutionary in presenting the client not simply as a person but as an energy field in constant interaction with the environment, which itself was also an irreducible energy field, coextensive with the universe (Meleis, 2007). According to Rogers, who based her theory on her interpretations of evolving ideas in physics, the role of nursing was to focus on the life process of a human being along a time–space continuum (Rogers, 1970). An early proponent of pattern recognition, Rogers believed that pattern gave the energy field its identity and its distinguishing characteristics (Meleis, 2007). The objective of nursing practice became one of helping clients reach their maximum health potential in the context of constant change and and to develop what Rogers referred to as homeodynamic unity within diversity.

Rosemarie Parse. Parse's (1981) theory of "man–living–health," later termed *human becoming* (Parse, 1997), was another view of the individual as a unitary being who is "indivisible, unpredictable, and everchanging" and "a freely choosing being who can be recognized through paradoxical patterns cocreated all-at-once in mutual process with the universe" (Parse, 2004, p. 293). According to Parse's perspective, the caring presences of nurses and their particular patterns of relating support individuals in the human "becoming" process. Within Parse's nursing theory, the goal of nursing is articulated not in traditional definitions of health but rather as the notion of people in a continuous process of making choices and changing health priorities. According to Parse's theory, nurses engage with people in their process of "becoming" through the application of three core processes referred to as explicating, dwelling with, and moving beyond (Parse, 1999).

Jean Watson. Watson (1979) considered the individual to be a totality who can be viewed as a transpersonal self. According to Watson, in contrast to depictions of the individual as a body and an ego, it is more useful to understand the individual as "an embodied spirit; a transpersonal transcendent evolving consciousness; unity of mindbodyspirit; person–nature–universe as oneness, connected" (Watson, 1999, p. 129). Watson therefore believed that nurses must do far more than deal with physical illness: they must attend to their primary function, which is caring. From Watson's perspective, caring infuses all aspects of a nurse's role and draws attention to nursing acts as embodying an esthetic that facilitates both healing and growth (see Chapter 19).

Each of the models just described attracts continual analysis and implementation. In some instances, nurses draw on them holistically as a coherent approach to guide all of their practices. More often, nowadays, nurses consider themselves informed by the intellectual structure that any good model provides, but typically expand their thinking beyond the limitations of a single model as their practice develops and progresses.

Theorizing in the Future

Theoretical knowledge leads us to reflect on "the basic values, guiding principles, elements, and phases of a conception of nursing" (Meleis, 2007). The goals of theoretical knowledge are to stimulate thinking and create a broad understanding of the science and practice of the nursing discipline (King & Fawcett, 1997). Although nurses today can appreciate the inherent complexity of these objectives, the creativity and vision modeled by these early theorists continue to inspire theorizing about the essence of nursing.

Nursing is solidly established as a distinct health care discipline with its own unique science. In addition, current theorists draw heavily from philosophy to resolve some of nursing's theoretical challenges. However, as Kikuchi (1999) pointed out, much of the theorizing about the purpose of nursing has confused rather than clarified thinking. As nursing scholarship evolves to include stronger philosophical and scientific inquiry, nursing practice must be conceptualized with increasing clarity (Silva et al., 1995). Nurse philosophers, as well as scientists, are continuing to use new ways of tackling nursing's most complex theoretical feature, which is applying expanding, dynamic, and multiple sources of knowledge to a diverse range of client situations. This problem of understanding the general and applying it to the particular appears in the work of many contemporary nursing scholars.

Meleis (1987), a scholar of nursing theory, challenged nurses to direct their theorizing away from the processes by which nurses use knowledge and toward the equally challenging issues associated with the substance of that knowledge. In accepting this challenge, many nursing scholars have shifted their theorizing about nursing to include both theoretical and substantive knowledge. Liaschenko (1997; Liaschenko & Fisher, 1999) oriented this theorizing into three levels of abstraction: knowing the case, knowing the client, and knowing the person. Engebretson (1997) positioned nursing theory in relation not only to biomedicine but also to Eastern and holistic understandings of health and illness. Starzomski and Rodney (1997) worked toward articulating the link between definitions of health and more philosophical notions of the greater social good. Campbell and Bunting (1991) explored the possibilities of using critical social and feminist theories for emancipatory theorizing in nursing. Watson (1990; see also Brenwick & Webster, 2000) developed the idea of embedding "caring" as a moral component into nursing theory. Yeo (1989) considered the implications of ethical reasoning for nursing theory.

The interrelationships between theory and practice are of increasing interest to nursing scholars. A dialogue representing the dynamic interaction between theorizing and clinical practice (termed **praxis**) has started to emerge (Clarke et al., 1996; Mitchell, 1995; Reed & Ground, 1997; Reed, 1995; Thorne, 1997). This newer theorizing does not seek static truths about nursing practice; rather, it creates a foundation upon which nurses can build, challenge, and integrate an infinite range of new knowledge and new ideas. As Levine (1995) wrote, "Theory is the poetry of science" (p. 14). Hence, theorizing brings familiar concepts of nursing together into bold new configurations, making disconnected aspects of human experience part of a greater whole. In so doing, it makes the discipline of nursing come alive.

✳ KEY CONCEPTS

- The hallmark of nursing practice is its unique body of knowledge and the way nurses use it.
- Nursing science has evolved in a historical and social context.
- Nursing theory represents the attempts by nursing scholars to articulate ways in which knowledge from various sources can be systematically applied in a wide variety of ways to guide professional, accountable, and defensible nursing practice.
- Much of the early theorizing about nursing practice was specifically designed to guide nursing curriculum development so that nursing education would be focused on the knowledge unique to nursing care.
- The nursing process is the fundamental problem-solving process by which new situations are assessed, plans are developed, and interventions are performed and evaluated.
- Nursing care requires the application of general knowledge to an infinite range of unique situations. Nursing process and nursing theory represent strategies to guide the process of such application.
- The major components of nursing theory, sometimes called the *metaparadigm concepts*, are person, environment, health, and nursing.
- Nurses' understanding of the role of science has changed as more complex forms of science have been articulated by philosophers of science; science is no longer limited to simple relationships such as cause and effect but instead provides strategies for understanding much more complex relationships and phenomena.
- Nursing knowledge derives from various sources in addition to science, including esthetics, personal knowing, sociocultural understanding, and ethics.

- Nursing theorists based their conceptual frameworks on various ways of thinking about human behaviour and experience; some drew their ideas from what they observed in excellent nursing practice, whereas others drew from theories of human behaviour, such as needs, interaction, or systems.
- Nursing conceptual frameworks include those for understanding both the person as the nurse's client and the nurse's role in relation to that client.
- Although each framework may have attempted to organize nursing knowledge and systematic reasoning processes in a different way, each was aiming for a very similar ideal of excellent decision making in nursing practice.
- Although nursing theoretical frameworks are no longer considered useful as prescriptive models for practice, they provide a way of conceptualizing nursing's interests and of identifying researchable nursing problems.
- As the practice of theorizing about nursing care evolves, the role of philosophy in helping nurses understand their relationship to knowledge has become increasingly relevant.

✳ CRITICAL THINKING EXERCISES

1. How do you think that different ways of conceptualizing the client might influence the kinds of decisions that nurses might make in their practice? Consider how understanding the person in terms of needs, system theory, or interaction might lead you to notice certain things and not others.

2. What sorts of gaps in information or misunderstandings might occur if nurses failed to use a systematic way of thinking about each individual client in their care?

3. How do you think that conceptual frameworks and nursing theories might be used to generate research questions for developing knowledge for evidence-informed practice?

4. Why is it useful for nurses to question how they know what they think they know?

✳ REVIEW QUESTIONS

1. A theory is a set of assumptions or propositions that is useful because it
   1. Helps people meet their self-care needs
   2. Isolates concepts
   3. Helps the nurse implement care
   4. Provides a systematic view of explaining, predicting, and prescribing phenomena

2. The drive for early theorizing about nursing practice was derived from
   1. Physicians
   2. Political leaders
   3. Nursing educators
   4. Policymakers

3. The nursing process originally involved which four basic steps?
   1. Assessment, planning, intervention, evaluation
   2. Assessment, nursing diagnosis, planning, intervention
   3. Nursing diagnosis, planning, intervention, evaluation
   4. Planning, assessment, intervention, evaluation

4. The metaparadigm concepts included
   1. The person, environment, health, and nursing
   2. The theories of Thomas Kuhn
   3. Chaos theory and games theory
   4. The grounded theory approach

5. The main question confronting early nursing theorists was about
   1. How to differentiate between nursing theories and medical theories
   2. How to reconcile the generalizations of the North American Nursing Diagnoses Association with the unique situations of each client
   3. How to organize and make sense of general nursing knowledge and apply this knowledge to an individual clinical case
   4. Whether to use theories from other disciplines such as philosophy and to apply them to nursing

6. According to Kuhn, scientific advances happen when creative individuals
   1. Approach a problem in a new way
   2. Use the cause-and-effect model to solve problems
   3. Use the work of other scientists to solve problems
   4. Use empirical evidence to solve problems

7. The McGill model
   1. Focuses on health rather than on illness or treatment
   2. Accounts for holistic aspects of the individual, rather than component parts
   3. Views the person as an energy field in constant interaction with the environment
   4. Considers the human experience to be based on behavioural drives

8. Hildegard Peplau considered the essence of nursing to be
   1. The role of the individual in health maintenance
   2. The relationship between the nurse and client
   3. Advancing nursing theories
   4. Caring

9. Theorist Evelyn Adam articulated the essence of nursing as
   1. A collaboration with health care professionals
   2. A helping process
   3. The management of clients and health care systems
   4. All of the above

10. Systems theorists considered the human being to be
    1. An irreducible whole
    2. A whole and component parts
    3. An embodiment of mind, body, and spirit
    4. All of the above

11. Parse's theory relies on
    1. A traditional definition of illness and health
    2. The idea of people engaging in a continuing process of making choices
    3. The notion of nursing as a caring profession
    4. All of the above

❋ RECOMMENDED WEB SITES

Department of Nursing, Clayton State University School of Nursing, "Nursing Theory Link Page": http://healthsci.clayton. edu/eichelberger/nursing.htm
This collection offers links to a wide range of nursing theories, including theories of nursing in general and theories about substantive fields within nursing.

Hahn School of Nursing and Health Science, University of San Diego, "The Nursing Theory Page": http://www.sandiego.edu/academics/nursing/theory/
This site orients the student to most of the major nursing theorists and resources to expand an understanding of their contributions.

7

Research as a Basis for Practice

Original chapter by Patricia A. Potter, RN, MSN, PhD, GMAC, FAAN

Canadian content written by Marilynn J. Wood, BSN, MSN, DrPH

objectives

Mastery of content in this chapter will enable you to:

- Define the key terms listed.
- Differentiate evidence-informed practice from traditional practice
- Identify methods of locating research findings
- Discuss how to implement evidence-informed practice
- Identify the various ways to acquire knowledge.
- Discuss methods for developing new nursing knowledge.
- Define nursing research.
- Discuss Canadian nursing research priorities.
- Identify ethical principles important in undertaking research.
- Explain how the rights of human research subjects are protected.
- Explain how to organize information from a research report.

key terms

Empirical data, p. 82
Ethnography, p. 84
Evidence-informed practice, p. 75
Grounded theory, p. 85
Hypothesis, p. 82
Informed consent, p. 85
Nursing research, p. 80
Phenomenology, p. 85
Qualitative nursing research, p. 84

Quantitative nursing research, p. 83
Quasi-experimental research design, p. 84
Research process, p. 82
Scientific method, p. 82
Scientific nursing research, p. 83
Subjects, p. 83
Surveys, p. 84
True experiment, p. 83

media resources

evolve Web Site

- Audio Chapter Summaries
- Glossary
- Multiple-Choice Review Questions
- Student Learning Activities
- Weblinks

Companion CD

- Glossary
- Interactive Learning Activities
- Fluids and Electrolytes Tutorial
- Test-Taking Skills

Rick has been a nurse in the emergency department for more than five years. During that time, the nurses have followed a policy of restricting the presence of family members when clients experience critical events that necessitate resuscitation. This policy allows staff to attend to the client and administer life-saving care without family interference. The nurses have assumed that the experience of watching a loved one undergoing resuscitation is too traumatic for family members. However, Rick has noticed for some time that the families of resuscitated clients experience significant stress when they are unable to stay with their loved one. Later, after the resuscitation, the families may express anger or resentment toward staff. Rick raises a question with the other nurses in the department: "What if we allowed family presence during resuscitation. What would be the outcomes for the families? Is it possible that families can benefit?"

Rick and the other emergency nurses have been practising according to what they know from their education and experience, as well as the policies and practices of their hospital. This type of practice may not be based on up-to-date information. Current evidence in the scientific literature is that family presence during resuscitation may have distinct benefits. The considerable number of studies that have been done all demontrate a positive outcome for the family. In spite of the evidence, however, health care practitioners continue to doubt the value of having families remain with the patient (Boudreaux et al., 2002; McGahey-Oakland et al., 2007). This doubt exemplifies the gap between research and practice.

Why Evidence?

Today, anyone can be an expert. The Internet opens up a world of information accessible to anyone. The public is more informed than ever before about individuals' own health and the issues facing society, as well as the types of errors that occur within health care insititutions across the country. Greater attention is paid to why certain health care approaches are used and which ones do and do not work. As a result, **evidence-informed practice** provides a safety net for nurses and other health professionals because it enables them to make accurate, timely, and appropriate clinical decisions. Evidence-informed practice is the integration of the most informative research evidence with evidence from expert clinical practice and other sources to produce the best possible care for clients.

Nursing knowledge must be expanded continuously to keep approaches to nursing care relevant and current. Without new knowledge, nursing cannot improve therapies such as infant care, pain management, grief counselling, or client education. The major source of new knowledge is research, which can provide a solid foundation for nursing practice. It is important to translate the best evidence into best practices at a client's bedside. Nurses need a sound knowledge base to support practice, and research is essential for building that knowledge.

Professional nurses must stay informed about current evidence. This is not easy to do. Students diligently read the assigned readings from texts and articles. A good textbook incorporates evidence into the practice guidelines it describes. However, it takes about two years for a book to be written, published, and in print; therefore, the scientific literature used in the book is often outdated by the time the book is published. Articles, particularly scientific ones, are more likely to be current, but the findings may not be easily applied. They may be inconclusive, or the particular practice may not have been studied yet. Moreover, these articles are not readily available to staff nurses at the bedside. It is a distinct challenge to obtain the best, most current evidence when you need it for client care.

The sources of information about evidence are well-designed, systematically conducted research studies, found in scientific journals; however, much of that evidence does not reach the bedside. Nurses currently have limited access to databases for scientific literature. When no evidence is available, tradition prevails.

Nonresearch evidence is another source of information to support practice. This includes quality improvement and risk management data; international, national, and local standards; infection control data; chart reviews; and clinical expertise. These sources can be valuable, but their value never approaches that of research evidence.

A third source of evidence that must be incorporated into good clinical decisions consists of individual clients and their values, beliefs, and experience. No efficacious clinical decision can be made without consideration of the uniqueness of the client.

Much current research focuses on ways to improve the use of new knowledge in practice. Steps to foster success are summarized in Box 7–1.

Researching the Evidence

Ask the Clinical Question

Clinical questions arise out of your practice and represent problems that you wonder about, or things that do not make sense to you. Titler et al. (2001) suggested using problem- and knowledge-focused triggers to think critically about clinical and operational nursing unit issues. A problem-focused trigger is a question you face while caring for a client or a trend you see on a nursing unit. For example, while caring for an unconscious client, you wonder, "What is the best cleaner to use when I provide mouth care to this client?" A problem-focused trend might be an increase in client falls or in the incidence of postoperative urinary tract infections. These trends lead you to ask, "How can I reduce falls on my unit?" or "What can I do to prevent urinary tract infections postoperatively?"

A knowledge-focused trigger is a question seeking new information available on a topic: for instance, "What is the current evidence to improve pain management in clients with migraine headaches?" Important sources of this type of information can be found in practice guidelines available from professional associations. All professions have focused on ensuring that service professionals understand practice guidelines. "Best practices" are guiding principles leading to the most appropriate courses of action in certain standard practice situations. They are based on the accumulated research findings, as

> ✱ BOX 7-1   STEPS FOR SUCCESSFUL EVIDENCE-INFORMED PRACTICE
>
> 1. Ask a question that clearly presents the clinical problem.
> 2. Identify and gather the most relevant and best evidence.
> 3. Critically appraise the evidence.
> 4. Integrate all evidence with clinical expertise, clients' preferences, and clients' values to make a practice decision or change.
> 5. Evaluate the outcome of the practice decision or change.
>
> From Melnyk, B. M, & Fineout-Overholt, E. (2005). *Evidence-based practice in nursing and health care. A guide to best practice.* Philadelphia: Lippincott Williams & Wilkins. Reprinted by permission of Lippincott Williams & Wilkins.

well as on evidence from practice. This sets best practices apart from the much more general nursing practice standards. Since 1999, the Ontario Ministry of Health and Long-Term Care has given substantial annual funding to the Registered Nurses Association of Ontario (RNAO) for a project to develop, vet, and disseminate "best practice guidelines" that identify actions in particular client situations. This is a multiyear project to assist nurses in providing informed and high-quality care (RNAO, 2008). These guidelines are available to all Canadian nurses (Box 7–2).

The questions you ask will eventually lead you to the evidence required for an answer. When you consult the scientific literature for an answer, you want to read the most informative four to six articles that address your practice question specifically, not be mired in hundreds of articles that might have some relationship to your question. This means that your question must be well stated and focused on just the relevant components of the issue. Unfocused questions ("What is the best way to reduce wandering?" "What is the best way to measure blood pressure?") are too vague and will lead to many irrelevant sources of information. Melnyk and Fineout-Overholt

(2005) suggested using a "PICO" format to state your question. A PICO question has four components:

P = Patient population of interest: What are the age, gender, ethnicity, and disease or health problem of the clients?

I = Intervention of interest: What is the best intervention (treatment, diagnostic test, prognostic factor)?

C = Comparison of interest: What is the usual standard of care or current intervention used now in practice?

O = Outcome: What result (e.g., change in client behavior, physical finding) do you want to achieve as a result of the intervention?

Do not be satisfied with clinical routines if they do not improve the patient's quality of life. Always question and use critical thinking to consider better ways to provide client care. The questions you raise by using a PICO format help you identify knowledge gaps within a clinical situation and assist you in making sound clinical decisions for change.

Collect the Best Evidence

Once you have a clear and concise PICO question, you are ready to search for evidence. You can find the evidence you need in a variety of sources: agency policy and procedure manuals, quality improvement data, existing clinical practice guidelines, or bibliographical databases. Always ask for help to find appropriate evidence. Nursing faculty are always a key resource, as are advanced practice nurses, staff educators, and infection control nurses.

> BOX 7-2   **Selected Nursing Best Practice Guidelines of the Registered Nurses Association of Ontario**

Adult Asthma Care Guidelines for Nurses: Promoting Control of Asthma
Assessment and Device Selection for Vascular Access
Assessment and Management of Foot Ulcers for People with Diabetes
Assessment and Management of Pain
Assessment & Management of Stage I to IV Pressure Ulcers—Revised 2007
Assessment and Management of Venous Leg Ulcers
Best Practice Guideline for the Subcutaneous Administration of Insulin in Adults with Type 2 Diabetes
Breastfeeding Best Practice Guidelines for Nurses
Care and Maintenance to Reduce Vascular Access Complications
Caregiving Strategies for Older Adults with Delirium, Dementia and Depression
Client Centred Care
Crisis Intervention
Enhancing Healthy Adolescent Development
Establishing Therapeutic Relationships
Integrating Smoking Cessation into Daily Nursing Practice
Interventions for Postpartum Depression
Nursing Care of Dyspnea: The 6th Vital Sign in Individuals with Chronic Obstructive Pulmonary Diseases (COPD)
Nursing Management of Hypertension
Prevention of Constipation in the Older Adult Population
Prevention of Falls and Fall Injuries in the Older Adult
Primary Prevention of Childhood Obesity
Promoting Asthma Control in Children
Promoting Continence Using Prompted Voiding
Reducing Foot Complications for People with Diabetes
Risk Assessment and Prevention of Pressure Ulcers
Screening for Delirium, Dementia and Depression in Older Adults
Stroke Assessment Across the Continuum of Care
Supporting and Strengthening Families Through Expected and Unexpected Life Events
Woman Abuse: Screening, Identification and Initial Response

See http://www.rnao.org/Page.asp?PageID=1110&SiteNodeID=190 for links to the abovementioned guidelines.

> BOX 7-3   **Searchable Scientific Literature Databases and Sources**

Database Sources

Cumulative Index of Nursing and Allied Health Literature (CINAHL): http://www.cinahl.com
Includes studies in nursing, allied health, and biomedicine

MEDLINE: http://medline/COS.com/
Includes studies in medicine, nursing, dentistry, psychiatry, veterinary medicine, and allied health

EMBASE: http://www.embase.com
Includes biomedical and pharmaceutical studies

PsycINFO: http://www.apa.org/psycinfo/
Contains information in psychology and related health care disciplines

Cochrane Database of Systematic Reviews: http://www.cochrane.org/reviews
Contains full text of regularly updated systematic reviews prepared by the Cochrane Collaboration; includes completed reviews and protocols

National Guideline Clearinghouse: http://www.guideline.gov
Contains structured abstracts (summaries) about clinical guidelines and their development; also includes condensed version of guideline for viewing

PubMed: http://www.nlm.nih.gov
Health science library at the US National Library of Medicine; offers free access to journal articles

OnLine Journal of Knowledge Synthesis for Nursing
Electronic journal; contains articles that provide a synthesis of research and an annotated bibliography for selected references

NurseOne Portal: http://www.nurseone.ca
Offers free access to all major databases; available to members of the Canadian Nurses Association (CNA)

When you go to the literature for evidence, a librarian can help you to locate the appropriate databases (Box 7–3). The databases contain published scientific studies, including peer-reviewed research. An article that has undergone peer review has been reviewed by a panel of experts before publication. The search process requires you to come up with key words or phrases from your PICO question that most accurately describe what you want from the search. The librarian can help you find the language that yields the most informative results. You usually need to adjust the wording of your search criteria until you get the results you want.

The best-known databases for nursing literature are MEDLINE and CINAHL. These are comprehensive databases containing articles from most nursing and health journals. These are usually available at no cost to students through the university or college library. Members of the CNA have free access to these and other databases through the NurseOne Portal (see Box 7–3).

The pyramid in Figure 7–1 represents the hierarchy of available evidence. At the top of the pyramid are systematic reviews and meta-analyses. These reviews have been conducted by experts in the clinical area, who review the evidence about a specific clinical question or issue and summarize the state of the science. Of primary importance in these reviews are the randomized controlled trials (RCTs) that have been conducted on the topic. On occasion, they include other types of research as well. Later in this chapter, the research process is examined more carefully, and you will find that the majority of nursing research is not at the level of the RCT. Nevertheless, the RCT is considered the "gold standard" in scientific research, in which the effect of a specific treatment or intervention is tested through the use of experimental and control groups. A systematic review of RCTs in which an intervention (such as computerized interactive patient teaching) is used would answer a PICO question about the effectiveness of this intervention in managing the blood glucose levels of clients with newly diagnosed diabetes.

Critique the Evidence

The most difficult step in the evidence-informed practice process probably is critiquing or analyzing the available evidence. The critiquing of evidence involves determining its value, feasibility, and utility for changing practice. When you critique evidence, first evaluate the scientific merit and clinical applicability of each study's findings. Then, with a group of studies and expert opinion, determine what findings have a strong enough basis for use in practice. After critiquing the evidence, you will be able to answer the questions, Do the articles together offer evidence to explain or answer your PICO question? Do the articles show that the evidence is true and reliable? Can you use the evidence in practice? Because you are a student and new to nursing, it will take time to acquire the skills to critique evidence like an expert. When you read an article from the literature, do not let the statistics or technical wording cause you to stop reading the article. Know the elements of an article, and use a careful approach when you review each one. Evidence-informed articles include the following elements:

- *Abstract:* An abstract is a brief summary of the article that quickly tells you whether the article is research or clinically based. An abstract summarizes the purpose of the study or clinical query, the major themes or findings, and the implications for nursing practice.
- *Introduction:* The introduction contains information about the purpose of the article and the importance of the topic for the audience who reads the article. Brief supporting evidence is usually presented as to why the topic is important from the author's point of view. Together, the abstract and introduction tell you

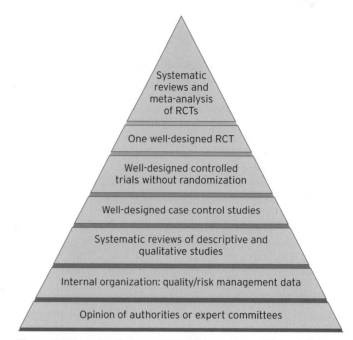

Figure 7-1 Hierarchy of evidence. RCT, randomized controlled trial. **Source:** Adapted from Guyatt, G., & Rennie, D. (2002). *User's guide to the medical literature.* Chicago: American Medical Association; and Melnyk, B. M., & Fineout-Overholt, E. (2005). *Evidence-based practice in nursing and healthcare: A guide to best practice.* Philadelphia: Lippincott Williams & Wilkins.

whether you want to read the entire article. You will know if the topic of the article is similar to your PICO question or related closely enough to provide you with useful information. Continue to read the next elements of the article:

- *Literature review or background:* A useful article has a detailed background of the existing level of science or clinical information about the topic of the article. Therefore, it offers an argument about what led the author to conduct a study or report on a clinical topic. This section of an article is valuable. Perhaps the article itself does not address your PICO question in the way you desire, but it may lead you to other articles that are more useful. A literature review of a research article indicates how past research led to the researcher's question. For example, an article about a study designed to test an educational intervention for older adult family caregivers reviews literature that describes characteristics of caregivers, the type of factors influencing caregivers' ability to cope with stressors of caregiving, and any previous educational interventions used with families.
- *Manuscript narrative:* "Middle sections," or narratives, of articles differ according to the type of evidence-informed article they are (Melnyk & Fineout-Overholt, 2005). A clinical article describes a clinical topic and often includes a description of a client population, the nature of a certain disease or health alteration, how clients are affected, and the appropriate nursing therapies. Some clinical articles explain how to use a therapy or new technology. A research article will contain several subsections within the narrative, including the following:
  - *Purpose statement:* A purpose statement explains the focus or intent of a study. It identifies what concepts were researched. This includes research questions or hypotheses: predictions made about the relationship or difference between study variables (concepts, characteristics, or traits that vary within subjects). An example of a research question is as follows: "What

characteristics are common among older adults who have annual breast screening?"

- *Methods or design:* The methods or design section explains how a research study is organized and conducted in order to answer the research question or to test the hypothesis. This explanation includes the type of study to be conducted (e.g., RCT, case control study, or qualitative study) and how many subjects or persons are in a study. In health care studies, "subjects" may include clients, family members, or health care staff. The language in the methods section is sometimes confusing because it contains details about how the researcher designs the study to minimize bias so as to obtain the most accurate results possible. Use your faculty member as a resource to help interpret this section.
- *Results or conclusions:* Clinical and research articles have a summary section. A clinical article explains the clinical implications for the topic presented, whereas a research article details the results of the study and explains whether a hypothesis is supported or how a research question is answered. If the study is quantitative, this section includes a statistical analysis . For a qualitative study, the article presents a thorough summary of the descriptive themes and ideas that arise from the researcher's analysis of data. Do not be stumped by the statistical analysis in an article. Read carefully, and ask whether the researcher describes the results and whether the results were significant. Have a faculty member assist you in interpreting statistical results. A helpful results section also discusses any limitations to a study. This information on limitations is valuable in helping you decide whether you want to use the evidence with your clients.
- *Clinical implications.* A research article includes a section that explains whether the findings from the study have clinical implications. This section also explains how to apply findings in a practice setting for the type of subjects studied. After you have critiqued each article for your PICO question, synthesize or combine the findings from all of the articles to determine the state of the evidence. Use critical thinking to consider the scientific rigor of the evidence and how well it answers your area of interest. Consider the evidence in view of your clients' concerns and preferences. Your review of articles offers a snapshot conclusion that is based on combined evidence about one focused topical area. As a clinician, judge whether to use the evidence for a particular client or group of clients, who usually have complex medical histories and patterns of responses (Melnyk & Fineout-Overholt, 2005). It is ethically important to consider evidence that benefits clients and does no harm. Decide whether the evidence is relevant, is easily applicable in your setting of practice, and has the potential for improving client outcomes.

Integrate the Evidence

Once you decide that the evidence is strong and applicable to your clients and clinical situation, incorporate the recommended evidence into practice. Your first step is to simply apply the research in your plan of care for a client. Use the evidence you find as a rationale for an intervention you plan to try. For instance, you learned about an approach for bathing older adults who are restless, and you decide to use the technique during your next clinical assignment. You use the bathing technique with your own assigned clients, or you work with a group of other students or nurses in revising a policy and procedure or in developing a new clinical protocol. In another example, after being concerned about the rate of intravenous catheter dislodgement, you consult the evidence to compare the efficacy of gauze dressings with that of transparent dressings. The literature suggests that fewer catheter dislodgements occur with transparent dressings

on peripheral intravenous sites than with gauze dressings, with no increase in phlebitis or infiltration rates (Melnyk & Fineout-Overholt, 2005; Tripepi-Bova et al., 1997). As a result of your findings, you meet with the policy and procedure committee of your institution to recommend the use of transparent dressings routinely. You then implement the use of transparent dressings in the routine care of peripheral intravenous catheters.

Evidence is useful in a variety of ways in formulating teaching tools, clinical practice guidelines, policies and procedures, and new assessment or documentation tools. Depending on the amount of change needed to apply evidence in practice, it becomes necessary to involve a number of staff from a given nursing unit. It is important to consider the setting in which you want to apply the evidence: Do all staff members support the change? Does the practice change fit with the scope of practice in the clinical setting? Are resources (time, administrative support, and staff) available to make a change? When evidence is not strong enough to apply in practice, your next option is to conduct a pilot study to investigate your PICO question. A pilot study is a small-scale research study or a study that includes a quality or performance improvement project. As a nursing student integrating evidence, your study begins with searching for and applying the most useful evidence to improve the care you provide directly to your clients. The evidence available within nursing literature gives you an almost unlimited access to innovative and effective nursing interventions. Using an evidence-informed practice approach helps you improve your skills and knowledge as a nurse and improve outcomes for your clients.

Evaluate the Practice Decision or Change

After applying evidence in your practice, your next step is to evaluate its effect. How does the intervention work? How effective was the clinical decision for your client or practice setting? Sometimes your evaluation is as simple as determining whether the expected outcomes you set for an intervention are met. For example, after the use of a transparent intravenous dressing, does the catheter dislodge, or does the complication of phlebitis develop? When you use a new approach to preoperative teaching, does the client learn what to expect after surgery?

When an evidence-informed practice change occurs on a larger scale, an evaluation is more formal. For example, evidence of factors that contribute to pressure ulcers might lead a nursing unit to adopt a new skin care protocol. To evaluate the protocol, the nurses track the incidence of pressure ulcers over a course of time (e.g., six months to a year). In addition, the nurses collect data to describe both the clients who develop ulcers and those who do not. This comparative information is valuable for determining the effects of the protocol and whether modifications are necessary.

Support for Evidence-Informed Practice

Nursing practice is based on theory, professional values, and evidence. Nurses base decisions on these factors, as well on other influences such as individual values, ethics, legislation, client choice, and practice environments. The CNA recommends evidence-informed decision making as an essential component of providing quality nursing care that optimizes the outcomes for patients. The evidence to be used in practice is derived through scientific evaluation of practice. Types of evidence include experimental studies of nursing interventions, meta-analysis of groups of studies on a particular topic, nonexperimental or observational studies, expert opinion through consensus documents, and historical information (CNA, 2002).

Knowledge Development in Nursing

Knowledge that provides the rationale for nursing practice is organized in a variety of ways. In her classic article on patterns of knowing in nursing, Carper (1978) identified four patterns: "empirics," or the science of nursing; esthetics, or the art of nursing; personal knowing; and ethics, or the moral component. A fifth type of knowing, emancipatory knowing, was later added by Chinn and Kramer (2008) (Table 7–1). These different types of knowledge focus on the meaning and value of nursing expertise. With evidence-informed practice, the evidence can be derived from any of these sources of knowledge.

Empirics: The Science of Nursing

Carper (1978) described empirics as "knowledge that is systematically organized into general laws and theories for the purpose of describing, explaining and predicting phenomena of special concern to the discipline of nursing" (p. 14). This pattern of knowing implies an objective reality; by studying this, you can interpret the meaning of particular phenomena and develop understandings of other similar phenomena. Fundamental to this model is the rational stance in which you can generalize from a sample to a population. The theoretical or conceptual models and frameworks help explain particular phenomena in health and illness and identify important questions for nursing research. The goal of scientific research is to produce this type of knowledge.

Esthetics: The Art of Nursing

Nursing incorporates an artistic, expressive component, which involves knowledge and understanding. As Carper (1978) noted, "The art of nursing involves the active transformation of the patient's behavior into a perception of what is significant in it—that is, what need is being expressed by the behavior" (p. 17). She further stated that perception is beyond mere recognition and, as such, moves nursing activities into the esthetic realm. Qualitative research often explores this area.

Personal Knowledge

This pattern of knowing can be the most difficult to understand and to teach. The nature of the relationship formed with the client and the depth and quality of the interpersonal experience are fundamental to the realm of personal knowledge. As Carper (1978) stated, "Personal knowledge is concerned with the knowing, encountering and actualizing of the concrete, individual self" (p. 18). Many investigators have attempted to understand the nature of therapeutic relationships. Through the rapport established with the client, how does a nurse succeed in assisting that client to reach health goals? Perhaps "the nurse in the therapeutic use of self rejects approaching the patient–client as an object and strives instead to actualize an authentic personal relationship between two persons" (Carper, 1978, p. 19). The knowledge gleaned from experience belongs to this pattern.

Ethics: The Moral Component

Nurses are faced with ethical questions that centre on what ought to be done in particular situations. Ethics goes beyond ethical theories, principles, and codes of professional conduct to include dilemmas such as choosing the better of two or more somewhat unsatisfactory actions. Now that technology can prolong life, ethical dilemmas have become more frequent and complex. As Carper (1978) stated, "The ethical pattern of knowing in nursing requires an understanding of different philosophical positions regarding what is good, what ought to be desired, and what is right; of different ethical frameworks devised for dealing with the complexities of moral judgements; and of various orientations to the notion of obligation" (p. 21).

Emancipatory Knowing: The Social, Economic, and Political Component

Emancipatory knowing makes it possible to create social and structural change (Chinn & Kramer, 2008). It represents the ability to recognize social and political problems of injustice or inequity, to picture how things could be different, and to figure out how to change a difficult situation into one that improves the lives of people. Nurses have dealt with emancipatory knowledge since the nineteenth century, when Florence Nightingale wrote passionately about the inequities in society affecting women. As described by Chinn and Kramer, "Emancipatory knowing is the capacity not only to notice injustices in a social order, but also to critically examine why injustices seem not to be noticed or remain invisible, and to identify social and structural changes that are required to right social and institutional wrongs" (p. 78).

> **TABLE 7-1** **Fundamental Patterns of Knowing in Nursing**

Empirics: the science of knowledge development in nursing	Knowledge developed through systematic research to describe and explain phenomena
Esthetics: the art of nursing	Creativity, with an artistic or expressive component
Personal knowledge	Knowledge derived from the depth and power of the interpersonal relationship with the client
Ethics: the moral component	Knowledge that emerges from ethical dilemmas and is based on what ought to be done in particular situations
Emancipatory knowing: the social, economic, and political component	Knowledge that allows change to occur

From Carper, B. A. (1978). Fundamental patterns of knowing in nursing. *Advances in Nursing Science, 1*(1), 13; and Chinn, P., & Kramer, M. (2008). Integrated theory and knowledge development in nursing (p. 78). St. Louis, MO: Mosby/Elsevier.

Nurses benefit from all these ways of knowing. According to the concept of evidence-informed practice, evidence gained from any and all of these means guides nurses to make sound clinical decisions. The knowledge gained from empirics is but one pattern of knowledge, but with it, you can build strength and confidence as you pursue research into nursing questions.

The Development of Research in Nursing

Research is the primary means by which new knowledge is discovered and brought into practice to improve the care that nurses provide to their clients. It is a systematic process in which questions that generate knowledge are asked and answered. This knowledge becomes part of the scientific basis for practice and may be used to validate interventions.

Nursing research is a systematic examination of phenomena important to the nursing discipline, as well as to nurses, their clients, and families. Its purpose is to expand the knowledge base for practice by answering nurses' questions. Nursing research addresses a range of issues related to actual and potential client populations and to individual and family responses to health problems. Some research tests nursing theories; other research generates theory from findings. This "back-and-forth" relationship between theory and research is the way knowledge develops in any discipline (Wood & Ross-Kerr, 2006). In the current health care environment, nursing research is frequently undertaken in multidisciplinary teams, in which nurses examine factors relevant to nursing in the context of the larger health care picture. The scientific knowledge needed for nursing practice is discovered, tested, and enhanced through nursing research. The multidisciplinary nature of nursing challenges nurses not only to keep up with nursing research but also to know the status of research in other health disciplines, as well as in the behavioural, social, and physical sciences.

The International Council of Nurses (ICN; 2007) is a staunch supporter of nursing research as a means to improve people's health and welfare. Research is a way to identify new knowledge, improve education and practice, and use resources effectively. In 1983, the National Center for Nursing Research in the United States and the ICN established priorities for nursing research. These priorities were to promote the in-depth knowledge base for nursing practice, to recognize nursing research as an integral part of nursing practice and education, to facilitate cross-cultural research, to ensure adequate preparation of nurse researchers, and to encourage all national nursing associations to establish ethical research standards (National Center for Nursing Research/ICN, 1990). These priorities are updated regularly. In 1999, the ICN established the ICN Research Network. The Network provides a means for sharing of research ideas, results, and progress around the world. Network members communicate with one another through the ICN Web site, as well as at annual conferences.

In 1995, the CNA, the Canadian Association of Schools of Nursing, and the Canadian Association for Nursing Research developed research priorities. These priorities identified the need to expand the knowledge base for nursing practice in Canada, including the study of contextual issues such as the social, political, and environmental predictors of health; specific clinical populations; and a range of interventions from health promotion strategies to specific clinical measures (Canadian Association of Schools of Nursing, 1997) (Box 7–4).

> **BOX 7-4**   **Canadian Nursing Research Priorities**

Priority 1: Nursing Practice

- Context (including determinants of health, health reform, and ethical issues)
- Populations (vulnerable groups, as well as specific clinical populations)
- Interventions (wide range, from health promotion to comfort measures)

Priority 2: Outcomes

- Development of valid measures for multiple dimensions
- Links with clinical judgement

Priority 3: Enhanced Links Between Research and Practice

- Development of body of nursing knowledge

Data from Canadian Association of Schools of Nursing. (1997). *Canadian nursing research priorities, results of Phase III of National Nursing Research Symposium.* Ottawa ON: Author. Retrieved November, 2008, from http://www.CAUSN.ca/Research/research.htm

---

Nursing research improves nursing practice, raising the profession's standards. Involvement in research takes many forms, including designing studies, being on a research team, collecting data, and using research findings to change clinical practice, improve client outcomes, and contain health care costs (Titler et al., 2001). Promoting research and using it in practice increases the scientific knowledge base for nursing practice. Clients benefit from these improvements to practice.

The History of Nursing Research in Canada

During the Crimean War, Florence Nightingale's detailed and systematic observation of nursing actions and outcomes resulted in major changes in nursing practice (Box 7–5). Her work demonstrated the importance of systematic observational research to nursing practice.

In Canada, the establishment of university nursing courses starting in 1918, followed by master's degree programs in the 1950s and 1970s and by doctoral programs in the 1990s and 2000s, was key to the development of nursing research. The first master's degree program, established at the University of Western Ontario in 1959, highlighted the need for Canadian research capacity in nursing.

The first nursing research journal, *Nursing Research*, was launched in the United States in 1952. The first nursing research journal published in Canada, *Nursing Papers* (later the *Canadian Journal of Nursing Research*), was established at McGill University in 1969. Other journals were later established, and today, nurses publish their research, both within nursing and in interdisciplinary fields, in dozens of journals.

Since the 1970s and 1980s, the two major factors in the development of nursing research have been the establishment of research training through doctoral programs and the establishment of funding to support nursing research. Throughout the 1970s and 1980s, university faculties and schools of nursing built their research resources so that they could establish doctoral programs. The first provincially

> **BOX 7-5** **Historical Milestones in the Development of Canadian Nursing Research**

1858	Florence Nightingale published *Notes on Matters Affecting the Health, Efficiency and Hospital Administration of the British Army* and *Notes on Hospitals.*
1918	The University of British Columbia launched the first baccalaureate nursing program in Canada.
1952	The American Nurses Association first published the journal *Nursing Research.*
1959	First Canadian Nursing master's degree program was launched at the University of Western Ontario.
1964–1965	The first nursing research project was funded by a Canadian federal granting agency; the *International Journal of Nursing Studies* and *International Nursing Index* were launched.
1969–1970	*Nursing Papers,* forerunner of the *Canadian Journal of Nursing Research,* was published at McGill University; Lysaught's (1970) report, *An Abstract for Action,* recommending increased research in education and practice, was published.
1971	McGill University launched Centre for Nursing Research; first national Canadian conference was held on nursing research; both were financed by the Department of National Health and Welfare.
1975	Commission on Canadian Studies noted that the slow start of graduate programs in Canada, and inadequate funding, resulted in few studies in nursing.
1978	Heads of university nursing schools and deans of graduate studies attended the Kellogg National Seminar on Doctoral Education in Nursing.
1982	The Alberta Foundation for Nursing Research, first funding agency for nursing research, was established; the Working Group on Nursing Research was established by the Medical Research Council (MRC).

1985	Report of the Working Group on Nursing Research was released by the MRC.
1988	The MRC and the National Health Research and Development Program established a joint initiative to structure nursing research grants.
1990	Francine Ducharme was the first nurse to graduate with a PhD in nursing from a Canadian university, through a special case program at McGill University.
1991	First Canadian nursing PhD program was launched at University of Alberta, followed by one at University of British Columbia
1992–1994	PhD programs in nursing were launched at McGill University, University of Toronto, and McMaster University
1992	The MRC mandate was revised to include health research.
1999	The Nursing Research Fund was launched with a $25 million grant over 10 years; the Canadian Health Services Research Foundation administered the funds. PhD program in nursing was launched at the University of Calgary.
2003–2008	PhD programs in nursing were initiated at Dalhousie University, the University of Victoria, the University of Western Ontario, the University of Ottawa, l'Université Laval, and l'Université de Sherbrooke.
2004	Forum on doctoral education held in Toronto under the auspices of Canadian Association of Schools of Nursing to develop a national position paper on the PhD in nursing for Canada.

approved doctoral nursing program was established at the University of Alberta Faculty of Nursing in 1991. Another was established at the University of British Columbia School of Nursing later that year, and programs at McGill University and the University of Toronto followed in 1993. Between 1993 and 2008, other programs were launched, which brought the total across Canada to 12.

Growing awareness of the importance of nursing research gradually led to the availability of research funds. The year 1964 marked the first time that a federal granting agency funded nursing research in Canada (Good, 1969). In 1999, 14 years after the US government had established funding for nursing research under the National Institutes of Health, the Canadian government established the Nursing Research Fund, budgeting $25 million for nursing research ($2.5 million over each of the following 10 years); the funds were to be administered by the Canadian Health Services Research Foundation. The research areas targeted for support included nursing policies, management, human resources, and nursing care. A total of $500,000 each year is designated for the Open Grants Competition, $500,000 to the Canadian Nurses Foundation for research on nursing care, $750,000 for training (postdoctoral fellowships and student grants), and $250,000 for knowledge networks and dissemination activities. Five chairs in nursing research, representing excellence in nursing research across Canada, were funded by this initiative. The incumbents were to develop research capacity in a particular area of nursing:

- Dr. Lesley Degner, University of Manitoba: Development of Innovative Nursing Interventions to Influence Practice and Policy in Cancer Care, Palliative Care, and Cancer Prevention
- Dr. Alba Dicenso, McMaster University: Evaluation of Nurse Practitioner/Advanced Practice Nurse Roles and Interventions
- Dr. Nancy Edwards, University of Ottawa: Multiple Interventions in Community Health Nursing Care
- Dr. Janice Lander, University of Alberta: Evaluating Innovative Approaches to Nursing Care
- Dr. Linda O'Brien-Pallas, University of Toronto: Nursing Human Resources for the New Millennium

More information about these five chairs is available at http://www.chsrf.ca/cadre/chair_awards_lca_e.php.

Nursing research has focused progressively on evidence-informed practice in response to demands to justify care practices and systems by improving client outcomes and controlling costs. The scope of nursing research has also broadened to include historical and philosophical inquiry. The establishment of the Institute for Philosophical Nursing Research at the University of Alberta and the Nursing History Research Unit at the University of Ottawa exemplify this new direction.

Three new training centres funded by the Nursing Research Fund at the Canadian Health Services Research Foundation were mandated in order to increase research capacity in nursing and related disciplines:

- The Centre FERASI (http://www.ferasi.umontreal.ca) in Quebec is a joint initiative among l'Université de Montréal, McGill University, and l'Université Laval to build research capacity in the administration of nursing services. It focuses on developing partnerships with health care decision makers in order to provide training opportunities and insights into the decision-making environment. Funding is provided for student scholarships.
- The Ontario Training Centre in Health Services and Policy Research (http://www.otc-hsr.ca) involves six Ontario universities for the purpose of enhancing health services and policy research. The centre is located at McMaster University and involves collaboration with the University of Toronto, York University, the University of Ottawa, Laurentian University, and Lakehead University.
- The Centre for Knowledge Transfer was designed as a national training centre at the University of Alberta providing funding for students and offering courses in knowledge utilization and transfer. This centre is now closed.

Nursing Research

In a mature discipline, practitioners use multiple research methods to develop a unique knowledge base (Wood and Ross-Kerr, 2006). A person continuously acquires knowledge, using critical thinking to interpret and evaluate complex information. Current research can be classified into one of two ways of thinking: scientific or qualitative (interpretive). Both have a great deal to offer when you are seeking evidence to support your practice.

The Scientific Paradigm

The term *paradigm* was introduced by Kuhn (1970) and can be loosely defined as a way of thinking (see Chapter 6). According to Kuhn, a dominant research paradigm can be identified during any one era. Eventually, this paradigm no longer provides solutions to research problems and is challenged by new ideas. It is then replaced by a new paradigm, and the process continues. The dominant paradigm for most of the nineteenth and twentieth centuries has been positivism. Positivism emphasizes tested and systematized experience, rather than speculation, and focuses on the search for cause-and-effect relationships to explain phenomena. In this paradigm, the **scientific method** arose as the major research approach.

Researchers who use the scientific method pose research questions and collect and analyze data to find answers to the questions. The process is rigorous and systematic and is guided by scientific principles, the most important of which is empiricism, which means that only things that can be observed by the human senses can be called *facts*. The focus is on deductive reasoning, in which a **hypothesis** is tested experimentally to confirm or reject theoretical explanations of phenomena.

The scientific method is characterized by systematic, orderly procedures that, although not without fault, are intended to limit the possibility of error and minimize the likelihood that any bias or opinion by the researcher might influence the results of research and, thus, the knowledge gained. Wood and Ross-Kerr (2006) described the **research process** as follows: The process begins with a researchable question. If properly stated, the question guides the rest of the process; thus, asking the question is a crucial step. Three levels of questions exist, and the appropriate level is chosen based on how much is known about the research topic. Once an initial question has been formulated, the literature is searched to discover what is already known about the topic and to determine whether the question must be revised in light of prior knowledge. The level of the question determines the research design needed to answer it. Table 7–2 describes the basic steps in planning nursing research.

The research design provides the ground rules for data collection and analysis, ensuring that the research question will have a valid answer. The design steps are systematic and precise in order to control unwanted influences that might affect the answer. For example, in a study of the relationship between diet and heart disease, influences such as stress or smoking must be controlled because they are known to influence heart disease. The design also specifies the type of sample and sample selection techniques that will provide the most useful data for the study.

Evidence that is part of experience (**empirical data**) is gathered from the sample through measurement techniques that quantify the variables in the research question. Techniques include interviews, tests of knowledge, and physiological measures such as heart rate and blood pressure. When the evidence is analyzed, the result answers the original question and becomes the basis for discovering new knowledge.

A goal of scientific research is to understand phenomena so that the knowledge gained can be applied generally, not just to isolated cases. Researchers achieve this goal by studying a sample that represents a larger population; this increases the likelihood that the results will apply across that population. In the scientific paradigm, researchers conduct studies that contribute to the testing or development of theories, thereby advancing knowledge that can be applied in nursing practice.

The Qualitative (Interpretive) Paradigm

Positivism has been criticized by those academics who believe that reality and people's perception of reality are so intertwined that they cannot be separated. Interpretivism is an alternative to positivism, representing the view that people construct their own world as they strive to make sense of their social environments (Speziale & Carpenter, 2006). The research that is driven by interpretivism can be broadly designated *qualitative research*. Qualitative research avoids the empirical notion of the study of people as objects and strives instead to understand human behaviour in the context of the people being studied. A qualitative researcher studies the behaviours, experiences, perceptions, and motives of individuals in social and cultural settings (Speziale & Carpenter, 2006).

Several approaches to qualitative research exist, and each is very different from the others. Unlike the scientific approach, many qualitative approaches have their own unique philosophic base, which makes comparisons difficult. Speziale and Carpenter (2006, p. 21) identified the following six characteristics common to all qualitative research:

- Belief in multiple realities.
- Commitment to identifying an approach to understanding that will support the phenomenon studied.
- Commitment to the participant's point of view.
- Conduct of inquiry in a way that does not disturb the natural context of the phenomena of interest.
- Acknowledged participation of the researcher in the research.
- Conveyance of the understanding of phenomena by reporting in a literary style rich with participants' commentary.

The idea of multiple realities is a challenge to positivist thinking, which proposes that researchers are searching for one reality or truth. Interpretivists say that because the experience of each individual is unique, each individual can come to know the world differently, which implies that many truths exist, rather than one. This

> **TABLE 7-2**   **Basic Steps in Planning Nursing Research**

Steps	Level I	Level II	Level III
Question	What?	What is the relationship?	Why?
Problem	Little known about topic	Conceptual base; variables have been studied before	Theoretical base
Purpose	Declarative statement	Question or hypothesis	Hypothesis
Design	Exploratory descriptive	Descriptive survey, correlational or comparative	Experiment
Sample	Convenience sample or total population	Probability sample	Random assignment to treatment and control groups
Methods	Qualitative, unstructured data; some quantitative descriptive data	Quantitative data collected by all methods	Quantitative data
Analysis	Content analysis; descriptive statistic	Correlation or tests of association; regression analysis	Differences between means: t test, analysis of variance (ANOVA)
Answer	Description of processes, concepts, or population	Explanation of relationship among variables	Test of theory

Adapted from Wood, M., & Ross-Kerr, J. (2006). *Basic steps in planning nursing research: From question to proposal.* Sudbury, MA: Jones & Bartlett. Copyright © 2006: Jones & Bartlett. Reprinted with permission.

belief leads qualitative researchers to seek multiple ways of understanding the world and to change methods and data collection strategies as needed, rather than following a single prescribed set of strategies. It follows that the participant's point of view would be the focus of the research and would guide the process. The researcher becomes a coparticipant in the process of understanding the participant's point of view.

Qualitative research is carried out in the participants' natural setting to maintain a natural context. The researcher is a participant and acknowledges that being a participant will affect the other participants and the setting. Objectivity is not a goal in qualitative research; rather, subjectivity from the participants' perspective is sought. Because of the nature of the data, rich with personal experience and example, the research is usually reported in a literary style, similar to storytelling. Liberal quotation from the participants adds to the detail of the report.

Research Designs

Nursing research approaches vary, depending on the specific problem to be studied. The paradigms of positivism and interpretivism lead to two research approaches, often categorized as quantitative (scientific method) and qualitative (interpretive). Neither is used exclusively in nursing research, although the scientific method is dominant. Nonetheless, interpretivism and qualitative methods have much to offer nursing research. The next section describes some common research designs in these two categories.

Scientific Nursing Research

Scientific nursing research (**quantitative nursing research**) is the investigation of nursing phenomena that can be precisely measured and quantified. Examples are pain severity, rates of wound healing,

and body temperature changes. These designs fall within the scientific paradigm and provide rigorous, systematic, objective examination of specific concepts and their relationships. The goal is to test theory and use numerical data, statistical analysis, and controls to eliminate bias (Polit & Beck, 2004; Wood & Ross-Kerr, 2006).

Experimental Research. Experimental design is the hallmark of scientific research. Experiments are appropriate designs for questions at level III (see Table 7–2), which concern why one variable causes a predictable change in another variable. In a **true experiment**, the conditions under which the variables are studied are tightly controlled to provide objective testing of hypotheses, which predict cause-and-effect relationships. Experimental research requires that the data be collected and quantified in a prescribed manner.

The requirements of a true experiment are as follows:

- The study usually includes at least one control or comparison group, which does not receive the nursing treatment or intervention being investigated. The results for this group are compared with those of the experimental group, which is the group that receives the treatment or intervention. The **subjects**—people selected for the comparison and experimental groups—are randomly assigned to these groups, so that the groups are as similar as possible to each other before the intervention. Random assignment of subjects ensures that all subjects have the same chance to be in the control or experimental (treatment) group and that variables that could affect the outcome of the study are randomly distributed between the groups and therefore are no more likely to affect experimental subjects than to affect control subjects.

- An experimental variable must be manipulated by the researcher. For example, in a study of the effect of preoperative teaching on postoperative anxiety, the researcher manipulates preoperative teaching by providing it for the experimental group but not for the control group. The expectation is that the differences in post-operative anxiety measures between the two groups can be attributed to the effect of preoperative teaching because all other factors are under control. However, the researcher cannot control subjects' prior experiences, such as hearing other clients' stories about surgery. Psychological factors, which cannot be controlled, may influence a subject's level of anxiety. If subjects are randomly assigned to the two groups, however, those with negative prior experiences should be distributed equally between the two groups, and these experiences would affect both groups equally. Thus, differences between the groups in postoperative anxiety can still be attributed to the preoperative teaching intervention.

- The researcher proposes theory-based and statistically tested hypotheses about the action of the variables to answer the research question. For example, in a study of preoperative teaching, the hypothesis might be as follows: "Clients who receive interactive preoperative teaching will have significantly lower postoperative anxiety levels than will clients who receive other teaching methods." The researcher must explain why a lower anxiety level is expected in a discussion of the theory behind the study.

A **quasi-experimental research design** is one in which groups are formed and the conditions are controlled, but the subjects are not randomly assigned to a control group or to treatment conditions. These designs also answer level III questions (Wood & Ross-Kerr, 2006). In many health care settings, assigning subjects randomly to experimental and control groups is not feasible. Quasi-experimental research is often carried out for practical reasons related to the subjects themselves. For example, to test the effect of a new intervention in the care of clients with Alzheimer's disease, carrying out two treatments on the unit at the same time might confuse the subjects. A quasi-experiment could entail the use of two care units: one as the experimental unit, in which all subjects receive the new intervention, and the second as the control group, in which subjects receive the usual care but not the new intervention. The two groups are compared before and after the intervention with regard to the outcome variable. The weakness in a quasi-experiment is that the researcher does not know whether the two groups were equivalent before the intervention. Unrecognized differences between the two units might exist that could influence the outcome of the study. For instance, subjects in one unit might have more cognitive impairment than do those in the other unit, and this difference could influence the outcome.

Descriptive Survey Designs.

Surveys are designed to answer level II questions about relationships among variables. The research question that leads to a survey design begins with "What is the relationship between . . . ?" and addresses two or more variables (Wood and Ross–Kerr, 2006): for example, the relationship between ethnicity and suicide among university students.

In many types of research, investigators use surveys in which people in a group are compared with regard to two or more variables. The purpose is to discover relationships among variables in the population. In a survey design, the sample determines whether the survey yields informative or uninformative results. The sample should be representative of the population so that generalizations can be made on the basis of the sample data. Surveys contain three key elements: First, a random sample of the population must be drawn, from which inferences can be made about the population. Second, the population sampled should be large enough to keep sampling error to a minimum. Third, the measurement tools (e.g., questionnaires, interviews) must yield accurate measurements of the study variables.

Exploratory Descriptive Designs.

Exploratory descriptive designs provide in-depth descriptions of populations or variables not previously studied. Level I (basic) questions are asked because not much is known about the topic. They typically begin with "what"; for example, "What are the health-promoting behaviours of older adults living in subsidized housing?" The results provide a detailed description of the variable or population. No relationships among variables are posited at this stage, although the results might indicate that relationships should be examined in subsequent research.

Data Analysis.

Except for some exploratory descriptive studies in which the outcome is a verbal description, all quantitative studies entail the use of statistical analysis. In experimental designs, researchers must discover whether the experimental and control groups are significantly different from each other after the intervention has been applied. Statistical tests that provide a test of group means are generally used for experiments.

Descriptive survey designs entail the use of statistical techniques to test for significant relationships among the variables. In general, these are correlational tests that indicate whether one subject's score on one variable (e.g., blood pressure) is related to the same subject's score on another variable (e.g., weight). The results of a correlational analysis of these two variables would reveal how much influence increased body weight has on blood pressure.

Exploratory descriptive studies entail the use of several techniques to analyze data, depending on the type collected. Unstructured data that do not lend themselves to numerical form are summarized verbally. If quantitative measures are used to collect the data, they can be described both numerically and verbally. Descriptions usually include measures of central tendency (mean, median, or mode) and dispersion (range, standard deviation).

Qualitative Nursing Research

Qualitative nursing research poses questions about nursing phenomena that cannot be quantified and measured. Examples are the study of the experience of pregnancy and the culture of a long-term care facility. To answer questions about these phenomena, researchers must understand the perspective of the person in the situation. Researchers using qualitative methods can choose one of many design strategies. Examples of three qualitative designs (ethnography, phenomenology, and grounded theory) are discussed in the following sections, but keep in mind that many other qualitative approaches, such as participatory action research, interpretive descriptive research, and narrative inquiry, are used in nursing research. As with scientific research, the research question is the basis for the choice of design. In addition, each of the various qualitative methods has its own unique underlying philosophy. Ethnography is chosen if the research question leads to the study of behaviour within a specific group or culture, phenomenology if the question relates to the lived experience of the participants, and grounded theory if the question is about a social process.

Ethnography.

Ethnography involves the observation and description of behaviour in social settings. It is derived from anthropology, and it provides the means to study the culture of groups of people. Anthropologists use participant observation as the major source of data collection, together with other sources such as artifacts and photographs. Nurse researchers use ethnography to study the behaviour of nurses and their clients in a variety of settings. The goal of ethnography is to understand the culture of the study population as the culture is practised in its own setting. The focus is on the cultural norms and social forces that shape behaviour in a given setting. The researcher becomes an accepted member of the community under study and collects data through repeated interviews of informants from the community. Data collection continues until understanding has been reached about why the members of the community behave as they do. Interview data are supplemented by other forms, such as artifacts and historical documents; the result is a detailed description of the culture. For example, Lauzon Clabo (2008) examined nursing pain assessment practice across two units, to seek variation that might exist and to examine the impact of the social context on pain assessment practice. The ethnographic analysis revealed a predominant pattern of pain assessment on each unit that was profoundly shaped by the social context of the unit.

Phenomenology. The focus of **phenomenology** is on the lived experience of a specific phenomenon from the perspective of the people who are in the situation. Phenomenology has its roots in German philosophy of the early twentieth century, stemming from the philosopher Edmund Husserl (1931/1962), who posited that only people who experience phenomena are capable of communicating these experiences. The researcher must learn to understand a phenomenon from the viewpoint of people experiencing it. For example, an investigator may want to study the impact of surrogate decision making regarding end-of-life decisions (Jeffers, 1998). The goal of this research is to describe fully the lived experience of surrogate decision makers, their perceptions of the surrogate role, the decision-making process, and the meaning of the decisions. The source of the data is the subject, and the data are the result of in-depth conversations. The units of analysis are the conversations, which are coded and analyzed to extract the meaning to the subjects of the phenomenon.

Grounded Theory. **Grounded theory** as a research method was developed by Glaser and Strauss (1967) as a means of generating hypotheses and theories about social processes inductively from the data. The grounded theory is "discovered," developed, and verified through a rigorous process of data collection and analysis. Glaser and Strauss advocated that researchers not review the literature before carrying out the study because they might be influenced by what others have found. The strength of the grounded theory approach comes from examining the situation afresh and opening up the possibility of a new perspective on an old problem.

For example, Mills et al. (2007) studied mentoring among rural nurses in the Australian workforce by using a grounded theory approach. The social process that was identified in this study was called "Live my work," stemming from the mentors' own histories of living and working in the same community. Personal strategies adapted to local context were the skills that these mentors passed on to neophyte nurses in rural areas through mentoring, which at the same time protected them through troubleshooting and translating local cultural norms.

Conducting Nursing Research

Nurses conduct research in a variety of settings. Student nurses and practitioners participate in investigations of client outcomes and nursing care, commonly called *quality assurance* or *improvement studies* (see Chapter 11). Data are collected to determine the influence of nurses on achievement of client care objectives in a particular clinical setting. Because the results usually apply only to one facility, this research is not scientific. However, it is important to the facility involved because the study can demonstrate the contributions made by nurses to client care and the facility can improve processes if necessary.

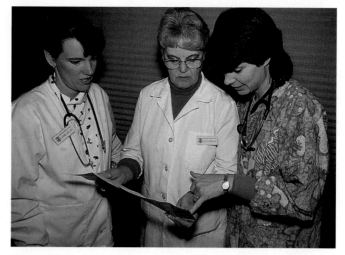

Figure 7-2 Nurses collaborating on research.

Clinical nursing research should be undertaken by nurses educated to conduct scientific investigations (Figure 7–2). An experienced researcher is usually more qualified than a beginner to undertake a complex, long-term project. Nurses new to research may, however, assist with data collection, conduct replication studies (studies previously performed elsewhere), or conduct less complex studies.

Ethical Issues in Research

Research must meet ethical standards in ways that respect the dignity and preserve the well-being of human research participants. In Canada, every health care facility and university receiving public funds for research must meet federal standards for protecting human research participants. The most recent standard is the *Tri-Council Policy Statement* (Canadian Institutes of Health Research et al., 2003), which requires that the institution have in place a research ethics board (REB) to review all research proposals to determine whether ethical principles are being upheld (Box 7–6). The REB focuses on **informed consent** and weighs benefits versus harms from the research. No research may be performed in a university or health care facility without the approval of the REB. All proposals are subject to review. However, if data collection processes (such as quality assurance studies) are a normal part of institutional business, performance reviews, or testing within normal educational requirements and are not for research purposes, they are exempt from REB review.

To refine existing knowledge and develop new knowledge, investigators in clinical research sometimes use new procedures whose outcome is doubtful or unknown. This research may seem to conflict with the purpose of nursing practice, which is to meet specific clients' needs. In such cases, the investigator must structure the research to avoid or minimize harm to the subjects. Although not all undesirable effects can be anticipated, investigators are obligated to inform everyone involved about the known potential risks. Other basic human rights must also be observed. These principles are set forth by the CNA (2008). Procedures for obtaining informed consent must be outlined in the study protocol. The consent form must describe in lay language the purpose of the study, the role of the subjects, types of data that are to be obtained, how the data are obtained, the duration of the study, subject selection, procedures, risks to the subject (including financial risks), potential benefits (including the possibility of no

> **BOX 7-6**   **Guiding Ethical Principles for Research in Canada**

1. *Respect for human dignity:* This principle is designed to protect the multiple and interdependent interests of the person (i.e., their bodily, psychological, and cultural integrity).
2. *Respect for free and informed consent:* This principle presumes that individuals have the capability and right to make free and informed decisions.
3. *Respect for vulnerable persons:* Children, institutionalized people, or others who are vulnerable are entitled, on grounds of human dignity, caring, solidarity, and fairness, to special protection against abuse, exploitation, or discrimination.
4. *Respect for privacy and confidentiality:* Standards of privacy and confidentiality protect the access, control, and dissemination of personal information and thus help protect mental or psychological integrity. These standards are consonant with values underlying privacy, confidentiality, and anonymity.
5. *Respect for justice and inclusiveness:* The ethics review process should be independent and use fair methods, standards, and procedures. No segment of the population should be unfairly burdened with the harms of research. Investigators have particular obligations to protect vulnerable individuals unable to protect their own interests. Individuals

and groups who may benefit from advances in research must neither be discriminated against nor be neglected.
6. *Balancing harms and benefits:* Research ethics require a favourable harms–benefit balance so that the foreseeable harms should not outweigh anticipated benefits.
7. *Minimizing harm:* Nonmaleficence (the duty to avoid, prevent, or minimize harms to others) is considered essential in research. No research subjects should be subjected to unnecessary risks of harm, and their participation in research must be essential to achieving important aims for science and for society.
8. *Maximizing benefit:* Beneficence, the duty to benefit others, in research ethics means a duty to maximize net benefits. In most research, the primary benefits produced are for society and for the advancement of knowledge, rather than for the individual research participant.

Adapted from Canadian Institutes of Health Research, the Natural Sciences and Engineering Research Council of Canada, & the Social Sciences and Humanities Research Council of Canada. (2003). *Tri-Council policy statement: Ethical conduct for research involving humans, 1998* (with 2000, 2002, and 2005 amendments). Retrieved August 20, 2008, from http://www.pre.ethics.gc.ca/english/policystatement/policystatement.cfm

benefit), alternatives to participation, and contact information concerning the principal investigator and local REB. The consent process gives subjects complete information regarding the study's risks, benefits, and costs so that they can make an informed decision.

The REB also determines whether the investigator has the necessary knowledge and skills to undertake the research, including familiarity with the clinical area in which the data will be collected and sufficient research training and experience. For example, a nurse planning a study of psychiatric clients should be familiar with psychiatric nursing principles and theory, as well as research procedures for data collection and analysis.

Rights of Other Research Participants

Student nurses and practising nurses may be asked to participate in research as data collectors or may be involved in the care of clients participating in a study. All participants, including health care professionals, have the right to be fully informed about the study, its procedures (including the consent process and risk factors), and physical or emotional injuries that clients could experience as a result of participation. Often, the physical risks are more obvious than the emotional risks. For example, clients may be asked to give highly personal, intrusive information; some may find this experience stressful. The researcher should prepare all participants, including nurses delivering care, for this possibility and assist them in coping with the effects. Participants also have the right to see review forms from the REB that certify approval of the study. Participants can refuse to perform research procedures if they are concerned about ethical aspects.

Applying Research Findings to Nursing Practice

Research evidence as a basis for scholarly, professional decision making in clinical practice is essential for providing competent, efficient, and state-of-the art nursing care (McCaughan et al., 2002). Advances

in care through research are meaningless unless they are accessible to nurses at the point of care. You make links between research findings and nursing care by reading relevant literature, identifying appropriate clinical problems, and incorporating **evidence-informed practice** activities into the nursing practice of your nursing unit or agency (Box 7–7).

In a policy statement, the CNA (2002) stated that evidence-informed decision making by registered nurses is key to quality nursing practice. Nurses need not only skills to access and appraise existing research but also scientific knowledge and skills to change practice settings and to promote evidence-informed decisions about client care.

Evidence-informed nursing practice deemphasizes ritual, isolated, and unsystematic clinical experiences; ungrounded opinion; and tradition as bases for nursing practice. It stresses the use of research findings and, as appropriate, quality improvement data, other evaluation data, and the consensus of recognized experts and affirmed experience to support a specific practice (Stetler et al., 1998). Many aspects of health care are not justly served by the research in only one discipline. The expertise of several disciplines must be brought to bear on complex health issues. Just as nurses play a vital role on the health care team, so they are crucial to multidisciplinary health research. Policymakers in the broader arena of health care must account for nursing practice, which is so essential to client care. Nurses need a sound knowledge base to support practice, and research is essential for building that knowledge.

✳ KEY CONCEPTS

- Nursing knowledge has five patterns: empirics, esthetics, personal knowledge, ethics, and emancipatory knowledge.
- A scientific investigation is an orderly, planned, and controlled study of real-life situations that tests theories and whose results can be applied to general situations.
- In nursing research, physical or psychosocial responses of people of all ages in various states of health and illness are examined.

✳ BOX 7-7   RESEARCH HIGHLIGHT

Comparison of Two Aerobic Training Programs on Outcomes for Women After a Cardiac Event

Research Focus

This study (Arthur et al., 2007) was carried out by a multidisciplinary team of researchers in cardiac rehabilitation, in an attempt to maximize the effect of exercise on the quality of life of women after myocardial infarction or cardiac surgery.

Research Abstract

The purpose of this study was to compare the effect and sustainability of a six-month combined aerobic and strength training program with those of aerobic training alone in women who had undergone coronary bypass graft surgery or who had experienced myocardial infarction. The primary outcome was improved health-related quality of life. Secondary outcomes were increases in perceived self-efficacy, strength, and exercise capacity.

The study was a two-group RCT. Ninety-two participants meeting the study criteria were randomly assigned to the two study groups. Measurements were taken at baseline, after two months, at the completion of the six-month exercise training program, and one year after discharge from the six-month program, which was 18 months after baseline measurements.

Participants were eligible to be in the study if (1) they were women, (2) they had undergone coronary artery bypass grafting or experienced myocardial infarction 8–10 weeks previously, (3) they were postmenopausal, (4) they were able to attend a supervised exercise program regularly, and (5) they were able to complete English-language questionnaires. Participants who exhibited negative responses to exercise were excluded from the study.

The study was approved by the Research Ethics Board of McMaster University and the Hamilton Health Sciences Centre.

Both groups attended an initial eight-week session of twice-a-week aerobics classes. Both groups were expected to attend supervised exercise seeions (separately) twice per week for six months. The sessions included 10–15 minutes of warm-up exercises, followed by aerobic interval training with stationary bicycles, treadmills, arm ergometers, and stair climbers. The total exercise time for both groups was 40 minutes per session, followed by a cool-down period of 10–15 minutes. After the initial eight weeks, 20–25 minutes of strength training was implemented in the treatment group in addition to aerobic exercise.

Results revealed no important baseline differences between groups with regard to demographics, medical history, peak volume of oxygen consumption (VO_2), peak metabolic equivalents level, or strength. The main outcome, health-related quality of life, improved over the six months of exercise training in both groups. However, one year after the completion of the intervention, scores differed significantly, in favor of the group with combined aerobic-strength training. Both groups experienced significant increases from baseline in both self-efficacy and strength, but these levels were not statistically significant between groups.

These findings demonstrate that strength training may be an important exercise intervention for female cardiac patients, inasmuch as most activities performed by persons in later life, especially after a cardiac event, require strength, not endurance. Both physical and psychological gains are apparent with either form of exercise, but it is likely that sustained or continued improvements may be achieved most efficiently through combined strength and aerobic training in woman with coronary artery disease.

Implications for Practice

- Women who have experienced a cardiac event should be encouraged to attend a supervised aerobic exercise program as part of their rehabilitation.
- A combined aerobic and strength-training program is likely to most effectively prepare these women to resume independent activities of daily living.

References: Arthur, H. M., Gunn, E., Thorpe, K. E., Ginis, K. M., Mataseje, L., McCartney, N., & McKelvie, M. (2007). Effect of aerobic vs. combined aerobic-strength training on 1 year post-cardiac rehabilitation outcomes in women after a cardiac event. Journal of Rehabilitation Medicine, 39(9), 730–735.

- In an experimental research study, investigators control factors that could influence the results, include comparison and experimental treatment groups of subjects, and use random means for selecting study subjects.
- In a qualitative research study, investigators organize information in narrative format so that phenomena can be described and patterns of relationships can be discovered.
- When human subjects participate in research, the researcher must obtain informed consent of study subjects, must maintain the confidentiality of subjects, and must protect subjects from undue risk or injury.
- When summarizing data reported in a research study, the nurse should note when, how, where, and by whom the investigation was conducted and who and what were studied.
- A researchable clinical nursing problem is one that is not satisfactorily resolved by current nursing interventions, occurs frequently in a particular group, can be measured or observed, and has a possible solution within the realm of nursing practice.
- To determine whether research findings can be used in nursing practice, the nurse considers the scientific worth of the study by substantiating evidence from other studies, the similarity of the research setting to the nurse's own clinical practice setting, the status of current nursing theory, and factors affecting the feasibility of application.

✳ CRITICAL THINKING EXERCISES

1. The nurse is concerned about learning to properly treat a pressure ulcer. Explain the benefits to the client if the nurse learns how to treat the sore by drawing from information in the research literature rather than using the scientific method.

2. The research literature reflects many different methods for treating pressure ulcers. If you wished to determine the best method for doing this, what type of research design would you use?

3. The nurses working on an orthopedic unit decide to study the factors that commonly result in clients' falling in their unit. How could they design a study to answer their questions?

✳ REVIEW QUESTIONS

1. The first provincially approved doctoral program in nursing was established in
   1. 1969
   2. 1974
   3. 1982
   4. 1991

2. Empirics is described by Carper (1978) as
   1. The artistic expression of knowledge
   2. Knowledge derived from the interpersonal relationship with the client
   3. Knowledge derived from ethical dilemmas
   4. Knowledge systematically organized into general laws and theories

3. The scientific method is characterized by
   1. Systematic procedures that seek to limit error and eliminate bias
   2. Studies of behaviours, experiences, perceptions, and motives
   3. A commitment to the participants' point of view
   4. The use of the participants' natural setting

4. If the research question leads to the study of behaviour within a specific culture, the design chosen is
   1. Phenomenology
   2. Grounded theory
   3. Ethnography
   4. Quantitative research

5. Subjectivity is the goal of
   1. Positivism
   2. Qualitative research
   3. True experiments
   4. The scientific method

6. Which research method is quantitative?
   1. Grounded theory
   2. Phenomenology
   3. Ethnography
   4. Quasi-experimental research

7. A sample in a survey design
   1. Is the main component of qualitative research
   2. Should be representative of the population surveyed
   3. Should be small enough to keep sampling error to a minimum
   4. Should be no different from the control group

8. Procedures for obtaining informed consent do *not* include
   1. Describing the purpose of the study
   2. Describing the role of the subjects
   3. Giving the names of other participants in the study
   4. Describing the risks that the subject may incur

9. In a quasi-experimental research design, subjects are assigned to
   1. An empirical group
   2. An ethnographic group
   3. Either a control group or a treatment condition, but not randomly
   4. An experimental group

10. Evidence-informed practice
    1. Enables the transfer of clinical practice techniques into a positivist paradigm
    2. Requires that evidence be always research based
    3. Is synonymous with research-based practice
    4. Entails the use of knowledge based on research studies and takes into account a nurse's clinical experience and client preferences.

✳ RECOMMENDED WEB SITES

Canadian Nurses Association: http://www.cna-aiic.ca/cna/
This Web site contains information about policies and position statements for nursing research in Canada, as well as information about research funding.

Canadian Nurses Foundation: http://www.cnf-fiic.ca/
This Web site provides information about available research funding and about scholarships for students.

The Canadian Health Services Research Foundation: http://www.chsrf.ca
This Web site contains information about funding for health services research and about the Nursing Research Fund.

Canadian Institutes of Health Research (CIHR): http://www.cihr.ca
This Web site contains pages for all 13 CIHR institutes.

8

Nursing Values and Ethics

Original chapter by Margaret Ecker, RN, MS

Canadian content written by Shelley Raffin Bouchal, RN, PhD

objectives

Mastery of content in this chapter will enable you to:

- Define the key terms listed.
- Discuss the role of values in the study of ethics.
- Examine and clarify personal values.
- Discuss how values influence client care.
- Explain the relationship between ethics and professional practice.
- Describe some basic ethical philosophies relevant to health care.
- Apply a method of ethical analysis to a clinical situation.
- Identify contemporary ethical issues in nursing practice.

key terms

media resources

evolve Web Site

- Audio Chapter Summaries
- Glossary
- Multiple-Choice Review Questions
- Student Learning Activities
- Weblinks

Companion CD

- Glossary
- Interactive Learning Activities
- Fluids and Electrolytes Tutorial
- Test-Taking Skills

Values and ethics are inherent in all nursing acts. A **value** is a strong personal belief and an ideal that a person or group (such as nurses) strives to uphold. **Ethics** is the study of the philosophical ideals of right and wrong behaviour. The term also commonly refers to the values and standards to which individuals and professions strive to uphold (e.g., health care ethics, nursing ethics). In other words, ethics are a reflection of what matters most to people or professions. Nurses and other health care professionals agree to national codes of ethics that offer guidelines for responding to difficult situations that occur in practice and demonstrate to the public an overview of professional practice standards. For example, the Canadian Nurses Association (CNA; 2008) publishes a **code of ethics** that outlines nurses' professional values and ethical commitments to their clients and the communities they serve.

Because of their prominent and intimate role in the provision of health care, nurses continually make decisions about the correct course of action in different circumstances. In many situations, no answer or course of action is best. To manage such difficult situations, nurses need a keen awareness of their values and those of their clients, a good understanding of ethics, and a sound approach to ethical decision making. They also must be guided by a broader understanding of ethics through the application of philosophies, theories, and sets of principles.

Values

Values are at the heart of ethics. Values influence behaviour on the basis of the conviction that a certain action is correct in a certain situation. An individual's values reflect cultural and social influences, relationships, and personal needs. Values vary among people, and they develop and change over time. In the context of beliefs about morality, values generate rights and duties.

In nursing, value statements express broad ideals of nursing care and establish reasonable directions for practice. The CNA (2008) *Code of Ethics* is organized around seven values that are central to ethical nursing practice. These values include providing safe, compassionate, competent, and ethical care; promoting health and well-being; being accountable; and preserving dignity. Each provincial nursing association also has shared values, such as those held in position statements and practice standards. These standards reflect the values of the profession and clarify what is expected of you as a practising nurse.

Because of the intimacy of the nurse–client relationship, you must be aware of your personal values, as well as the values of clients, physicians, employers, or other groups. To understand the values of others, it is important to understand your own values: what they are, where they came from, and how they relate to others' values.

Values Formation

People acquire values in many ways, beginning in early childhood. Throughout childhood and adolescence, people learn to distinguish right from wrong and to form values on which to base their actions. This is known as *moral development* (see Chapter 23). Family experiences strongly influence value formation.

Values are also learned outside the family. A person's culture, ethnic background, and religious community strongly influences that person's values, as do schools, peer groups, and work environments. **Cultural values** are those adopted as a result of a social setting (see Chapter 10). A basic task of the young adult is to identify personal values within the context of the community. Over time, the person acquires values by choosing some values that are strongly upheld in the community and by discarding or transforming others. A person's experience as well as lack of experience also influences his or her values.

Values Clarification

Within the context of nursing, several layers of values inform the ethical questions and actions that you consider in your practice. Clarifying your values helps you articulate what matters most and what priorities are guiding your life and decision making. Values influence how you interpret confusing or conflicting information. As you mature and experience new situations, your values change. You may reorder your values or replace old values with new ones. As a result, you may modify your attitudes and behaviour. The willingness to change reflects a healthy attitude and an ability to adapt to new experiences.

To adopt new values, you must be aware of your existing values and how they affect behaviour. **Values clarification** is the process of appraising personal values (Box 8–1). It is not a set of rules, nor does it suggest that certain values should be accepted by all people; rather, it is a process of personal reflection. When you clarify your values, you make careful choices. The result of values clarification is greater self-awareness and personal insight.

By understanding your personal values, you will better understand your clients' and colleagues' values. In *value conflict*, personal values are at odds with those of a client, a colleague, or an institution. Values clarification plays a major role in resolving these dilemmas. In addition, you can better advocate for a client when you can identify your personal values and the values of the client.

> **BOX 8-1   Values Clarification Questions**

- Describe a situation in your personal or professional experience in which you felt uncomfortable, in which you believed that your beliefs and values were being challenged, or in which you believed your values were different from others.
- As you record the situation, mention how you felt physically and emotionally at the time you experienced the situation.
- Write down your feelings as you remember the situation. Are your current reactions any different from those when you were actually in the situation?
- What personal values do you identify in the situation? Try to remember where and from whom you learned these values. Do you completely agree with the values, or do you question some aspect of the values, or do you wonder about their validity?
- What values do you think were being expressed by others involved? Are they similar to or different from your own values?
- What do you think you reacted to in the situation?
- Can you remember having similar reactions in other situations? If you do, how were the situations similar or different?
- How do you feel about your response to the situation? If you could repeat the scenario, would you change something about it? Rewrite the scenario with the same changes. What might be the consequences of these same changes?
- How do you feel about the new scenario?
- What do you need to do to reinforce behaviours, ideals, beliefs, and qualities that you have identified as personal values in this situation? When and how can you do this?

From Burkhardt, M.A., & Nathaniel, A. K. (2007). *Ethics and issues in contemporary nursing* (3rd ed.). Albany, NY: Thomson Delmar Learning. © Delmar, a part of Cengage Learning, Inc. Reproduced by permission (www.cengage.com/permissions).

Once you master the skill of clarifying personal values, you can help clients identify their personal priorities, values, and emotions. This may help clients resolve conflicts between values and behaviours. The goal of values clarification with clients is effective nurse–client communication. As the client becomes more willing to express problems and feelings, you can collaborate with the client in developing an individualized plan of care.

Structured communication is a useful way in which to clarify values with a client. Simple strategies that promote the process of sharing feelings can be effective. For example, responding to a client by repeating the client's sentence as a question ("You wish you could be at home?") encourages the client to continue the story. Instead of asking questions that can be answered by only "yes" or "no," you can encourage the client to answer in greater detail. For example, rather than asking, "Do you want to live at home with your daughter?" the nurse might say, "Tell me how you feel about living at home with your daughter."

Your response can motivate the client to examine personal thoughts and actions. When you make a clarifying response, it should be brief and nonjudgemental. For example, when talking with a client who exercises only rarely, you might ask, "What is your understanding of the purpose of exercise?" An effective clarifying response encourages the client to think about personal values after the exchange is over and does not impose your own values onto the client. In this way, you respect the client's self-direction and avoid inappropriately introducing personal values into the conversation.

Values clarification plays a key role in communication. In particular, when the topic concerns issues of personal health, private habits, and quality of life, participants in a discussion benefit from clarity of values. In appreciating values, you can identify differences between personal opinion and the values that others embrace. Through values clarification, you can better serve the needs of clients, especially when values differ. By demonstrating respect for the client's differences and helping the client to clarify values, you are better able to teach and to heal.

Ethics

Ethics is the study of good conduct, character, and motives. It is concerned with determining what is good or valuable for all people. Often the terms *ethics* and *morals*, or **morality**, are used interchangeably (Johnstone, 2004), inasmuch as both words are derived from an original meaning of "custom or habit." Johnstone suggested that it is not incorrect to use these terms interchangeably and that the choice is a matter of personal preference rather than of philosophical debate. The classic textbook definition of *ethics* is a "generic term for various ways of understanding and examining the moral life" (Beauchamp & Childress, 2001, p. 1). Essentially, ethics requires you to be critically reflective exploring your values, behaviours, actions, judgements, and justifications (Beauchamp & Childress, 2001, p xii). In this chapter, the terms *ethics* and *morals* are used interchangeably.

Professional Nursing and Ethics

Codes of Ethics. A "code of ethics serves as a foundation for nurses' ethical practice" (CNA, 2008, p. 3) and is accepted by all members of a profession. The code is a statement of the ethical values of nurses and of nurses' commitments to clients with health care needs and clients who receive care. It is intended for nurses in all contexts and domains of practice and at all levels of decision making. The code is relevant for all nurses in their practices with individuals, families, communities, and public health care systems. The code developed by nurses for nurses serves the profession when questions arise about practising ethically and working through ethical challenges (CNA, 2008). The nursing code of ethics, as in other professions, sets forth ideals of conduct.

"The code provides guidance for ethical relationships, responsibilities, behaviours and decision-making and it is to be used in conjunction with professional standards, laws and regulations that guide practice" (CNA, 2008, p. 4). It does not provide rules of behaviour for every circumstance. Situations are unique to the context in which they occur. The environment or institution can greatly influence the values that you are encouraged to uphold. Furthermore, a code does not offer guidance as to which values should take priority or how to balance them in practice.

The CNA and the International Council of Nurses (2006) have established widely accepted codes for nurses that reflect the principles of responsibility, accountability, and advocacy (Boxes 8–2 and 8–3).

► BOX 8-2 Canadian Nurses Association Code of Ethics

The following is the CNA's statement of the seven values that must be upheld in nursing practice. The complete code of ethics also includes responsibility statements outlining how nurses can incorporate these values into their practice; it can be found on the CNA Web site (see the "Recommended Web Sites" section at the end of this chapter).

Providing Safe, Compassionate, Competent, and Ethical Care

Nurses provide safe, compassionate, competent, and ethical care.

Promoting Health and Well-Being

Nurses work with clients to enable them to attain their highest level of health and well-being.

Promoting and Respecting Informed Decision Making

Nurses recognize, respect, and promote a client's right to be informed and make decisions.

Preserving Dignity

Nurses recognize and respect the intrinsic worth of each client.

Maintaining Privacy and Confidentiality

Nurses recognize the importance of privacy and confidentiality, and they safeguard personal, family, and community information obtained in the context of a professional relationship.

Promoting Justice

Nurses uphold principles of justice by safeguarding human rights, equity, and fairness in promoting the public good.

Being Accountable

Nurses are accountable for their actions and answerable for their practice.

Adapted from Canadian Nurses Association. (2008). *Code of ethics for registered nurses.* Ottawa, ON: Author.

> **BOX 8-3** **International Council of Nurses: The Code of Ethics for Nurses**

Nurses have four fundamental responsibilities: to promote health, to prevent illness, to restore health, and to alleviate suffering. The need for nursing care is universal. Inherent in nursing care is respect for human rights, including cultural rights, the right to life and choice, the right to dignity, and the right to be treated with respect. Nursing care is respectful of and unrestricted by considerations of age, creed, culture, disability or illness, gender, sexual orientation, nationality, politics, race, economic status, or social status. Nurses render health services to the individual, the family, and the community, and they coordinate their services with those of related groups.

Nurses and People

The nurse's primary professional responsibility is to clients who require nursing care.

In providing care, the nurse promotes an environment in which the human rights, values, customs, and spiritual beliefs of the individual client, family, and community are respected.

The nurse ensures that the individual client receives sufficient information on which to base consent for care and related treatment.

The nurse keeps the client's personal information confidential, sharing it only with appropriate other professionals.

The nurse shares with society the responsibility for initiating and supporting action to meet the health and social needs of the public, particularly those of vulnerable populations.

The nurse also shares responsibility to sustain and protect the natural environment from depletion, pollution, degradation, and destruction.

Nurses and Nursing Practice

The nurse carries personal responsibility and accountability for nursing practice and for maintaining competence by continual learning.

The nurse maintains a standard of personal health in such a way that the ability to provide care is not compromised.

The nurse uses judgement regarding individual competence when accepting and delegating responsibility.

The nurse at all times maintains standards of personal conduct that reflect positively on the profession and enhance public confidence.

In providing care, the nurse ensures that the use of technology and scientific advances is compatible with the safety, dignity, and rights of clients.

Nurses and the Nursing Profession

The nurse assumes the major role in determining and implementing acceptable standards of critical nursing practice, management, research, and education.

The nurse is active in developing a core of research-based professional knowledge.

The nurse, acting through the professional organization, participates in creating and maintaining equitable social and economic working conditions in nursing.

Nurses and Coworkers

The nurse sustains a cooperative relationship with coworkers in nursing and other fields.

The nurse takes appropriate action to safeguard clients when their care is endangered by a coworker of the nurse or by any other person.

Adapted from International Council of Nurses. (2006). *ICN code of ethics for nurses.* Geneva, Switzerland: Author. Reprinted by permission of International Council of Nurses.

Responsibility. **Responsibility** refers to the characteristics of reliability and dependability. It implies an ability to distinguish between right and wrong. In professional nursing, responsibility includes a duty to perform actions adequately and thoughtfully. When administering a medication, for example, you are responsible for assessing the client's need for the drug, for administering it safely and correctly, and for evaluating the client's response to it. By agreeing to act responsibly, you gain trust from clients, colleagues, and society.

Nurses in all domains of practice uphold responsibilities related to all the values in the code of ethics. You are responsible in your interactions with individual clients, families, groups, populations, communities, and society, as well as with students, nursing colleagues, and other health care colleagues. These responsibilities serve as the foundation for articulating nursing values to employers, other health care professionals, and the public (CNA, 2008).

Accountability. **Accountability** means being able to accept responsibility or to account for one's actions and refers to being answerable to someone for something one has done. **Answerability** means being able to offer reasons and explanations to other people for aspects of nursing practice. You balance accountability to the client, the profession, the employer, and society. For example, you may know that a client who will be discharged soon is confused about how to self-administer insulin. The action that you take in response to this situation is guided by your sense of accountability. The client, the institution, and society rely on your judgement and trust you to take action in response to this situation. You may request

more hospitalization to provide further teaching, or you may arrange home care to continue teaching at home. The goal is the prevention of injury to the client. Your sense of accountability guides actions that achieve this goal.

According to the CNA (2008), nurses who are enacting professional accountability are (1) keeping up with professional standards, laws, and regulations; (2) ensuring that they have the skill to provide these practices; (c) maintaining their fitness to practise, ensuring that they have the necessary physical, mental, and emotional capacity to practise safely and competently; (d) sharing their knowledge with other nurses through mentorship and giving feedback to other nurses when appropriate.

Professional accountability is also the mandate of professional associations. Professional associations both check unethical practice in a profession and support conscientious professionals who may be under pressure to act unethically or to overlook unethical activity by colleagues. Professional nursing associations have the authority to register and discipline nurses. They also set and maintain professional standards of practice and communicate them to the public. These standards, developed by nursing clinical experts, provide a basic structure against which nursing care is objectively measured. They do not eliminate the need for individualized care plans; rather, the nurse incorporates the standards into each client's care plan.

Advocacy. The ethical responsibility of **advocacy** means acting in behalf of another person, speaking for persons who cannot speak for themselves, or intervening to ensure that views are heard. The CNA

(2008) advises nurses to advocate for all clients in their care. This includes protecting the client's right to choice by providing information, obtaining informed consent for all nursing care, and respecting clients' decisions. Nurses should protect clients' right to dignity by advocating for appropriate use of interventions in order to minimize suffering, intervening if other people fail to respect the dignity of the client, and working to promote health and social conditions that allow clients to live and die with dignity. Nurses should protect a client's right to privacy and confidentiality by helping the client access his or her health records (subject to legal requirements), intervening if other members of the health care team fail to respect the client's privacy, and following policies that protect the client's privacy. According to the *Code of Ethics,* nurses should also advocate for the discussion of ethical issues among health care team members, clients, and families, and nurses should advocate for health policies that enable fair and inclusive allocation of resources.

Advocacy requires that you have a strong awareness of the context in which situations arise, as well as an understanding of the influence of power and politics on how you make decisions. If you experience **constrained moral agency**—that is, if you feel powerless to act for what you think is right, or if you believe your actions will not effect change—then you will have difficulty being an effective advocate.

Ethical Theory

Ethics concern the examination of the moral basis for judgements, actions, duties, and obligations. For centuries, moral philosophers have tried to answer two questions: "What is the meaning of right and good?" and "What is the morally right thing to do in a given situation?" You are mainly concerned with the second question because you are often in situations in which you must make decisions that affect client well-being.

Philosophical discussion about health care issues has progressed over time, just as developments in health care and society itself have progressed. The philosophical constructions that shape the discussions have also changed. Ethics began as a standard reference point for the determination of right action. It has grown into a field of study filled with differences of opinion, competing systems of values, and deeply meaningful efforts to understand human interaction through new technologies. Some knowledge of ethical theories that have shaped philosophical thinking is necessary to understand the development of nursing ethics. The following section introduces a variety of contemporary ethical theories. It is neither exclusive nor comprehensive.

Deontology.

A traditional ethical theory, **deontology** is the system of ethics that is perhaps most familiar to practitioners in health care. Its foundations are often associated with the work of the eighteenth century philosopher Immanuel Kant (1724–1804). In deontology, actions are defined as right or wrong on the basis of their "right-making characteristics such as fidelity to promises, truthfulness, and justice" (Beauchamp & Childress, 2001). The essence of right or wrong is located within deontological principles. Deontologists specifically do not look to consequences of actions to determine rightness or wrongness. Instead, they critically examine a situation for the existence of essential rightness or wrongness. Ethical principles such as justice, allowing free choice (autonomy), and doing the greatest good (beneficence) serve to define right or wrong. If an act is just, respects autonomy, and provides good, then the act is ethical. The process depends on a mutual understanding and acceptance of these principles.

Difficulty arises when you must choose among conflicting principles, which is often the case in ethical dilemmas concerning health care. For example, applying the principle of respect for autonomy can be confusing when dealing with the health care of children. The health care team may recommend a treatment, but a parent may disagree with or refuse the recommendation. In discussion of the dilemma, you may refer to a guiding principle such as respect for autonomy. However, questions remain: Whose autonomy should receive the respect? The parent's? Who should advocate for the child's best interest? Society often struggles to understand who should be ultimately responsible for the well-being of children. A commitment to respect autonomy does not guarantee that controversy can be avoided.

Utilitarianism.

According to a utilitarian system of ethics, the value of something is determined by its usefulness. This philosophy, **utilitarianism,** may also be known as **consequentialism** because its main emphasis is on the outcome or consequence of action. A third term associated with this philosophy is **teleology** (from the Greek word *telos,* meaning "end"), which is the study of ends or final causes. Its philosophical foundations were first proposed by John Stuart Mill (1806–1873), a British philosopher and social commentator. The greatest good for the greatest number of people is the guiding principle for determining the correct action in this system. As with deontology, this theory relies on the application of a certain principle, namely: measures of "good" and "greatest" (Beauchamp & Childress, 2001). The difference between utilitarianism and deontology is in the focus on consequences or outcomes. Utilitarianism concerns the effect that an act will have; deontology concerns the presence of principle, regardless of outcome.

Individuals or groups may have conflicting definitions of "greatest good." For example, research suggests that education regarding safer sex practices may reduce the spread of the human immunodeficiency virus. Some scholars argue, however, that education about sex should be provided by the family and that sex education in public schools diminishes the role and the value of the family. For them, the greater good is the preservation of family values and the protection of individual choices regarding sex education of children. For other scholars, however, the "greater good" is defined as educating the greatest number of people in the most effective way possible. The concepts of utilitarianism provide guidance, but they do not invariably provide for universal agreement.

Bioethics.

In the 1970s, a group of ethics scholars concluded that then-current ethical theories were not sufficient for the health care field because they did not provide specific guidance for important moral questions that arose in the context of medicine. **Biomedical ethics** came to denote ethical reasoning for physicians, whereas **bioethics** became the general term for principled reasoning across health care professions. The central idea of bioethics is that moral decision making in health care should be guided by four principles: autonomy, beneficence, nonmaleficence, and justice. According to this theory, health care providers should examine each situation, determine which of the principles has priority, and use that principle to guide action.

Autonomy.

Autonomy refers to your ability to make choices for yourself that should be based on full understanding, free of controlling influences (Beauchamp & Childress, 2001). Respect for another person's autonomy is fundamental to the practice of health care. It is the reason why clients should be included in all aspects of decision making regarding their care. The agreement to respect autonomy involves the recognition that clients have the right to be respected and supported by you with regard to their health care decisions. For example, the purpose of the preoperative consent that clients must read and sign before surgery is to ensure in writing that the health care team respects the client's independence by obtaining permission to proceed. The consent process implies that a client may refuse treatment, and in most cases, the health care team must agree to follow the client's wishes. Health care professionals agree to abide by a standard of respect for the client's autonomy.

Beneficence. **Beneficence** means doing or promoting good for others. It involves taking positive actions to help others. Commitment to beneficence helps guide difficult decisions concerning whether the benefits of a treatment may be challenged by risks to the client's well-being or dignity. For example, vaccination may cause temporary discomfort, but the benefits of protection from disease, both for the client and for society, outweigh the client's discomfort. The agreement to act with beneficence also requires that the best interests of the client remain more important than self-interest. For example, you do not simply follow medical orders; you act thoughtfully to understand client needs and then work actively to meet those needs.

Nonmaleficence. *Maleficence* refers to harm or hurt; thus **nonmaleficence** is the avoidance of harm or hurt. In health care ethics, ethical practice involves not only the will to do good but also the equal commitment to do no harm. The health care professional tries to balance the risks and benefits of a plan of care while striving to cause the least harm possible. This principle is often helpful in guiding discussions about new or controversial technologies. For example, a new bone marrow transplantation procedure may provide a chance for cure. The procedure, however, may entail long periods of pain and suffering. These discomforts should be considered in view of the suffering that the disease itself might cause and in view of the suffering that other treatments might cause. The commitment to provide least harmful interventions illustrates the term *nonmaleficence*. The standard of nonmaleficence promotes a continuing effort to consider the potential for harm even when it may be necessary to promote health.

Justice. **Justice** refers to fairness. The term is often used during discussions about resources: When competition for a scarce resource exists, justice mandates that decisions be fair and, to the greatest extent possible, unbiased. In decisions about which client receives an available lung for transplantation, for example, it is understood that the lung will be allocated as fairly as possible. Understandings of fairness depend on community values. In Canadian society, community standards dictate that the decision should not depend on who has the higher intellect or larger salary; instead, the decision must be based on need alone. Of course, the definition of need can be debated, and when two people have equal need, nothing in the theory helps health care professionals decide between them. These are ethical questions that require further exploration of values, principles, and priorities to guide decisions in resource allocation.

The literature also mentions other prevalent forms of justice that you need to understand, such as **social justice**. Social justice is often related to a concern for the eqitable distribution of benefits and burdens in society (Boutain, 2005) and has also been discussed as changing social relationships and institutions to promote equitable relationships (Drevdahl et al., 2001). According to the "Ethical Endeavours" section of the CNA (2008) *Code of Ethics,* your moral obligations extend to recognizing "the need for change in systems and societal structures in order to create greater equity for all. You should endeavour as much as possible, individually and collectively, to advocate for and work toward eliminating social inequities . . . ." (p. 16). This section of the *Code of Ethics* is somewhat visionary, inasmuch as its statements extend beyond just "what is" to "what ought to be" in nursing as a profession. It makes clear that if the status quo in health care is inefficacious, you must be an active participant in effecting change. This means you must recognize that part of your role is to work for change at the broader systems level, agitating for revisions to social policy, legislation, and institutional structures. This

section of the *Code of Ethics* emphasizes the advocacy role for you and the need to work to bring about a system that is more focused on prevention, takes more account of the social determinants of health, is more accessible, and is more sustainable. This is a daunting task, but you have the educational preparation and theoretical base to assume a leadership role in making the reality of Canadian health care match the vision (Oberle & Raffin Bouchal, in press).

Feminist Ethics. Feminist ethicists consider their work a critique of conventional ethics, as well as a critique of social values. Their work focuses on continuing inequalities between people (Lindemann, 2006). They look to the nature of relationships between people for guidance in working out ethical dilemmas. The underlying values, according to a group of noted feminist nursing scholars, are social justice, relationships, and community (Peter et al., 2004).

Changes in attitudes toward women reflect new perspectives in women's relationship with family, with work, with science, and with society (Sherwin, 1992). For example, until the early 1980s, moral development was thought to reach the highest stages more often in men than in women. According to this thinking, moral development occurred in predictable stages. The most complex stage involved a sense of justice, and young girls did not reach this stage as often as did young boys (Kohlberg, 1981). Findings of research in the early 1980s disputed this conclusion. Gilligan (1982) proposed that Kohlberg's tools to measure moral development were gender biased. Gilligan went on to build a revised theory of moral development from her findings. She attempted to accommodate gender differences. Specifically, she concluded that young girls tend to pay attention to community and to individual circumstances and that young boys tend to process dilemmas through ideals or principles determined abstractly.

Feminist ethicists value the role of relationships and stories about relationships. They emphasize the importance of stories and the role of community over an attention to universal principles. In fact, they argue that it is impossible to be unbiased or not influenced by relationships to people. They propose that the natural human urge to be influenced by relationships is a positive value (Wolf, 1996).

This system of ethics also addresses issues of gender-based inequality. Feminists propose that an inequality of attention to women can be remedied by routinely asking, in the midst of any ethical dilemma, how bioethical decisions affect women (Sherwin, 1992). For example, in a discussion regarding the ethics of fetal surgery (surgical intervention in an unborn child), **feminist ethics** would propose that questions about the effects of the intervention on the mother are at least as important as questions about the effects on the fetus. Hilde Lindemann Nelson (2000), a noted feminist scholar in the United States, provided a history of the development of feminist ethics and bioethics. She noted that the feminist attention to gender and gender-related issues gave rise to an important perspective called **care theory**, which is about a type of virtue ethic that gives moral weight to caring for others (see Chapter 19). This was an important development in thinking about ethics because it moved attention away from the traditional masculine virtues towards those that had traditionally been considered more feminine.

Relational Ethics. It is becoming increasingly apparent that relationships are the basis of ethics in nursing. According to **relational ethics** theory, ethical understandings are formed in, and emerge from, a person's relationships with others, whether those others are clients, families, communities, or colleagues (Bergum, 2004; Bergum, & Dossetor, 2005; Hartrick Doane & Varcoe, 2007). Relational ethics refers not only to individual relationships but also to a person's relationships within an institutional structure. It is important that you understand the concept of relational ethics because many ethics scholars believe it is the foundation of your moral understanding of nursing. According to Bergum (2004), relational ethics is a way of "being," displayed in everyday interactions rather than a mode of decision making. It is how you insert a needle, how you enter into conversation, how you show respect, or how you behave with other people.

Relational ethics focuses on the role of relational context or the experience of the relationships in shaping moral choices (Bergum, 2004). In research on relational ethics, Bergum (2004) identified four themes: environment, embodiment, mutual respect, and engagement. **Environment** concerns critical elements or characteristics of the health care system within which you work and how the nature of your relationships is affected by this system. Bergum encouraged nurses to consider the entire health care arena as a network or matrix, in which each part is connected, either directly or indirectly, to the other. An awareness of this connectedness encourages you to look beyond the immediate situation and to try to envision a broader context. It also makes you conscious of how power and politics affect your entire system of care (Oberle & Raffin Bouchal, 2009).

In relational ethics, **embodiment** means recognizing that the mind–body split is artificial and that healing for both client and family cannot occur unless "scientific knowledge and human compassion are given equal weight [and it is recognized that] emotion and feeling are as important to human life as physical signs and symptoms" (Bergum, 2004, p. 492). Such recognition requires you to become truly aware of what other people may be experiencing. You must make this awareness a part of your own experience. The nurse–client relationship requires that you value clients and treat them with respect. It goes far beyond just being "nice" to them; in addition, it requires a commitment to care about clients and their experience.

Within the nurse–client relationship, you use nursing knowledge to enhance the client's health and well-being. You always consider the unique needs of the client as an individual. Mutual respect is created, with attention to both your and the client's needs, wishes, expertise, and experience (Bergum & Dossetor, 2005). **Mutuality**, loosely defined as a relationship that benefits both you and the client and harms neither, requires your and the client's willingness to participate in a relationship that embraces the values and ideas of one another as a means of developing new understandings, rather than judging the other person's values and ideas.

Engagement means connecting with another person in an open, trusting, and responsive manner. Bergum (2004) suggested that it is through this connection that you develop a meaningful understanding of the other person's experience. Engagement takes skill and practice, inasmuch as it requires a commitment to keeping the relationship caring and respectful. Bergum asserted that engagement "does not ask for *selflessness* on the part of you, but for both you and the patient to be recognized as *whole beings*" (p. 498). Engagement requires that you connect with the client but, at the same time, set boundaries in such a way that the relationship remains on a professional level. Knowing how much to engage with another person is one of the greatest challenges in nursing.

How to Process an Ethical Dilemma

An **ethical dilemma** is a conflict between two sets of human values, both of which are judged to be "good" but neither of which can be fully served. Ethical dilemmas can cause distress and confusion for clients and caregivers. You may well be faced with ethical questions that have not been examined previously and for which no practical

wisdom exists. You must be able to examine issues and apply experience and wisdom in each situation. The CNA (2008) *Code of Ethics* identified the responsibility of nurses to maintain their "fitness to practice" as having the "necessary physical, mental or emotional capacity to practice safely and competently" (p. 15). Such fitness requires you to be knowledgeable and skillful as you engage in problem solving. Ethical issues must be processed carefully and deliberately. An ethical decision is not based solely on emotions or on what people want and feel; however, the process promotes the free expression of feelings. Ethical decision making is a negotiating process that evolves over time, not in a straight line with a beginning and an end.

To resolve an ethical dilemma—in a committee setting, at the client's bedside, or in a family conference—you apply a careful, critical reflection of the dilemma. Resolving an ethical dilemma requires deliberate, critical, and systematic thinking. It also requires negotiation of differences (between beliefs, values, opinions, and so forth), incorporation of conflicting ideas, and an effort to respect differences of opinion. The process of negotiating ethical dilemmas may be in part the process of understanding ambiguities. You need to be knowledgeable and adept in making logical, fair, and consistent decisions. Ethical decision-making models offer a variety of methods for making informed conclusions (Box 8–4).

Each step in the processing of an ethical dilemma resembles steps in critical thinking. You begin by gathering information and move through assessment and identification of the problem, planning a solution, implementation of a solution, and evaluation of the results. The first step guides you in determining whether the problem is an ethical one. Not all problems are ethical in nature. You learn to distinguish ethical problems from questions of procedure, legality, or medical diagnosis. To distinguish an ethical problem from other problems, Curtin and Flaherty (1982) recommended that you decide whether the problem has one or more of the following characteristics:

- It cannot be resolved solely through a review of scientific data. To make this determination, you must gather detailed information about the situation. This information may come from medical records, health care literature, or consultation with colleagues or with the client and the client's family.
- It is perplexing. It is hard to think logically or make a decision about the problem, or you may disagree with a decision that other people are making, and the difference of opinion is perplexing.
- The answer to the problem is profoundly relevant to several areas of human concern.

A part of gathering information includes an examination of your own values as they relate to the issues. The distinction between personal opinion and the facts of the case, or the opinions of others, is essential for resolution to proceed. To clarify the true ethical issues in any situation, you need to be aware of personal responses.

After reviewing relevant information and personal values, a clear statement of the ethical problem becomes the groundwork to begin negotiation. Discussions are more likely to remain focused and constructive when all parties agree on the statement of the dilemma. The group then lists possible courses of action. Possibilities may occur at any time during deliberations. After alternatives are considered, people in an ethical conflict come to a point of resolution or agreement, and action is taken. Decisions are made that can be evaluated in an ongoing manner (Box 8–5).

Documentation of the ethical process can take a variety of forms. Whenever the process involves a family conference or results in a change in the plan of care, the process should be documented in the medical record. At some institutions, the ethics committee may use

> BOX 8-4   **Two Ethical Decision-Making Frameworks**

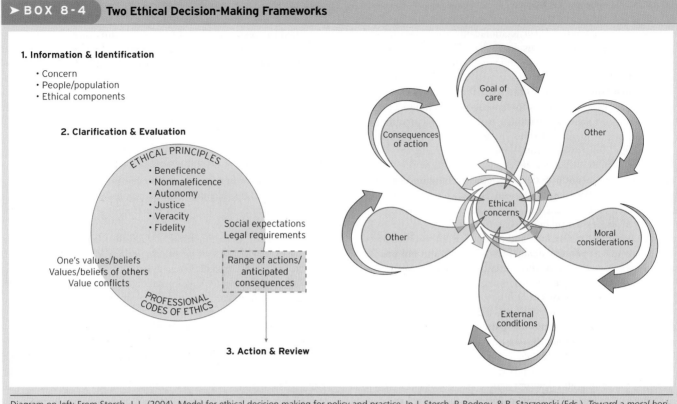

1. Information & Identification

- Concern
- People/population
- Ethical components

2. Clarification & Evaluation

ETHICAL PRINCIPLES
- Beneficence
- Nonmaleficence
- Autonomy
- Justice
- Veracity
- Fidelity

Social expectations
Legal requirements

One's values/beliefs
Values/beliefs of others
Value conflicts

Range of actions/
anticipated
consequences

PROFESSIONAL
CODES OF ETHICS

3. Action & Review

Goal of
care

Consequences
of action

Other

Ethical
concerns

Other

Moral
considerations

External
conditions

Diagram on left: From Storch, J. L. (2004). Model for ethical decision making for policy and practice. In J. Storch, P. Rodney, & R. Starzomski (Eds.), *Toward a moral horizon: Nursing ethics for leadership and practice* (p. 515). Toronto, ON: Pearson Education. Diagram on right: From Alberta College and Association of Registered Nurses (1996). A model for questioning. In *Ethical decision-making for registered nurses in Alberta: Guidelines and recommendations* (p. 13). Edmonton, AB: Author. Reprinted by permission of College and Association of Registered Nurses of Alberta.

a formal consultation format whenever a request for discussion arises. If the ethical dilemma does not directly affect client care, however, discussion may be documented by minutes from a meeting or in a memorandum to affected parties. In the following case study, the nursing concerns and the family conferences would be recorded in the medical record and in nursing flow sheets.

On your unit, a 35-year-old woman has been hospitalized in the final stages of brain cancer. She is a single mother with two young children. Although she has been treated by both conventional and experimental treatments, the tumour continues to grow, and the medical team has agreed that further treatment would be futile. You have cared for this client during past hospital admissions, and during an especially open discussion, she expressed wishes to explore "do not resuscitate" (DNR) orders. During the current admission, her primary physician is out of town. The attending physician does not know the client personally, but he has spent time with her. He has reviewed the clinical data and agrees that the client is entering the terminal stage of the disease. In his opinion, however, the client is not ready to discuss end-of-life issues. He states that the client has declined to discuss DNR orders with him. You ask the physician to convene a family conference about the issues. He refuses, stating that he believes the client is not ready to participate.

Step 1: Is this an ethical dilemma? What may at first appear to be a question of ethics may be resolved by clarifying your knowledge base about clinical facts. A review of policy and procedure, or of standards of care, may reveal legal obligations that determine a course of action, regardless of personal opinion. If the question remains perplexing, and

> BOX 8-5   **How to Process an Ethical Dilemma**

Step 1:   Determine whether the issue is an ethical dilemma.
Step 2:   Gather all the information relevant to the case.
Step 3:   Examine and determine your own values on the issues.
Step 4:   Verbalize the problem.
Step 5:   Consider possible courses of action.
Step 6:   Reflect on the outcome.
Step 7:   Evaluate the action and the outcome.

the answer will be profoundly relevant to several areas of human concern, then an ethical dilemma may exist.

The single mother's situation meets the criteria for an ethical dilemma. Further review of scientific data will probably not contribute to a resolution of the dilemma, but it is important to review the data carefully to make this determination. The disagreement does not revolve around whether the client is in a terminally ill state, so further clinical information will not change the basic question: Should the client have an opportunity to discuss DNR orders at this time? The question is perplexing. Two professional team members disagree on an assessment of a client's readiness to confront the difficult issues related to dying. The answer to the question "Is this client ready to discuss end of life?" has important implications. If she is not ready, then raising the issue may cause anguish and fear in the client and her family. If she is ready and the team avoids discussion, she may suffer unnecessarily in silence. If she is very close to death, then in the absence of a DNR order, necessitate cardiopulmonary resuscitation (CPR) will be performed in a futile situation. You know that CPR can cause pain. If applied in a situation in which the client's life is unlikely to be extended or improved, then CPR could prolong her suffering and reduce her dignity.

Step 2: Gather as much information as possible that is relevant to the case. Because resolution to dilemmas may arise from unlikely sources, incorporate as much knowledge as possible at every step of the process. At this point, the information could include laboratory and test results, the clinical state of the client, and current literature about the diagnosis or condition of the client. It may include investigation of the psychosocial concerns of the client, as well as those of her significant others. The client's religious, cultural, and family orientations are part of the nurse's assessment.

You obtain all the clinical information that is pertinent to the question. It may be helpful to determine whether the client retains most cognitive functions, even though her tumour is aggressive. You review the chart and discuss this aspect with the physician, and you agree that the client is fully competent but afraid and overwhelmed by the prognosis. Because two professionals disagree on a client's state of mind, it may be helpful to reassess the client or request that an independent person assess the client's readiness to discuss end-of-life issues. Sometimes family members or significant others hold important clues to a client's state of mind.

Step 3: Examine and determine your own values on the issues. This step is important for all participants in the discussion. At this stage, you and the other participants practice values clarification, and you differentiate between your own values and the values of the client and of other health care team members. Essential parts of the goal are to form your own opinion and to respect others' opinions.

At this point, you stop to reflect on your own values. Your own religious practices may allow you to decide to forgo further treatment if you were in the client's condition. You also may not yet have family members who rely on you, such as children or elderly parents. This client's religious practices may be more strictly constructed than your own. Her religion discourages actions that diminish life in any way, and you realize that she may have come to see a DNR order as giving up, or as "acting like God." In addition, you understand that the attending physician has not had time to know this client as her own physician has or as you have. You continue to believe that the client would be capable of a discussion, despite her statements to the physician. In fact, you believe that she would benefit from a discussion, because perhaps the presence of an unfamiliar caretaker, combined with declining physical health, has silenced her, even though her fears and concerns persist.

Step 4: Verbalize the problem. Once all relevant information has been gathered, accurate definition of the problem may proceed. It is helpful to state the problem in a few sentences. By agreeing to a statement of the problem, the health care team, the patient, and the family can proceed with discussion in a focused way.

Here, the problem seems to be this: whether this client should discuss DNR at this time. Determine the benefits and risks of a DNR order at this time. Other important questions relate to the client's current state of mind: Is she afraid to speak? Is she feeling cut off from her normal network (a primary physician)? Are these feelings contributing to confusion about DNR decisions?

Step 5: Consider possible courses of action. What options are available within the context of the situation and the client's values?

Once you have asked the basic question, other questions and possible courses of action arise. Should you initiate a discussion with the client independently of the physician? Would you be outside your professional role if you facilitated a DNR order? What if your assessment were incorrect? Would you contribute not to the dignity but to the distress of the client? The answers to these questions may be elusive, because they depend on an understanding of the client's feelings and values that are not necessarily obvious. Even if the nurse cannot legally write a DNR order, the nurse can influence a physician's or client's decision regarding DNR; therefore, troubling questions remain.

Step 6: Reflect on the outcome. This is the most important and delicate step of the process. These negotiations may happen informally at the client's bedside or in the charting room, or a formal ethics meeting may be necessary. Your point of view represents a unique contribution to the discussion.

In an ethics committee meeting, the discussion is usually multidisciplinary. A facilitator or chairperson ensures that all points of view are examined and that all pertinent issues are identified. A decision or recommendation is the usual outcome of discussion and the result of a successful discussion. In the best of circumstances, participants discover a course of action that meets criteria for acceptance by all. On occasion, however, participants may leave the discussion disappointed or even opposed to the decision.

The discussion focuses on the disagreement between your assessment and the physician's regarding the client's readiness to discuss end-of-life issues. The principles involved during the discussion include beneficence and nonmaleficence: Which plan would provide the most good for this client—a DNR order or no order? A separate question addresses the client's point of view: Would a discussion with the client promote well-being or promote anguish? Furthermore, according to the principle of autonomy, a troublesome question remains: Does the client want something different from the desire she is expressing?

With several members of the health care team present, the discussion proceeds. You present your point of view. You continue to sense that the client is ready to discuss DNR orders but that she may be reluctant to trust the circumstances of this admission. But you also respect the attending physician and his analysis and continue to be concerned that the client may have experienced a change of mind between the last admission and this one. In the end, the team proposes the following: a formal meeting with the client, in which you, the attending physician, and a supportive family member are all present. You support this proposal because you sense that it will maximize the support of the client's existing network. In addition, you recognize that in a trusting environment, the client is more likely to express her fears, insecurities, and wishes. Team members agree to keep the discussion open ended and exploratory. You suggest that rather than asking whether the client wants a DNR order, perhaps the team could wait for her to bring up the issue. In this way, the team could be assured of her consent and willingness to participate in the discussion.

Step 7: Evaluate the action and the outcome.

At the meeting, the client in fact opens up. She expresses relief at the chance to explore her options and feelings. Pain management issues are clarified. She wants to discuss a DNR order but requests a visit from her priest before she must make a final decision.

Ethical Issues in Nursing Practice

With increased professional responsibility and accountability, and with changes in the workplace and health care system, you are increasingly facing a myriad of ethical issues. You face ethical issues daily while caring for clients and families, while relating to other health care professionals, institutions, and global societal issues. The following section explores current issues in which ethical issues arise.

Client Care Issues

Informed Consent. The intimacy and integrity of the nurse–client relationship mandate that you protect the rights of their clients. You achieve this mandate as you follow standards, policies, guidelines, and legislation regarding consent to treatment. **Informed consent** is consent to treatment on the basis of accurate and complete information (see Chapter 9). The goal of informed consent is to protect the client's right to autonomy. The CNA (2008) *Code of Ethics* (p. 11) asserts that to promote and respect informed decision making, some of the nurse's ethical responsibilities are as follows:

- Building trusting relationships to ensure that the client's choice is understood, expressed, and advocated.
- Providing the desired information and support so that clients can make informed decisions.
- Assisting clients in obtaining the most accurate current knowledge about their health condition.
- Being sensitive to the inherent power differentials between health care professionals and clients: nurses must not misuse power to influence decision making.
- Recognizing that the client has the right to refuse or withdraw consent.
- Respecting the informed choices of capable persons, including choice of lifestyles or of treatment not conducive to good health.

Many unethical scenarios can involve consent: a client's signing consent forms without understanding what treatment entails; a nurse's mistaken assumption that a physician has explained a medical procedure to a client before obtaining the client's consent; obtaining consent from a client who does not speak the health care team's language without the assistance of an interpreter; or a client's consenting to a procedure without knowing about associated risks or potential adverse side effects.

Although obtaining informed consent for medical procedures is not a nursing duty, you may witness the client's signature on the consent form. When you provide consent forms for clients to sign, your main responsibility lies with ensuring that the client fully understands the nature of the treatment or procedure. If not, notification of the physician must occur so that the physician can clarify or provide additional information.

Futile Care. In the early 1980s, issues such as enhanced life-sustaining technologies, clients rights movements, and growing concerns about using health care resources in a cost-effective and efficient manner led to academic discussions, debates, and practice policies on medical futility. **Medical futility** is defined as a medical treatment that is considered nonbeneficial because it is believed to offer no reasonable hope of recovery from or improvement in the client's condition (CNA, 2001). Clients often worry, in the event of their becoming incapacitated and unable to express their wishes, that they will be "hooked up to machines" and receive treatment that

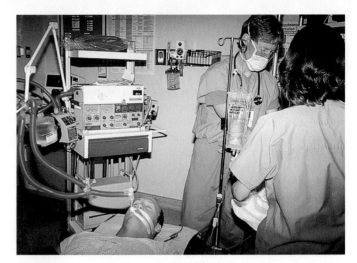

Figure 8-1 Nurses often struggle when clients are receiving care that they believe is prolonging their suffering and their life.

they do not desire (Figure 8–1). At issue is whether clinicians are sufficiently objective to establish that a given intervention is futile and that they are therefore authorized to withhold or withdraw its use (Callahan, 1991).

Although health care professionals are best equipped to determine the physical benefits of treatment, only the client or people who know the client best can determine whether treatment is advancing the client's overall well-being. Bennett Jacobs and Taylor (2005a) identified this issue as "qualitative" futility or subjective determination, in which not just medical facts but also values lead the client or the client's surrogate decision makers to conclude that the treatment has no benefit according to those values.

Achieving holistic outcomes of care must be based on an interplay of physical facts and subjective values. Taylor (1995) suggested the following four classifications of futility: (1) not futile: beneficial to both physical and overall well-being; (2) futile: nonbeneficial to either physical or overall well-being; (3) futile from the client's perspective: medically indicated but not valued by the client; and (4) futile from the clinicians' perspective and not medically indicated but valued by the client (p. 301). It is evident that these classifications have objective and subjective dimensions, as well as quantitative and qualitative dimensions, and constitute a more complete way of viewing the complex notion of futility.

The issue of who has priority in health care decision making remains complex and often troublesome. The potential for futility conflicts is high in situations of critically and chronically ill clients. What then, is your role? Taylor (1995) suggested that nurses play a leading role in working toward pursuing negotiated compromise between health care professionals and clients equally, for the best possible outcome for the particular client. She suggested that this may be accomplished "by identifying patients, families, and health care teams at risk of experiencing conflict about futile care, and then initiating dialogue that may prevent or resolve conflict" (p. 303).

Advance directives are one way to address this problem (see Chapter 9). They are "the means used to document and communicate a person's preferences regarding life-sustaining treatment in the event that they become incapable of expressing those wishes for themselves" (CNA, 1998, p. 1). Advance directives are commonly expressed in two ways: (1) an instruction directive, or living will, that identifies what life-sustaining treatment a client desires in certain situations, and (2) a proxy directive, or power or attorney for personal care, that explains who is to make health care decisions if the client becomes incompetent (CNA, 1998). A routine part of any admission to a hospital now usually includes inquiry about the client's advance directives; if they exist, they are included as part of the medical record. It has become necessary for nurses to be aware of the legal status of all types of advance directives in their province or territory.

You have several roles regarding advance directives. You may be involved in helping clients plan an advance directive by discussing its uses and helping clients to clarify their values and wishes for end-of-life treatment. Your role also includes following the advance directive, alerting other health care professionals to changes in the client's wishes, and advocating on behalf of the client or substitute decision maker if the client's wishes or advance directive are not being followed.

Withdrawal of Food and Hydration. Maintaining nutrition is a natural life-sustaining measure and common part of the nursing role. A change in the client's ability to drink and eat raises many issues. When food and hydration are administered for a prolonged period to a client whose condition is not expected to improve, some nurses may view this care as extraordinary or heroic, whereas others see this as humane.

Current literature suggests that fluids should not be routinely administered to dying individuals or automatically withheld from them; rather, they should be given on the basis of the goals of care and a careful assessment of the client's comfort. A position statement by the CNA (2001) on futility stresses the importance of the health care team to determine whether food and fluid are most beneficial or harmful to a client. The following questions may aid health care professionals in reflecting on the goals of care: Will the client's well-being be enhanced by administration of nutrition? Does the client have symptoms that could be relieved or aggravated by administration of nutrition? Could hydration enhance the client's mental status or level of consciousness? Will it prolong the client's life? Is that the wish of the client and family? (Bennett Jacobs & Taylor, 2005b; Ganzini, 2006).

Administration of hydration may raise dilemmas when its use is intended merely to maintain physical life (e.g., when the client is in a vegetative state or is near death). You should know that during the natural dying process, the body starts to "shut down," and the client may lose the desire for food and fluids. Force-feeding a dying client may sometimes do more harm than good. Withholding or withdrawing nutrition or hydration from a client is no different from the decision to forgo any other medical treatment that may prolong the dying process. It is considered appropriate to withhold or discontinue life-sustaining medical interventions if they are not benefiting the client or are contrary to the client's wishes. Furthermore, it is important to stress to families that dying individuals who are not receiving artificial nutrition or hydration will still be provided with adequate overall care.

Issues of Safety in the Work Environment

Nurses are responsible for providing safe, compassionate, competent, and ethical care (CNA, 2008). In ensuring safety, care must be such that harm is minimized. Lack of control over important aspects of the environment can lead to ethically ambiguous situations (Austin et al., 2003). Complex life-and-death events, multiple role responsibilities, loyalties and expectations, reduced numbers of skilled health care professionals, minimal clinical nursing leadership, interdisciplinary team conflict, and autocratic organizational

decision making may create personal moral conflict for you (Aiken et al., 2002; Canadian Health Services Research Foundation, 2006).

Causing harm to clients in the form of pain and suffering from continuing treatment is a source of **moral distress** for nurses that they often believe could be avoided. "Moral distress arises when there is inconsistency between one's beliefs and one's actions" (Hardingham, 2004, p. 128). Sometimes nurses find it hard to care for a client when other health care professionals, usually physicians, make choices that nurses think are causing more harm than good. For example, the situation of a client in intensive care who is comatose but seems to experience great pain when turned over can be very upsetting for nurses. They may experience moral distress if they feel that they are, in effect, torturing the client each time they turn him or her over. Keeping clients safe from harm can be difficult, and sometimes it requires great ethical sensitivity to be aware of harms that are being caused. In these situations, nurses may lose their sense of **moral integrity** or "wholeness" when they are committed to certain values and beliefs that are not upheld because of situational constraints. If these situations continue and integrity is compromised, nurses may experience **moral residue**, a long-lasting discomfort that arises whenever they face moral distress (Webster & Baylis, 2000). Relational ethics helps you know what the client considers harm, and it is crucial to engage in discussions with your clients and colleagues.

Other kinds of harm can come to clients because of inadequate or inappropriate caregiving. Sometimes harm results from mistakes that can be explained; sometimes it results from carelessness or incompetence. For example, when you have a lot of very ill clients to care for and you have many demands on your time, medication errors can occur because you are distracted and feeling rushed. These kinds of errors are unfortunate, but they are not breaches of ethics as such. On the other hand, if you make a medication error because you have been out partying all night before your shift and you were not fit to practice that day, the error would be considered unethical. Either way, you need to monitor your own competence to practice, and you must admit to your mistakes. Regardless of the cause, if you make a mistake, not admitting it is considered unethical.

In a multidisciplinary environment, all health care professionals must take responsibility for the care that is provided (Box 8–6). You need to be aware of what other professionals are doing for and with their clients. If **adverse events** occur—that is, "unexpected, undesirable incidents resulting in injury or death that are directly associated with the process of providing health care or services to a person receiving care" (CNA 2008, p. 18)—then you must report them, regardless of who is responsible. The person who is most directly involved when an adverse event occurs should be the one to report it, but sometimes that does not happen. In that situation, if you observe the event, you must report it. It is your obligation to ensure client safety, but it is not easy because it can mean exposing the incompetence of a colleague. Imagine, for example, that you observe another nurse drop a frail elderly client during transfer. The client does not seem hurt, and the other nurse does not seem to plan to report the incident. Should you report it yourself? Your obligation is to speak to the other nurse and ensure that the incident is reported. If the nurse does not report it, then you must, inasmuch as this is a clear issue of client safety, and your obligations are clear. **Whistleblowing** (i.e., reporting a colleague's errors, incompetence, unsafe or negligent practice, or abuse of clients) is one of the most difficult actions you must take in ensuring that safe, compassionate, competent, and ethical care is met (Oberle & Raffin Bouchal, 2009).

✳ BOX 8-6 RESEARCH HIGHLIGHT

Ethics in Nursing Practice

Research Focus

Rodney et al. (2006) were interested in exploring ethical nursing practice in a large emergency department and a medical oncology unit located in separate regions of British Columbia, Canada. Rodney et al.'s goal was to describe the moral climate of nurses' workplaces and how the nurses acted to improve it.

Research Abstract

This participatory action research study involved participant observation, interviews, focus groups, meetings, workshops, and everyday work in the two practice settings. The research team at each site included a team of staff nurses (clinical nurse researchers), academic investigators, and research assistants, all of whom worked in partnership. Qualitative data were collected in focus groups, interviews, and regular meetings with staff to discuss, debrief, and plan for change. The research process supported staff in initiating changes in their workplaces aimed at improving the environment for ethical practice.

Evidence-Informed Practice

- Strong evidence must influence the everyday practice of individual nurses and the moral climate in which nursing care takes place.

- Many factors influence nurses' difficulties in practising ethically: deficiencies in resources; how nurses feel about themselves; how they treat other nurses and health care professionals, clients, and clients' families; and how they are treated by other professionals who also adhere to the often unspoken values that reflect their practices.

Reporting the wrongdoing of a colleague can be distressing. You worry about how to report or deal with unacceptable practice and still maintain healthy relationships with other colleagues. You need to examine relative risks and benefits and then decide on appropriate action (Box 8–7). You must be prepared to struggle with difficult questions and reflect on the facts and your internal values and perspectives. Such concerns, in addition to having elements of a classic dilemma, reveal the complexity and effect of relational issues within the workplace. When positive professional relationships are absent, both the profession and the professionals suffer.

References: Rodney, P., Hartrick Doane, G., Storch, J., & Varcoe, C. (2006). Ethics in action: Strengthening nurses' enactment of their moral agency within the cultural context of health care delivery. *Canadian Nurse, 102*(8), 25–26.

✳ BOX 8-7 FOCUS ON PRIMARY HEALTH CARE

How to Encourage Nurses Individually and Collectively to Work Toward Eliminating Social Inequities

- Utilize the principles of primary health care for the benefit of the public and clients receiving care.
- Understand that some groups in society are systemically disadvantaged, which leads to poorer health and diminished well-being. Nurses work to improve the quality of lives of people who are part of disadvantaged and vulnerable groups and communities, and they take action to overcome barriers to health care.
- Recognize and work to address organizational, social, economic, and political factors that influence health and well-being within the context of your role in the delivery of care.

✳ KEY CONCEPTS

- Values clarification helps nurses explore personal values and feelings and to decide how to act on personal beliefs. It also facilitates nurse-client communication.
- Ethics is the study of philosophical ideals of what is beneficial or valuable for all.
- A code of ethics provides a foundation for professional nursing. Such a code promotes accountability, responsibility, and advocacy.
- Theories of bioethics refer to ethical issues specific to the delivery of health care. They are based on the principles of autonomy, beneficence, nonmaleficence, and justice.
- Relational ethics theory encompasses more than bioethics: It addresses the role of relationship in the ethical delivery of health care. It maintains that the nurse-client relationship is the foundation of nursing ethics.
- Ethical problems arise from differences in values, from technological advances, from end-of-life experiences, and from changes in work environments.

- A standard process for thinking through ethical dilemmas, including critical thinking skills, helps health care professionals resolve conflict or uncertainty about correct actions.

✳ CRITICAL THINKING EXERCISES

1. Complete the values clarification exercise (Box 8-1) with your classmates or others. Compare the answers and discuss the differences.

2. You are a clinic nurse in a small community clinic. A 17-year-old female client has been coming to the clinic for treatment for and support with a sexually transmitted disease. During recent months, she has lost her support from a close friend. In addition, her parents are divorced, and she has little contact with them. Her health and well-being are of concern. Her appearance is unkempt, her nutritional status is not balanced, and she has admitted to being depressed. She asks for your help in planning her suicide. Discuss your response to her request. Begin by acknowledging the laws related to assisted suicide in Canada. Examine your personal feelings about suicide. Include a discussion about your understanding of sexually transmitted diseases: Where do they come from? Who gets these diseases? Why do people get these diseases? What are your feelings and opinions about people with sexually transmitted diseases? Construct your response, keeping in mind the theory of relational ethics. Discuss your role in this situation. What are your possible courses of action?

3. You have been assigned the care of a 98-year-old woman who was recently admitted with a diagnosis of pneumonia. She has a history of cardiac disease and takes a number of medications. She had been fairly active until the past few days, when her cough worsened and a fever developed. You note that her pulse has become weak and threadlike and that her respirations are increasingly laboured. The client is now too weak to respond to you. When you mention to the family that you may need to call the physician and even take heroic lifesaving measures, the client's son and daughter become distraught, saying that they do not want their mother to be kept alive on "machines." They report that they have discussed this situation with their mother.

You find that her wishes have not been documented in her chart. The family members have not discussed this situation with the client's primary physician. What actions would you consider taking at this moment? Take into account the ethical principles of autonomy and beneficence and the idea of futile care. What are your personal values about interventions at the end of life?

✽ REVIEW QUESTIONS

1. Values clarification plays a major role in:
   1. Creating a set of rules for conduct
   2. Identifying values that should be accepted by all
   3. Resolving issues of "value conflict"
   4. Developing a code of ethics

2. In Canada, equitable access to health care means that all citizens have equal access to medically necessary services. Many jurisdictions have implemented private magnetic resonance imaging clinics. A discussion about the ethics of this situation would involve predominately the principle of
   1. Accountability
   2. Autonomy
   3. Relational ethics
   4. Justice

3. It may seem redundant when health care professionals, including professional nurses, agree to "do no harm" to their clients. The point of this agreement is to reassure the public that in all ways, not only will the health care team work to heal clients but they also agree to do this in the least painful and harmful way possible. The principle that describes this agreement is called
   1. Beneficence
   2. Accountability
   3. Nonmaleficence
   4. Respect for autonomy

4. Vaccination may cause temporary discomfort, but the benefits of protection from disease, both for the individual and for society, outweigh the client's discomfort. This involves the principle of
   1. Beneficence
   2. Fidelity
   3. Nonmaleficence
   4. Respect for autonomy

5. If a nurse assesses a client for pain and then offers a plan to manage the pain, the principle that encourages the nurse to monitor the client's response to the plan is
   1. Beneficence
   2. Justice
   3. Nonmaleficence
   4. Respect for autonomy

6. Including clients in decision making regarding their care and respecting their choices of treatment demonstrate the principle of:
   1. Beneficence
   2. Autonomy
   3. Justice
   4. Veracity

7. Nurses agree to be advocates for their clients. Practice of advocacy calls for the nurse to
   1. Seek out a nursing supervisor in situations involving conflict
   2. Work to understand the law as it applies to the client's clinical condition
   3. Assess the client's point of view and prepare to articulate this point of view
   4. Document all clinical changes in the medical record in a timely manner

8. Which of the following is *not* part of the nurse's role as client advocate?
   1. Intervening if other people fail to respect the client's dignity
   2. Protecting the client's right to confidentiality and privacy
   3. Making nursing care decisions for the client
   4. Advocating for appropriate use of interventions to minimize suffering

9. The philosophy of relational ethics suggests that ethical dilemmas can best be solved by attention to
   1. Relationships
   2. Ethical principles
   3. Clients
   4. Code of ethics for nurses

10. Ethical dilemmas often arise over a conflict of opinion. Once the nurse has determined that the dilemma is ethical, a critical first step in negotiating the difference of opinion is to
    1. Consult a professional ethicist to ensure that the steps of the process occur in full
    2. Gather all relevant information regarding the dilemma
    3. List the ethical principles that inform the dilemma so that negotiations agree on the language of the discussion
    4. Ensure that the attending physician has written an order for an ethics consultation to support the ethics process

✽ RECOMMENDED WEB SITES

Canadian Bioethics Society: http://www.bioethics.ca
Founded in 1988 through the amalgamation of the Canadian Society of Bioethics and the Canadian Society for Medical Bioethics. Members include health care administrators, lawyers, nurses, philosophers, physicians, theologians, and other professionals concerned with the ethical and humane dimensions of health care. The Web site offers information about the annual CBS conference, national and international ethics organization links, and relevant ethics journals from a variety of disciplines.

Canadian Nurses Association–Code of Ethics: http://www.cna-aiic.ca/CNA/documents/pdf/publications/ Code_of_Ethics_2008_e.pdf
Provides a link to the CNA and the *Code of Ethics for Registered Nurses* (CNA, 2008).

W. Maurice Young Centre for Applied Ethics: http://www.ethics.ubc.ca
Established by the University of British Columbia in 1993; primarily an interdisciplinary research centre in which a variety of ethics topics are studied. The Web site has links to other ethics organizations and ethics resources. The centre's newsletter is also available on the Web site.

Nursing Ethics.ca: http://www.nursingethics.ca/
Has links to Canadian resources that support ethical nursing practice.

Provincial Health Ethics Network of Alberta (PHEN): http://www.phen.ab.ca/
Established as a society in 1995; provides information for all Albertans about ethics and access to health ethics resources. Its mission is to facilitate examination, discussion, and decision making with regard to ethical issues in health and health care.

9

Legal Implications in Nursing Practice

Written by Carla Shapiro, MN, RN

Based on the original chapter by Janis Waite, RN, MSN, EdD

objectives

Mastery of content in this chapter will enable you to:

- Define the key terms listed.
- Explain legal concepts that apply to nurses.
- Describe the legal responsibilities and obligations of nurses.
- List sources for standards of care for nurses.
- Define legal aspects of nurse–client, nurse–physician, nurse–nurse, and nurse–employer relationships.
- List the elements needed to prove negligence.
- Give examples of legal issues that arise in nursing practice.

media resources

evolve Web Site

- Audio Chapter Summaries
- Glossary
- Multiple-Choice Review Questions
- Student Learning Activities
- Weblinks

Companion CD

- Glossary
- Interactive Learning Activities
- Fluids and Electrolytes Tutorial
- Test-Taking Skills

Safe nursing practice includes knowledge of the legal boundaries within which nurses must function. Nurses must understand the law to protect themselves from liability and to protect their clients' rights. Nurses need not fear the law; rather, they should view it as representing what society expects from them. Laws are continually changing to meet the needs of the people they are intended to protect. As technology has expanded the role of the nurse, the ethical dilemmas associated with client care have increased and often become legal issues as well. As health care evolves, so do the legal implications for health care. Although federal laws apply to all provinces and territories, nurses must also be aware that laws do vary across the country. It is important for nurses to know the laws in their province or territory that affect their practice. Being familiar with the law enhances nurses' ability to be client advocates.

Legal Limits of Nursing

Nurses have a fiduciary relationship with their clients. A fiduciary relationship is one in which a professional (the nurse) provides services that, by their nature, cause the recipient (the client) to trust in the specialized knowledge and integrity of the professional. In the fiduciary relationship, nurses are obligated to provide knowledgeable, competent, and safe care.

Although legal actions against nurses were once rare, the situation is changing. The public is better informed now than in the past about their rights to health care and are more likely to seek damages for professional negligence. The courts have upheld the concept that nurses must provide a reasonable standard of care. Thus, it is essential that nurses understand the legal limits influencing their daily practice.

Sources of Law

The Canadian legal system can be divided into two main categories: public law and private law. Public law is chiefly concerned with relations between individuals and the state or society in general and includes constitutional, tax, administrative, human rights, and criminal law. Private law involves disputes between individuals and covers issues such as wills, contracts, marriage and divorce, and civil wrongs (e.g., negligence). Whereas public law is addressed in the same manner across the country, two systems deal with private law issues—**civil law** (based on Roman law) in Quebec and **common law** (based on British common law) throughout the rest of the country. These two systems differ primarily in their legal processes. In each system, courts interpret the rules made by the legislature in the context of specific disputes.

When either a civil or a criminal case goes to court, decisions are based on previous case rulings. How courts rule on the circumstances and facts surrounding the case is called a *precedent*. If a case is decided on the basis of certain facts, the court is bound to follow that decision in subsequent similar cases. Not every jurisdiction has case law on a given issue. For example, cases regarding a client's right to refuse treatment are not found in every province. In such situations, other jurisdictions are consulted for guidance. In general, breaches of private law result in the payment of money to compensate the aggrieved party for damages incurred. Violations of public law may result in a range of remedies, including fines or imprisonment.

Statute law is created by elective legislative bodies such as Parliament and provincial or territorial legislatures. Federal statutes apply throughout the country, and provincial and territorial statutes apply only in the province or territory in which they were created. Examples of provincial statutes are the *Regulated Health Professions Act* (1991) in Ontario and nursing practice acts throughout the country, which describe and define nursing practice within each province.

Examples of federal statutes are the new *Assisted Human Reproduction Act* (2004), the *Controlled Drugs and Substances Act* (1996), and the *Food and Drugs Act* (1985).

Professional Regulation

Like all self-governing professions in Canada, nursing is regulated at the provincial or territorial level. Each province and territory has legislation that grants authority to a nursing regulatory body. These regulatory bodies are accountable to the public for ensuring safe, competent, and ethical nursing care. Regulatory bodies are responsible for granting certificates of registration, offering practice support, ensuring continuing competence of its members, investigating complaints against members' conduct, and disciplining members when necessary. Regulatory bodies are also responsible for developing codes of ethics, setting standards of practice, and approving nursing education programs (McIntyre et al., 2006).

Separate regulatory bodies exist for registered nurses and practical nurses. Some provinces also have regulatory bodies for registered psychiatric nurses. These regulatory bodies are called either the *provincial association* or the *college of nursing* (e.g., the Alberta Association of Registered Nurses; the College of Licensed Practical Nurses of Alberta; the College of Nurses of Ontario). The trend appears to be a move to the college model, with a stronger focus on regulation of practice and accountability to the public.

Nurses must be registered by the professional nursing association or college of the province or territory in which they practise. The requirements for registration (or licensure, as applicable) varies across the country, but most provinces and territories have minimum education requirements and require the nurse to pass an examination. All provinces and territories (except Quebec) use the Canadian Registered Nurse Examination. Quebec has created its own examination. Registration (or licensure) enables people to practise nursing and use the applicable nursing title and initials: registered nurse (RN) or registered practical nurse (RPN). All nurses' credentials must be verified, either by the listing of their names on a register or by their holding a valid licence to practise.

Registration can be suspended or revoked by the regulatory body if a nurse's conduct violates provisions in the registration statute. For example, nurses who perform illegal acts, such as selling controlled substances, jeopardize their registration status. Due process must be followed before registration can be suspended or revoked. *Due process* means that nurses must be notified of the charges brought against them and have an opportunity to defend themselves against the charges in a hearing. Such hearings do not occur in courts but are usually conducted by the regulatory body. If a nurse loses his or her professional licence, or if the nurse's name is removed from the provincial or territorial register, and if the case involves civil or criminal wrongs, then further legal consequences may follow.

Standards of Care

Standards of care are legal guidelines for nursing practice. Standards establish an expectation of nurses to provide safe and appropriate client care. If nurses do not perform duties within accepted standards of care, they may place themselves in jeopardy of legal action and, more important, place their clients at risk for harm and injury. Nursing standards of care arise from a variety of sources, including statutes and laws of broad application, such as the statutes and common law relating to human rights, privacy, and negligence; provincial statutes that specifically apply to health care professionals or nurses only; and the detailed regulations, practice standards, and codes of ethics that are generated by the professional associations. Nursing standards are also outlined in the written policies and procedures of employing institutions.

All provincial and territorial legislatures have passed health professions, **nursing practice acts**, or both that define the scope of nursing practice. These acts set educational requirements for nurses, distinguish between nursing and medical practice, and generally define nursing practice. The rules and regulations enacted by the provincial or territorial regulatory body help define the practice of nursing more specifically. For example, a nursing association may develop a rule regarding intravenous therapy. All nurses are responsible for knowing the provisions of the nursing practice act for the province or territory in which they work, as well as the rules and regulations enacted by the regulatory administrative bodies of their province or territory.

Professional organizations are another source for defining standards of care. The Canadian Nurses Association (CNA) has developed standards for nursing practice, policy statements, and similar resolutions. The standards delineate the scope, function, and role of the nurse in practice. Nursing specialty organizations also have standards of practice defined for certification of nurses who work in specific specialty areas, such as the operating room or the critical care unit. The same standards also serve as practice guidelines for defining safe and appropriate nursing care in specialty areas.

The Canadian Council on Health Services Accreditation requires that accredited health care institutions have nursing policies and procedures in writing that detail how nurses are to perform their duties. These internal standards of care are usually quite specific and are found in procedural manuals on most nursing units. For example, a procedure or policy that outlines the steps that should be taken when a dressing is changed or medication is administered gives specific information about how nurses are to perform these tasks. Nurses must know the policies and procedures of their employing institution because they all must follow the same standard of care. Institutional policies and procedures must conform to laws and cannot conflict with legal guidelines that define acceptable standards of care.

In a negligence lawsuit, these standards are used to determine whether the nurse has acted as any reasonably prudent nurse in a similar setting with the same credentials would act. A nursing expert is called to testify about the standards of nursing care as applied to the facts of the case (Box 9–1). The expert may be called to define and explain to the court what a reasonably prudent nurse would have been expected to do in view of the facts of the case in any similar setting around the country. It is recognized and understood that nursing practice differs according to the rural or urban nature of the institutional setting. In addition, home health care, occupational health nursing, and other community-based clinical settings require that the expert be familiar with the standards of care in these settings, as opposed to the traditional hospital or institutional setting. The expert must have the appropriate credentials, the appropriate experience, and an understanding of what the standard of care should have been in the specific case. The expert witness is distinguished from the fact witness. Staff nurses may testify in a court proceeding as fact witnesses if they have first-hand personal experience with the facts of the case. The expert witness evaluates the defendant's professional judgements and behaviour under the circumstances being reviewed.

General duty nurses are often legally responsible for meeting the same standards as other general duty nurses in similar settings. However, specialized nurses, such as nurses in a critical care unit or nurses who perform dialysis, are held to standards of care and skill that apply to all professionals in the same specialty. All nurses must know the standards of care that they are expected to meet within their specific specialty and work setting. Ignorance of the law or of standards of care is not a defence against negligence, nor is being asked by an employer to perform an out-of-scope procedure. The law as written overrules any agency policy or procedure.

> ▶ **BOX 9-1** Anatomy of a Lawsuit

Pleadings: Statements of Claim and Defence

- The plaintiff outlines what the defendant or defendants did wrong and how that action caused injury.
- The statement of claim is then issued by the court and served on the defendant or defendants.
- Statements of claim are often very broad and may be served on the employer, institution, and all members of the health care team involved in the client's care at the relevant time.
- The defendant or defendants must deliver a statement of defence to the allegations. The defendant or defendants can admit or deny each allegation in the petition.

Procedures of Discovery

Pretrial proceedings enable each side to gather legally relevant information from the other side and usually lead to a settlement between the parties before a trial.

1. *Examination for discovery:* The plaintiff's lawyer is permitted to question each defendant under oath. Examination for discovery usually takes place in private offices, with only the plaintiffs and defendants, their lawyers, and a reporter present to record a transcript of the testimony. Questioning can be wide-ranging and detailed in order to reveal useful information. Answers given to questions will be available for trial.
2. *Discovery of documents:* Each side can be forced to produce all documents relevant to the litigation. Medical records and nurses' notes may be of particular value.
3. *Independent medical examination of the plaintiff:* This examination is conducted to determine the extent of the plaintiff's injuries. Negligence cannot be charged without proof of damage.
4. *Discovery by interrogatories:* Similar to the examination for discovery, interrogatories involves a series of written questions, which must be answered under oath.

Expert Witnesses

An expert witness is an individual who, because of education, experience, or both, has knowledge that can assist decision makers in establishing whether the nursing care that was provided met the expected standard of practice. Each side usually selects experts to help explain and interpret the evidence as it emerges.

Pretrial Conference

The purpose of the pretrial conference is to identify points of contention, narrow down the issues, and encourage settlement out of court. In some jurisdictions, the pretrial conference may be mandatory. A pretrial conference is presided over by a judge and attended by counsel for the various parties. Most settlements take place without any admission of liability.

Trial

A trial usually occurs several years after the initial statement of claim is filed. Most nursing negligence cases are heard and decided by a judge alone. Damages are usually assessed at trial.

Legal Liability Issues in Nursing Practice

Torts

A **tort** is a civil wrong committed against a person or property. Torts may be classified as intentional or unintentional. **Intentional torts** are willful acts that violate another person's rights (Keatings & Smith, 2000). Examples are assault, battery, invasion of privacy, and false imprisonment. Negligence is example of an unintentional tort.

Intentional Torts

Assault. **Assault** is conduct (such as a physical or verbal threat) that creates in another person apprehension or fear of imminent harmful or offensive contact. No actual contact is necessary in order for damages for assault to be awarded (Fridman, 2003; Osborne, 2003). Threats by a nurse to give a client an injection or to restrain a client for an x-ray procedure when the client has refused consent constitute assault. The key issues are whether the client was afraid of being harmed in the situation and whether the client consented to a procedure. In a lawsuit wherein assault is alleged, the client's consent would negate the claim of assault against a nurse.

Battery. **Battery** is any intentional physical contact with a person without that person's consent. The contact can be harmful to the client and cause an injury, or it can be merely offensive to the client's personal dignity (Sneiderman et al., 2003). In the example of a nurse's threats to give a client an injection without the client's consent, if the nurse actually gives the injection, it is considered battery. Battery could even be life-saving, as in the Ontario case of *Malette v. Shulman* (1990). In that case, the plaintiff was unconscious and bleeding profusely. The physician determined that she needed a life-saving blood transfusion. Before the transfusion, a nurse found a signed card in the plaintiff's purse that identified the client as a Jehovah's Witness and stated that under no circumstances was she to receive blood. Despite this, the physician chose to administer the blood to preserve the client's life. The plaintiff survived, recovered from her injuries, and successfully sued the physician for battery (Sneiderman et al., 2003).

In some situations, consent is implied. For example, if a client gets into a wheelchair or transfers to a stretcher of his or her own volition after being advised that it is time to be taken for an x-ray procedure, the client has given implied consent to the procedure. A client has the right to revoke or withdraw consent at any time.

Invasion of Privacy. The tort of invasion of privacy protects the client's right to be free from unwanted intrusion into his or her private affairs. Clients are entitled to confidential health care. Nursing standards for what constitutes confidential information are based on professional ethics and the common law. The ideals of privacy and sensitivity to the needs and rights of clients who may not choose to have nurses intrude on their lives, but who depend on nurses for their care, guide the nurse's judgement. The nurse's fiduciary duty requires that confidential information not be shared with anyone else except on a need-to-know basis.

One form of invasion of privacy is the release of a client's medical information to an unauthorized person, such as a member of the press or the client's employer. The information that is contained in a client's medical record is a confidential communication. It should be shared with health care providers only for the purpose of medical treatment.

A client's medical record is confidential. The nurse should not disclose the client's confidential medical information without the client's consent. For example, a nurse should respect a wish not to inform the client's family of a terminal illness. Similarly, a nurse should not assume that a client's spouse or family members know all of the client's history, particularly with regard to private issues such as mental illness, medications, pregnancy, abortion, birth control, or sexually transmitted infections.

Confidentiality is not an absolute value, however, and in certain circumstances, breaching confidentiality is justifiable. At times, a nurse may be required by law (statutory duty) to breach confidentiality and disclose information to a third party. For example, each province and territory has laws that require health care workers to report suspected child abuse to a local child protection agency. Nurses may also be required to release information about a client when they receive a subpoena (a legal order) to testify in court.

Nurses are under no legal obligation to release confidential information to the police except in rare cases in which the life, safety, or health of the client or an innocent third party is in jeopardy (such as when a client tells a nurse that he or she intends to hurt or kill someone; Tapp, 1996). Such a statement should be reported to the authorities of the institution and to the police. Other admissions made by a client to a nurse about past or future criminal activity may not have to be disclosed unless the nurse is compelled to do so by a court of law. The conflict between confidentiality and risk of public harm is not always clear. When a nurse has serious concerns about the welfare of others (e.g., if a client is infected with human immunodeficiency virus [HIV] and admits to having unsafe sex or donating blood), the nurse should first suggest and strongly encourage the client to disclose this information. If the client refuses, then the nurse should seek consultation with professional colleagues and supervisors. A careful balancing of the need for privacy and confidentiality of privileged communication would need to be weighed carefully.

Computers and Confidentiality. Most health care facilities use computer systems to maintain client records. "Computerization in health care raises major legal concerns related to confidentiality of health records because of the potential for unauthorized access and data sharing" (Tapp, 2003). Access to confidential client information is generally controlled by means of a variety of technological safeguards, including magnetized cards and passwords. It is important that these security devices not be shared with other people and that access cards be used to retrieve files only when warranted. The improper use of a magnetized card and password to seek out confidential information could lead to legal repercussions or disciplinary action.

Likewise, the use of e-mail messages carries a potential legal risk because they are susceptible to unauthorized access by third parties. E-mail messages may also be introduced as evidence in any court or legal proceedings (Tapp, 2001).

False Imprisonment. The tort of false imprisonment serves to protect a person's individual liberty and basic rights. Preventing a client from leaving a health care facility voluntarily may constitute the tort of false imprisonment. The inappropriate or unjustified use of restraints (e.g., by confining a person to an area, or by using physical or chemical restraints) may also be viewed as false imprisonment. Nurses must be aware of their facility's policies and specific legislation in their jurisdiction (e.g., under the *Mental Health and Consequential Amendments Act,* 1998) relating to when and how restraints can be used (Canadian Nurses Protective Society [CNPS], 2004a).

Unintentional Torts

Negligence. When nurses are sued, most often the proceedings against them are for the tort of negligence, also referred to as *malpractice* (Sneiderman et al., 2003). **Negligence** in nursing is conduct that does not meet a standard of care established by law. No intent is needed for negligence to occur. It is characterized chiefly by inadvertence, thoughtlessness, or inattention. Negligence may involve carelessness, such as not checking an identification bracelet, which results in administration of the wrong medication. However, carelessness is not always the cause of misconduct. If nurses perform a procedure for which they have not been educated and do so carefully but still harm the client, a claim of negligence can be made. In general, courts define nursing negligence as the failure to use the degree of skill or learning ordinarily used under the same or similar circumstances by members of the nursing profession (Box 9–2).

Nurses can be found liable for negligence if the following criteria are established: (1) The nurse (defendant) owed a duty to the client (plaintiff); (2) the nurse did not carry out that duty; (3) the client was injured; and (4) the nurse's failure to carry out the duty caused the injury.

The ability to predict harm (i.e., the foreseeability of risk) is evaluated in negligence cases. The circumstances surrounding the injury are evaluated to determine whether it was likely that the injury or harm to the client could have been expected from the care that was or was not provided. The cause of the injury is also investigated through the evaluation of the actual and the nearest causes of the injury. Had it not been for what the nurse did or did not do, could an injury have been prevented?

The case of *Downey v. Rothwell* (1974) is an example of nursing negligence. This case involved a plaintiff who suffered a severe arm injury when she fell off an examining table while under the care of a nurse. The client, who had a history of epilepsy, informed the nurse that she was about to have a seizure. The nurse left the client unattended on an examining table while she left the room for a few moments. During this time, the client had a seizure, fell onto the floor, and broke her arm. The nurse should have anticipated that the client could have fallen during a seizure and ensured her safety either by moving her to the floor or by putting up guard rails on the examining table. This case involved an undertaking by the nurse to provide care, a reliance by the client on this nurse, and a foreseeable risk. The nurse was found negligent in this case, and her employers were held vicariously liable. "Vicarious liability is a legal doctrine that applies in situations where the law holds the employer legally responsible for the acts of its employees that occur within the scope and course of their employment" (CNPS, 1998).

In the case of *Granger v. Ottawa General Hospital* (1996), two nurses (a staff nurse and her team leader) were found negligent in the care they provided to a woman in labour. During labour, the plaintiff's fetal heart monitor strip showed deep, persistent, variable decelerations. The staff nurse did not appreciate that these were a sign of fetal distress and did not immediately report these findings to other members of the obstetrical team. The ensuing delay in care resulted

in severe and permanent brain injury in the baby, leaving her severely disabled. In this case, the nurses breached their duty to exercise appropriate skill in making an assessment and to communicate the information to the physicians.

Preventing Negligence. The best way for nurses to avoid being negligent is to follow standards of care; give competent health care; insist on appropriate orientation, continuing education, and adequate staffing; communicate with other health care providers; develop a caring rapport with the client; and document assessments, interventions, and evaluations fully.

The health care record, or "chart," is a permanent record of the nursing process. The courts consult the patient's chart for a chronological record of all aspects of care provided from admission to discharge. "Courts use nursing documentation at trial to reconstruct events, establish times and dates, refresh memories of witnesses and . . . resolve conflicts in testimony" (CNPS, 2007a). As a legal document, it is the most comprehensive record of the care provided. Careful, complete, and thorough documentation is one of the best defences against allegations of negligence or violations of nursing standards (see Chapter 16). The record can show that even in the event of an adverse patient outcome, the nursing care that was provided met the expected standards. An institution has a legal duty to maintain nursing records. Nursing notes contain substantial evidence needed in order to understand the care received by a client. If records are lost or incomplete, the care is presumed to have been negligent and therefore the cause of the client's injuries. In addition, incomplete or illegible records undermine the credibility of the health care professional.

In the case of *Kolesar v. Jeffries* (1976), the Supreme Court of Canada addressed the issue of poor record keeping. In that case, a client underwent major spinal surgery and was transferred to a surgical unit, where he was nursed on a Stryker frame. The client was found dead the following morning. No nursing notes were recorded from 2200 hours the previous evening until 0500 hours, when he was found dead. Although at trial several nurses and nursing assistants testified that they had tended to the client multiple times throughout the night, the court inferred that "nothing was charted because nothing was done." One of the nurses was held negligent for this client's death.

It is very important for documentation to be accomplished in a timely manner. Any significant changes in the client's condition must be reported to the physician and documented in the chart (see Chapter 16). Recording nursing care notes in a notebook and then transferring them to the chart at the end of the shift can be a dangerous practice. If this practice is followed, other health care professionals may administer medications or provide care to the client without up-to-date information. Harm may come to a client whose record is not accurate and current. Nurses must always follow the particular style of charting adopted by their employer (Phillips, 1999a).

Truthful documentation is also essential. If an error is made in the documentation, it is important to follow the policies and procedures of the institution to correct it. Obliterating or erasing errors may appear to be concealing misconduct and lead to charges of fraud. The credibility of a nurse who goes to court is negatively affected if it appears that the nurse's initial charting has been changed after an injury has occurred to a client. This scenario is exemplified in the case of *Meyer v. Gordon* (1981). Nurses did not adequately monitor a woman in labour, and their notes were sloppy and vague. The fetus experienced severe distress, required resuscitation on delivery, and was transferred to another hospital. When a nurse realized that the documentation was deficient, she altered it. However, the original chart had already been photocopied and sent to the second hospital. At trial, it was obvious that the original document had been tampered

> **► BOX 9-2   Common Negligent Acts**

Medication errors that result in injury to clients

Intravenous therapy errors that result in infiltrations or phlebitis

Burns caused by equipment, bathing, or spills of hot liquids and foods

Falls resulting in injury to clients

Failure to use aseptic technique as required

Errors in sponge, instrument, or needle counts in surgical cases

Failure to give a report, or giving an incomplete report, to an incoming shift of health care staff

Failure to monitor a client's condition adequately

Failure to notify a physician of a significant change in a client's status with. The court held that the nursing staff had been negligent in several ways, and the judge severely condemned the nurse's tampering with the evidence. The court commented as follows: "My criticism of the defendant hospital is not confined to the lack of care of its nursing staff. The hospital chart contains alterations and additions which compel me to view with suspicion the accuracy of many of the observations which are recorded."

Nurses should also be familiar with the current nursing literature in their areas of practice. They should know and follow the policies and procedures of the institution in which they work. Nurses should be sensitive to common sources of injury to clients, such as falls and medication errors. Nurses must communicate with the client, explain the tests and treatment to be performed, document that specific explanations were provided to the client, and listen to the client's concerns about the treatment.

Nurse–client relationships are very important not only in ensuring quality care but also in minimizing legal risks. Trust develops between a nurse and client. Clients who believe that the nurses performed their duties correctly and were concerned with their welfare are less likely to initiate a lawsuit against the nurses. Sincere caring for clients is an essential role of the nurse and is an effective risk-management tool. However, caring does not protect nurses completely if negligent practice occurs. When a client is injured, the investigation into the incident may implicate the nurses even if the client feels kindly toward them.

Criminal Liability

Although most nursing liability issues involve private law matters (e.g., torts), the criminal law is also relevant. Canadian nurses have been charged with criminal offences such as assault, administering a noxious substance, and criminal negligence that causes death (a category of manslaughter). The difference between the tort of negligence and criminal negligence charges is the degree to which the act deviated from the standard of a reasonably competent practitioner. For example, in the case of criminal negligence, the courts must prove that the nurse was extremely careless, indicating "wanton or reckless disregard for the lives or safety of other persons" (*Criminal Code*, 1985, Part VIII, Section 219 [1]).

Consent

A signed consent form is required for all routine treatment, procedures such as surgery, some treatment programs such as chemotherapy, and research involving clients. A client signs general consent forms when admitted to the hospital or other health care facility. The client or the client's representative must sign a special consent or treatment form before each specialized procedure or treatment. "If a person receiving care is clearly incapable of consent, the nurse respects the law on capacity assessment and substitute decision-making in his or her jurisdiction" (CNA, 2008, p.11; see also CNPS, 2004b). Provincial and territorial laws describe what constitutes the legal ability to give consent to medical treatment. Nurses should know the law in their own jurisdiction and be familiar with the policies and procedures of their employing institution with regard to consent.

In general, the following factors must be verified for consent to be legally valid:

• The client must have the legal and mental capacity to make a treatment decision.
• The consent must be given voluntarily and without coercion.
• The client must understand the risks and benefits of the procedure or treatment, the risks of not undergoing the procedure or treatment, and any available alternatives to the procedure or treatment.

If a client is deaf, is illiterate, or does not speak the language of the health care professionals, an official interpreter must be available to explain the terms of consent. A family member or acquaintance who is able to speak a client's language should not be used to interpret health information except as a last resort. A client experiencing the effects of a sedative is not able to clearly understand the implications of an invasive procedure. Every effort should be made to assist the client in making an informed choice.

Nurses must be sensitive to the cultural issues of consent. The nurse must understand the way in which clients and their families communicate and make important decisions. It is essential for nurses to understand the various cultures with which they interact. The cultural beliefs and values of the client may be very different from those of the nurse. It is important for nurses not to impose their own cultural values on the client (see Chapter 10).

Informed Consent.

"Nurses ensure that nursing care is provided with the person's informed consent. Nurses recognize and support a capable person's right to refuse or withdraw consent for care or treatment at any time." (CNA, 2008, p. 11).

Informed consent is a person's agreement to allow a medical action to happen, such as surgery or an invasive procedure, on the basis of a full disclosure of the likely risks and benefits of the action, alternatives to the action, and the consequences of refusal (Black, 1999). Informed consent creates a legal duty for the physician or other health care professional to disclose material facts in terms that the client can reasonably understand in order to make an informed choice (Sneiderman et al., 2003). The explanation should also describe treatment alternatives, as well as the risks involved in all treatment options. Failure to obtain consent in situations other than emergencies may result in a claim of battery. In the absence of informed consent, a client may bring a lawsuit against the health care professional for negligence, even if the procedure was performed competently. Informed consent requires the provision of adequate information for the client to form a decision and the documentation of that decision.

The following materials are required for informed consent (Sneiderman et al., 2003):

• A brief, complete explanation of the procedure or treatment.
• Names and qualifications of people performing and assisting in the procedure.
• A description of any possible harm, including permanent damage or death, that may occur as a result of the procedure.
• An explanation of therapeutic alternatives to the proposed procedure/treatment, as well as the risks of doing nothing. Clients also need to be informed of their right to refuse the procedure/treatment without discontinuing other supportive care and of their right to withdraw their consent even after the procedure has begun.

Informed consent is part of the physician–client relationship. Because nurses do not perform surgery or direct medical procedures, obtaining clients' informed consent is not usually one of nurses' duties. Even though the nurse may assume the responsibility for witnessing the client's signature on the consent form, the nurse does not legally assume the duty of obtaining informed consent. The nurse's signature witnessing the consent means that the client voluntarily gave consent, that the client's signature is authentic, and that the client appears to be competent to give consent (Sneiderman et al., 2003). When nurses provide consent forms for clients to sign, the clients should be asked whether they understand the procedures to which they are consenting. If they deny understanding, or if the nurse suspects that they do not understand, the nurse must notify the physician or nursing supervisor. Some consent forms also have a line for the physician to sign after explaining the risks and alternatives to a client. Such a form is helpful in a court case when a client alleges that consent was not informed. If a client refuses treatment, this rejection should also be written, signed, and witnessed.

If a client participates in an experimental treatment program or submits to use of experimental drugs or treatments, the informed consent form must be even more detailed and stringently regulated. An organization's institutional review board should review the information in the consent form for research involving human subjects. The client may withdraw from the experiment at any time (see Chapter 8).

Many procedures that nurses perform (e.g., insertion of intravenous or nasogastric tubes) do not require formal written consent; nonetheless, clients' right to give or refuse consent to treatment must be protected. Implied consent to treatment is often involved in nursing procedures. For example, when the nurse approaches the client with a syringe in hand and the client rolls over to expose the injection site, consent is implied. If the client resists the injection either verbally or through actions, the nurse must not proceed with the injection. Forcing or otherwise treating a client without consent could result in criminal or civil charges of assault and battery. Many advanced practice nurses are now autonomously treating clients. It is therefore likely that formal written consent for nursing procedures will also be expected for the treatment received from advance practice nurse specialists.

Parents are usually the legal guardians of pediatric clients, and, therefore, consent forms for treatment must be signed by parents. If the parents are divorced, the form must be signed by the parent with legal custody. On occasion, a parent or guardian refuses treatment for a child. In those cases, the court may intervene in the child's behalf. The practice of making the child a ward of the court and administering necessary treatment is relatively common in such cases.

The example of 13-year-old Tyrell Dueck from Saskatchewan illustrates such a case. The teenager received a diagnosis of cancer in 1998. He completed part of the chemotherapy treatment when he decided that he did not want more treatment or the recommended amputation of his leg, believing that he had been "cured by God" and that further treatment was unnecessary. His statements were consistent with his family's Christian value system. Following his parents' advice, the boy wished to undergo alternative therapy at a clinic in Mexico. The treating physicians maintained that without further conventional treatment, Tyrell would die within a year. A judge concluded that Tyrell had been given inaccurate information by his father about the benefits and risks of the proposed alternative therapy and, therefore, was unable to make an informed consent or refusal. Thus, the family's wishes to forgo conventional treatment were legally overruled, and the boy's grandparents were to take him for treatments. Before the enforced treatment could be started, however, tests revealed that the cancer had already spread and the treatment would no longer be helpful. The teenager was returned to the care of his parents, and he died a short time later.

In some instances, obtaining informed consent is difficult or simply not possible. If, for example, the client is unconscious, consent must be obtained from a person legally authorized to give consent on the client's behalf. Other surrogate decision makers may have legally been delegated this authority through proxy directives or court guardianship procedures. In emergency situations, if it is impossible to obtain consent from the client or an authorized person, the procedure required to benefit the client or save the client's life may be undertaken without liability for failure to obtain consent. In such cases, the law assumes that the client would wish to be treated. This is referred to as the *emergency doctrine.*

Clients with mental health problems and frail older adults must also be given the opportunity to give consent. They retain the right to refuse treatment unless a court has legally determined that they are incompetent to decide for themselves.

Nursing Students and Legal Liability

Nursing students must know their own capabilities and competencies and must not perform nursing actions unless competent to do so. "However, if a student nurse performs a nursing action which is one an RN would perform (e.g. administration of an I.M. [intramuscular] injection), that student will be held to the standard of an RN. Student nurses, like all other nurses, are accountable for their own actions" (Phillips, 2002). In a few reported cases in Canada, nursing students were sued for negligence in their care of patients. A nursing student in Nova Scotia who caused permanent injury in a client through an improperly administered intramuscular injection was found negligent, and the hospital was found vicariously liable for the student's actions (CNPS, 2007b; *Roberts v. Cape Breton Regional Hospital,* 1997). Thus, nursing students are liable if their actions cause harm to clients. However, if a client is harmed as a direct result of a nursing student's actions or lack of action, the liability is generally shared by the student, the instructor, the hospital or health care facility, and the university or educational institution. Nursing students should never be assigned to perform tasks for which they are unprepared, and they should be carefully supervised by instructors as they learn new skills. Although nursing students are not considered employees of the hospital, the institution has a responsibility to monitor their acts. Nursing students are expected to ensure that their student status is known to clients and to perform as professional nurses would in providing safe client care. Faculty members are usually responsible for instructing and observing students, but in some situations, staff nurses serving as preceptors may share these responsibilities. Every nursing school should provide clear definitions of student responsibility, preceptor responsibility, and faculty responsibility (Phillips, 2002).

When students are employed as nursing assistants or nurses' aides when not attending classes, they should not perform tasks that do not appear in a job description for a nurses' aide or assistant. For example, even if a student has learned to administer intramuscular medications in class, this task may not be performed by a nurses' aide. If a staff nurse overseeing the nursing assistant or aide knowingly assigns work without regard for the person's ability to safely conduct the task as defined in the job description, that staff nurse is also liable. If students employed as nurse's aides are requested to perform tasks that they are not prepared to complete safely, this information should be brought to the nursing supervisor's attention so that the needed help can be obtained.

The Web site of the CNPS (http://www.cnps.ca/ through its members-only section) is an excellent resource available to nursing students, providing information about legal risks nurses face in practice. However, nursing students are not entitled to receive legal consultation services or financial assistance from the CNPS; these services are provided only for the benefit of eligible registered nurses.

Professional Liability Protection

Most nurses in Canada are employed by publicly funded health care facilities that carry malpractice insurance. These facilities are considered employers and therefore are vicariously liable for negligent acts of their employees as long as the employees were working within the normal scope and course of practice (Keatings & Smith, 2000).

Because of this legal principle, if an employee is found liable in a civil lawsuit, the employer is generally ordered to pay the damages (CNPS, 1998). A nurse who exceeds the bounds of acceptable practice or is self-employed is fully liable for his or her own negligence. All nurses should be aware of their employment status and professional liability coverage.

The CNPS is a nonprofit society established in 1988 to provide legal support and liability protection to nurses. The services of CNPS are available free as a benefit of membership in a subscribing provincial or territorial professional association or college. The only two jurisdictions in Canada not included in CNPS are British Columbia and Quebec. Registered nurses in British Columbia are covered by their own insurance corporation, and those in Quebec have commercial insurance available through the Order of Nurses of Quebec. CNPS services are available to nurses in a variety of work settings, including independent practice and volunteer settings. Eligible nurses can obtain confidential assistance from a nurse lawyer by contacting the CNPS toll-free by telephone, Monday to Friday from 0845 to 1630 hours Eastern Standard Time or Eastern Daylight Time at 1-800-267-3390. A nurse providing emergency assistance at an accident scene would not be covered by an employer's insurance policy because the care given would not be the responsibility of the employer. However, some provinces have passed "Good Samaritan" laws (e.g., Alberta's *Emergency Medical Aid Act*, 2000) that prevent voluntary rescuers from being sued for wrongdoing unless it can be proved that they displayed gross negligence. Nurses must be familiar with these laws in their own province or territory (Phillips, 1999b).

Abandonment, Assignment, and Contract Issues

Short Staffing. During nursing shortages or periods of staff downsizing, the issue of inadequate staffing may arise. Legal problems may result if the number of nurses is insufficient or if an appropriate mix of staff to provide competent care is lacking. If assigned to care for more clients than is reasonable, nurses should bring this information to the attention of the nursing supervisor. In addition, a written protest such as a workload or staffing report form should be completed to document the nurse's concerns about client safety. Most provinces and territories have some reporting mechanism in place to document heavy workload or staffing situations. Although such a protest may not relieve nurses of responsibility if a client suffers injury because of inattention, it would show that they were attempting to act reasonably. Whenever a written protest is made, nurses should keep a copy of this document in their personal files. Most administrators recognize that knowledge of a potential problem shifts some of the responsibility to the institution.

Nurses should not walk out when staffing is inadequate, because charges of abandonment could be made. A nurse who refuses to accept an assignment may be considered insubordinate, and clients would not benefit from having even fewer staff available. It is important to know the institution's policies and procedures and the nursing union's collective agreement on how to handle such circumstances before they arise.

Floating. Nurses are sometimes required to "float" from the area in which they normally practise to other nursing units. Nurses must practise within their level of competence. Nurses should not be floated to areas where they have not been adequately cross-trained. Nurses who float should inform the nursing supervisor of any lack of experience in caring for the type of clients on the nursing unit. They should also request and be given orientation to the unit. A nursing supervisor can be held liable if a staff nurse is given an assignment he

or she cannot safely perform. In one case (*Dessauer v. Memorial General Hospital*, 1981), a nurse in obstetrics was assigned to an emergency room. A client entered the emergency room, complaining of chest pain. The obstetrical nurse gave the client too high a dosage of lidocaine, and the client died after suffering irreversible brain damage and cardiac arrest. The nurse lost the negligence lawsuit.

Physicians' Orders. The physician is responsible for directing medical treatment. Nurses are obligated to follow physicians' orders unless they believe the orders are in error, violate hospital policy, or would harm clients. Therefore, all orders must be assessed, and if an order is found to be erroneous or harmful, further clarification from the physician is necessary. If the physician confirms the order and the nurse still believes it is inappropriate, the supervising nurse should be informed. A nurse should not proceed to perform a physician's order if harm to the client is foreseeable. The nursing supervisor should be informed of and given a written memorandum detailing the events in chronological order; the nurse's reasons for refusing to carry out the order should also be written, to protect the nurse from disciplinary action. The supervising nurse should help resolve the questionable order. A medical or pharmacy consultant may be called in to help clarify the appropriateness or inappropriateness of the order. A nurse carrying out an inaccurate or inappropriate order may be legally responsible for any harm suffered by the client.

In a negligence lawsuit against a physician and a hospital, one of the most frequently litigated issues is whether the nurse kept the physician informed of the client's condition. To inform a physician properly, nurses must perform a competent nursing assessment of the client to determine the signs and symptoms that are significant in relation to the attending physician's tasks of diagnosis and treatment. Nurses must be certain to document that the physician was notified and to document his or her response, the nurse's follow-up, and the client's response. For example, nurses noticed that a client with a cast on his leg was experiencing poor circulation in his foot. The nurses recorded these changes but did not notify the physician. Gangrene subsequently developed in the client, and an amputation was required. The hospital, physician, and nursing staff were all charged with negligence.

The physician should write all orders, including "do not resuscitate" (DNR) orders, which many physicians are reluctant to write out because they fear legal repercussions for criminal neglect or failure to act. The nurse must make sure that orders are transcribed correctly. Verbal orders are not recommended because they increase the possibilities for error. If a verbal order is necessary (e.g., during an emergency), it should be written and signed by the physician as soon as possible, usually within 24 hours. The nurse should be familiar with the institution's policy and procedures regarding verbal orders.

Dispensing Advice Over the Phone. Providing advice over the telephone is a high-risk activity because diagnosing over the phone is extremely difficult. The nurse is legally accountable for advice given over the phone. The most common allegations of negligence in this area are provision of inadequate advice, improper referrals, and failure to refer (CNPS, 1997). It is essential that nurses precisely follow institutional guidelines and policies and thoroughly document each call to avoid serious repercussions for all parties.

Contracts and Employment Agreements. In Canada, most nurses belong to unions or associations that engage in collective bargaining on behalf of a group. The collective agreements between employers and union members are written contracts that set out the conditions of employment (e.g., salary, hours of work, benefits, layoffs, and termination). Many laws, including labour laws, apply to nurses. For example, laws outline eligibility for and details of workers' compensation and maternity benefits. It is important for nurses to understand the employment laws in the province or territory where they work.

By accepting a job, a nurse enters into an agreement with an employer. The nurse is expected to perform professional duties competently, adhering to the policies and procedures of the institution. In return, the employer pays for the nursing services and ensures that facilities and equipment are adequate for safe care.

Legal Issues in Nursing Practice

Abortion

In the 1988 case of *R. v. Morgentaler,* the Supreme Court of Canada ruled that the *Criminal Code* (1985) regulations on legal access to abortion were unconstitutional. The *Criminal Code* had required a woman seeking abortion to secure the approval of a hospital-based committee before the procedure could be performed. By rejecting the *Criminal Code* provisions, the Supreme Court in effect referred the abortion issue to Parliament, but Parliament has not rewritten a criminal law policy on abortion. Abortion is thus unregulated by law, which is tantamount to its legalization. However, the legal entitlement to abortion does not mean abortion services are readily available. Because health care facilities are not obliged to offer abortions, many do not do so. Thus, access remains a continuing issue.

Drug Regulations and Nurses

Canadian law closely regulates the administration of drugs. Two federal acts control the manufacture, distribution, and sale of food, drugs, cosmetics, and therapeutic devices in Canada: the *Food and Drugs Act* (1985) and the *Controlled Drugs and Substances Act* (1996). The *Food and Drugs Act* lists the drugs that can be sold only by prescription (e.g., antibiotics) and drugs that are subject to stringent controls (e.g., barbiturates, amphetamines). The distribution of these drugs requires specific handling and record keeping. The *Controlled Drugs and Substances Act* controls the manufacture, distribution, and sale of narcotics (e.g., morphine, codeine). However, it also regulates other drugs that are controlled in the same manner as narcotics, such as cocaine and marijuana. Most institutions have policies about medication administration and record keeping, especially for controlled drugs and narcotics. Nurses must be aware of their employer's policies.

Nurses are not legally entitled to prescribe drugs. However, in several jurisdictions, nurse practitioners may prescribe certain nonnarcotic drugs specific to their area of practice.

The administration of medications in accordance with a physician's prescription is a basic nursing responsibility. A competent nurse is expected to know the purpose and effect of any drug administered, as well as potential side effects and contraindications. It is also a nurse's responsibility to question any physician's orders that may be incorrect or unsafe. A nurse who follows a physician's order that is unclear or incorrect may be found negligent.

Communicable Diseases

The care of people with communicable conditions such as HIV infection, acquired immunodeficiency syndrome (AIDS), hepatitis, or severe acute respiratory syndrome (SARS) or during a possible influenza pandemic has legal implications for nurses. Health care workers are at risk for exposure to communicable diseases because of the nature of their work. Despite the best attempts to protect oneself

against communicable diseases through the proper and consistent use of protective gear (e.g., latex gloves or masks), accidental needlestick injuries or life-threatening illnesses such as SARS can occur. Nurses have an ethical and legal obligation to provide care to all assigned clients, and employers have an obligation to provide their employees with necessary protective gear. However, there may be "some circumstances in which it is acceptable for a nurse to withdraw from care provision or to refuse to provide care" (College of Registered Nurses of British Columbia [CRNBC], 2007, p. 1; see also College of Registered Nurses of Nova Scotia, 2006). "Unreasonable burden is a concept raised in relation to duty to provide care and withdrawing from providing or refusing to provide care. An unreasonable burden may exist when a nurse's ability to provide safe care and meet professional standards of practice is compromised by unreasonable expectations, lack of resources, or ongoing threats to personal well-being" (CNA, 2008; see also CRNBC, 2007, p. 1).

In all cases involving privacy, confidentiality, and disclosure, the rights of the clients with a communicable disease must be balanced with the rights of the public or of health care professionals. Both civil and criminal liability can result if private information is disclosed without authorization. Nurses must understand the reporting laws in the province or territory in which they practise. Courts can order disclosure of the records of clients with AIDS in situations that are not addressed by a statute, even without the client's consent. Whenever information about a client is requested by any third parties, including insurance companies or employers, nurses must obtain a signed release from the client before releasing confidential information. Not every health care professional who comes in contact with a client has a need to know the client's HIV status. Confidential information must be protected.

The courts have upheld the employer's right to fire a nurse who refuses to care for a client with AIDS. Nurses who flatly refuse to care for HIV-infected clients or possibly a client with SARS may be reprimanded or fired for insubordination. According to the CNA's (2008) *Code of Ethics for Registered Nurses,* nurses must not discriminate in the provision of nursing care on the basis of factors such as a person's sexual orientation, health status, or lifestyle (p. 13). One limitation outlined in the code regarding a nurse's right to refuse care to a client is that nurses are not obligated to comply with a client's wishes when those wishes are contrary to the law (e.g., assisting the client to commit suicide). If the care requested is contrary to the nurse's personal values, such as assisting with an abortion, the nurse must provide appropriate care until alternative care arrangements are arranged.

Nurses must be concerned with balancing the right to protect themselves with protection of the client's rights. Both are afforded protection against discrimination and protection of privacy by human rights legislation. Most current legal cases involving nurses and communicable diseases are related to the protection needed for nurses as employees. Strict compliance with standard precautions and routine practices and the use of transmission-based precautions (e.g., against airborne or droplet transmission) for clients known or suspected of having other serious illnesses is the nurse's wisest strategy (see Chapter 33).

Death and Dying

Many legal issues surround the event of death, including a basic definition of when a person is considered dead. The only province that has a statutory definition of death is Manitoba, which defines it as "the irreversible cessation of all brain function" (*Vital Statistics Act,* 1987). However, this "brain death" definition has become standard medical practice across Canada. Until the 1960s, death was defined as the irreversible cessation of cardiopulmonary function. However, two developments at that time necessitated a shift to consideration of the brain: (1) the emergence of artificial life-support devices that could maintain cardiopulmonary functioning in a brain-dead person and (2) the emergence of organ transplantation. Death had to be redefined so that organs could be donated.

Ethical and legal questions are raised by the related issues of euthanasia and assisted suicide. **Euthanasia** is an act undertaken by one person with the motive of relieving another person's suffering and the knowledge that the act will end the life of that person (Downie, 2004). In Canada, euthanasia is illegal. It is legally irrelevant whether the client has consented to the act because according to Section 14 of the *Criminal Code* (1985), "no person can consent to have death inflicted on him." Furthermore, according to Section 241 of the *Criminal Code,* it is an offence to "aid a person to commit suicide, whether suicide ensues or not."

On the other hand, the law draws a distinction between "killing" and "letting die." Euthanasia and assisted suicide are considered "killing." Withholding or withdrawing life-prolonging treatment is considered "letting die." The disease process causes the client to die a natural death. Thus, a mentally competent client has the legal right to refuse life-prolonging treatment. If, for example, such a client requests that a ventilator be disconnected, understanding that she will die as a result, her wishes must be honoured in accordance with the principle of "no treatment without consent."

In the case of *Nancy B. v. Hôtel-Dieu de Québec* (1992), a young, mentally competent client who was totally and permanently paralyzed by a neurological disease had twice asked that her ventilator be disconnected. After the second refusal, she sought a court order to enforce her will. The order was granted by the Quebec Superior Court, which ruled that as a mentally competent client, she could not be treated without consent. Also, even if a client has not asked for the termination of life-prolonging treatment (either directly or by way of an advance directive), physicians are still allowed, after consultation with family members, to terminate such treatment when it no longer offers any reasonable hope of benefit to the person.

When clients reject life-prolonging treatment, the nurse focuses on the goal of caring versus curing. Nurses have a legal obligation to treat the deceased person's remains with dignity (see Chapter 29). Wrongful handling of a deceased person's remains could cause emotional harm to the surviving family members and other loved ones.

Advance Directives and Health Care Surrogates

The **advance directive** is a mechanism enabling a mentally competent person to plan for a time when he or she may lack the mental capacity to make medical treatment decisions. It takes effect only when the person becomes incompetent to speak for himself or herself. The advance directive is a more sophisticated concept than that of the living will, although the two terms are often confused. A **living will** is a document in which the person makes an anticipatory refusal of life-prolonging measures during a future state of mental incompetence. An advance directive, in contrast, is not restricted to the rejection of life-support measures; its focus is on treatment preferences, which may include both requests for and refusals of treatment. The advance directive assumes two forms: the instructional directive (in which the maker of the document spells out specific directions for governing care, in more detail than is generally found in the living will); and the proxy directive (in which the person appoints someone as a health care agent to make treatment decisions in his or her behalf). Legislation in British Columbia, Alberta, Saskatchewan, Manitoba, Ontario, Prince Edward Island, Newfoundland and Labrador, and the Yukon gives full legal effect to both kinds of directives; the proxy directive is also recognized in Quebec and Nova Scotia. Even in provinces and territories that do not recognize an instructional directive, nothing prohibits a physician from following a directive.

If nurses know about the existence of a health care directive, they are required to follow it. Nurses are also required to follow the wishes of a validly appointed proxy (assuming these instructions are legal). A proxy has the right to receive all medical information concerning the client's condition and proposed plan of care. Failure to comply with a proxy's directions could result in charges of battery.

If a physician ignores the advance directive, the nurse must bring the advance directive to the physician's attention and document that he or she did so, along with the physician's response to this information. The nurse should also notify the nursing supervisor, who can then give direction regarding institutional policies and guidelines for such circumstances.

The psychiatric advance directive is a new type of advance directive. An individual with mental health problems completes this type of directive during periods of mental stability and competence. The directive outlines how the client wishes to be treated in the future if the underlying mental illness causes him or her to lose decision-making capacity. For example, it may specify preferences for and against certain interventions (e.g., electroconvulsive therapy) or medications. The psychiatric advance directive can also designate a surrogate decision maker to act on the person's behalf in the event of an incapacitating mental health crisis.

Organ Donation

Legally competent people are free to donate their bodies or organs for medical use. Every province and territory has human tissue legislation that provides for both the *inter vivos* (live donor) and post-mortem (cadaveric) donation of tissues and organs. For example, a mentally competent adult is allowed to donate a kidney, a lobe of the liver, or bone marrow. Statutes provide that adults may consent to organ donation after death. If the deceased has left no direction for post-mortem donation, then consent may be obtained from the person's family. In two provinces—Manitoba and Nova Scotia—the statutes contain "required request" provisions that take effect when a deceased person did not consent to organ removal but is considered a good donor candidate. In such an event, the physician is legally obliged to seek permission from the family. In many hospitals, a nurse transplantation coordinator performs this function.

Mental Health Issues

Treating clients with mental health problems raises legal and ethical issues. Provincial mental health legislation such as the *Mental Health and Consequential Amendments Act* (1998) provides direction for health care professionals, protects client autonomy, and recognizes that some individuals with severe mental health problems may lack the ability to appreciate the consequences of their health condition.

A client can be admitted to a psychiatric unit involuntarily or on a voluntary basis. Clients admitted on a voluntary basis should be treated no differently than any other client. They have the right to refuse treatment and the right to discharge themselves from hospital. However, provincial mental health legislation provides that if the client may cause harm to self or others, police officers (or other authorized parties) may bring the client to a health care facility for examination and treatment without the client's consent (Morris et al., 1999).

Potentially suicidal clients may be admitted to psychiatric units. If the client's history and medical records indicate suicidal tendencies, the client must be kept under supervision. A lawsuit may result if a client attempts suicide within the hospital. The allegations in the lawsuits would be that the institution failed to provide adequate supervision or safeguard the facilities. Documentation of precautions against suicide is essential.

Public Health Issues

It is important that nurses, especially those employed in community health settings, understand the public health laws. Public health acts, which have been enacted in all provinces and territories, are directed toward the prevention, treatment, and suppression of communicable disease (Sneiderman et al., 2003). Community health nurses have the legal responsibility to follow the laws enacted to protect the public health. These laws may include reporting suspected abuse and neglect, such as child abuse, elder abuse, or domestic violence; reporting communicable diseases; and reporting of other health-related issues enacted to protect the public's health.

Some provinces (e.g., Ontario and New Brunswick) have legislation that requires proof of immunization for school entry. In these provinces, however, exceptions are permitted on medical or religious grounds and for reasons of conscience (Health Canada, 1997). Although a signed consent form is not required for an immunization, nurses are advised to obtain some documentation (evidence) that they discussed the risks and benefits with the parent or legal guardian. Nurses should be aware of their employer guidelines for documentation.

Every province and territory has child abuse legislation that requires health care professionals, such as nurses, to report witnessed or suspected child abuse or neglect directly to child protection agencies. To encourage reports of suspected cases, the laws offer legal immunity for the reporter if the report is made in good faith. Health care professionals who do not report suspected child abuse or neglect maybe held liable for civil or criminal action. Several provinces and territories also have laws that require health care workers to report witnessed or suspected abuse of clients within facilities (e.g., *The Protection of Persons in Care Act*, 2000, in Manitoba). These reports must be made directly to a public authority. Even if public reporting is not required, nurses should report all suspicions of client abuse to their nursing supervisors. It is essential for nurses to know their provincial or territorial laws and employer policies regarding the reporting of abuse.

Risk Management

Risk management is a system of ensuring appropriate nursing care by identifying potential hazards and eliminating them before harm occurs (Guido, 2006). The steps involved in risk management include identifying possible risks, analyzing them, acting to reduce them, and evaluating the steps taken.

One tool used in risk management is the **incident report**, or **adverse occurrence report**. When a client is harmed or endangered by incorrect care, such as a drug error, a nurse completes an incident report (see Chapter 16). Such reports are analyzed to determine how future problems can be avoided. For example, if incident reports show that drug errors commonly involve a new intravenous pump, the risk manager must ensure that staff members have been properly trained in its use. In-service education may be all that is necessary to prevent future errors.

The underlying rationale for quality assurance in risk-management programs is the highest possible quality of care. Some insurance companies and medical and nursing organizations require the use of quality assurance and risk-management procedures. Quality care is the responsibility of both the employer and the individual provider.

Risk management requires sufficient documentation. The nurse's documentation can be the evidence of what actually was done for a client and can serve as proof that the nurse acted reasonably and safely. Documentation should be thorough, accurate, and performed in a timely manner. When a lawsuit is being evaluated, the nurse's notes are very often the first record to be reviewed by the plaintiff's counsel. If the nurse's credibility is questioned because of these documents, the risk of greater liability exists for the nurse. The nurse's notes are risk-management and quality assurance tools for the employer and the individual nurse.

Professional Involvement

Nurses must be involved in their professional organizations and on committees that define the standards of care for nursing practice. If current laws, rules and regulations, or policies under which nurses must practise do not reflect reality, nurses must become involved as advocates to see that the scope of nursing practice is accurately defined. Nurses must be willing to represent the nursing profession's perspective, as well as the client's perspective in the community. Nurses can be powerful and effective when the organizing focus is the protection and welfare of the public entrusted to their care.

✳ KEY CONCEPTS

- With increased emphasis on client rights, nurses in practice today must understand their legal obligations and responsibilities to clients.
- The civil law system is concerned with the protection of a person's private rights, and the criminal law system deals with the rights of individuals and society.
- A nurse can be found liable for negligence if the following criteria are established: the nurse (defendant) owed a duty of care to the client (plaintiff), the nurse did not carry out that duty, the client was injured, and the nurse's failure to carry out the duty caused the client's injury.
- Clients are entitled to confidential health care and freedom from unauthorized release of information.
- Under the law, practising nurses must follow standards of care, which originate in nursing practice acts and regulations, the guidelines of professional organizations, and the written policies and procedures of employing institutions.
- Nurses are responsible for confirming that the client has given informed consent to any surgery or other medical procedure before the procedure is performed.
- Nurses are responsible for performing all procedures correctly and exercising professional judgement as they carry out physicians' orders.
- Nurses are obligated to follow physicians' orders unless they believe the orders are in error or could be detrimental to clients.
- Staffing standards determine the ratio of nurses to clients, and if the nurse is required to care for more clients than is reasonable, a formal protest should be made to the nursing administration.
- Legal issues involving death include documenting all events surrounding the death and treating the deceased client's remains with dignity.
- A competent adult can legally give consent to donate specific organs, and nurses may serve as witnesses to this decision.
- All nurses should know the laws that apply to their area of practice.
- Depending on provincial statutes, nurses are required to report suspected child abuse and certain communicable diseases.
- Nurses are client advocates and ensure quality of care through risk management and lobbying for safe nursing practice standards.
- Nurses must file incident reports in all situations when someone could or did get hurt.

❋ CRITICAL THINKING EXERCISES

1. Nurse Rossi and Nurse Kao are getting on an elevator to go down to the cafeteria. Several visitors are present in the elevator, as are hospital personnel. Nurse Rossi and Nurse Kao are talking about a client who is in the intensive care unit who has just tested positive for HIV infection. They identify the client as "the man in Room 14B." One of the visitors on the elevator who overhears this information is a woman who is engaged to the client in Room 14B.
   a. Have Nurse Rossi and Nurse Kao breached a client's right to confidential health care?
   b. Would the client in Room 14B have any legal cause of action against the nurses?
   c. Even though the client's fiancée may have a right to know the HIV status of her future husband, do the nurses have any duty to disclose confidential information to the fiancée?

2. While transporting a client down the hall on a stretcher, Nurse Reyes stops to chat with an orderly. The side rails on the stretcher are down, and while Nurse Reyes has her back to the stretcher, the client rolls over, falls off the stretcher, and fractures his hip. In a lawsuit by the client against Nurse Reyes, what must the client establish to prove negligence against the nurse?

❋ REVIEW QUESTIONS

1. The nursing practice acts are an example of
   1. Statute law
   2. Common law
   3. Public law
   4. Criminal law

2. Treating a client without his or her consent is considered
   1. Battery
   2. Negligence
   3. Implied consent
   4. Expressed consent

3. The nurse restrains a client without the client's permission and without a physician's order. The nurse may be guilty of
   1. Assault
   2. False imprisonment
   3. Invasion of privacy
   4. Neglect

4. The situation in which a confused client fell out of bed because side rails were not used when they were ordered is an example of which type of liability?
   1. False imprisonment
   2. Assault
   3. Battery
   4. Negligence

5. What should you do if you think the client does not understand the procedure for which he or she is being asked to give consent?
   1. Do not be concerned if the consent is already signed.
   2. Notify the physician or nursing supervisor.
   3. Send the client for the procedure and discuss it afterward.
   4. Ask a family member to give consent.

6. When a client is harmed as a result of a nursing student's actions or lack of action, the liability is generally held by
   1. The student alone
   2. The student's instructor or preceptor
   3. The hospital or health care facility
   4. All of the above

7. When the nurse stops to help in an emergency at the scene of an accident, if the injured party files suit and the nurse's employing institution's insurance does not cover the nurse, the nurse would probably be covered by
   1. The nurse's automobile insurance
   2. The nurse's homeowner's insurance
   3. The Patient Care Partnership, which may grant immunity from suit if the injured party consents
   4. The Good Samaritan laws, which grant immunity from suit if no gross negligence is involved

8. The nurse is obligated to follow a physician's order unless
   1. The order is a verbal order
   2. The physician's order is illegible
   3. The order has not been transcribed
   4. The order is in error, violates hospital policy, or would be detrimental to the client

9. If a third party (e.g., insurance company of employer) requests health information on a client, the nurse must
   1. Provide the information
   2. Refuse to provide the information
   3. Obtain a signed release by the client before releasing the information
   4. Contact the client's family or lawyer

❋ RECOMMENDED WEB SITES

Canadian Nurses Association–Provincial/Territorial Members: http://www. cna-aiic.ca/CNA/about/members/provincial/default_e.aspx
This CNA site offers up-to-date Weblinks and contact information for all provincial and territorial nursing colleges and associations.

The Canadian Nurses Protective Society: http://www.cnps.ca
The Canadian Nurses Protective Society (CNPS) helps nurses manage their professional legal risks by offering legal support and liability protection. The members-only section of the Web site (the user name is the acronym of your professional association or college, and the password is "assist") provides information on a variety of legal topics affecting Canadian nursing practice.

The College of Licensed Practical Nurses of Nova Scotia: http://www.clpnns.ca/provincial_links/outofprovincelinks.html
This site provides links to all provincial licensing authorities.

Department of Justice Canada: http://laws.justice.gc.ca/en/
This site provides links to consolidated statutes, including the *Criminal Code* (1985) of Canada.

The Health Law Institute of Dalhousie University: The End of Life Project: http://as01.ucis.dal.ca/dhli/cmp_welcome/default.cfm
This site contains information about the Canadian law pertaining to various aspects of end-of-life care, including advance directives and withholding of life-sustaining treatment.

10

Culture and Ethnicity

Written by Barbara J. Astle, RN, PhD,

and Sylvia Barton, RN, PhD

Based on the original chapter by Anahid Kulwicki, RN, DNS, FAAN

objectives

Mastery of content in this chapter will enable you to:

- Describe the key terms listed.
- Describe the enthocultural diversity of the Canadian population.
- Define key cultural concepts related to health, illness, and ethnicity.
- Describe the historical development of transcultural nursing, cultural competence, and cultural safety in relation to nursing practice.
- Describe social and cultural influences on healing, well-being, and caring patterns.
- Analyze components of cultural assessment to understand the values, beliefs, and practices critical in the nursing care of people experiencing ethnocultural transitions.
- Apply selected components of cultural assessment to a particular cultural group as an example.
- Examine nursing obligations that underpin relational practice and the way in which relational inquiry can enhance contemporary nursing practice.
- Apply research findings to the provision of culturally competent care with considerations for cultural safety and relational practice.

key terms

media resources

evolve Web Site

- Audio Chapter Summaries
- Glossary
- Multiple-Choice Review Questions
- Student Learning Activities
- Weblinks

Companion CD

- Glossary
- Interactive Learning Activities
- Fluids and Electrolytes Tutorial
- Test-Taking Skills

Ethnocultural Diversity

Canada has always been a multicultural nation. At the time of Confederation, more than 50 Aboriginal groups—each with their own language and culture—lived in Canada, in addition to the founding, British and French settlers and other settlers migrating from primarily European countries. Canada is well known as a country that embraces ethnic diversity, relying heavily on immigration for population growth (Adams, 2007). As a result, the societal landscape changes continuously, integrating people from many ethnic groups who have migrated to this country and formed a cultural mosaic that is uniquely Canadian (Statistics Canada, 2007a, 2008b).

The ethnocultural profile of Canada is continually evolving. More than 200 ethnic orgins were reported by the total population in Canada in the 2006 census. After Canadian, the other most frequently reported origins in 2006, either alone or with other origins, were English, French, Scottish, Irish, German, Italian, Chinese, North American Indian, and Ukrainian. According to the 2006 census, visible minorities acccounted for 16.2% of Canada's total population, up from 13.4% in 2001 and 11.2% in 1996 (Statistics Canada, 2008b; Figure 10–1). Between 2001 and 2006, the visible minority population increased at a much faster rate than did the total population (Statistics Canada, 2008b). For the purposes of the 2006 census, the *Employment Equity Act* defines visible minorities as persons, other than Aboriginal peoples, who are non-Caucasian in race or nonwhite in colour (Statistics Canada, 2008b). The increase in the visible minority population was largely attributable to the high proportion of newcomers who belonged to visible minorities.

Figure 10–2 shows the most common visible minority groups in Canada. The three largest visible minority groups are South Asians, Chinese, and Blacks. South Asians surpassed Chinese as the largest visible minority group in 2006 (Statistics Canada, 2008b). Both the populations of South Asians and Chinese were well over 1 million. In Canada in 2006, South Asians represented 24.9% of all visible minorities and 4.0% of the total population; Chinese accounted for about 24.0% of the visible minority population and 3.9% of the total population; and Blacks accounted for 15.5% of the visible minority population and 2.5% of the total population (Statistics Canada, 2008b).

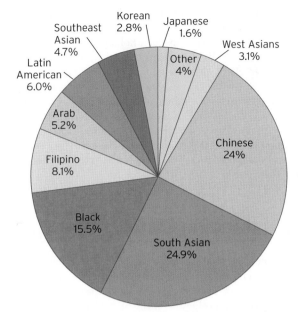

Figure 10-2 The composition of Canada's visible minority population, 2006. **Source:** Adapted from Statistics Canada (2008b). *Canada's ethnocultural mosaic, 2006 census.* Retrieved April 2, 2008, from http://www12.statcan.ca/english/census06/analysis/ethnicorigin/index.cfm

Immigration continues to play a pivotal role in shaping Canada's ethnocultural profile (Statistics Canada, 2007a). According to the 2006 census, approximately 19.8% (one per five) of Canada's total population were born outside of the country, reaching its highest level in 75 years (Statistics Canada, 2007a). For the purposes of the 2006 census, a *foreign-born population* is also known as an *immigrant population* and is defined as persons who are, or who have been, landed immigrants in Canada (Statistics Canada, 2007a). Canada ranks second only to Australia as the country with the highest proportion of foreign-born citizens. In addition, Canada per capita receives more immigrants than does the United States (Statistics Canada, 2007a). The largest groups of immigrants to Canada are from Asian and Middle Eastern countries; this fact has remained virtually unchanged since the 2001 census. In contrast, during 1971, only 12.1% of immigrants to Canada were born in Asian and Middle Eastern countries, and 61.6% were born in Europe. By 2006, 58.3% of recent immigrants were Asian and only 16.1% were European. Immigration has now outpaced the natural birth rate of the country, as revealed by Statistics Canada (2007a) between 2001 and 2006. It indicates that Canada's foreign-born population increased by 13.3%, which was four times higher than the increase in the Canadian-born population of 3.3%. Thus, immigrants and refugees come to Canada from many places, representing more than 200 ethnocultural groups across the country (Statistics Canada, 2007a).

Two other significant parts of Canada's cultural mosaic are the Aboriginal population and the population of French ancestry. In the 2006 census, more than 2 million people, representing 3.8% of the total population, reported having at least some Aboriginal ancestry (Statistics Canada, 2008a). Further details of the Aboriginal population are given later in this chapter. In the 2006 census, population by knowledge of official language by province and territory revealed that citizens who spoke only French totaled more than 4 million, of a total of more than 31 million Canadians (Statistics Canada, 2007b).

In response to Canada's ethnocultural mosaic, nurses require an understanding of difference in order to perceive, critically, the diversity influences that shape healing, well-being, and caring patterns

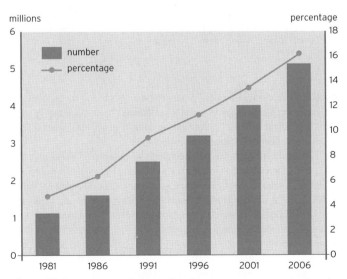

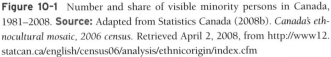

Figure 10-1 Number and share of visible minority persons in Canada, 1981–2008. **Source:** Adapted from Statistics Canada (2008b). *Canada's ethnocultural mosaic, 2006 census.* Retrieved April 2, 2008, from http://www12.statcan.ca/english/census06/analysis/ethnicorigin/index.cfm

(Racher & Annis, 2008). As a nurse who attends to the significance of culture, you must approach clients from a relational standpoint, providing care that is sensitive and holistic (Box 10–1). You will then begin to recognize that clients bring their own cultural values and beliefs to client–nurse relations. You need not impose these restrictions on clients; instead, you should take steps toward creating a relationship in which each person respects the other person's differences. With this understanding between you and your clients, care can be mutually effective and respectful (Canadian Nurses Association [CNA], 2004). With the ever-changing demographics of a multicultural population, you are obliged to provide effective care to all Canadians.

Understanding Cultural Concepts

Clarification of key concepts related to culture and ethnicity will help you understand their complexity and differentiate between them. It is important, however, to emphasize that these concepts are continuing to be examined critically for their strengths and limitations in the interpretation of social reality (Gustafson, 2005). When you think critically, you analyze and evaluate thinking with the goal of improving it. The CNA (2004) describes **culture** broadly as shared patterns of learned values and behaviours that are transmitted over time and that distinguish the members of one group from another. Culture can include language, ethnicity, spiritual and religious beliefs, socioeconomic class, gender, sexual orientation, age, group history, geographic origin, education, as well as childhood and life experiences. According to the CNA's (2008) *Code of Ethics*, "When providing care, nurses do not discriminate on the basis of a person's race, ethnicity, **culture**, political and spiritual beliefs, social or marital status, gender, sexual orientation, age, health status, place of origin, lifestyle, mental or physical ability or socioeconomic status or any other attribute" (p. 14).

Culture has both **visible** (easily seen) and **invisible** (less observable) components. The invisible value and belief system of a particular culture is the major driving force behind visible practices. Although a Sikh man can be easily identified by visible symbols (uncut hair with wooden comb, beard, turban, steel bracelet, and steel dagger), for example, the meanings and beliefs associated with these artifacts are not readily apparent. These artifacts symbolize a devotee's allegiance to the pillars of Sikhism, and removal of them without expressed consent of the individual or his family is considered sacrilegious, violating the ethnoreligious identity of the person. Conversely, an Arab woman who wears a veil may not believe in the reasons for wearing it, but she does so because of her cultural norms.

Any society can be viewed traditionally as being more homogeneous, both linguistically and religiously, than the rest of the country (Adams, 2007). Issues of migration and pluralism, however, are present in each Canadian province. It is important to acknowledge that unique concerns and discussions that characterize the homogeneous societies' approach to new immigrants need to be examined critically. Although **subcultures** may have similarities with the homogeneous culture, their unique life patterns, values, and norms are maintained. In Canada, the prevalent cultures are Anglophones and Francophones with origins from Western Europe. Subcultures such as the Ukrainian and Acadian cultures represent various ethnic, religious, and other groups with characteristics distinct from those of the prevalent cultures. **Ethnicity** refers to groups whose members share a social and cultural heritage. Members of ethnic groups, for example, may share common values, language, history, physical characteristics, and geographical space. The most important characteristic of an ethnic group is that its members feel a sense of common identity. People may

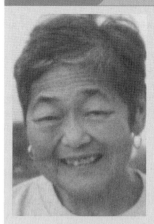

> ► **BOX 10-1**   **Milestones in Canadian Nursing History**

May Aiko Watanabe Yoshida, 1930–2000

Born in Vancouver, British Columbia, May Aiko Watanabe Yoshida was a clinical nurse, teacher, and researcher. She focused her professional life on the need to understand clients and their families in light of their cultural heritage. Not surprisingly, her respect for the cultures and traditions of others grew out of her early personal experiences of discrimination as a Japanese Canadian.

Racist attitudes toward Japanese were rampant in Canada from the time the first immigrants arrived in the late nineteenth century. Laws excluded Asians from most professions, the civil service, and teaching. All Japanese Canadians—including the Canadian-born children of immigrants—were denied the right to vote. Anti-Japanese feeling peaked after Japan attacked Pearl Harbor in 1941; the Canadian government used the *War Measures Act* to order the removal of all Japanese Canadians living within 160 km of the Pacific Coast. Approximately 21,000 men, women, and children of Japanese ancestry—75% of whom were Canadian citizens—were stripped of their property and transported to detention camps. May Watanabe Yoshida and her family were among them.

After the war ended in 1945, Japanese Canadians were forced to choose between deportation to Japan or dispersal east of the Rocky Mountains. May's family chose to relocate in southern Ontario. May, a brilliant student, entered the nursing program at McMaster University in Hamilton and graduated in 1953. She went on to earn a master's degree in 1959.

As a clinician, May Watanabe Yoshida was well known for her work with immigrant families. Specializing in parent–child nursing, she focused on the child-bearing and child-rearing practices of various ethnic groups. She came to believe that people's cultural traditions were central to their health and well-being. Professor May Watanabe Yoshida's many research projects on a range of cultural issues, together with her compelling teaching style, made her a popular speaker internationally. Her work on caring for people of diverse cultures was groundbreaking and continues to be influential.

declare their ethnic identity, for instance, as Scottish, Vietnamese, or Colombian. A term that is usually contrasted with ethnicity is **race**, which is limited to the common biological attributes shared by a group, such as skin colour (Spector, 2004).

Cultural pluralism is a perspective that appreciates "another group for being different and promotes respect for the rights of others to have different beliefs, values, behaviours, and ways of life" (Racher & Annis, 2008, p. 172). **Cultural relativism** "fosters awareness and appreciation of cultural differences, rejects assumptions of superiority of one's culture and adverts ethnocentrism" (Racher & Annis, 2008, p. 172). In any intercultural encounter, nurses "are challenged to be open and responsive to cultural differences, while respecting, protecting, and promoting the rights and well-being of those people and groups with whom they work" (Racher & Annis, 2008, p. 172). As a nurse, for example, you may be baffled by a Korean woman's request for seaweed soup for her first meal after she gives birth. Your personal view of professional postpartum care may not include understandings of the

Korean culture, and so you may be unaware of the significance of the client's traditional cultural practices. Conversely, the Korean client who has an alternative view of Canadian professional care may assume that seaweed soup should be available in the hospital, because it cleanses the blood and promotes healing and lactation (*Korean Health Beliefs*, 2003). Unless you seek to learn your client's ethnocultural views, you are likely to offer inappropriate suggestions, such as another choice of soup.

The processes of enculturation and acculturation facilitate cultural learning. Socialization into one's primary culture during childhood is known as **enculturation**. The process of adapting to and adopting characteristics of a new culture is **acculturation** (Cowan & Norman, 2006). Acculturation outcomes may result in varying degrees of affiliation with the mainstream culture (Spector, 2004). **Assimilation** is a process whereby a minority group gradually adopts the attitudes and customs of the mainstream culture (Srivastava, 2007a).

In contrast to assimilation, **multiculturalism**, regarded as a fundamental characteristic of Canadian society, is a process whereby "many cultures co-exist in society and maintain their cultural differences. Multiculturalism also refers to the public policy of managing cultural diversity in a multi-ethnic society, emphasizing tolerance and respect for cultural diversity" (Srivastava, 2007b, p. 328). In 1971, Canada became the first country in the world to officially adopt a multiculturalism policy. Since then, various laws have been passed to protect and promote the rights of minorities in Canada (Box 10–2). As expressed in the spirit of the multicultural policy, citizens are able to retain their unique ethnocultural traditions within a Canadian context.

Cultural Conflicts

Culture provides the context for valuing, evaluating, and categorizing life experiences. As values, morals, and norms are transmitted from one generation to another, members of ethnic groups may display **ethnocentrism**, a tendency to view their own way of life as more valuable than others'. Health care practitioners who do not understand cultural differences often resort to **cultural imposition**, in which they use their own values and ways of life as the absolute guides in providing services to clients and interpreting their behaviours. Hence, if a nurse believes that pain is to be borne quietly as a demonstration of strong moral character, that nurse may be annoyed by a client's insistence on being given pain medication and, in denying the client's discomfort, may exacerbate the client's pain.

Ethnocentrism is the root of stereotypes, biases, and prejudices against other people perceived to be different from the valued group. You must avoid **stereotypes**, which are generalizations about any particular group that prevent further assessment of unique characteristics. When a person acts on his or her prejudices, **discrimination**—treating people unfairly on the basis of their group membership—occurs. **Racism** involves specific actions and an attitude whereby one group exerts power over others on the basis of either skin colour or racial heritage; its effects are to marginalize and oppress some people and to endow others with privileges (Srivastava, 2007a). Often people do not realize that they are displaying prejudice or discrimination; such displays may be simply negative or fearful reactions to cultural differences (see Chapter 11, description of Ethel Johns's work on racism).

Cultural Awareness

You must be tolerant and nonjudgemental about clients' beliefs and practices. It is important to realize that you will bring your own personal cultural perspectives to the nurse–client relationship and to be aware of how your own culture influences your provision of care (CNA, 2004; Vollman et al., 2008). A strategy for achieving **cultural awareness** is to conduct a self-assessment in order to reflect on your biases and feelings. A set of questions for personal reflection is suggested for this purpose in Box 10–3. Another strategy is to observe nurses who are considered to be exemplary relational practitioners and to notice the particular qualities or characteristics they display when handling of cultural aspects of relationships (Box 10–4).

Historical Development of the Nursing Approach to Culture

It is important to review historically the emergence of transcultural nursing in relation to shifts in thinking about the provision of culturally competent care and cultural safety. Framed primarily within the Canadian context, this history is also best discussed in terms of culturally appropriate nursing practice and education. The importance of being culturally sensitive and aware of a diverse society has been acknowledged by nurses and continues to evolve. Nurses became aware of the conceptual limitations of culture, partly by studying the complexities of race (Ramsden, 2002). Through a critical cultural analysis of the significance of power relations and structural constraints on health and health care, nurses are conceptualizing new ways to provide culturally competent and culturally safe care (Anderson et al., 2003; Browne & Varcoe, 2006; Ramsden, 2002; Smith et al., 2006). A critical historical view of transcultural nursing, cultural competence, and cultural safety is important for understanding the strengths and limitations of these approaches in nursing practice and education (Gustafson, 2005). Increasingly, nurse scholars are questioning whether the health needs of ethnocultural groups are being equitably met (Anderson et al., 2003; Baker, 2007; Smith et al., 2006). Equity may be considered one of the prerequisites and conditions for health. Mill et al. (2005) revealed how "nurses can provide valuable support to the realization of the goal of global health by becoming informed advocates and integrating these concepts, in nursing practice, education and research" (p. 22). Furthermore, in a second article (Ogilvie et al., 2005),

---

> ► **BOX 10-2** | **Legislation Recognizing Diversity in Canada**

Official Languages Act (1969; Updated 1988)

This act recognizes English and French equally as Canada's official languages. The 1988 amendment to this act outlines the obligations of Canadian federal institutions to be committed to promoting full recognition and use of both English and French in Canadian society, as well as supporting the development of the Anglophone and Francophone communities across the country.

Canadian Constitution Act (1982)

This act replaced the *British North America Act* as Canada's Constitution, outlining how Canada governs and structures its society. It also recognizes the Aboriginal peoples of Canada as Indians (Status and Non-Status), Inuit, and Métis.

Canadian Charter of Rights and Freedoms (1982)

Written into the Canadian Constitution in 1982, this charter is a statement of the basic human rights and freedoms of all Canadians.

Canadian Multiculturalism Act (1988)

In recognition of Canada's cultural diversity, this act enshrines the enhancement and preservation of multiculturalism in Canada.

> BOX 10-3   Questions for Reflection and Building Awareness in Community Practice

Personal Self-Awareness

What is my ethnic background? How does my knowledge of my ethnicity affect my identity? What meaning do I ascribe to my ethnic origins? How have they shaped who I am today? What cultural groups do I belong to? What are the rules, customs, and rituals that have been passed on to me and that I will pass on to the next generation of my family? How were these passed on to me, and what meaning do I give to them now? How do the rules and customs passed on to me inform how I engage with others?

Professional Self-Awareness

In my work, how do I relate to others of different cultures? What taken-for-granted assumptions am I prepared to make in the name of efficiency and time constraints? What stereotypes do I hold? How do these beliefs influence my practice? How do I maintain an attitude of cultural attunement in my work with groups and organizations? How do I bridge the differences between ethnic backgrounds in my work? What action might I take to improve my cultural attunement?

Organizational Awareness

What are the values and principles of my organization for working cross-culturally? How does my organization reflect behaviours, attitudes, policies, and structures when working cross-culturally? How does my organization value diversity, manage the dynamics of difference, acquire and institutionalize cultural knowledge, and adapt to diversity and the cutural contexts of the communities it serves?

Community Awareness

How do the dynamics of the community, such as racial tensions, enter into my work with community groups and organizations? When does difference make a difference? How does this community influence feelings of belonging among its residents? What actions do we take to be inclusive? How do we celebrate and honour cultural diversity? What do we need to do differently to be more inclusive and generate feelings of belonging among residents from all cultures?

Adapted from Hoskins, M. L. (1999). Worlds apart and lives together: Developing cultural attunement. *Child and Youth Care Forum, 28*(2), 73–85; Kirkham, S. (2003). The politics of belonging and intercultural health care. *Western Journal of Nursing Research, 25*(7), 762–780; Goode, T. (2004). *Cultural competence continuum.* Washington, DC: National Center for Cultural Competence. Retrieved November 30, 2006, from http://www11.georgetown.edu/research/gucchd/nccc/projects/sides/dvd/continuum.pdf; and Racher, F. E., & Annis, R. C. (2008). Honouring culture and diversity in community practice. In A. R. Vollman, E. T. Anderson, & J. McFarlane (Eds.), *Canadian community as partner: Theory & multidisciplinary practice* (2nd ed., p. 185). Philadelphia, PA: Lippincott Williams & Wilkins.

> BOX 10-4   An Exemplary Relational Practitioner

1. *Identify* someone who you would say is "good at relationships." Why did you identify that person? What qualities or characteristics stand out?
2. Now *identify* someone who is a nurse and is good at relationships. Think of someone with whom you have worked—perhaps a fellow student, a colleague, an instructor. What makes [this person] good at relationships? How is this person perceived by his or her colleagues?
3. *Compare notes* with someone else. Talk to someone who has thought about this question, or talk to someone who knows the person or people you have identified. Do you both value similar attributes and qualities?

From Doane, G. H., & Varcoe, C. (2005). *Family nursing as relational inquiry: Developing health-promoting practice* (p. 192). Philadelphia, PA: Lippincott Williams & Wilkins.

2002a). According to Leininger, the goals of transcultural nursing are to provide *culturally congruent* and *culturally competent* care.

Culturally congruent care is "the use of sensitive, creative, and meaningful care practices to fit with the general values, beliefs, and lifeways of clients" (Leininger & McFarland, 2002, p. 12). In other words, you need to determine how to provide care that does not conflict with clients' valued life patterns and sets of meanings, which may be distinct from your own (Leininger, 2002b).

Leininger and McFarland (2002) defined **culturally competent care** as "the explicit use of culturally based care and health knowledge in sensitive, creative, and meaningful ways to fit the general lifeways and needs of individuals or groups for beneficial and meaningful health and well-being or to help them face illness, disabilities, or death" (p. 84). To provide culturally competent care, you must bridge cultural gaps in care, work with cultural differences, and enable clients and families to receive meaningful care. You need to exhibit specific ability, knowledge, sensitivity, openness, and flexibility toward the appreciation of cultural difference (Suh, 2004). You are then able to develop effective and meaningful interventions that promote optimal health for clients, families, and communities.

The work of Leininger in promoting culturally competent care with people from diverse cultures has been the prevailing model identified in the nursing literature. It has been used as a guide in nursing curricula and practice policies in North America for several decades. In addition, other scholars have developed models of cultural competency in which they have expanded Leininger's work. Davidhizar and Giger (1998; Giger & Davidhizar, 2004) developed a **transcultural assessment model** with a focus on cultural competency that is used in nursing practice. The underlying premise of their model is that each person is culturally unique and should be assessed according to six cultural phenomena: communication, space, social organization, time, environmental control, and biological variations. The model suggests that these phenomena are apparent in all cultural groups, but their application to practice settings varies. Giger and Davidhizar's transcultural assessment model offers a means for you to assess clients' unique health care needs, including their specific cultural health practices.

Campinha-Bacote (2002) further defined cultural competence as an ongoing process, whereby you continuously strive to work within the client's cultural context. As a result, you develop cultural competence rather than possess it. This ongoing process involves integrating cultural awareness, knowledge, skill, encounters, and desire, as depicted in Figure 10–3. *Cultural awareness* is insight into one's own background, and it involves an in-depth self-examination to

the same scholars explained how "nurses can play a pivotal role by becoming informed advocates, challenging their organizations to incorporate a global health mandate and exercising their rights as citizens to influence policy" (p. 25).

The discipline of anthropology and seminal work by Leininger (2002a) relative to cultural nursing have highly influenced the establishment of a theoretical foundation of transcultural nursing (Glittenberg, 2004). Leininger defined **transcultural nursing** as a comparative study of cultures, an understanding of similarities (culture universal) and differences (culture specific) across human groups in order to provide meaningful and beneficial delivery of health care (Leininger, recognize biases, prejudices, and assumptions about other people. *Cultural knowledge* is knowing about the client's culture. It involves learning about diverse groups, including their values, health beliefs, care practices, and world views. As a nurse assigned to a female Egyptian-Canadian client, for example, you decide to seek information about the Egyptian culture. Upon learning that female modesty and gender-congruent care are valued in the culture, you encourage the client's female relatives to assist with her hygiene needs. *Cultural skills* include assessment of social, cultural, and biophysical factors that influence client care. *Cultural encounters* involve engaging in cross-cultural interactions that can teach about other cultures. *Cultural desire* is the motivation and commitment to learn from other people, to accept the role as learner, to be accepting of cultural differences, and to build relationships based on cultural similarities.

Narayanasamy (2002), a nurse scholar in Britain, also developed a framework for cultural competence: the ACCESS model (A for **a**ssessment; C for **c**ommunication; C for **c**ultural negotiation and compromise; E for **e**stablishing respect and rapport; S for **s**ensitivity; and S for **s**afety). The focus of this model is on developing cross-cultural communication, cultural negotiations, diversity, and celebrations, and on fostering cultural safety (Narayanasamy & White, 2005).

In Canada, the CNA (2004) advocated in its position paper that culturally competent care can and should be practised in all clinical settings. Although nurses are responsible for providing culturally competent care, nursing regulatory bodies, professional associations, educational institutions, governments, health service agencies, and accreditation organizations share the responsibility of supporting culturally competent care. You are in a position to build partnerships with other health care professionals, clients, and funding agencies in order to establish culturally diverse practices that optimize clients' health outcomes.

The provision of culturally competent care has been promoted since the 1960s. Only since 2000, however, have Canadian nurse scholars begun to question the limitations of such an approach (Anderson et al, 2003; Kirkham, 2003) and to examine, critically, the concept of **cultural safety** as another approach to providing care to diverse groups, in contrast to the conceptual notion of transcultural nursing (Ramsden, 2002). The College of Registered Nurses of British Columbia's (2006) profile of newly graduated registered nurse practice focuses on the establishment and maintenance of therapeutic caring and culturally safe relationships between clients and health care team members. The cultural safety literature is framed within a critical social theory and postcolonial framework. The concept of cultural safety evolved over a number of years in New Zealand, as nurses tried to identify a way in which health care professionals could more effectively address the inequity in the health status of Maori people. This was combined with an analysis of the historical, political, social, and economic situations influencing the health of Maori people (Ramsden, 2002). Cultural safety involves considering the redistribution of power and resources in a relationship. The notion "is based on the premise that the term 'culture' is used in its broadest sense to apply to any person or group of people who may differ from the nurse/midwife because of socio-economic status, age, gender, sexual orientation, ethnic origin, migrant/refugee status, religious belief or disability" (Ramsden, 2002, Chapter 8, p. 3). In contrast to transcultural nursing, the term *culture* refers to ethnicity. As a result, the philosophy of cultural care has shifted from a notion of cultural sensitivity underpinning the provisions of care irrespective of culture to one of cultural safety with the recognition of power imbalances, the understanding of the nature of interpersonal relationships, and the awareness of institutional discrimination (Browne, & Fiske, 2001; Polaschek, 1998) (Box 10–5).

Ramsden (2002) articulated that *cultural awareness* and *cultural sensitivity* are separate concepts and that those terms are not interchangeable with *cultural safety.* Achieving cultural safety is a stepwise progression from cultural awareness through cultural sensitivity to cultural safety (see Figure 10–4). The outcome of cultural safety is that safe care, defined as such by clients who receive the care, is provided. According to Ramsden (2002), **cultural sensitivity** "alerts students to the legitimacy of difference and begins a process of self-exploration as the powerful bearers of their own life experience and realities which can have an impact on others" (Ramsden, 2002, Chapter 8, p. 4). *Cultural awareness* "is a beginning step toward understanding that there is difference. Many people undergo courses designed to sensitize them to formal ritual and practice rather than the emotional, social, economic and political context in which people exist" (Ramsden, 2002, Chapter 8, p. 4). In terms of achieving cultural safety in nursing practice, Ramsden stated that "the skill for nurses does not lie in knowing the customs or even the health related beliefs of ethno-specific groups. The step before that lies in professional acquistion of trust. . . . Rather than the nurse determining what is culturally safe, it is consumers or patients who decide whether they feel safe with the care that has been given, that trust has been established, and that difference between the patient, the nurse and the institutions that underpin them, can then be identified and negociated" (Ramsden, 2002, Chapter 8, p. 4), as depicted in Figure 10–4.

Cultural Context of Health and Caring

Healing, well-being, and caring are phenomena embedded in a culture (Leininger, 2002a). Culture is the context in which groups of people interpret and define their experiences relevant to life transitions, such as birth, illness, and death. It is the system of meanings by which people make sense of their experiences. Culture is the framework used in defining social phenomena, such as when a person is healthy or requires medical intervention.

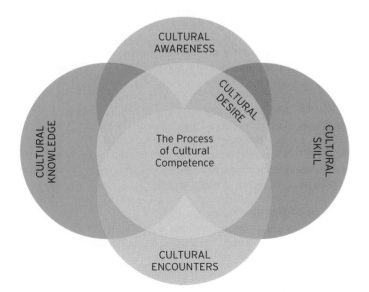

Figure 10-3 The process of cultural competence. **Source:** From Campinha-Bacote, J. (2002). The process of cultural competence in the delivery of health-care services: A model of care. *Journal of Transcultural Nursing, 13*(3), 181. Printed with permission from Transcultural CARE Associates, Cincinnati, OH.

✳ BOX 10-5   RESEARCH HIGHLIGHT

Globalization and the Cultural Safety of an Immigrant Muslim Community

Research Focus

The social health of Muslims who reside in smaller areas of Canada is not clearly understood by health care professionals. The concept of cultural safety has been used in studies of both Aboriginal peoples and immigrants to understand the health of Aboriginal peoples and immigrants in a large metropolitan centre, but the dichotomy between culturally safe and unsafe groups was found to be blurred. To further understand the concept of cultural safety, Baker (2007) focused on the social health of a small immigrant community of Muslims in a relatively homogeneous region of Canada after the terrorist attacks in the United States on September 11, 2001 ("9/11").

Research Abstract

Many Muslims living in North America and Western Europe were negatively affected by the events of 9/11. A qualitative approach based on the constructivist paradigm was used to guide the study, and 26 in-depth interviews were conducted with Muslims (10 women and 16 men) of Middle Eastern, Pakistani, or Indian origin. The participants resided in the province of New Brunswick, Canada, between 2002 and 2003. Data collection and analysis were conducted simultaneously. Steps of unitizing, categorizing, and pattern seeking were used to dissect the interviews until saturation was obtained. Many participants reported that after 9/11, their Islamic faith and experiences of being Muslim suddenly became significant to society at large. The research findings revealed that these participants talked about a sudden transition from cultural safety to cultural risk after 9/11. Their positive experiences of cultural safety included invisibility as a minority and a sense of social integration in the community. Cultural risk was found to stem from intensive international media attention that highlighted their now-visible minority status.

Evidence-Informed Practice

In this study, the findings indicated that globalization does not necessarily blur the distinction between culturally safe and culturally unsafe groups. Cultural risk may be generated by outside forces rather than by long-term inequities in relationships between groups within the community, which did not necessarily originate in historical events. Such findings suggest that you need to think about cultural safety in Muslims within the context of globalization. In addition, you should be cognizant about the cultural safety of your practice when providing care to members of socially disadvantaged cultural groups and how this may influence the heath care received.

References: Baker, C. (2007). Globalization and the cultural safety of an immigrant Muslim community. *Journal of Advanced Nursing, 57,* 296–305.

Table 10–1 provides comparative cultural contexts of health and illness in Western and non-Western cultures. As noted, attributed causes of illness are highly influenced by cultural beliefs. Among the Hmong refugees (a group of people who originated from the mountainous regions of Laos), for example, epilepsy is believed to be caused by wandering of the soul; hence, treatment includes intervention by a shaman who can perform the ritual to retrieve the client's soul (Helsel et al., 2005). The Hmong refugees' beliefs are distinct from those of the scientific community which determine that neurological abnormality causes seizures.

In the Hmong refugee example, the biomedical orientation of Western cultures, which emphasizes scientific investigation and views the human body as reduced into distinct parts, is in conflict with the holistic conceptualization of health and illness in non-Western cultures. Holism is evident in the belief of continuity between humans and nature and between human events and metaphysical and magical–religious phenomena. Hence, epilepsy as conceived by the Hmong people is caused by the loss of one's spirit to the magical and supernatural forces in nature. Establishing a diagnosis of epilepsy in Western cultures requires scientifically proven techniques and confirmed criteria for the abnormality. Such medical criteria are meaningless to the Hmong, who believe in the global causation of the illness that goes beyond the mind and body of the person to forces in nature. The choice of healers or health care practitioners is conditioned by the attributed cause. Whereas a Hmong client may seek a shaman, a Westerner may seek a qualified neurologist. A shaman, unlike a neurologist, has an established reputation in the Hmong community, and the shaman's qualifications are neither determined by standardized criteria nor confined to specific bodily systems. A shaman uses rituals symbolizing the supernatural, spiritual, and naturalistic modalities of prayers, herbs, and incense burning.

The prevailing value orientation in North American society is individualism and self-reliance in achieving and maintaining health. Caring approaches generally promote the client's independence and ability for self-care. In collectivistic cultures that value group reliance and interdependence, such as traditional South Asian culture, caring behaviours are manifested by actively providing physical and psychosocial support for family members. Adult clients are not expected to be solely responsible for their care and well-being; rather, family members are relied upon to make decisions and provide for the care

Cultural safety
is an outcome of nursing education that enables safe service to be defined by those who receive the service.

Cultural sensitivity
alerts nurses to the legitimacy of difference and begins a process of self-exploration as powerful bearers of their own realities which can have an impact on others.

Cultural awareness
is a beginning step toward understanding that there is difference. Many people undergo courses designed to desensitize them to formal ritual and practice rather than the emotional, social, economic, and political context in which people exist.

Figure 10-4 Steps toward achieving cultural safety in nursing practice. **Source:** Adapted from Ramsden, I.M. (2002). *Cultural safety and nursing education in Aotearoa and Te Waipounamu* [Unpublished PhD thesis]. Wellington, New Zealand: Victoria University of Wellington. Retrieved March 31, 2009, at http://culturalsafety.massey.ac.nz.

➤ TABLE 10-1	Comparative Cultural Contexts of Health and Illness	
Characteristic	**Western Cultures**	**Non-Western Cultures**
Cause of illness	Biomedical causes	Imbalance between humans and nature Supernatural Magical–religious
Method of diagnosis	Scientific, high-tech Specialty focused Organ-specific manifestations	Naturalistic, magical–religious Holistic Mixed (e.g., magical–religious, supernatural herbal, biomedical) Observation of global, nonspecific symptoms
Treatment	Specialty specific Pharmacological Surgery	Holistic Mixed
Practitioners/healers	Uniform standards and qualifications for practice	May be learned through apprenticeship Nonuniform criteria for practice Reputation established in community
Caring pattern	Self-care Self-determination	Caring provided by others Group reliance and interdependence

Data from Foster, G. (1976). Disease etiologies in non-Western medical systems. *American Anthropology, 78,* 773; Kleinman, A. (1979). *Patients and healers in the context of culture.* Berkeley, CA: University of California Press; and Leininger, M., & McFarland, M. (2002). *Transcultural nursing: Concepts, theories, research and practice* (3rd ed.). New York: McGraw-Hill.

of clients (Pacquiao, 2003). For example, an older Chinese woman's refusal to independently perform rehabilitation exercises after hip surgery, until her daughter is present to assist her, may be misconstrued by you as a lack of responsibility and motivation for self-care. In contrast, she may interpret your insistence on self-reliance as uncaring behaviour.

Cultural Healing Modalities and Healers

Foster (1976), an anthropologist, identified two distinct cross-cultural categories of healers. **Naturalistic practitioners** attribute illness to natural, impersonal, and biological forces that cause alteration in the equilibrium of the human body. Healing emphasizes naturalistic modalities with the use of herbs, chemicals, heat, cold, massage, and surgery. In contrast, **personalistic practitioners** believe that health and illness can be caused by the active influences of an external agent, which can be human (i.e., a sorcerer) or nonhuman (e.g., ghosts, evil, or a deity). Personalistic beliefs emphasize the importance of humans' relationships with other people, both living and deceased, and with their deities. A voodoo priest, for example, uses modalities that combine supernatural, magical, and religious beliefs through the active facilitation of an external agent or personalistic practitioner. A Haitian woman who believes in voodoo may attribute her illness to a curse that has been placed on her and may then seek the services of a voodoo priest to remove the curse. Personalistic approaches also include naturalistic modalities such as massage, aromatherapy, and herbs (see Chapter 35). Some clients seek both types of practitioners to achieve health and treat illness.

Because clients may use both healing systems simultaneously, you must avoid making judgements about clients' practices. To prevent cultural imposition, you need to gain knowledge and understanding of folk remedies used by clients. Many Southeast Asian cultures, for example, practise folk remedies such as coining, cupping, pinching, and burning to relieve aches and pains and to remove bad winds or noxious elements that cause illness. Other groups,

including Eastern Europeans, also use cupping to treat respiratory ailments. These folk remedies leave peculiar visible markings on the skin in the form of ecchymosis, representing superficial burns, strap marks, or local tenderness. Cultural ignorance may lead a health care practitioner to call authorities for suspicion of abuse. Instead of dismissing the herbal therapy as dangerous and incompatible with Western medicine, you need to inquire further into whether the practice needs to be changed. By consulting and collaborating with herbalists and other naturalistic practitioners, you can prevent unwarranted distress for clients.

Culture and the Experience of Grief and Loss

Dying and death bring a resurgence of traditions that have been meaningful to groups of people most of their lives (see Chapter 29). Societies assign different meanings to death of a child, death of a young person, and death of an older adult. In Western cultures with strong time orientation toward the future and in which children are expected to survive their parents, death of a young person is devastating. In cultures in which infant mortality rates are high, however, the emotional distress over a child's death may be tempered by the reality of the commonly observed risks of growing up. Hence, the untimely death of an adult may be mourned more deeply.

In societies that hold a belief in the concept of reincarnation, such as those of devout Hindus and Buddhists, people may view death as a step toward rebirth. Hence, care of the dying is focused on supporting the client's preparation for a good death. The family may pray and read religious scriptures to the client to improve his or her chances for a good next life. Buddhists generally believe that suffering is a part of life and is mitigated when a person moves beyond the earthly desires and atones for past misdeeds. A dying Hindu man may prepare for a good death by refusing nourishment and medications, concentrating all his energies on the spiritual aspects of the journey for the next life cycle (Pacquiao, 2002).

Culture also strongly influences pain expression and need for pain medication. Whereas most people in Western culture desire freedom from pain and suffering, other groups accept discomfort. As a nurse, you should not assume that pain relief is valued equally across groups. Clients may experience cultural pain when their valued way of life is disregarded by practitioners (Leininger & McFarland, 2002). Because of limitations on the number of visitors allowed at a dying client's bedside. Orthodox Jews may not be permitted to pray in groups there, and this restriction can cause emotional pain to the client and family. Working with the family and its religious or spiritual leader facilitates culturally congruent care (Pacquiao, 2003).

Regulatory mandates and organizational policies intended to benefit clients should be implemented with sensitivity and understanding of clients' cultural life patterns. The high value that Western society places on personal autonomy and self-determination may be in direct conflict with the values of diverse groups. Advanced care directives, informed consent, and consent for hospice are examples of mandates that may violate clients' values. Informed consent and advanced care directives protect the right of the individual to know and make decisions, ensuring continuity of these rights even to the time when the person is incapacitated. Other cultures, however, are organized so that in these situations, the group assumes decision making for a family member and is trusted to make the right decision for the person. Indeed, some groups such as Asian Canadians and South Asian Canadians may expect their family to make decisions for them, and family members may prefer to protect the person from unnecessary suffering caused by knowing that death is imminent. These cultures value group interdependence and view personal autonomy as an unnecessary burden for a loved one who is ill (Pacquiao, 2002, 2003).

The meaning and expression of grief also vary among cultures. Among the usually reserved East Asians, the social position and status of the deceased reflects the extent to which mourners publicly express grief. Korean families, for example, sometimes hire people to lead the open grieving. Religious beliefs also affect attitudes toward cremation, organ donation, and the treatment of body parts. Devout Muslims may refuse an autopsy or organ donation for fear of desecrating the dead and because of their belief that one be whole to appear in front of the creator.

Cultural Assessment

A comprehensive cultural assessment is the basis for providing culturally competent care. A cultural assessment, combined with critical thinking skills, provides the knowledge necessary for transcultural nursing care (Andrews & Boyle, 2003). Cultural assessment is a systematic and comprehensive examination of the cultural care values, beliefs, and practices of individuals, families, and communities. The goal of cultural assessment is to generate from the clients themselves significant information that enables culturally congruent care (Leininger & McFarland, 2002). Several models of cultural assessment exist, each involving different levels of skill and knowledge. Leininger's Sunrise Model (Leininger & McFarland, 2002) depicted in Figure 10–5, demonstrates the inclusiveness of culture in everyday life and helps explain why cultural assessment must be comprehensive. According to the Sunrise Model, cultural care values, beliefs, and practices are embedded in the cultural and social structural dimensions of society, which include environmental contexts, language, and ethnohistory (i.e., significant historical experiences of a particular group). For older adults, for example, the experience of the Great Depression has sometimes resulted in a tendency to be frugal. You must encourage clients to share stories about their lives that reveal how they think and the cultural lifestyle they embrace. Leininger's model differentiates folk care, which is caring as defined by the people, from the health care professions, which is based on the scientific, biomedical system of care.

Whichever assessment model is used, you begin cultural assessment by knowing population demographic changes in the practice setting. You anticipate the client populations that use their own methods of care and gain some knowledge about their cultures before they come to the clinical setting. Background knowledge about a culture assists you in conducting a focused assessment when time is limited. Demographic information can be gathered from the local and regional census data, as well as from the clients themselves. Population demographic information might include the distribution of ethnic groups, education, occupations, and incidence of the most common illnesses. Comprehensive cultural assessment requires skill and time; hence, preparation and anticipation of needs are important.

A challenge in cultural assessment is the lack of ability to assess multiple perspectives of clients and to interpret the assessment information elicited. It helps to use open-ended questions (e.g., "What do you think caused your illness?"), focused questions (e.g., "Have you had this problem before?"), and contrast questions (e.g., "How different is this problem from the one you had previously?"). The aim is to encourage clients to describe values, beliefs, and practices that are significant to their care, which may be taken for granted unless otherwise revealed. Culturally oriented questions are by nature broad and require a lot of description. Table 10–2 provides a list of guiding questions (a **cultural assessment guide**) that focuses on social and cultural dimensions of assessment.

According to some health care professionals, the idea of a specific cultural assessment model or tool further marginalizes those from particular cultures by placing emphasis on the difficulties with difference. It is important to remember that the many questions used in the cultural assessment tool and culturally sensitive communication tool are just as suitable for Canadians within the dominant group, such as white Anglo-Saxons. The question to be raised is this: Why not just have one assessment tool for everyone? For instance, everyone might be asked what their preference for touch is or how they like to be addressed.

Selected Components of Cultural Assessment

Cultural assessment is important in the total care of any client. Over time, you will learn various skills needed to gather an accurate and comprehensive assessment. The following sections describe certain components of cultural assessment which provide information that can be useful in planning and providing nursing care. You may use the following information as a starting point to assess the similarities and differences of clients and families. However, you must not assume that because any two clients come from the same region or country, they share similar values, beliefs, attitudes, and experiences. Other elements to consider are socioeconomic, educational background, family heritage, work or occupation, length of time in Canada, urban or rural origin, and other individual characteristics, such as a disability, sexual orientation, and sociocultural identity (St. Hill et al., 2003).

Ethnohistory

Knowledge of a client's country of origin and its history and ecological contexts is significant to health care. Haitian immigrants, for example, have linguistic and communication patterns distinct from

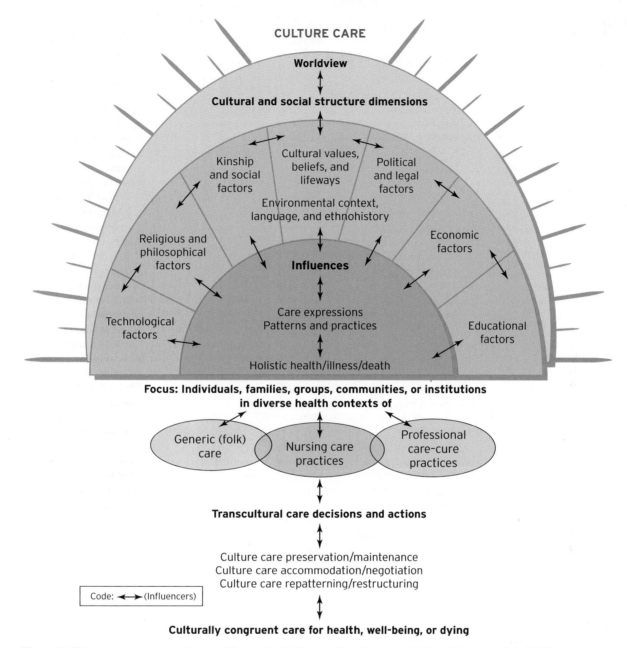

CULTURE CARE

Worldview

Cultural and social structure dimensions

Kinship and social factors

Cultural values, beliefs, and lifeways

Political and legal factors

Environmental context, language, and ethnohistory

Religious and philosophical factors

Economic factors

Influences

Technological factors

Care expressions
Patterns and practices

Educational factors

Holistic health/illness/death

**Focus: Individuals, families, groups, communities, or institutions
in diverse health contexts of**

Generic (folk) care

Nursing care practices

Professional care-cure practices

Transcultural care decisions and actions

Culture care preservation/maintenance
Culture care accommodation/negotiation
Culture care repatterning/restructuring

Code: ◄—► (Influencers)

Culturally congruent care for health, well-being, or dying

Figure 10-5 Leininger's culture care theory and Sunrise Model. **Source:** From Leininger, M. M., & McFarland, M. R. (2002). *Transcultural nursing: Concepts, theories, research and practice* (3rd ed., p. 80). New York: McGraw-Hill.

those of Jamaicans, even though both groups come from the Caribbean region and may have a common history of oppression. Differences can be traced to their colonial history and intermingling with the local indigenous people. Cultural characteristics of Hindu immigrants from Jamaica are different from those of Hindu immigrants from India because of the cultural contexts of the different regions. The nutritional, communication, and health patterns of Hindus from Jamaica may be more similar to those of African Jamaicans than to those of South Asian Hindus. When caring for a Hindu client of Indian descent who grew up in Jamaica, you may expect that he or she will interact more like a Jamaican, although he or she may look South Indian.

You should be aware that people immigrate to another country for various reasons and have different motivations for doing so. Refugees may be relocated without having chosen their new location, in contrast to immigrants who are able to choose where they live. Refugees

tend to experience greater dislocation and deprivation than do immigrants who enter Canada with specialized skills and education and who have the option to return to their homeland. Age at immigration may determine the level of acculturation: Younger immigrants acculturate faster than do their older counterparts. Similarities shared by an immigrant group with the prevailing culture in society are strong predictors of how easily the members of that group adjust. Although acculturation and length of residence in the new country are related, outcomes may be affected by other factors, such as education, racial characteristics, and familiarity with language and religion. You may ask clients about the circumstances that brought them to Canada and how they believe they are adjusting. You need to understand, for instance, any problems the client may have (such as becoming comfortable with routines or the language used to arrange medical appointments), in order to make reasonable and appropriate adjustments to care.

> **TABLE 10-2**   **Cultural Assessment Guide**

Subject	Suggested Questions
Cultural identity/ancestry/heritage	Where were you born? Where were your parents born?
Ethnohistory	How long have you or your parents resided in this country? What is your ethnic background or ancestry? How strongly are you influenced by your culture? Why did you leave your homeland?
Social organization	Who lives with you? Whom do you consider members of your family? Where do you live? Where do other members of your family live? How do you contact them? How often do you have contact with your family members? Who makes the decisions for you or your family? Whom do you go to outside of your family for support? What do you expect your family members to do for you? How different are your expectations of them now from your expectations at other times? What expectations do you have of your family members who are male, female, old, or young?
Socioeconomic status	What do you do for a living? What did you do back in your homeland? Where did you go to school? What level did you finish in school? How different is your life here from your life back in your homeland? Do you have a primary health care professional? What other health care professionals have you seen?
Biocultural ecology and health risks	What is your purpose for coming here? What caused your problem? Have you had this problem before? Does this problem affect your life and your family? How? Do other members of your family have this kind of problem? How do you treat this problem at home? Whom do you go to for this kind of problem? What other plans do you have for dealing with this problem? What do you think we should do for you? What other problems do you have? Have these problems occurred with any other member of your family?
Language and communication	What language(s) do you speak at home? What language(s) are you most comfortable speaking? In what language(s) can you read and write? How do you want us to talk to you? How should we address you, or what should we call you? What kinds of communication upset or offend you? What words would you use to describe how you feel? Do you need an interpreter? Would you prefer a female or male interpreter?
Religion/spirituality	What is your religion? Who is your religious or spiritual leader? Do you want to be in touch with your religious leader? How do we contact your spiritual leader? What are some of the things we need to do within your religion? How do you practise your religion? Do you follow specific dietary practices?

> **TABLE 10-2** **Cultural Assessment Guide** *continued*

Caring beliefs and practices	What do you do to keep yourself well?
	What do you do to show someone you care?
	How does your family or you take care of sick family members?
	Which caregivers do you seek when you are sick?
	How do you decide when to go to a caregiver and which one to go to?
	How different is what we do from what your family does for you when you are sick?
	Are we doing what you think we should be doing for you?
	How should we give you care?
Experience with professional health care	Since you came to this country, have you had contact with doctors or hospitals?
	How do you compare your past health care experience is with those of the present?
	What were some of the problems that you encountered?
	How were they resolved?
	What were the positive experiences you had?
	What type of health care professional do you prefer? Why?
	If you have a choice, what changes do you wish to see?

You should also be aware that newly arrived immigrants and refugees, depending on the geographic location from which they originate, are vulnerable to a variety of health conditions, including tuberculosis, hepatitis B, anemia, dental caries, intestinal parasites, nutritional deficiencies, incomplete immunization, and mental and emotional concerns such as depression and post-traumatic stress disorder (Kemp, 2004). New immigrants and refugees also frequently experience language barriers, social isolation, separation from family, loss and grief, and a lack of information about available resources. It is important that you explore the historical and sociopolitical background of a client with regard to the specific immigrant community; this knowledge assists you in formulating a plan of care (Lo & Pottinger, 2007). Therefore, you should be aware of, and advocate for, primary health care programs in the community for these vulnerable clients (Box 10–6).

Social Organization

Cultural groups consist of units of organization delineated by kinship, status hierarchy, and appropriate roles for their members. In the prevailing Western society, the most common unit of social organization is the nuclear family, in which adult children are expected to establish residences separate from those of their parents. In collectivistic cultures, family composition may be extended to distant blood relatives across generations and non–blood-related kin. Kinship may be extended to both the father's and mother's side of the family (bilineal) or limited to the side of either the father (patrilineal) or the mother (matrilineal). Patrilineally extended families—in which a woman is expected to move into her husband's clan after marriage and kinship ties with her family of orientation (her own parents and siblings) are minimized—are observed among Chinese and Hindus. You must consider all options when determining a client's next of kin. This is especially relevant to new immigrants and refugees, who may have relocated without intact families. Collectivistic groups may regard members of their ethnic group as closest kin and might want to consult them for health care decisions, as well as permit them to speak on their behalf.

The status of a client within the social hierarchy is generally linked with qualities such as age and gender, as well as with achievements such as education and position. The mainstream culture in Canada emphasizes achievement as the determinant of status, whereas most collectivistic cultures give higher priority to age and gender. In many

---

✳ BOX 10-6 **FOCUS ON PRIMARY HEALTH CARE**

Providing Primary Health Care to Canadian Immigrants

Responsiveness to community needs is a key element of primary health care and refers to an approach to health and a spectrum of services beyond those provided by the traditional health care system. New immigrants and refugees in Canada often need assistance overcoming the language, cultural, and information service barriers that prevent them from using health and social services. Across the country, many community health centres respond to these needs; for example, the New Canadian Clinic in Surrey (NCCS) is overcoming barriers to provide better primary health care access to immigrants who have recently arrrived in the lower mainland of British Columbia. The NCCS is an excellent example of innovation in action that is effectively addressing a pressing community need to ensure that all community members have access to timely and appropriate medical care. Its goal is to augment and integrate existing Fraser Health services with the social supports of the immigrant network in Surrey, British Columbia, in order to provide a coordinated continuum of care. The benefits of this new health care model include shorter lengths of stay in hospitals, fewer visits to emergency departments, and improvement in the overall health of immigrants.

The NCCS uses a multidisciplinary and multilingual team approach to assist new immigrants in integrating more quickly into the mainstream health care system. The team, led by a nurse practitioner, includes a nurse, a mental health counsellor, a medical office assistant, and a community health liaison worker, each of whom has the skills necessary to address the complex needs of recently arrived immigrants. The services of interpreters are readily used, and the clinical team focuses mainly on providing health management, education, and self-management support for new immigrants with multiple chronic diseases, such as heart disease, lung disease, diabetes, and renal disease.

Modified from Ministry of Health, Fraser Health, British Columbia. (2008, January 23). *Innovation helping to meet health needs of immigrants* [news release]. Retrieved September 4, 2008, from http://www2.news.gov.bc.ca/news_releases_2005-2009/2008HEALTH0006-000079.htm

Asian and African cultures, for instance, the eldest son is next in line after his father in terms of authority. Therefore, a Korean mother is subject to the authority of her oldest son in the absence of her husband. Older adults generally occupy higher status in some societies, so that grandparents may impose their decisions regarding the care of grandchildren over the decisions of their married children. You may be required to facilitate and support the negotiations for determining who has the responsibility for family decision making. Think of a nurse you have observed who acted as negotiator, advocate, and facilitator in a situation in which family roles needed to be clarified.

Role expectations of family members may be defined by culture and differentiated by gender. Devout female Muslims, for example, tend to be caregivers, and male Muslims tend to be providers and major decision makers. Some Muslim women may insist on staying at the bedside of an unwell child, in-laws, or husband, but the assumption that she can be relied on to make decisions independently as the primary caregiver may be unrealistic. An understanding of the social hierarchy of the family must be determined as soon as possible, in order to avoid offending clients and their families.

Socioeconomic Status, Biocultural Ecology, and Health Risks

The identification of health risks related to sociocultural and biological history can be assessed on admission of clients. Distinct health risks can be attributed to the ecological context of the culture. Immigrants from the region near the Nile River, for example, are generally predisposed to parasitic infestations endemic to that region. Immigrants from developing countries with poor sanitary conditions and water supply may have infections such as hepatitis that they can pass on to others. In addition, biological variations exist between people from different ethnic groups. As a result, some groups have greater risk of developing certain health conditions. Some genetic disorders, for example, are linked with specific groups, such as Tay-Sachs disease among Ashkenazi Jews and malignant hypertension among Black Canadians.

Language and Communication

Distinct linguistic and communication patterns are associated with different cultural groups. These patterns reflect the core cultural values of a society. In Western cultures that uphold individualism, assertive communication is valued because it demonstrates autonomy and self-determination. People are expected to say what they mean and to mean what they say. In collectivistic cultures, communication is shaped by the context of relationships among participants. Group harmony is the priority, so that participants interact on the basis of their expected positions and relationships within the social hierarchy. People are more likely to remain respectful and show deference to older adults or family leaders, even though they may disagree on an issue. Differences in status and position, age, and gender determine the content and process of communication (Box 10–7). Among Asian cultures, for example, face-saving communication promotes harmony by indirect, ambiguous communication and by conflict avoidance. Messages spoken may have little to do with their meanings. Saying "no" to a superior or older person may not be permitted; hence, an affirmative response of a subordinate may mean only "I heard you," rather than full agreement.

In cultural groups with distinct linear hierarchy, conflict is negotiated between people with the same level of position or authority. Identifying and working with family members of an established hierarchy may prevent miscommunication. In cultures with highly differentiated gender roles, some clients may place more value on the

✳ BOX 10-7 FOCUS ON OLDER ADULTS

Culturally Sensitive Communication

- Ask older adults how they like to be addressed. If you are in doubt, address them formally (e.g., "Mr. Lin").
- Determine the client's preferences where touch is concerned. For example, US citizens often greet each other with a firm handshake. Many Native Americans, however, may see this as a sign of aggression, and touch outside of marriage is sometimes forbidden for older adults from the Middle East.
- Investigate the client's preferences vis-à-vis silence. In general, silence is valued in Eastern cultures, whereas in Western cultures, people are uncomfortable with silence.
- Be aware of the client's beliefs about eye contact during conversation. Direct eye contact in European American cultures may be a sign of honesty and truthfulness. However, eye contact with other groups, such as older Native Americans, may not be allowed. Older Asian adults sometimes avoid eye contact with authority figures because this is considered disrespectful, and direct eye contact between genders in Middle Eastern cultures is sometimes forbidden except between spouses.

Data from Meiner, S. E., & Leuckenotte, A. G. (2006). *Gerontologic nursing* (3rd ed.). St. Louis, MO: Mosby.

advice of a male nurse than on that of a female nurse. By recognizing and working within a particular cultural context, the nurse can become more effective in achieving appropriate outcomes.

Nonverbal communication is also shaped by communication. Culture influences the distance between participants in an interaction, the extent of touching, the degree of eye contact, and how much private information the client shares. Clients use less distance when speaking to trusted affiliates and persons of the same gender, age, and social position. Members of many ethnic groups tend to speak their own dialect with each other in order to feel ease and to secure privacy. To minimize the distance when communicating with clients, you need to consider taking up a relational approach to cultural nursing that greatly enhances the ability to know and respond to people (Hartrick Doane & Varcoe, 2005). A relational approach to nursing allows you not only to connect across differences but also to recognize cultural similarities and differences more intently. Such an approach provides opportunities "to attend to issues of meaning, experience, race, history, culture, health, and sociopolitical systems. In addition, as we relationally honor and attend to such differences the potential for growth, change, and knowledge development is enhanced" (Hartrick Doane & Varcoe, 2005, p. 9).

Religion and Spirituality

Religious and spiritual beliefs have major influences on the person's attitudes toward health and illness, pain and suffering, and life and death. The distinction between religion and spirituality is often blurred. It is advisable for you to understand the multiple perspectives of clients. Many cultures do not separate religion and spirituality, whereas many others have totally distinct concepts of the two. To a Hmong animist, spirits could be those of dead ancestors or forces external to the person. To an Anglo-Canadian, spirituality may mean an inner, personal relationship with a higher being. Although a discussion of religious and spiritual philosophies is difficult in a hospital setting, you must assess what is important to the spiritual well-being of clients and learn as much as possible about their spiritual and religious practices (see Chapter 28).

Caring Beliefs and Practices

Caring beliefs and practices incorporate a client's perception of his or her ability to control circumstances or factors in the environment. Specifically, it may refer to a client's perception of how he or she can influence causes of illness and use cultural healing modalities and healers. During cultural assessment, you should identify the health practices of the client and respect them (Box 10–8). Obtain information about folk remedies used and cultural healers employed by the client. Unless these practices are harmful, they should be incorporated into the client's plan of care.

Experience with Professional Health Care

All cultures have concepts of past, present, and future dimensions of time. An aspect of a client's experience with professional health care, for instance, may be your understanding of the client's orientation of time. This information can be useful in planning care, arranging appointments for procedures, and helping a client plan self-care activities at home. Differences exist in the concepts of time that cultures emphasize and in how time is expressed. Communication concerning time may be indirect and circular in order to avoid offending and disrespecting other people.

Present time orientation, for instance, may conflict with the policies of a health care institution that emphasizes punctuality and adherence to appointments. Improving clients' access to health services may be achieved by mutually negotiating schedules and by accommodating cultural patterns.

Application of Cultural Assessment Components to Aboriginal Peoples of Canada

Aboriginal peoples represent an important and growing group within Canada. In 2006, the number of people who identified themselves as Aboriginal (i.e., North American Indian [First Nations], Métis, and Inuit) surpassed one million (Statistics Canada, 2008a). Since the mid-1990s, the Aboriginal population has increased significantly. Between 1996 and 2006, it grew by 45%, nearly six times faster than the 8% rate of increase for the non-Aboriginal population (Statistics Canada, 2008a). In 2006, Aboriginal peoples accounted for almost 4% of the total population of Canada (Statistics Canada, 2008a). Of the three Aboriginal groups in Canada, the Métis population increased the most. Aboriginal peoples in Canada also increasingly live in urban centres. In 2006, 54% lived in urban areas (including large cities or census metropolitan areas and smaller urban centres); this proportion increased from 50% in 1996 (Statistics Canada, 2008a). Furthermore, the Aboriginal population is, on average, younger than the non-Aboriginal population. Almost half (48%) of the Aboriginal population consists of children and youth aged 24 and younger, in comparison with 31% of the non-Aboriginal population (Statistics Canada, 2008a).

The three Aboriginal groups—First Nations, Métis, and Inuit—have their own unique languages, heritages, cultural practices, and spiritual beliefs. These groups contain many subgroups, each with its own unique culture. The term *Indian* describes all the Aboriginal peoples in Canada who are not Métis or Inuit. These include the nations or groups of people who were originally living in Canada before the European explorers began to arrive in the 1600s. Three legal definitions are used to describe Indians in Canada: Status, Non-Status, and Treaty Indians. Status Indians are registered under the *Indian Act* (Indian and Northern Affairs Canada, 2004), which regulates the management of reservations and sets out certain federal obligations. Non-Status Indians are not registered under the *Indian Act* (Indian and Northern Affairs Canada, 2004). A *Treaty Indian* is a Status Indian who belongs to a First Nation that signed a treaty with the United Kingdom (Indian and Northern Affairs Canada, 2004).

Many Aboriginal people find the term *Indian* offensive and outdated; in the 1970s, the term *First Nation* became preferred to *Treaty Indians*. In addition, many Indian people adopted the term *First Nation* to replace the word *band,* and also amended the term *First Nation* to the name of their community, such as the *Nuxalk First Nation* (Indian and Northern Affairs Canada, 2004; Wasekeesikaw, 2006). Some Aboriginal people prefer the more inclusive term *First Peoples* rather than the word *Nation* because in English, *Nation* does not fit with the Aboriginal social structure. The first European explorers to arrive in North America used the term *Indian* because they thought they had reached India (Canadian Health Network, 2004). First Nations peoples claim that the roots of the term *Indian* reflect a history of colonialism and that the term is, therefore, inappropriate (Wasekeesikaw, 2006).

The following sections describe the variations from the non-Aboriginal culture that exist among Canadian Aboriginal peoples. Bear in mind that these discussions are general in nature, and each client must be assessed as an individual.

✳ **BOX 10-8**   **NURSING STORY**

Identifying the Client's Health Care Practices

A Chinese immigrant who recently arrived in Canada has given birth to her first child. Once the newborn has been cared for and is resting, you ask the new mother if she would like to take a shower. The mother refuses politely. Her belief is that if she takes a shower, she could contract rheumatism in old age. Then the mother's food tray arrives, and she does not touch or eat anything. For this newcomer to Canada, the hospital food may seem different and served in an unfamiliar manner. Her family brings plain rice and salted pork into the hospital. They also bring two different soups, which are thought to bring heat, the "yang," into her body, thereby removing the impurities from her system.

In traditional Chinese culture, good health means achieving a balance between yin and yang. The belief is that all body systems interact with each other and with the environment to produce a balanced state of wellness. In consultation with the mother, you are able to assess and understand why she is refusing to shower and eat the hospital food. With this increased understanding, you are able to mutually negotiate with the mother some alternatives for her care to accommodate her needs, without jeopardizing her care or causing her distress. You appropriately assess that rather than showering, the mother would prefer a basin of water and a cloth that she could use to clean herself. In terms of her dietary requests, you determined that she can eat the food from home as long as it does not interfere with or jeopardize her health status. As a result, your sensitivity and respect for the new mother's cultural beliefs enable her to relax and recover in a culturally appropriate manner. You were open to learning about the cultural beliefs of the new mother and then collaborating with her on decisions about care.

Ethnohistory

"I am an Indian. I am proud to know who I am and where I originated. I am proud to be a unique creation of the Great Spirit. We are part of Mother Earth . . . .
We have survived, but survival by itself is not enough.
A people must also grow and flourish."
(Snow, Chief John. [1977]. *These mountains are our sacred places.* Toronto, ON: Samuel Stevens.)

An understanding of specific cultural Aboriginal groups in Canada is important in order to appreciate contemporary health issues affecting Aboriginal peoples. The First Nations of Canada are exceptionally diverse, culturally, linguistically, socially, economically, historically, and in other ways. As Waldram et al. (2006) emphasized, "the recognition and acceptance of such diversity is essential to an appreciation of developments in the health care field and to an appreciation of the myriad processes that have affected the health status of Aboriginal people in both the pre-contact and post-contact periods" (p. 23).

Pre-European contact refers to the history of Aboriginal people before exploration and settlement of the Americas by Europeans. During that period, Aboriginal people were composed of distinct cultures from the Arctic, Western Subarctic, Easter Subarctic, Northeastern Woodlands, Plains, Plateau, and Northwest Coast. Traditional health beliefs, shamans, herbalists, and folk medicine were aspects of how Aboriginal communities experienced healing and well-being. **European contact** began on Canada's east coast, where French explorers and fur traders settled and introduced diseases such as smallpox, tuberculosis, and measles, which killed thousands of Aboriginal people. Scarce resources diminished Aboriginal livelihoods, and malnutrition, starvation, and alcohol consumption made circumstances worse (Dickason, 2006). During **post-European contact,** Europeans established relationships with Aboriginal people, and colonization influenced Aboriginal systems of government, trade, and health care. Over the years, the Canadian government displaced Aboriginal people from their traditional lands and developed policies to isolate them, "civilize" them, and assimilate them into Canadian society, which resulted in the destruction of Aboriginal cultures. These oppressive and suppressive policies, and the acts that followed, had extensive negative effects on Aboriginal cultural identities and governances (Wasekeesikaw, 2006). The Indian residential school system, for instance, which no longer exists in Canada, left a multi-generational legacy of physical and psychological abuse that "lives on in the form of significant pain and suffering among residential school survivors and their families" (Barton et al., 2005b, p. 295).

Social Organization

Many First Nations peoples live on reserves and in communities in each of the Canadian provinces and territories, and many Inuit live in settlements throughout the territories. The reserves are easily accessible in the southern regions but remote and isolated in the northern regions. Métis live in communities across Canada and in settlements set aside for them in Alberta. For many Aboriginal people, the biological family is the traditional centre of social organization and includes all members of the extended family. The principles that guide family and community social organization by which they live their lives include the notion of wholeness, whereby "all things are interrelated, and everything in the universe is part of a signal whole. Everything is connected in some way to everything else, and it is only possible to understand something if one understands how it is connected to everything else" (Hunter et al., 2004, p. 274).

Socioeconomic Status

Cultural disorganization resulting from colonization underpins the culture of poverty, circumstances that are experienced by many Aboriginal people in contemporary Canadian society. Large proportions of the Aborginal population live in remote communities (Statistics Canada 2008a) and travel back and forth between rural and urban environments. In general, the Aboriginal population experiences both poorer health and reduced access to health services in comparison with most Canadians living in rural and urban locations. Along with other inequities and social injustices that contribute to their vulnerability, they are socially, economically, and politically marginalized from mainstream society. "Thus, there is a complex interplay between geographical context and the historical socio-economic and political context of Aboriginal people's health, and it has profoundly influenced the health and social status of Aboriginal Canadians" (Tarlier et al., 2007, p. 129).

Biocultural Ecology and Health Risks

Since the 1950s, dramatic changes in lifestyle have affected the social, environmental, and health status of Aboriginal people (Waldram et al., 2006). The disease patterns in many First Nations and Inuit communities continue to resemble those found in low-income countries, despite improvements since the 1990s (Health Canada, 2003). In addition, the prevalence of major chronic diseases, including diabetes, cardiovascular disease, cancer, arthritis, and rheumatitis, appears to be increasing in this population (Vollman et al., 2008). Rates of unintentional injuries, deaths from drowning, and other accidents are also high among children and families in Aborginal communities (Vollman et al., 2008).

Tuberculosis. Although the overall incidence of tuberculosis has dropped steadily since the 1960s, the incidence among First Nations and Inuit people is almost seven times higher than the national rate, according to 1998 statistics (Health Canada, 2008a). Factors contributing to such a high rate include overcrowding and unsafe or unreliable water supplies in these communities.

Hepatitis A. The rate of hepatitis A virus infection among First Nations and Inuit people tends to be significantly higher than the overall Canadian rate (Minuk & Uhanova, 2003). The major factors believed to contribute to these periodic outbreaks are poor housing, poor water supplies, and lack of sewage treatment.

Diabetes Mellitus. Diabetes is considered to be an epidemic in progress for Canadian Aboriginal peoples, with a prevalence of diabetes of three to five times higher, according to location, than that in non-Aboriginal communities (Health Canada, 2003). The factors contributing to this rate appear to be a combination of genetic susceptibility, a change from a physically active lifestyle to a sedentary lifestyle, and a diet high in sugar, fats, and salt. Type 2 diabetes is diagnosed with increasing frequency in Aboriginal children (Health Canada, 2003). Earlier onset of the disease leads to an earlier onset of complications, as well as excessive mortality rates among young and middle-aged adults. In Inuit communities, the rate of diabetes is still relatively low, but concerns have been raised that this may change if the Inuit alter their traditional eating patterns and lifestyle (Health Canada, 2003).

HIV and AIDS. Human immunodeficiency virus (HIV) infections and cases of acquired immune deficiency syndrome (AIDS) among Canadian Aboriginals have increased steadily since the 1990s, whereas the annual number of AIDS cases has levelled off in the rest of the population. The proportion of Aboriginal people who tested positive for HIV infection increased from 19% in 1998 to 24% in 2002. This number may be misleadingly low, however, inasmuch as ethnic identity is unknown for about 15% of clients with AIDS. Aboriginal clients with AIDS differ significantly from non-Aboriginal clients with AIDS. Among Aboriginal clients, for example, the proportion of female clients is much higher than that of male clients (25% in comparison with 9%), and the proportion of intravenous drug users is higher among non-Aboriginal clients (38% in comparison with 7%) (Waldram et al., 2006).

Alcohol and Substance Abuse. It is difficult to collect accurate data, but the abuse of alcohol and other substances is perceived to be common in some Aboriginal communities (Health Canada, 2008b). Alcohol and substance abuse can be viewed as part of a set of complex issues affecting the social and physical well-being of the client, the family, and the community. The National Native Alcohol and Drug Abuse Program was established to assist First Nations and Inuit community members in instituting and operating programs aimed at reducing the level of alcohol, drug, and solvent abuse among target groups on reserves. The program emphasizes prevention and treatment, as well as training, research, and development.

Suicide. The suicide rates in Inuit and First Nations communities are five to six times higher than the rates found in the non-Aboriginal population (Statistics Canada, 2008c). Possible factors contributing to the suicide rate include psychobiological factors (pre-existing mental illness, personality disorders, dysfunctional cognitive style), situational life history factors (early childhood trauma, family dysfunction, substance abuse, conflict with authority, absence of spirituality), socioeconomic factors (poverty, unemployment), and cultural stress (low self-esteem, lack of cultural heritage) (Waldram et al., 2006).

Language and Communication

Approximately 53 Aboriginal languages exist, with Algonquian being the largest and most widespread language family in Canada (Dickason, 2006). Many of these languages have identifiable dialects. Interpreters who can speak the various dialects within a language are invaluable, but locating them poses challenges to the health care system. Knowledgeable interpreters, however, not only understand and translate the clients' words but also interpret the culture and make relevant the concepts underlying it as well. For some Aboriginal Canadians, for instance, it is important to realize that reflection may lead to gaps, and thus long silences, in the conversaton (Watts & McDonald, 2007).

Religious and Spiritual Practices

The spiritual approaches of Aboriginal peoples incorporate a mind–body–spirit connection that is harmonious with nature. For some, the circle of life is often viewed as having four aspects or directions: spiritual, physical, mental, and emotional. The presence of all components together enables the person to heal the self and restore well-being. It is in the understanding of wholeness that the spiritual, physical, mental, emotional, and relational parts of the self are integrated. Transcending these dimensions, however, is the spiritual component, which assists the person in discovering his or her human potential (Hunter et al., 2004).

Caring Beliefs and Practices

Aboriginal peoples subscribe to a holistic concept of health but exemplify tremendous diversity of background and experience in terms of culture, language, and traditions (Wasekeesikaw, 2006). The caring beliefs and practices of various groups are linked to being alive and well, which may be understood as the interconnected relationship people create with the land and the plants and animals of nature. Aboriginal health and healing incorporates many aspects within the circle of life that includes, for instance, being human, stewarding the land, hunting wild animals, eating traditional foods, and practising herbal medicine. In a study that focused on the experience of diabetes among Aboriginal people living in a rural Canadian community (Barton et al., 2005a), the findings revealed cultural themes associated with Western and traditional medicines; dietary changes, exercise, and weight loss; culturally relevant communication; Aboriginal life choices and the responsibility to choose; and a belief in living day by day. Within this particular First Nations community, the researchers found that "(i) consultative meetings with community members; (ii) the use of a cultural awareness program for health professionals; and (iii) the involvement of Aboriginal people in the development of their own diet, exercise and prevention strategies would greatly enhance [diabetes] programs in the future. [Such initiatives] could contribute not only to the culturally safe management of diabetes, but also encourage its early detection now and in the future" (Barton et al., 2005a, p. 245).

Experience With Professional Health Care

Although cultural sensitivity frameworks will guide you in your relationships with clients, systematized and taxonomic descriptions of characteristics particular to a cultural group do not always "accommodate peoples' diet preferences, communication styles, family dynamics, and culturally-based responses to pain, child-birth, childrearing, etc." (Browne & Varcoe, 2006, p. 158). You need to ask yourself how you can think about notions of culture without stereotyping or thinking simplistically about Aboriginal people and without inciting hurtful and nonconstructive assumptions about cultural difference. In contemplating this question, Dion Stout and Downey (2006) described the conceptual links between nursing, Aboriginal peoples, and cultural safety. They contended that (1) "the caring spaces that are occupied by Indigenous people and nurses are also potentially the new arenas of struggle for both sides"; (2) "attention between the totality of self and the totality of one's environment is inherent in cultural safety affecting both nurses and Indigenous people"; and (3) "an overemphasis on culture as a health determinant can bring about an abdication of responsibility over all other health determinants by health determiners like Indigenous people and nurses" (p. 327).

Implications for Nursing Practice

The importance of cultural competency and safety for health care administrators, practitioners, and educators has been recognized by the National Aboriginal Health Organization (NAHO). NAHO's (2008) document describes the origins of cultural competency and cultural safety; a theoretical and methodological approach to cultural safety, an approach that originated with Aboriginal peoples; and the importance of its application to health care.

Increasingly, nurse scholars are researching the health challenges faced by Aboriginal peoples and discovering how to provide culturally competent care (Majumdar et al., 2004; Smith, 2003). Smith et al. (2006) focused on establishing safety and responsiveness as a mainstay of care for pregnant and parenting Aborginal people. Their findings revealed "that safety and healthcare relationships and settings, and responsiveness to individuals' and families' experiences and capacities must be brought into the forefront of care. [These] results suggest that the intention of care must be situated in a broader view of colonizing relations to improve early access to, and relevance of, care during pregnancy and parenting for Aboriginal people" (p. E27).

One reason why people become nurses is a desire to "act in ways that are respectful, compassionate, and equitable and that leaves [nurses] feeling that [they] have somehow 'done good'" (Hartrick Doane & Varcoe, 2005, p. 16). A relational approach to nursing shapes the places of inquiry and practice that determine how to find your way through relationships, culture, safety, ethics, diversity, power, economics, communication, and history. A deep consideration of **relational practice** and nursing obligations offers you the means to understand experience and to imagine how you might incorporate reflexivity, intentionality, and openness into practice, education, and research.

In regard to practice, Hartrick Doane and Varcoe (2007) presented an example of a nurse recalling the interaction with an elderly woman in the emergency department who needed to be invited to reveal her "whole" experience. The woman's story "exemplifies the significance of a nurse–patient relationship and the profound difference it can make in promoting health and healing" (p. 195). In terms of education, Smith et al. (2007) described "community-based stakeholders' views of how safe and responsive care 'makes a difference' to health and well-being for pregnant and parenting Aboriginal people." Smith et al. concluded that "design and evaluation of care based upon community values and priorities and using a strengths-based approach can improve early access to a relevance of care during pregnancy and parenting for Aboriginal people" (p. 321). In considering research, Barton (2004) focused on a form of narrative inquiry as a relational method of critically analyzing its appropriateness as an innovative approach to researching Aboriginal people's experience of living with diabetes. By locating Aboriginal epistemology in a relational method such as narrative inquiry, "the ability to adapt a methodology for use in a cultural context, preserve the perspectives of Aboriginal peoples, maintain the holistic nature of social problems, and value co-participation in respectful ways are strengths of an inquiry partial to a responsive and embodied scholarship" (p. 519).

✳ KEY CONCEPTS

- Culture is the context for interpreting human experiences such as health and illness and provides direction for decisions and actions.
- Transcultural nursing is a comparative study and understanding of cultures to identify culture-specific and culture-universal caring constructs across ethnic groups.
- Culturally congruent care is meaningful, supportive, and facilitative because it conforms to valued life patterns of clients; it is achieved through cultural assessment.
- Culturally competent care requires knowledge, attitudes, and skills supportive of implementation of culturally congruent care.
- Cultural safety is an outcome of nursing education that enables safe service to be defined by clients who receive the service.
- Cultural assessment requires a comprehensive inquiry into the client's cultural values, beliefs, and practices; it may involve assessing ethnohistory, social organization, socioeconomic status, biocultural ecology and health risks, language and communication, religion and spirituality, caring beliefs and practices, and experiences with professional health care.
- Relational practice is the nursing obligation to examine relationships, ethics, and effective nursing practice, and the personal and contextual elements that continuously shape and influence nursing relationships.

✳ CRITICAL THINKING EXERCISES

1. You are about to begin giving an Arab Muslim man his morning care when he states, "I don't want a bath now." He becomes annoyed when you try to explain that you must give him a bath at this time. Before you leaqve the room, he asks you to leave a basin of water and towel by his bedside. He also asks you to get his prayer rug from his closet.
   a. How should you respond to the client?
   b. What may be the reasons for his refusal and annoyance?

2. A 50-year-old Chinese woman is hospitalized with a respiratory condition. She insists that you give her warm water and rub her back with Tiger balm liniment. When she receives her lunch, consisting of a turkey sandwich, tossed salad, and milk, she keeps the turkey sandwich and tossed salad but asks that you take the milk away.
   a. How should you respond to the client's requests?
   b. What is the significance of her requests?
   c. Why does she refuse her lunch?

3. You are assigned to a 60-year-old South Asian Hindu widow who is admitted with chest pain and shortness of breath. The client recently arrived from India to visit her son and pregnant daughter-in-law. She can speak only Gujarati and understands very little English. She is accompanied by her son.
   a. What areas should you include in your focused cultural assessment?
   b. How should you communicate with the client?
   c. Identify ways to preserve and accommodate the client's culture in her care.
   d. What aspects of the client's way of life may need repatterning?

✳ REVIEW QUESTIONS

1. Socialization into one's primary culture during childhood is known as
   1. Enculturation
   2. Acculturation
   3. Assimilation
   4. Multiculturalism

2. Multiculturalism results when a person
   1. Has an experience with a new or different culture that is extremely negative
   2. Maintains his or her culture and interacts peacefully with people of other cultures
   3. Gives up his or her ethnic identity in favour of the dominant culture
   4. Adapts to and adopts a new culture

3. Cultural awareness involves an in-depth self-examination of one's
   1. Background, recognizing biases and prejudices
   2. Social, cultural, and biophysical factors
   3. Engagement in culturally safe interactions
   4. Motivation and commitment to caring

4. Culturally competent care is the process of
   1. Learning about vast cultures
   2. Delivering care that is based on knowledge of the client's cultural heritage, beliefs, and attitudes
   3. Influencing treatment and care of clients
   4. Motivation and commitment to caring

5. Ethnocentrism is the root of
   1. Stereotypes, biases, and prejudices
   2. Meanings by which people make sense of their experiences
   3. Cultural beliefs
   4. Individualism and self-reliance in achieving and maintaining health

6. When a person acts on his or her prejudices,
   1. Discrimination occurs
   2. Sufficient comparative knowledge of diverse groups is obtained
   3. Delivery of culturally congruent care is ensured
   4. Effective intercultural and relational communication develops

7. The prevailing value orientation in Western society is
   1. Use of rituals symbolizing the supernatural
   2. Group reliance and interdependence
   3. Healing emphasizing naturalistic modalities
   4. Individualism and self-reliance in achieving and maintaining health

8. Disparities in health outcomes between rich and poor clients illustrate
   1. The attribution of illness to natural, impersonal, and biological forces
   2. Biological and sociocultural health risks
   3. Influence of socioeconomic factors in morbidity and mortality
   4. Combination of naturalistic, religious, and supernatural modalities

9. Culture strongly influences pain expression and need for pain medication. However, cultural pain
   1. May be suffered by a client whose valued way of life is disregarded by practitioners
   2. Is more intense, thus necessitating more medication
   3. Is not expressed verbally or physically
   4. Is expressed only to others of similar culture

10. The prevailing values in Western society on individual autonomy and self-determination
    1. Rarely have an effect on other cultures
    2. Do not have an effect on health care
    3. May hinder ability to get into hospice programs
    4. May be in direct conflict with the values of diverse groups

✳ RECOMMENDED WEB SITES

Canadian Ethnocultural Council: http://www.ethnocultural.ca/
This Web site explains the purposes of the Canadian Ethnocultural Council, which is a nonprofit, nonpartisan coalition of national ethnocultural organizations representing ethnocultural groups across Canada. Links to other related publications and sites related to ethnocultural groups are included.

Citizenship and Immigration Canada: Cultural Profiles Project: http://www.settlement.org/cp/
This Web site provides an overview of the life and customs of immigrants to Canada. Each profile includes a summary fact sheet and information about their culture, food, health, landscape, climate, arts, holidays, and literature.

Aboriginal Nurses Association of Canada: http://www.anac.on.ca/
This Web site offers a valuable resource of information regarding this association, founded by Jean Goodwill and Jocelyn Bruyere. Similar to provincial groups in existence, the association is available to provide support to Aboriginal nurses and Aboriginal student nurses, and it recognizes the need for increased numbers of Aboriginal nurses in Canada. It is also a valuable resource for students in nursing programs who do not self-identify as Aboriginal people.

11

Nursing Leadership, Management, and Collaborative Practice

Original chapter by Patricia A. Stockert, RN, BSN, MS, PhD

Canadian content written by Susan M. Duncan, RN, PhD

All nurses must be leaders, and nurses assume positions of leadership in health care delivery much earlier in their careers today than in previous generations. As you develop the knowledge and skills to enter the nursing workforce, you also learn how to become a leader among colleagues for the delivery of care in many health care settings. It is therefore important that you develop an understanding of **leadership and management** roles in nursing early in your educational program because this is one of the competencies required of entry-level nurses. You can see from the list of competencies required of entry-level nurses in Box 11–1 that leadership begins with a strong professional identity and accountability. For optimal nursing care, managers and leaders are needed to ensure both the vision for quality care and the management skills required for best practices and quality care (Hibberd et al., 2006). Whereas *leadership* refers to a shared vision, values, organizational strategy, and relationships, *management* most often refers to the competencies required to ensure the day-to-day delivery of nursing care according to available resources and standards of professional practice. To be effective in promoting a healthy work environment, leaders and managers must demonstrate leadership practices that honour the importance of relationships, values, and culture (Cummings, 2004; Gifford et al., 2006). Figure 11–1 provides a conceptual model of transformational leadership practices that have been identified as contributing to health **outcomes**.

In the current context of health care in which qualified health care professionals are in short supply, competencies related to leadership in nursing relate to creating environments for healthy working relationships and teamwork. A healthy work environment is most likely to retain nurses in practice settings in which they are both satisfied and able to provide high-quality care. RNs must work collaboratively with other members of the nursing team, as well as with

professionals from other disciplines and with clients and their families. The importance of such work is most often discussed as **collaborative practice**, defined as working together toward mutually identified goals while valuing different perspectives and accountabilities of individual team members (Gardner, 2005; RNAO, 2006b; Tschannen, 2004). This chapter therefore focuses on current thinking in nursing leadership and management, including definitions, roles and relationships, shifts to collaborative practice models, and the role of leaders in ensuring healthy practice environments and best practices. The ideas and examples included in this chapter apply to the different practice settings in which nurses work: in homes, in institutions, and in communities.

Management and Leadership Roles for Nurses

Nurses assume a wide variety of management and leadership roles in health care organizations in order to ensure that clients receive safe and high quality care. Research has revealed that nurses must provide leadership to ensure that nursing care takes place in quality practice environments. (Aiken et al., 2002; Canadian Nursing Advisory Committee, 2002; Scott et al., 1999; Silas, 2007) and that these work environments are essential for health, high-quality client care, and client safety (Estabrooks et al., 2005). A high-quality practice environment is also a healthy work environment, defined as "a practice setting that maximizes the health and well-being of nurses, quality client outcomes, organizational performance and societal outcomes" (RNAO, 2006a, p. 13).

A **healthy practice environment** begins with the senior nurse leader in the organization, who most often holds the title of Chief Nurse Executive, Chief Nursing Officer, or Director or Vice President of Nursing or of Patient Care (Canadian Nurses Association [CNA], 2002). In 1999, the government of Canada instituted the first Office of Nursing Policy with Dr. Judith Shamian, RN, Executive Director, hired to provide leadership needed to ensure that attention was paid in government to the nursing perspective on programs and policies (Health Canada, n.d.). Since then, several provinces have followed suit, instituting provincial nursing policy offices led by nurses in executive positions. These positions are key to ensuring that nurses influence the policy directions that governments take to ensure high-quality nursing services for Canadians. In policy roles, nurses act as policy advocates, by which they have made a difference throughout history and continue to advocate today for progressive public policy in primary health care and population health (Spenceley et al., 2006; see Unit I in this text). As a student, you will learn the skills involved in nursing advocacy and assume the role of advocate in order to promote the health of people. Advocacy is key to nursing leadership at all levels. Nurses today "stand on the shoulders of giants"; the nurse leaders of the past held a powerful vision for the development of nursing as a profession and advocated tirelessly to bring this vision to fruition ("A century of progress," 2005). One such leader was Ethel Johns, Director of the University of British Columbia's first nursing school. She inspired other nurses with her vision and challenged them to think for themselves (Boxes 11–2 and 11–3).

As in the past, a strong nurse executive unites the strategic direction of the organization with the values and goals of nursing. Nurse executives must also build teams of leaders who work across the organization to implement best practices and develop high-quality work environments in which nursing practice can flourish. Although it takes a strong senior nursing leader to inspire a healthy work

---

> **BOX 11-1**   **Entry-Level Staff Nurse Competencies Related to Leadership and Management**

- Is accountable and responsible for own actions and decisions, including personal safety.
- Demonstrates leadership in providing client care by promoting healthy and culturally safe work environments.
- Displays initiative, self-confidence, and self-awareness, and encourages collaborative interactions within the nursing and health care team.
- Organizes own workload and develops time-management skills for meeting responsibilities.
- Integrates quality improvement principles and activities into nursing practice.
- Uses relational knowledge and ethical principles when working with students and other health care team members to maximize collaborative client care.
- Participates in and contributes to nursing and health care team development.
- Supports professional efforts in the field of nursing to achieve a healthier society (e.g., lobbying, conducting health fairs, and promoting principles of the *Canada Health Act*).
- Demonstrates an awareness of healthy public policy and social justice.
- Develops support networks with registered nurse (RN) colleagues, health care team members, and community suppports.

Adapted from College of Registered Nurses of British Columbia (2006). *Competencies in the context of entry-level registered nurse practice in British Columbia. Leadership and management practices for healthy work environments.* Vancouver: Author.

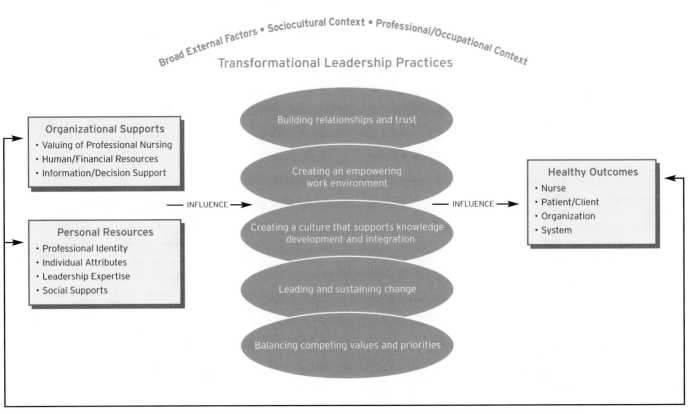

Figure 11-1 Conceptual model for developing and sustaining leadership. This model organizes and guides the discussion of the Registered Nurses Association of Ontario (RNAO) recommendations. It provides a framework for understanding the leadership practices needed to achieve healthy work environments and the organizational supports and personal resources that enable effective leadership practices. **Source:** From Registered Nurses Association of Ontario. (2006a). *Healthy work environments best practices guidelines: Developing and sustaining nursing leadership* (p. 22). Toronto, ON: Author.

➤ BOX 11-2   **Milestones in Canadian Nursing History**

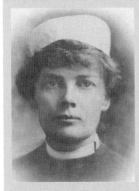

Ethel Johns, 1879–1968

A 1902 graduate of the Winnipeg General Hospital School of Nursing, Ethel Johns served as head nurse of several units at this hospital before becoming the first staff nurse to oversee its X-ray department. In 1907, she assumed editorship of its *Nurses Alumnae Journal* and began contributing to *Canadian Nurse*. Her literary talent, combined with her ability to challenge nurses to think independently, led to her nomination for membership in the Canadian Women's Press Club in 1911.

In 1913, Johns took a position as head surgical nurse at Good Samaritan Hospital in Los Angeles. After returning to Manitoba in 1915, she assumed the post of superintendent of the Children's Hospital of Winnipeg. She also worked tirelessly for the registration of nurses in Manitoba.

Johns held strong convictions about social issues and nursing, and she supported needed reforms. During the Winnipeg General Strike of 1919, her pro-labour views led her into conflict with the Children's Hospital board of directors, and she resigned.

Subsequently, Johns was appointed director of the Department of Nursing at the University of British Columbia, which offered the first Canadian university degree program in nursing. In 1929, she became director of nursing studies at New York Hospital–Cornell Medical College. She also worked on a landmark study of nursing education in the United States.

In 1933, Johns became editor of *Canadian Nurse,* which enabled her to communicate with a wide audience of nurses. Dr. Rae Chittick, president of the CNA during Johns's tenure as editor, praised Johns for bringing to the position "a world perspective on nursing, a hospitality of the mind from her rich experience . . . . She . . . reached out to challenge nurses to think for themselves and to create a body of nursing opinion on the changes essential to meet the health needs of a rapidly expanding nation." In 1947, Johns helped establish a new journal, *Just Plain Nursing,* which continued publication for the next 13 years. Also in 1947, Johns Hopkins Hospital asked her to write a history of its School of Nursing; this history was published in 1953. Later, she published the *Winnipeg General Hospital School of Nursing, 1887–1953*.

The CNA awarded Johns the Mary Agnes Snively Memorial Medal in 1940 and an honorary life membership in 1958 in recognition of her leadership in Canadian nursing.

Based on Street, M. M. (1973). *Watch-fires on the mountains: The life and writing of Ethel Johns.* Toronto, ON: University of Toronto Press.

environment, the role and responsibility of every nurse is to be a leader (CNA, 2002), displaying attributes such as articulating a vision, enabling others to act, encouraging others, and taking initiative. The leader and nursing staff must share a philosophy of care that integrates purpose, best practices, and concern for relationships, including how staff will work together and with clients and families (Box 11–4).

Nursing Care Delivery Models, Collaborative Practice, and Nursing Teams

Integral to the philosophy of care is the selection of a nursing care delivery model and a management structure that support professional nursing practice. Ideally, the vision for client care should drive the selection of a care delivery model (RNAO, 2006a). However, scarcity of resources and business initiatives from the health care organization influence this selection (Smith et al., 2006). The care delivery model must help nurses achieve desirable client outcomes. Key factors contributing to success are strong nursing leadership, decision-making authority for nurses who provide direct care, and effective respectful communications with colleagues, physicians, and other

health care professionals (Canadian Nursing Advisory Committee, 2002; Canadian Patient Safety Institute, 2007; Hinshaw, 2008; Manojlovich et al., 2008).

Nursing care delivery models are designs that determine how nurses provide care. Historically, the choices of a nursing care delivery models have been influenced by the social and economic conditions, and this is the case today when care models are changing because of a shortage of nurses and other health care professionals (Manojlovich et al., 2008). **Continuity of care** is an extremely important concept in determining the choice of a nursing care delivery model. *Continuity of care* is defined as "a seamless continuous implementation of a plan of care that is reviewed and revised to meet the changing needs of the client" (RNAO, 2006b, p. 61). It refers to continuity of information or knowledge, continuity of relationships between a client and one or more health care professionals over time, and continuity of management of care across organizational boundaries (Smith et al., 2006). In the choice of nursing care delivery models, it is important to consider how nurses ensure that a client's plan of care is as consistent as possible. Functional, team, total client care and primary nursing, and case management models have been used. As change occurs in health care delivery and nursing practice, new care delivery models are evolving (Kimball et al., 2007). In the current context, a client care model known as the *collaborative practice model*, which includes nurses and others; it incorporates some of the features of earlier models.

Nursing care delivery models entail higher staff ratios of unregulated care providers (UCPs) in many settings of practice, including home care, institutional acute care, and residential long-term care, than do other models. The title of the UCP typifies the role of providing front-line personal and delegated care to increasing numbers of clients across different health care settings in Canada. UCP practice is not defined by qualifications or established standards. The title of the role differs from province to province, as does its requirement for training or educational programs. In British Columbia, for example, UCPs are referred to as *home support/resident care attendants* (HSRCAs), and they are required to take a preparatory six-month certification program offered in public and private post-secondary educational institutions. This is not the case in all provinces; for example, in Alberta, UCPs are not required to have educational preparation, and they are referred to as *patient care attendants* (PCAs).

Functional Nursing. **Functional nursing** became popular during World War II in response to a nursing shortage. This model is task focused, not client focused. Tasks are divided; for example, one nurse may assume responsibility for hygiene and dressing changes, and another nurse may assume responsibility for medication administration. A lead nurse on a shift assigns tasks to staff members according to their qualifications, their abilities, and the tasks required. Nurses become highly competent with tasks that they perform repeatedly. The disadvantages of functional nursing are problems with continuity of care, absence of a holistic view of clients, and the possibility that care will become mechanical (Dadich, 2003). A task-focused approach does not ensure that clients' needs are met from shift to shift. Communication is not always clear, because one nurse is not responsible for the overall care of the client. The task-focused approach and ineffective communication lead to fragmented care and client dissatisfaction (Dadich, 2003).

Team Nursing. **Team nursing** developed in response to the nursing shortage after World War II (Marriner Tomey, 2004). It involves the delivery of nursing care by various staff members. An RN leads a team of other RNs, registered psychiatric nurses (RPNs), licensed practical nurses (LPNs), UCPs, or a combination of these professionals. The team leader, an experienced RN, develops client care plans, coordinates care delivered by the nursing team, and provides care that requires complex nursing skills. The team leader also performs problem solving with physicians and members of other disciplines and assists the team in evaluating the effectiveness of their care (Wywialowski, 2004). One of the limitations of the model is that the team leader does not spend a large amount of time with clients. Depending on the mix of staff members, this sometimes means that clients interact with any RN infrequently. Risks exist if an RN is unable to make necessary client assessments and cannot be involved in important clinical decision making. The task orientation of the model and the fact that nurses do not always interact with the same clients each day can result in a lack of continuity of care. An advantage of team nursing is the collaborative style that encourages each member of the team to help the other members. This model has a high level of autonomy for the team leader and is an example of decision making at a clinical level (Marriner Tomey, 2004).

Total Client Care. **Total client care** delivery was the original care model developed in the nineteenth century, during Florence Nightingale's time. It became popular in the 1970s and 1980s, when the numbers of RNs were increasing. In this model, an RN is responsible for all aspects of care for one or more clients. The RN may assign or delegate aspects of care to an RPN, an LPN, or a UCP but remains accountable for care of all assigned clients. The nurse works directly with the client, family, physician, and health care team members. The model typically has a shift-based focus. The same nurse does not necessarily care for the same client over time. Continuity of care from shift to shift or day to day is compromised if staff members do not clearly communicate the client's needs to one another.

Primary Nursing. The **primary nursing** model aimed to place RNs at clients' bedsides and improve nursing accountability for client outcomes and relationships among staff (Ritter-Teitel, 2002). The model was popular in the 1970s and early 1980s, when hospitals employed more RNs. Primary nursing supports a philosophy of strong nurse–client relationships. An RN assumes responsibility for a caseload of clients (Smith et al., 2006). Typically, the RN selects the clients and cares for the same clients during their stay in the health care setting. The RN assesses clients' needs, develops care plans, and ensures that appropriate nursing care is delivered. Primary nursing maintains continuity of care across shifts, days, or visits. It can be applied in any health care setting. When a primary nurse is off duty, associate nurses, including RPNs, LPNs, or other RNs, follow the care plan. If differences in opinion occur, associate and primary nurses collaborate to redefine the plan as necessary. Although primary nursing requires more RNs, the model is not necessarily more costly than others. The strengths of this model may be realized in case management and the collaborative practice model.

Case Management. The **case management** model coordinates health care services and links them to clients and their families while streamlining costs and maintaining quality (Dadich, 2003). The term *case managers* has been criticized because clients and families are not "cases" to be managed (Smith et al., 2006). In view of the importance of language and discourse in denoting the values of care, the term *case management* may, in the future, more appropriately refer to care or service coordination, or another descriptive label may communicate the value of client-centredness. Case management, as it has evolved, is "a collaborative process which assesses, plans, implements, coordinates, monitors, and evaluates the options and services required to meet an individual's health needs, using communications and available resources to promote quality, cost-effective outcomes" (Case Management Society of America, 2008). Clinicians, as individuals or in teams, care for clients with specific conditions and associated care needs (e.g., clients with complex nursing and medical problems) and are usually held accountable for quality and cost management. Many case managers use critical pathways, or "care maps," which are multidisciplinary treatment plans for clients with specific case types (see Chapter 13). The plans help in the delivery of timely, coordinated care.

Roles of case managers vary across health care settings, including long-term care, home care, community mental health, and acute care institutions, and these professionals increasingly coordinate and integrate care across these settings. Roles and responsibilities of case managers across settings include those of clinical experts, advocates, educators, facilitators, negotiators, managers, and researchers (Smith et al., 2006).

Collaborative Practice Model. The collaborative practice model is increasingly used by **intraprofessional nursing teams** (teams whose members provide nursing care) and by other health care professionals who are members of the **interprofessional team**. A call for interprofessional team and collaborative practice development has been sounded across Canada because this model is viewed as the way to ensure that all professionals and providers can practice to the full potential of their role and competencies. Collaborative practice is therefore also the best way to ensure that health human resources are used most effectively during a time of shortage. It is important for students in nursing and other professional health care programs to learn the competencies associated with collaborative practice during their educational programs. As a student, you are an integral member of both nursing and interprofessional teams that cross health care settings, including acute care, mental health care, community and home care, and public and population health care (RNAO, 2006b). One of first and most important responsibilities is to learn about the roles and responsibilities of other team members. Central to the collaborative practice model are the client, family, and population as full participants in care or service delivery. Nurse leaders in the Vancouver Coastal Health Authority (2007) launched an important initiative to support the shift in thinking required for collaborative practice among teams of nurses and health care professionals and across disciplines. This initiative provides opportunities for RNs, LPNs, UCPs, and members of other health care professions to learn from each other and to understand and respect their different roles and responsibilities. It also provides educational sessions in which team members learn about the competencies necessary in collaborative practice on a day-to-day basis in the work setting.

The RNAO (2006b) developed evidence-informed **best practice guidelines** for collaborative practice. These guidelines show how teamwork and collaborative practice can be supported at individual, team, organizational, and system levels of nursing practice. These guidelines are comprehensive and indicate the need for transformational leadership to support a culture of teamwork and collaboration. Thus, a collaborative practice model potentially incorporates the best of other care delivery models, including team, primary, and case management models previously discussed. It is important for students and entry-level nurses to acquire competencies that promote collaboration among teams as identified in Box 11–5.

> **BOX 11-5**   **RNAO Best Practice Guideline: Nursing Collaborative Practice**

Guideline 1.4: Nursing teams establish clear processes and structures that promote collaboration and teamwork that leads to quality work environments and outcomes for clients by
- Establishing processes for conflict resolution and problem solving
- Establishing processes to develop, achieve, and evaluate team performance
- Developing systems and processes to recognize and reward success
- Incorporating nonhierarchical, democratic working practices to validate all contributions from team members
- Incorporating processes that support continuity of care with clients to enhance staff satisfaction, staff self-worth, and client satisfaction
- Developing and implementing processes that clarify their understanding of the unique and shared aspects of roles within the teams
- Ensuring that the composition of the team is adequate to achieve their goals and meet their responsibilities to the needs of the client population
- Establishing processes for decision making for a variety of circumstances such as
  - Emergencies
  - Day-to-day functioning
  - Long-term planning
  - Policy development
  - Care planning

From Registered Nurses Association of Ontario. (2006b, November). *Healthy work environments best practices guidelines: Collaborative practice among nursing teams* (p. 33). Toronto: Author.

Nurses are well situated to provide leadership for collaborative practice in many health care settings. One example may be found in the home care setting, in which nurses work closely with UCPs, who provide a large amount of the continuous day-to-day care for clients who have been discharged from hospitals after undergoing surgery or who have chronic illnesses and disabilities. UCPs must have opportunities to meet and communicate regularly with the nurses and other professionals involved in the care of the clients, to ensure that they understand the client situation and receive support for the challenges they face in providing care. Nurses can also aid UCPs by providing education and other supports so that they are able to contribute to best practices in important areas such as safety, emotional support, and wound healing. In this way, UCPs are recognized and valued for their role, and the continuity of care to a single client or family is supported by UCPs, nurses, and other health care professionals. Nurses who are employed in long-term or residential care settings may also provide leadership for collaborative practice by ensuring opportunities for communication and learning among professionals involved in teams or systems of care.

Home care delivery also often includes social workers, physicians, nutritionists, physiotherapists, and other health care professionals, as well as nurses and UCPs. At the centre of the collaborative practice model is the client and family; research is just beginning into how health care professionals and other caregivers include clients as part of the team or the social network of care (Cott et al., 2008). A nurse in home care or another practice setting is well situated to provide leadership for collaborative practice by providing opportunities for clients and families to meet with caregivers and and by ensuring that the client's voice is heard in his or her care planning.

Decentralized Decision Making

One of the most important recommendations to achieve healthy practice environments is that staff at all levels be involved in decision making about nursing practice. Of equal importance is that the most senior nurse in the organization be included in the executive decision-making level of the organizations and agencies, including those responsible for the delivery of home care, mental health care, public health care, or hospital care. The nurse executive supports managers and staff by creating a management structure that helps achieve organizational goals and provides support for democratic decision making and collaborative practice models. With a vision for nursing established, the manager helps staff realize that vision.

Decentralized management, in which decision making occurs at the staff level, is common in health care organizations. The advantage of this structure is that managers and staff are actively involved in shaping an organization's identity and determining success. Decentralized management requires workers to be empowered to accept greater responsibility for the quality of client care (Ellis & Hartley, 2005). A decentralized structure has the best potential to lead to positive outcomes, such as increased collaboration among staff, best practice implementation, and client satisfaction (Table 11–1).

The nurse manager is crucial for the successful functioning of nursing units and systems. Figure 11–2 illustrates the responsibilities and competencies of nurse managers, including supervising, planning, scheduling and staffing, as situated within a framework of leadership competencies.

For decentralized decision making to work, managers must enable decision making by the professionals who are most involved and must encourage inclusion rather than exclusion of staff (RNs, RPNs, LPNs, UCPs, unit administrators, and secretaries). Key elements in organizational decision making are responsibility, autonomy, authority, and accountability (Anders & Hawkins, 2006). CNA (2003b) outlined principles and criteria for decentralized decision making (Box 11–6).

> **TABLE 11-1**   **Examples of Management Structures**

Structural Approach	Characteristics
Centralized management	A single administrator leads the organization, and directors oversee departments or programs. Decisions are made by the leader and directors, with little staff input. Managers have minimal responsibility or accountability for operation of nursing unit. Staff do not feel involved in care processes, and collaborative practice is not supported.
Decentralized management	Structure may be similar to that of centralized management. Often, the number of directors is lower. Staff members with the most knowledge about an issue make decisions. Managers often have 24-hour accountability and responsibility for staff, budget, and day-to-day management of work unit.
Matrix	Traditional units are reorganized into business units. Staff may report to multiple managers—such as one with responsibility for professional practice (e.g., nursing) and another with responsibility for a specific program (e.g., child and family health)—who may be from a variety of professional practice backgrounds.

Responsibility refers to the duties and activities that an individual is employed to perform. A professional nurse's responsibilities in a given role are outlined in a position description of the nurse's duties in client care and of participation as a member of the nursing team. Managers must be sure that staff members understand their responsibilities, particularly during change. For example, when hospitals restructure and client care delivery models change, the manager must clearly define the nurse's role within the new care delivery model. If decentralized decision making is in place, professional staff can help shape the new nurse role. All nurses are responsible for knowing their role.

Autonomy is the freedom of choice and responsibility for choices (Marriner Tomey, 2004). With autonomy, a nurse can make independent decisions about client care according the role and scope of practice. Innovation by nurses, increased productivity, higher employer retention of nurses, and greater client satisfaction are results of autonomy in nursing practice (Canadian Nursing Advisory Committee, 2002; Estabrooks et al., 2005; Hicks, 2003).

Authority to act is the right to act in areas in which a nurse has been given and accepts responsibility according to legislation, standards,

and the code of ethics governing the professional practice of nursing. Nurses have authority to act and to question actions concerning the practice of other professionals in relation to this scope of responsibility. For example, a nurse who as a case manager finds that the nursing team did not follow a discharge teaching plan for an assigned client has the authority to consult with other nurses to learn why the plan was not followed. The nurse as case manager has accepted responsibility for the care of a group of clients and therefore has the final authority in selecting the best course of action for the client's care, while collaborating with others to ensure quality outcomes.

Accountability means being answerable for one's actions. It means that as a nurse, you accept the commitment to provide excellent client care and the responsibility for the outcomes of actions in providing that care (Anders & Hawkins, 2006). A nurse is accountable for clients' outcomes. In the example just described, the nurse as case manager is accountable for the client's health outcomes by ensuring a continuity of care across hospitalization and home care.

A successful decentralized nursing unit exercises the four elements of decision making: responsibility, autonomy, authority, and accountability. The staff must meet routinely to discuss how to maintain an

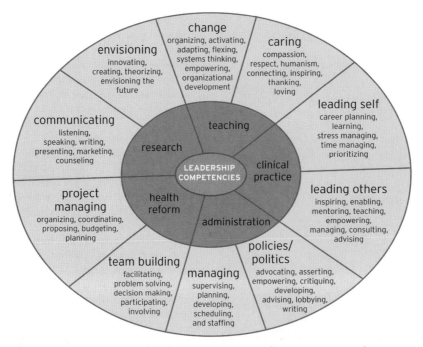

Figure 11-2 Management and leadership competencies. **Source:** From Canadian Nurses Association. (2005). *Nursing leadership development in Canada* (p. 28). Ottawa, ON: Author.

> **BOX 11-6** **Principles of Decentralized Decision Making**

- Decision making is based on having the appropriate number of positions and the competencies required to ensure safe, competent, and ethical care.
- Nurse administrators and managers (including supervisors, middle managers, and senior managers) are responsible for ensuring the appropriate staff mix.
- Legislative, professional, and organizational parameters are respected.
- The safety of clients must never be compromised by substituting less qualified workers when the competencies of an RN are required.
- The staffing decision-making process recognizes the unique and shared competencies of each health care professional group.
- Responsibility and accountability of health care professionals are clear.
- RNs at all levels in the organization are involved in decision making that affects nursing practice, client care, and the work environment.
- Staffing decisions are evidence informed.
- Organizations and other stakeholders, including RNs, ensure that the elements necessary for a high-quality professional practice environment are in place.
- RNs are leaders in implementing collaborative practice and promoting effective communication among all members of the health care team.

Adapted from Canadian Nurses Association. (2003b). *Staffing decisions for the delivery of safe nursing care—Position statement.* Ottawa, ON: Author.

equality and balance in these elements. Individuals should be comfortable in expressing differences in opinion and in challenging the status quo, while understanding their own responsibility, autonomy, authority, and accountability.

Supporting Staff Involvement. In decentralized decision-making structures, all staff members actively participate in unit or agency activities (Figure 11–3). Staff members benefit from the knowledge and skills of the entire team. If the staff members value knowledge and their colleagues' contributions, client care improves. The nursing manager supports staff involvement through the following approaches.

Establishment of Nursing Practice or Professional Shared Governance Councils. Chaired by senior clinical staff, these councils are empowered to maintain care standards for nursing practice (Gokenbach, 2007). The councils review and establish standards of care, develop policy and procedures, resolve client satisfaction issues, or develop new documentation tools. Mechanisms are established to empower all staff to contribute input on practice issues. Managers might not sit on the council, but they receive progress reports. The types of work in the nursing unit determines council membership. Professionals from other disciplines (e.g., pharmacy, respiratory therapy, social work, medicine, or clinical nutrition) might participate in these councils. Professional practice councils can advocate for resources and conditions necessary for healthy practice environments and safety.

Interprofessional Collaboration. As previously described, collaborative practice among professionals from different disciplines is essential to ensuring that health human resources are used in the best possible way. Whenever systems or programs are redesigned, interprofessional involvement is crucial because most health care processes involve more than one discipline (CNA, 2003a). Nurses must recognize the importance of prompt referrals and timely communication with other health care professionals. Inclusion of professionals from various disciplines in practice projects, in-service programs, conferences, and staff meetings fosters interprofessional collaboration.

Staff Communication. Communication with staff is one of the manager's greatest challenges, especially in a large work group in which change is constant. It is difficult to ensure that all staff members receive the correct messages. In the current health care environment, staff quickly become uneasy and distrusting if they fail to hear about planned changes in their work unit. A manager cannot be responsible for all communication but can use several approaches to communicate quickly and accurately with all staff: increasing presence on work units, circulating newsletters, posting minutes of committee meetings, and using list servers and e-mail. Of most importance is that staff members have the opportunity to meet and to discuss issues pertinent to their role and ability to provide care. Professional councils must be valued and invited to provide advice on emerging issues.

Developing a Learning Organization. Nurses must continually update their knowledge and incorporate best practices that are evidence informed (Cullum et al., 2008). Leaders and managers are challenged to develop the conditions for learning to flourish in what has been described as a *learning organization* (Senge, 2006). In learning organizations, many forms of knowledge are shared. Leadership strategies are needed to help nurses incorporate evidence-informed best practice guidelines into their nursing practice. These strategies include "support, role modelling commitment to best practices and reinforcing organizational policies and goals consistent with evidence based care" (Gifford et al., 2006, p. 73).

Leadership Skills for Nursing Students

Nursing students prepare for leadership roles. This does not mean you must quickly learn how to lead a nursing team; rather, you first learn to become an accountable and competent health care professional. Leadership development is ongoing throughout a career, and individual leadership styles are influenced from a variety of sources including theories, best practices, mentors, role models, and experiences. You learn leadership by making good clinical decisions, advocating for public health and quality care, learning from mistakes, seeking guidance, engaging in collaborative practice with nursing teams and other professionals, seeking mentors, and striving to improve during each client interaction. Your nursing education program provides you with the opportunity to develop leadership competencies: advocacy, conflict management, collaborative practice, client centredness, delegation, and evidence-informed decision making.

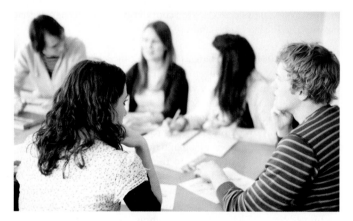

Figure 11-3 Students in nursing and other health care professional programs learning about their roles and contributions to collaborative practice. **Source:** © Renè Mansi, iStockPhoto.

Clinical Care Coordination

As a nursing student, you develop the skills necessary to ensure timely and effective client care. At first, you may have only one client, but eventually you will coordinate the care of groups of clients. Clinical care coordination includes decision making, priority setting, use of organizational skills and resources, time management, and evaluation.

Clinical Decisions. Leadership and decision-making skills are required as the nurse engages in the complex interactions—collaboration, negotiation, conflict resolution, and delegation—necessary to elicit the involvement of other people. You learn to value and practice client centredness in every interaction. You will adopt a critical thinking approach, applying understanding of clients' perspectives, your knowledge, evidence-informed best practice guidelines, and experience to the decision-making process (see Chapter 12).

Priority Setting. You must establish priorities of care as they relate to actions taken to meet clients' needs. This is particularly important in caring for groups of clients with health challenges involving immediate needs and actions to be taken. Hendry and Walker (2004) classified client problems in three priority levels on the basis of the time frame in which you must act:

- *High (first-order) priority:* An immediate threat to a client's survival or safety, such as a physiological episode of obstructed airway, loss of consciousness, injury, or an anxiety attack.
- *Intermediate (second-order) priority:* Nonemergency, non–life-threatening actual or potential needs that the client and family members are experiencing, such as anticipating teaching needs of clients with regard to a new drug, wound care, or measures to decrease falls among older adults.
- *Low (third-order) priority:* Actual or potential problems that may or may not be directly related to the acute phase of the client's health challenge. This means that they are not as time sensitive; however, they should be viewed as important to the health outcomes over the slightly longer term. Examples include promoting family members' understanding of a diabetic diet or other aspects of chronic illness management.

Many clients can have all three types of priorities, which requires you to use careful judgement in choosing a course of action. First-order priority needs require your immediate attention and, most often, immediate assistance in meeting these needs. Setting priorities also requires that you know the priority needs of each client, assessing each client's needs as soon as possible, including the client and family determination of priorities, and addressing needs in a timely manner (Wywialowski, 2004). You consider resources, recognize that priority needs can change, and use your time wisely.

Time Management. Changes in health care delivery and increasing complexity in all settings of care can create time management challenges for nurses as they work to meet clients' needs (Marriner Tomey, 2004). Time management skills can help you manage stress. These skills include reflecting on how you use time, planning effectively, and being aware of competing priorities. Because of the complexity of practice, nurses are often required to juggle priorities and respond to multiple demands on their time. It is therefore most important to track these demands and ensure that resources are in place that allow you to focus on priorities in a timely manner. Technology such as e-mail correspondence has increased demands on nurses' time, which often require immediate responses to issues. It is therefore important for you to to realize and reflect on the impact of technology and other forces and to acquire the ability to set limits and refuse demands that are unreasonable.

Evaluation. Evaluation is one of the most important aspects of clinical care coordination. Evaluation is an ongoing process that provides focus and direction for each phase of nursing care. Once you begin to provide care, you should also learn to immediately evaluate its effectiveness and the client's response. In the evaluation process, you compare expected client outcomes with actual outcomes. For example, a clinic nurse assesses a diabetic client's foot ulcer to determine whether healing is progressing and expected outcomes are met. Evaluation reveals the need to revise approaches to care and introduce new therapies. Focusing on evaluation of a client's progress and outcomes, rather than on tasks, lessens the chance of distraction. You learn to keep the client at the centre of the care by asking the client for his or her ideas and evaluation of how he or she is experiencing the care plan.

Delegation. Changes in staff mix have resulted in more UCPs delivering care to clients (CNA, 2005b; McGillis Hall, 2004). In the new working environment, a nurse must understand the evolving role of nursing and delegated care responsibilities in order to ensure the safety and quality of nursing care delivery. **Delegation** refers to the transferring of responsibility for the performance of an activity or task while retaining accountability for the outcome (College of Registered Nurses of British Columbia, 2005). Delegated tasks are those that are outside of the role description of the UCP. As a student, you will work with teams of nurses and UCPs during your practica in many health care settings, including home care, residential care, community health care, and acute care settings. As you develop in your role, it is important to learn about the roles and scopes of practice of UCPs in different practice settings. You will learn about how your role relates to that of the UCP and how the principles of delegation are applied in practice. Students and nurses also have access to valuable resources such as nursing practice consultants and practice guidelines to assist them in making complex decisions about delegation. The nurse may also assume responsibility for the education, supervision, and support of UCPs as they perform delegated nursing activities (Box 11–7).

Provincial regulations define the scope of an RN's practice, including activities that only RNs can perform (e.g., client assessment and planning care). Although most provinces identify the delegation and supervision of work as an RN's responsibility, each province addresses the specifics of delegation differently. In Ontario, British Columbia, and Alberta, for example, legislation that applies to all regulated health care professions identifies specific tasks or activities that can be performed by only certain professions. In British Columbia, these authorized tasks are known as *reserved acts;* in Ontario, they are called *controlled acts;* and in Alberta, they are known as *restricted activities.* UCPs are not allowed to perform actions authorized for RNs unless those actions have been properly delegated by an RN and only if they are within the UCP's job description and employer policy (Sorrentino, 2004).

An institution's policies, procedures, and job descriptions for UCPs provide specific guidelines regarding which tasks or activities can be delegated. The job description should specify any required education and the types of tasks UCPs can perform, either independently or under an RN's direct supervision. Institutional policy helps in defining the amount of training required of UCPs while they are employed. Procedures specify who is qualified to perform a given nursing procedure, whether supervision is necessary, and the type of reporting required. Job descriptions, policies, and procedures should comply with provincial laws and regulations. Nurses should have a means of accessing policies easily or have supervisory staff who can inform them about the UCP's job duties.

Effective delegation requires trust between the RN and UCPs. It also requires constant communication: sending clear messages and

> **BOX 11-7**   **The Five Rights of Delegation**

Right Task

The right task is one that can be delegated for a specific client, such as tasks that are repetitive, require little supervision, and are relatively non-invasive (bathing, toileting, feeding, some oral medication administration, positioning, and assisting with mobility).

Right Circumstances

The appropriate client setting, available resources, and other relevant factors are considered. In an acute care setting, clients' conditions can change quickly. Good clinical decision making is needed to determine what to delegate.

Right Person

The right person (e.g., the nurse) is delegating the right tasks to the right person (e.g., the UCP) to be performed on the right person (the correct client).

Right Direction or Communication

A clear, concise description of the task, including its objective, limits, and expectations, is given. Communication must be ongoing between RN and UCPs during a shift of care.

Right Supervision

Appropriate monitoring, evaluation, intervention as needed, and feedback are provided. UCPs should feel comfortable asking questions and seeking assistance.

Modified from National Council of State Boards of Nursing. (1995). *Delegation: Concepts and decision-making process.* Chicago, IL: Author; National Council of State Boards of Nursing. (1997). *The five rights of delegation.* Chicago, IL: Author; and American Nurses Association (ANA) and National Council State Boards of Nursing. (2006). *Joint statement on delegation.* Retrieved April, 2008, from http://www.ncsbn.org/pdfs/joint_statement.pdf.

listening so that all participants understand expectations regarding client care. An RN should provide clear instructions when delegating tasks. These instructions may initially focus on the procedure itself, as well as on the unique needs of the client. As the RN becomes more familiar with a staff member's scope of practice, trust builds and fewer instructions may be needed, but clarification of clients' specific needs is always necessary.

A key step in delegation is evaluation of the staff member's performance and the client's outcomes. When UCPs do a good job, it is important to provide praise and recognition. If the staff member's performance is unsatisfactory, the RN must give constructive feedback, specifically discussing mistakes and how they could have been avoided. Giving feedback in private in a professional manner preserves the staff member's dignity. A UCP may fail to meet expectations because of inadequate training or assignment of too many tasks. The RN may need to review or demonstrate a procedure with staff or schedule additional training with the education department. The delegation of too many tasks might be a nursing practice issue. All staff should discuss delegation on their unit because UCPs may need help in learning how to prioritize and RNs may need to ensure that they are not overdelegating.

A few tips for nurses on appropriate delegation (College of Registered Nurses of British Columbia, 2006; Keeling et al., 2000) are as follows:

- *Assess the knowledge and skills of the delegate.* Nurses should determine what the UCP knows and what he or she can do by

asking open-ended questions that will elicit conversation and details; for example, "Can you tell me what you would observe in Mr. S when you visit him today that would alert you to call me immediately?"

- *Match tasks to the delegate's skills.* Nurses need to know what skills are included in the UCP training program at their facility and to determine whether personnel have learned critical thinking skills, such as knowing the difference between normal clinical findings and changes to report.
- *Communicate clearly.* Nurses should provide unambiguous directions by describing a task, the desired outcome, and the time period for completion of the task. Rather than giving instructions through another staff member, nurses should make the delegate feel part of the team. For example, "I'd like you to help me by getting Mr. Floyd up to ambulate before lunch. Be sure to check his blood pressure before he stands and write your finding on the graphic sheet. OK?"
- *Listen attentively.* Nurses should listen to the UCP's responses as they give directions. Is the UCP comfortable asking questions or requesting clarification? Nurses need to be especially attentive if the UCP has a deadline assigned by another nurse and to help sort out priorities.
- *Provide feedback.* Nurses should give feedback about performance, regardless of outcome. They must tell the person about a job well done or, if an outcome is undesirable, find a private place to discuss what occurred, any miscommunication, and how to achieve a better outcome in the future.

Quality Care and Client Safety

As discussed throughout this chapter, safe and high-quality care is delivered when leadership, staffing models, and collaborative practice are in place to support it. Studies reveal that high-quality practice environments produce better client outcomes and more satisfied clients and staff (Aiken et al., 2001, 2002; CNA, 2005b; Tourangeau et al., 2002). Initiatives such as the College of Nurses of Ontario's (2004) *Quality Assurance Practice Consultation Program* and the Registered Nurses Association of British Columbia's (2003) *Quality Practice Environment Program* assess organizational attributes that enhance practice. The assessment is voluntary, but response by health care agencies is encouraging.

Organizational programs such as total quality management (TQM) and **continuous quality improvement (CQI)** were developed to encourage staff to reflect on how to improve work. In quality management, the client's or customer's definition of quality is recognized (Wendt & Vale, 2003). Most organizations have moved away from programs identified as TQM or CQI and focus instead on the more generic and pervasive concept of **quality improvement (QI)**, defined by the Canadian Council on Health Services Accreditation (2003) as "an organizational philosophy that seeks to meet clients' needs and exceed their expectations by using a structured process that selectively identifies and improves all aspects of service" (p. 1). This council describes quality as responsiveness, system competency, client or community focus, and work life. QI focuses on improving organizational performance related to processes.

Quality in Nursing Practice

Quality Defined. Standards or guidelines define the meaning of quality. For example, to judge whether rehabilitation has been delayed, a standard of when rehabilitation should begin must exist. Quality of care in nursing practice is not arbitrarily defined. A definition of quality begins with the mission, vision, philosophy, and values of the nursing department. These statements define how all nurses within an organization are to perform and which services must be provided. Written values give direction for professional standards and care guidelines that lead to positive client outcomes.

Professional Standards. Professional standards are authoritative statements used by the profession in describing the responsibilities for which its practitioners are accountable (Peters, 1995). They include the policies and position descriptions that identify performance expectations within an organization. Standards are an organization's interpretation of the professional's competency. The adherence to professional standards is measured through professional outcomes.

Care and Best Practice Guidelines. Care guidelines encompass best practice guidelines, which are statements to assist in providing care according to the best evidence available (RNAO, 2003). Guidelines can be developed by single disciplines or can be multidisciplinary in focus. Examples of nursing practice guidelines are found on the RNAO Web site encompassing some of the examples referred to in this chapter, including wound care and prevention of falls. The effectiveness of nursing practice is measured through client outcomes and the accumulation of evidence (Graham & Harrison, 2008).

Nurse-Sensitive Outcomes.

Outcomes are conditions to be achieved as a result of care. It is important that the outcomes selected to measure the effectiveness of nursing care are related to the work that nurses do. A **nurse-sensitive outcome** reveals whether interventions are effective, whether clients progress, how well standards are being met, and whether changes are necessary. Examples of outcomes related to the implementation of best practice guidelines may include incidence of pressure sores, falls in elderly clients, and hypertension control measures.

To judge whether standards of care are met, processes and outcomes are measured. For example, a staff measures its success in implementing a new process of diabetes instruction and also measures the outcome: Can clients administer insulin correctly? When selecting quality indicators, teams should consider processes and related outcomes that are most likely to improve nursing practice. Processes to improve may include the following:

- A weak process that is causing problems (e.g., poor pain management for clients with cancer who are at home).
- A stable process that is adequate but can improve (e.g., access to education and support for people with diabetes in rural communities).
- A process linked to negative outcomes (e.g., care of intravenous access sites with the occurrence of phlebitis).

Building a Culture of Safety

Client safety has been recognized as a crucial component of health care delivery. The Canadian Patient Safety Institute (2007) defined client safety as "the reduction and mitigation of unsafe acts within the health care system, as well as through the use of best practices shown to lead to optimal patient safety." Issues such as staff shortages, new technology, and other demands on health care systems have prompted a re-examination of how errors and adverse events for clients can be prevented. Increasingly, the emphasis is on enabling health care professionals and providers to communicate effectively and to acknowledge and receive timely assistance for errors. This assistance includes the education of nursing and other health care professional students to view mistakes as learning, to know and prevent conditions that lead to unsafe practices, and to develop the **competencies for safe practice** (Canadian Association of Schools of Nursing, 2006; Davidson Dick

et al., 2006). The Canadian Patient Safety Institute (2007) identified seven core domains of abilities for all health care professionals, including their contributions to developing a culture of client safety as a most important foundation (Box 11–8).

Coming Full Circle: Leadership for a High-Quality Work Life and High-Quality Health Care. Leaders and managers at all levels of health care organizations must do what they can to improve the quality of work life in health care in order to ensure client safety and quality health care; evidence and awareness of this need are growing. A forward thinking and exciting partnership of 10 leading health care organizations in Canada, including the CNA and the Canadian Council on Health Services Accreditation (now known as "Accreditation Canada"), have formed the Quality Worklife–Quality Healthcare Collaborative (QWQHC) with the mandate and a guiding conceptual framework to "improve the health of health workplaces." The foundational belief of the QWQHC is that "A fundamental way to better healthcare is through healthier health care workplaces; it is unacceptable to work in, receive care in, govern, manage and fund unhealthy workplaces" (QWQHC, n.d.).

Transformational leadership, including the concepts and competencies discussed in this chapter, is needed to shift the current culture of health care to achieve the vision of health care professionals delivering high-quality health care, adopted by the collaborative. This means that nurses and other professionals working directly with clients and the midlevel managers have key roles to play in leading change. They must be inspired and supported through mentoring and by the implementation of leadership best practices guidelines and collaborative practice. Senior leaders must ensure adequate staffing and support for the culture of a healthy workplace. The way forward is to inspire lifelong learning at all levels of the organization and provide access and resources to education that enables staff to work with the client and the client's family at the centre of health care delivery and decision making.

Nurses working at all levels of organizations can contribute by making a commitment to this vision and being part of the change that is required to transform Canadian health care. Indeed, the CNA in its centenary year inspires the theme of leadership for a transformed

> ### ▶ BOX 11-8   The Safety Competencies

Domain 1: "Creating a Culture of Patient Safety" (http://www.patientsafetyinstitute.ca/education/safetycompetencies.html)

Health care professionals must be enabled to contribute to health care organizations, large or small, in ways that promote client safety in their structure and function. Content in this domain could include but is not limited to the following aspects:

- Understanding of client safety concepts, epidemiology, and basic theories
- Awareness of health care error
- Promotion of a systems approach to care and safety
- Promotion of staff empowerment to resolve unsafe situations
- Role modelling and demonstration of a commitment to leadership in safe practice
- Ensuring feedback on safety issues
- Integration of safe practices into daily activities
- Commitment to communication, teamwork, and quality
- Reporting of adverse events
- Commitment to a just, nonpunitive culture

Canadian health care system and calls for Canadian Nurses to "be the change" required to sustain quality health care for all. As a student and as as a qualified nurse, you have the opportunity and the challenge to effect positive change in nursing practice and Canadian health care (Box 11–9).

✳ BOX 11-9   NURSING STORY

Leadership for Best Practices in Falls Prevention

Kaley Hart is a recently graduated RN working in a residential care facility. Ann Best, the nurse manager of the facility, is aware of Kaley's interest in leadership for best practices. As a fourth-year student, Kaley had completed a special project on falls prevention in the facility, using local statistics on falls and evidence-informed practice guidelines. Ann wishes to enroll the long-term care facility in the *National Collaborative on Falls in Long-Term Care* (RNAO, 2007a). This program requires the commitment of an improvement team consisting of five to seven staff members. Ann's vision is that the improvement team would be supported by the educational and research resources of this national program and by access to national experts in falls prevention. She sees this as an excellent opportunity for Kaley to be involved and to continue to develop her leadership skills in the areas of collaborative practice and best practices implementation.

At Ann's invitation, Kaley becomes involved with the quality improvement team, which also includes a nurse researcher from the university. Kaley begins her work by inspiring other nurses to become involved with the initiative, and she advocates for UCPs and other professionals to become members of the team in order to achieve a broad perspective on the changes required to prevent falls. She refers to the Canadian statistic that 50% of elderly residents in nursing homes fall every year (RNAO, 2007a), which results in a negative impact on their quality of life and increased costs to the health care system. Kaley inspires a vision of changes to be made in the interest of preventing falls and achieving the best possible health outcomes for the residents in the facility. She advocates for residents' and their families' involvement in the initiative and seeks input from all clients and professionals as to how the learning sessions should take place, in order to promote engagement as a learning community.

As a member of the team, Kaley contributes her knowledge of the RNAO (2007b) *Falls Prevention* Best Practices Guidelines and helps develop a practical approach to identifying residents who are at risk for falls. Drawing on her knowledge of collaborative practice, Kaley ensures that other team members, including the physiotherapist, UCP, recreation therapist, nutritionist, and housekeeping manager, are able to contribute their experiences and ideas about risk management and participate in the learning sessions. Kaley takes the opportunity to praise the contributions of diverse team members and to facilitate input and participation from the residents.

An evaluation of the quality improvement team reveals high levels of participation and interest within the facility. The experience of being involved in a national initiative has contributed to the capacity for best practices implementation and evidence-informed practice. Kaley has been inspired by the experience and has further developed her management and leadership competencies in the areas of inspiring a vision, leading change, facilitating collaborative practice, and developing respectful and supportive relationships among team members. She has worked with the nurse researcher at the local university to develop the plan for studying the impact of the changes on the incidence of falls, over time. Of most importance is that Kaley looks forward to the next opportunity to make a difference in the health outcomes of the residents through the exercise of progressive management and leadership initiatives.

✳ KEY CONCEPTS

- A leader must set a vision or philosophy for a work unit, ensure appropriate staffing, mobilize staff and institutional resources to achieve objectives, motivate staff members to carry out their work, set standards of performance, and make the right decisions to achieve objectives.
- Management and leadership are related processes; both are essential to nursing practice and health care delivery.
- Healthy practice environments are key to quality nurse and client care outcomes.
- Leadership plays a key role in ensuring healthy practice environments.
- An empowered nursing staff has decision-making authority to change how they practise.
- Nursing care delivery models vary by the responsibility of the RN in coordinating care delivery and the roles other staff members play in assisting with care.
- Continuity of nursing care can be compromised in total client care delivery, functional nursing practice, and team nursing.
- Best practice guidelines are evidence informed and contain recommendations for developing and sustaining collaborative practice models and leadership.
- For decentralized decision making to succeed, staff members must be aware that they have the responsibility, authority, autonomy, and accountability for the care they give and the decisions they make.
- A nurse manager can foster decentralized decision making by establishing nursing practice committees, supporting collaborative practice, implementing quality improvement plans, and maintaining timely staff communication.
- Clinical care coordination involves accurate clinical decision making, establishing priorities, efficient organizational skills, appropriate use of resources and time management skills, and an ongoing evaluation of care activities.
- To promote an enriching professional environment, each member of a nursing work team is responsible for open, professional communication.
- Delegation involves transferring responsibility for performing an activity while retaining accountability for the outcome.
- When accomplished correctly, delegation can improve job efficiency and job enrichment.
- An important responsibility for the nurse who delegates nursing care is evaluation of the staff member's performance and client outcomes.
- In a quality improvement-oriented environment, every staff member becomes involved in finding ways to improve or change work processes so as to promote client safety and quality care outcomes.
- The QWQHC was developed to transform Canadian health care delivery systems.

✳ CRITICAL THINKING EXERCISES

1. John, an RN, is working with Tammy, a UCP, to manage care for five clients. John has completed morning assessments and rounds on the assigned clients and is giving Tammy directions for what she needs to do in the next hour. John says to Tammy, "Why don't you go to Room 415 and see what Mr. Thomas needs, and go to Room 418 to check if Mrs. Landry is doing all right." Based on what you know about delegation, were these appropriate or inappropriate delegations to Tammy? Provide a rationale for your answer.

2. You are a recently graduated RN working in a home care setting. The manager of the nursing program asks you to assist with the implementation of a collaborative practice model. She asks you to help her set the agenda for the first meeting to discuss the concept and principles of collaborative practice. What ideas and resources would you contribute to the agenda?

3. You have just received morning shift reports on your clients. You have been assigned the following clients:
   - A 52-year-old man who was admitted yesterday with a diagnosis of angina. He is scheduled for a cardiac stress test at 0900.
   - A 60-year-old woman who was transferred out of intensive care at 0630 today. She underwent uncomplicated coronary bypass surgery yesterday.
   - A 45-year-old man who experienced a myocardial infarction three days ago and is complaining of chest pain, which he rates as 5 on a scale of 0 to 10.
   - A 76-year-old woman who had a permanent pacemaker inserted yesterday and is complaining of incision pain, which she rates as 7 on a scale of 0 to 10.

   Which one of these clients do you need to see first? Explain your answer.

✳ REVIEW QUESTIONS

1. The nursing model of client care in which specific tasks are divided (e.g., one nurse assumes responsibility for hygiene and dressing changes, and another nurse assumes responsibility for medication administration) is
   1. Team nursing
   2. Total client care
   3. Functional nursing
   4. Primary nursing

2. Collaborative practice models aim to
   1. Improve delegation between staff
   2. Improve communication between staff
   3. Place the client at the centre of care delivery
   4. Ensure that health care professionals can cover for one another

3. The type of care management approach that coordinates and links health care services to clients and their families while streamlining costs and maintaining quality is
   1. Case management
   2. Total client care
   3. Functional nursing
   4. Primary nursing

4. The type of management structure that has a potential for greater collaborative effort, increased competency of staff, and ultimately a greater sense of professional accomplishment and satisfaction is
   1. Case management
   2. Primary nursing
   3. Total client care
   4. Decentralized

5. While administering medications, the nurse realizes she has given the wrong dose of medication to a client. The nurse acts by completing an incident report and notifying the client's physician. The nurse is exercising
   1. Authority
   2. Responsibility
   3. Accountability
   4. Decision making

6. A manager who wishes to improve client safety in the health care organization should focus on
   1. Problem-solving committees
   2. Staffing models and ratios
   3. Systems for reporting mistakes
   4. Staff communication

7. A home care nurse is working with three UCPs who were recently hired and are new to their roles. For the first two weeks of their employment, the UCPs have been providing care for clients at home with complex wounds and caring for families in palliative care situations. The nurse believes in the principles of collaborative practice and wishes to support the UCPs in their development. An important first step would be to
   1. Provide an opportunity for the UCPs to talk about their experiences, questions, and roles
   2. Provide an educational session on palliative care
   3. Set up a mentoring system among the UCPs
   4. Discuss the role of the RN in home care

8. A client is experiencing an anxiety attack. This is which priority nursing need for this client?
   1. First-order priority
   2. Second-order priority
   3. Third-order priority

9. The nurse checks on a client who was admitted to the hospital with pneumonia. He has been coughing profusely and has required nasotracheal suctioning. He has an intravenous infusion of antibiotics. He is febrile. The client asks the nurse whether he can have a bath because he has been perspiring profusely. The nurse may delegate to the UCP working with her today the task of
   1. Assessing vital signs
   2. Changing intravenous dressing
   3. Nasotracheal suctioning
   4. Administering a bed bath

10. An example of a nurse-sensitive outcome based on best practice guidelines is
    1. Rates of emergency room readmission after postsurgical discharge
    2. Percentage of time it takes to count narcotics by nursing staff every shift
    3. Number of falls among residents in a long-term care setting
    4. Time it takes for a client to be transported from the emergency department to an inpatient nursing unit

✳ RECOMMENDED WEB SITES

Academy of Canadian Executive Nurses (ACEN): http//www.acen.ca

This is an association of nurses in leadership positions across the spectrum of health services. ACEN activities support leadership, advocacy and policy intitiatives, and mentorship for emerging nurse leaders and executives.

Accreditation Canada: http//www.cchsa.ca/default.aspx

Accreditation Canada, formerly known as the Canadian Council on Health Services Accreditation, is a national, nonprofit, independent organization whose role is to help health services organizations, across Canada and internationally, examine and improve the quality of care and service they provide to their clients.

Canadian Association of Schools of Nursing (CASN): http://www.casn.ca

The Canadian Association of Schools of Nursing (CASN) is the national voice for nursing education, research, and scholarship and represents baccalaureate and graduate nursing programs across Canada.

Canadian Health Services Research Foundation: http://www.chsrf.ca

The Web site of the Canadian Health Services Research Foundation contains research resources for policymakers and for health system leaders and managers pertaining to staffing models, high-quality health work life, and high-quality health care.

Canadian Nurses Association (CNA): http//www.cna-nurses.ca/cna

The CNA is a federation of 11 provincial and territorial nursing associations representing more than 120,000 RNs. The CNA's mission is to advance the quality of nursing in the interest of the public.

Canadian Nursing Students Association (CNSA): http//www.cnsa.ca/

The CNSA is the national voice of nursing students in Canada. For more than 30 years, the CNSA has represented the interests of nursing students to federal, provincial, and international governments and other nursing and health care organizations.

Canadian Patient Safety Institute: http://www.patientsafetyinstitute.ca/index.html

The Canadian Patient Safety Institute (CPSI) is an independent not-for-profit corporation, operating collaboratively with health professionals and organizations and with regulatory governments and bodies to build and advance a safer health care system for Canadians.

International Council of Nurses (ICN): http://www.icn.ch/

The ICN is a federation of national nurses' associations, representing nurses in more than 120 countries. Operated by nurses for nurses, ICN works to ensure quality nursing care for all clients, sound health policies globally, and the advancement of nursing knowledge.

Interprofessional Network of BC (In-BC): http:/www.in-bc.ca

The Interprofessional Network of BC promotes the development of interprofessional development and education for collaborative practice. Its Web site contains resources that include information about interprofessional competencies.

Interprofessional Rural Program of BC (IRPbc): http://www.bcahc.ca/irpbc/

The IRPbc offers a unique opportunity for students from various health care professional programs to experience life and work in a rural community in British Columbia and to participate in a number of interprofessional team activities. The Web site offers access to a 10-minute film, *Learning Together in Rural Communities,* which highlights the voices of the students about their experiences.

Registered Nurses Association of Ontario (RNAO): http://www.rnao.org

This Web site offers a complete and up-to-date inventory of best practice guidelines, including implementation and evaluation.

Quality Worklife-Quality Healthcare Collaborative (QWQHC): http://www2.cchsa.ca/qwqhc

This Web site describes the national interprofessional coalition of health care leaders who work together to develop an integrated action-oriented strategy to transform the quality of work life for Canada's health care professionals. According to the QWQHC, this strategy enables client safety and high-quality client care and system outcomes.

12

Critical Thinking in Nursing Practice

Original chapter by Patricia A. Potter, RN, MSN, PhD, GMAC, FAAN

Canadian content written by Donna M. Romyn, RN, PhD

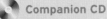

As a nurse, you will face many complex situations involving clients, family members, and other health care workers. To deal with these experiences effectively, you need to develop sound **critical thinking** skills so that you can approach each new problem involving a client's care with open-mindedness, creativity, confidence, and wisdom. When a client develops a new set of symptoms, asks you to provide comfort, or requires a procedure, it is important to think critically and make prudent clinical judgements so that the client receives the best nursing care possible. Critical thinking is not a simple, step-by-step linear process that you can learn overnight. Your ability to think critically will increase as you gain experience and progress from novice to expert nurse (Benner, 1984). Critical thinking is central to professional nursing practice because it allows you to test and refine nursing approaches, learn from successes and failures, apply new knowledge (e.g., nursing research findings), and ensure holistic client-centred care.

Critical Thinking Defined

Most definitions of critical thinking emphasize the use of logic and reasoning (Di Vito-Thomas, 2005) to make accurate clinical judgements and decisions. Accordingly, nurses recognize that an issue (e.g., client problem or health-related concern) exists, analyze information about the issue (e.g., clinical data about the client), evaluate information (e.g., reviewing assumptions and evidence), and draw conclusions (Settersten & Lauver, 2004). In consultation with clients, nurses consider what is important in a situation, imagine and explore alternative solutions, consider ethical principles, and then make informed decisions about how to proceed. Consider the following case example:

> Mr. Jacobs is a 58-year-old client who had a radical prostatectomy for prostate cancer yesterday. His nurse, Tonya, finds him lying supine in bed with his arms extended along his sides and his hands clenched. When Tonya checks his sugical wound and drainage device, she notes that he winces when she gently palpates over the incisional area. She asks Mr. Jacobs when he last turned onto his side, and he responds, "Not since sometime last night." Tonya asks Mr. Jacobs if he is having incisional pain and he nods, saying, "It hurts too much to move." Tonya considers her observations and the information she has learned from the client to determine that his pain is severe and his mobility is reduced because of it. Together, she and Mr. Jacobs decide to take action to relieve Mr. Jacob's pain so he can turn more frequently and begin to get out of bed to aid his recovery.

Critical thinking requires purposeful and reflective reasoning during which you examine ideas, assumptions and beliefs, principles, conclusions, and actions within the context of the situation (Brunt 2005a, 2005b). When you care for a client, you begin to think critically by asking questions such as "What do I know about the client's situation?" "How do I know it?" "What is the client's situation now? How might it change?" "What else do I need to know to understand this situation better or improve it? How can I obtain that information?" "In what way will a specific therapy affect the client?" "Are other options available?" By answering these questions, you are able to identify alternative solutions to resolve the client's health-related concerns.

As you gain experience in nursing, avoid letting your thinking become routine or standarized. Instead, learn to look beyond the obvious in any clinical situation, explore the client's unique responses to actual or potential health alterations, and recognize what actions are needed to benefit the client. Over time, your experience with many clients will help you recognize patterns of behaviour, see commonalities in signs and symptoms, and anticipate reactions to nursing interventions. Reflecting on your experiences will allow you to better anticipate clients' needs and recognize problems when they develop. It will also help you determine how the knowledge you gained working with one client may be applicable to another client's situation.

In Tonya's case, she knows that the client is likely to have pain because the surgery was extensive. Her review of her observations and the client's report of pain confirm that pain is a problem. Her options include giving Mr. Jacobs an analgesic and then waiting until it takes effect so that she can help him find a more comfortable position. Once his pain is less acute, Tonya might also ask Mr. Jacobs whether he would like to try some relaxation exercises and mobilization techniques she learned while caring for another postoperative client that may be effective in increasing his mobility.

You can begin to learn to think critically early in your practice. For example, as you learn about administering bed baths and other hygiene measures to your clients, take time to read this book and the nursing literature about the concept of comfort. What are the criteria for comfort? How do clients from other cultures perceive comfort? What are the many factors that promote comfort? Learning and thinking critically about the concept of comfort prepares you to better anticipate your clients' needs. You will also identify comfort problems more quickly and offer appropriate care. The use of **evidence-informed knowledge**—knowledge based on research or clinical expertise—makes you an informed critical thinker.

Critical thinking requires not only cognitive skills, such as interpretation, analysis, inference, evaluation, explanation, and self-regulation, but also a nurse's habit (disposition) to ask questions, to be well informed, to be honest in facing personal biases, and to always be willing to reconsider and think clearly about issues. Without these dispositions, sound critical thinking is unlikely to occur (Facione, 1990; Facione & Facione, 1996; Profetto-McGrath, 2003). When applied to nursing, these core critical thinking skills and critical thinking dispositions reveal the complex nature of the **clinical decision-making process** (Table 12–1). Being able to apply all of these skills and acquiring all of these critical thinking habits take time and practice. You also need to have a sound knowledge base and thoughtfully consider the knowledge you gain when caring for clients.

Nurses who apply critical thinking in their work consider all aspects of a situation and make well-reasoned judgements about a variety of possible alternative actions rather than hastily and carelessly implementing solutions (Kataoka-Yahiro & Saylor, 1994). For example, nurses who work in crisis situations such as child abuse and suicide prevention programs act quickly when client problems develop. These nurses must, however, exercise discipline in decision making to avoid premature and inappropriate decisions. Learning to think critically helps you to care for clients as their advocate and to make better informed choices about their care. Critical thinking is more than just problem solving; it is an attempt to continually improve how you apply knowledge when faced with problems in client care.

Levels of Critical Thinking in Nursing

Your ability to think critically grows as you gain new knowledge and experience in nursing practice. Kataoka-Yahiro and Saylor (1994) developed a critical thinking model that incorporates three levels of critical thinking in nursing: basic, complex, and commitment. As a beginning nursing student, you apply the critical thinking model at the basic level. As you advance in practice, you adopt complex critical thinking and commitment.

> **TABLE 12-1**   **Critical Thinking Skills and Dispositions**

Elements of Decision-Making Process	Critical Thinking Behaviour
Skill	
Interpretation	Be orderly in data collection. Look for patterns to categorize data (e.g., formulate nursing diagnoses [see Chapter 13]). Clarify any data about which you are uncertain.
Analysis	Be open-minded as you look at information about a client. Do not make careless assumptions. Ask whether the data reveal what you believe is true or whether other scenarios are possible.
Inference	Examine meanings and relationships in the data. Form reasonable hypotheses and conclusions, on the basis of the patterns observed.
Evaluation	Assess all situations objectively. Use criteria (e.g., expected outcomes) to determine the effectiveness of nursing actions. Identify required changes. Reflect on your own behaviour.
Explanation	Support your findings and conclusions. Use knowledge and experience to select the strategies you use in the care of clients.
Self-regulation	Reflect on your experiences. Adhere to standards of practice. Apply ethical principles in your nursing practice. Identify in what way you can improve your own performance.
Dispositions or Habits	
Truth seeking	Learn what is actually happening in a situation. Be courageous about asking questions. Consider scientific principles and evidence, even if they do not support your preconceptions or personal beliefs.
Open-mindedness	Be receptive to new ideas and tolerant of other points of view. Respect the right of other people to hold different opinions. Be aware of your own prejudices.
Analyticity	Determine the significance of a situation. Interpret meaning. Anticipate possible results or consequences. Value reason. Use evidence-informed knowledge in your nursing practice.
Systematicity	Be organized and focused in data collection. Use an organized approach to problem solving and decision making.
Self-confidence	Trust your own reasoning processes. Seek confirmation from experts when uncertain.
Inquisitiveness	Actively seek new knowledge. Value learning for learning's sake.
Maturity	Accept that multiple solutions are possible. Reflect on your own judgements; be willing to consider other explanations. Use prudence in making, suspending, or revising judgements.

Modified from Facione, P. (1990). *Critical thinking: A statement of expert consensus for purposes of educational assessment and instruction. The Delphi report: Research findings and recommendations prepared for the American Philosophical Association* (ERIC Doc No. ED 315-423). Washington, DC: Educational Resources Information Center (ERIC).

Basic Critical Thinking

At the basic level of critical thinking, a learner trusts that experts have the right answers for every problem. Thinking is concrete and based on a set of rules or principles. For example, as a student nurse, you use a hospital's procedure manual to confirm how to insert a Foley catheter. In completing this procedure for the first time, you will probably follow the procedure step by step without adjusting the procedure to meet a client's unique needs (e.g., positioning to minimize the client's pain or mobility restrictions) because you do not have enough experience to know how to individualize the procedure. At this level, answers to complex problems are seen to be either right or wrong (e.g., the Foley catheter balloon contains too much or not enough air), and you may believe that one right answer exists for each problem. As you gain more experience in nursing, you will begin to explore the diverse opinions and values of experts (e.g., instructors and role models among staff nurses) and engage in more complex critical thinking.

Complex Critical Thinking

When you engage in complex critical thinking, you begin to separate your thinking processes from those of authorities and to analyze and examine choices more independently. Your thinking abilities and initiative to look beyond expert opinion begin to change, as you realize that alternative, and perhaps conflicting, solutions to a problem or issue exist.

Consider the following case study:

Mr. Rosen is a 36-year-old man who injured his back in a skiing accident. He suffers from chronic pain but is refusing to take a prescribed analgesic. While discussing the importance of rehabilitation with Mr. Rosen, the nurse, Edwin, learns that Mr. Rosen practises meditation at home. In complex critical thinking, Edwin recognizes that for pain relief, the client has options other than accepting analgesics. Edwin decides to discuss meditation and other nonpharmacological interventions with Mr. Rosen and his other health care professionals as pain control options.

In complex critical thinking, you are willing to consider other options in addition to routine procedures when complex situations develop. As a nurse, you learn to weigh the benefits and risks of each potential solution before making a final decision. Thinking becomes more creative and innovative as you explore a broad range of perspectives and alternative solutions.

Commitment

The third level of critical thinking is commitment. You anticipate the need to make choices without assistance from other professionals, and then you assume responsibility and accountability for those choices. As a nurse, you do more than just consider the complex alternative solutions that a problem poses. At the commitment level, you choose an action or belief on the basis of the alternative solutions available, and you stand by your choice. Sometimes an action is to not take action, or you may choose to delay an action until a later time as a result of your experience and knowledge. Because you take accountability for the decision, you give attention to the results of the decision and determine whether it was appropriate.

A Critical Thinking Model for Clinical Decision Making

Thinking critically is becoming the benchmark or standard for professional nursing competence. To help you in the development of critical thinking, this text offers a model for critical thinking. Because critical thinking in nursing is complex, a model helps explain what is involved as you make clinical decisions and judgements about your clients. Kataoka-Yahiro and Saylor (1994) developed a model of critical thinking for nursing judgement based in part on previous work by Paul (1993), Glaser (1941), Perry (1979), and Miller and Malcolm (1990) (Figure 12–1). The model defines the outcome of critical thinking: nursing judgement that is relevant to nursing problems in a variety of settings. According to this model, critical thinking consists of five components: knowledge base, experience, competencies, qualities, and standards. The elements of the model combine to explain how nurses make clinical judgements that are necessary for safe, effective nursing care (Box 12–1).

Throughout this text, this model is used for applying critical thinking during the nursing process. Each clinical chapter of the text (Chapters 31 to 49) is organized by the steps of the nursing process and includes both scientific and nursing knowledge. It is your knowledge base (the first critical thinking component) that prepares you to make clinical judgements as a nurse. Figure 12–1 demonstrates how to apply elements of critical thinking in assessing clients, in planning the interventions you provide, and in evaluating your results. If you learn to apply each element of this model in the way you think about clients, you will be become a confident and effective professional.

Specific Knowledge Base

To think critically, establish accurate clinical judgements and decisions, and improve clinical practice (Di Vito-Thomas, 2005), nurses must possess a sound knowledge base. Your knowledge base includes

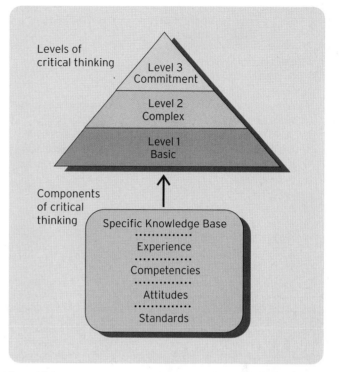

Figure 12-1 Critical thinking model for nursing judgement. **Source:** Redrawn from Kataoka-Yahiro, M., & Saylor, C. (1994). A critical thinking model for nursing judgment. *Journal of Nursing Education, 33*(8), 351. Adapted from Glaser, E. (1941). *An experiment in the development of critical thinking.* New York: Bureau of Publications, Teachers College, Columbia University; Miller, M., & Malcolm, N. (1990). Critical thinking in the nursing curriculum. *Nursing & Health Care, 11,* 67; Paul, R.W. (1993). The art of redesigning instruction. In Wilsen, J., Blinker, A.J.A. (Eds.). *Critical thinking: How to prepare students for a rapidly changing world.* Santa Rosa, California: Foundation for Critical Thinking; and Perry, W. (1979). *Forms of intellectual and ethical development in the college years: A scheme.* New York: Holt, Rinehart, & Winston.

information and theory from the basic sciences, humanities, behavioural sciences, and nursing. Nurses use their knowledge base in a different way than other health care professionals because they think holistically about client problems and health-related matters. For example, a nurse's broad knowledge base offers a physical, psychological, social, moral, ethical, and cultural view of clients and their health concerns. The depth and breadth of knowledge influences your ability to think critically about nursing problems. Consider this scenario:

Robert Perez previously earned a bachelor's degree in education and taught high school for one year. He has successfully completed the required courses in his nursing program in the sciences, health ethics, fundamental nursing concepts, and communication principles. His first clinical course focuses on health promotion with a clinical assignment in an outpatient primary care clinic. Although he is still new to nursing, his experiences as a teacher and his preparation and knowledge base in nursing will help him know how to begin to make clinical decisions about clients' health promotion practices.

Experience

Nursing is a practice discipline. Clinical nursing experiences are necessary for you to acquire clinical decision-making skills (Roche, 2002). In clinical situations, you learn from observing, sensing, talking with

> **BOX 12-1**   **Components of Critical Thinking in Nursing**

I. Specific knowledge base
II. Experience in nursing
III. Critical thinking competencies
    A. General critical thinking competencies (scientific method, problem solving, and decision making)
    B. Specific critical thinking competencies in clinical situations (diagnostic reasoning, clinical inference, and clinical decision making)
    C. Specific critical thinking competency in nursing (use of nursing process)
IV. Qualities for critical thinking
V. Standards for critical thinking
    A. Intellectual standards
    B. Professional standards
      1. Ethical criteria for nursing judgement
      2. Criteria for evaluation
      3. Professional responsibility

Adapted from Kataoka-Yahiro, M., & Saylor, C. (1994). A critical thinking model for nursing judgment. *Journal of Nursing Education, 33*(8), 351. Data from Paul, R. W. (1993). The art of redesigning instruction. In Willsen, J., & Blinker, A. J. A. (Eds.). *Critical thinking: How to prepare students for a rapidly changing world.* Santa Rosa, CA: Foundation for Critical Thinking.

clients and families, and then reflecting actively on your experiences. Clinical experience is the laboratory for testing nursing knowledge. You learn that "textbook" approaches form the basis for nursing practice, but you make safe adaptations or revisions in approaches to accommodate the setting, the unique qualities of the client, and the experience you gained from caring for previous clients. With experience, you begin to understand clinical situations, recognize cues of clients' health patterns, and interpret cues as relevant or irrelevant (Tanner, 2006). You also learn to seek new knowledge as needed, act quickly when events change, and make quality decisions that promote the client's well-being. It is important for you to admit to any limitations in your knowledge and skills. Critical thinkers admit what they do not know and try to acquire the knowledge needed to make proper decisions. A client's safety and welfare are at risk if you do not admit your inability to deal with a practice problem. You must rethink the situation, acquire additional knowledge, and then use new information to form opinions, draw conclusions, and take appropriate action. Perhaps the best lesson to be learned by a new nursing student is to value all client experiences, which enable you to build new knowledge and inspire innovative thinking.

During the previous summer, Robert worked as a nurse assistant in a long-term care facility. This experience provided him with valuable experience in interacting with older adults and in giving basic nursing care. Specifically, he has been able to develop good interviewing skills and understand the importance of the family in an individual's health, and he has learned how nurses advocate for clients. He has also learned that older adults require more time to perform activities such as eating, bathing, and grooming, and so he has adapted skill techniques for dealing with this requirement. His time in the physical assessment laboratory and the time he worked in the nursing home helped him begin to be a careful observer. As he reflects on his experiences, Robert also knows that much of what he learned can be applied in promoting health, wellness, and independence among the older clients who attend the outpatient clinic for routine follow-up visits.

Becoming familiar with practice standards developed by clinical experts also assists you in enhancing your knowledge base. For example, the *Nursing Best Practice Guidelines* developed by the Registered Nurses Association of Ontario (RNAO; n.d.) include standards for nursing care for a number of clinical conditions, such as asthma, chronic obstructive pulmonary disease, diabetes, and depression. Other standards focus on nursing practice issues such as embracing cultural diversity and fostering collaborative practice. Visit the RNAO's Web site (http://www.rnao.org/bestpractices/), as well as the Web site of the professional nursing association in the province or territory in which you reside, to learn more about the wide range of practice guidelines and to develop a sound knowledge base for your nursing practice.

Critical Thinking Competencies

Kataoka-Yahiro and Saylor (1994) described critical thinking competencies as the cognitive processes that a nurse uses to make judgements about the clinical care of clients. They include general critical thinking, specific critical thinking in clinical situations, and specific critical thinking in nursing. General critical thinking competencies are not unique to nursing. They include the scientific method, problem solving, and decision making. Specific critical thinking competencies in clinical situations include diagnostic reasoning, clinical inference, and clinical decision making. The specific critical thinking competency in nursing involves use of the nursing process.

General Critical Thinking Competencies

Scientific Method. The **scientific method** is a systematic, ordered approach to gathering data and solving problems that is used in nursing, medicine, and various other disciplines. Nurse researchers use the scientific method to verify that a set of facts is true when testing research questions in nursing practice situations. Research incorporating the scientific method contributes to evidence-informed nursing practice and the development of best practice guidelines.

The scientific method has five steps:

- Identification of the problem
- Collection of data
- Formulation of a research question or hypothesis
- Testing of the question or hypothesis
- Evaluation of the results of the test or study

Consider the following example of the scientific method in nursing practice:

A nurse caring for clients who receive large doses of chemotherapy for ovarian cancer detects a pattern whereby these clients develop severe inflammation of the mouth (mucositis) (identifies the problem). The nurse reads research articles (collects data) about mucositis and learns about evidence that cryotherapy, in which clients keep ice in their mouths during the chemotherapy infusion, reduces the severity of the mucositis after treatment. The nurse asks (forms research question), "Can ovarian cancer clients who receive chemotherapy have less severe mucositis when given cryotherapy instead of standard mouth rinse in the oral cavity?" The nurse then designs a study that compares the incidence and severity of mucositis in a group of clients who use cryotherapy with those in clients who use traditional mouth rinse (tests the question). The nurse hopes that the results from the study will give oncology nurses a better approach for reducing the frequency and severity of mucositis in cancer clients. A nurse in another oncology setting critically analyzes the study before implementing its recommendations for client care (evaluates the results of the study).

Problem Solving. Everyone faces problems every day. When a problem arises, people obtain information and then use the information, in addition to what they already know, to find a solution. Clients routinely present problems in nursing practice. For example, a home care nurse visits a client and learns that the client cannot describe what medications she has taken for the past three days. The nurse must solve the problem of why the client is not adhering to her medication schedule. The nurse knows the client was recently discharged from the hospital, and five medications were prescribed. When the nurse asks the client to show the medications that she takes in the morning, the nurse notices that the client has difficulty reading the medication labels. The client is able to tell the nurse the names of the medications she is to take but is uncertain about the times of administration. The nurse recommends having the client's pharmacy relabel the medications in larger lettering. In addition, the nurse shows the client examples of pill organizers that will help her sort her medications by time of day for a period of 7 days.

Effective **problem solving** also involves evaluating the solution over time to be sure that it is still effective. It becomes necessary to try different options if a problem recurs. As a continuation of the example just described, the nurse finds during a follow-up visit that the client has organized her medications correctly and is able to read the labels without difficulty. The nurse obtained information that correctly clarified the cause of the client's problem, and the nurse tested a solution that proved successful. Having solved a problem in one situation adds to the nurse's experience in practice and allows the nurse to apply that knowledge in future situations with clients.

Decision Making. When you face a problem or situation and need to choose a course of action from several options, you are making a decision. **Decision making** is a product of critical thinking that focuses on problem resolution. Following a set of criteria helps you make a well-reasoned decision. For example, decision making occurs when a person chooses a fitness consultant. To make a decision, the person has to recognize and define the problem (need for a physical activity), assess all options (consider recommended trainers or choose one on the basis of proximity to the person's home). The person has to weigh each option against a set of criteria (e.g., credentials, reputation, experience), test possible options (interview potential trainers; assess safety of equipment), consider the consequences of the decision (increased fitness; risk of injury), and then make a final decision. Although the criteria follow a sequence of steps, decision making involves moving back and forth between steps when all criteria are considered. Decision making leads to informed conclusions that are supported by evidence and reason. Examples of decision making include deciding on a choice of dressings for a client with a surgical wound or selecting the best approach for teaching a family how to assist a client who is returning home after a stroke. You learn to make sound decisions by approaching each clinical situation thoughtfully and by applying each component of the decision-making process described previously.

Specific Critical Thinking Competencies in Clinical Situations

Diagnostic Reasoning and Inference. As soon as you receive information about a client in a clinical situation, you begin **diagnostic reasoning**, a process of determining a client's health status after you make physical and behavioural observations and after you assign meaning to the behaviours, physical signs, and symptoms exhibited by the client. The information that you collect and analyze leads to a diagnosis of the client's condition. An expert nurse sees the context of a client situation (e.g., recognize that a client who is feeling lightheaded, has blurred vision, and has a history of diabetes is experiencing a problem with blood glucose levels), observes patterns and themes (e.g., symptoms including weakness, headache, hunger, and visual disturbances that suggest hypoglycemia), and chooses an appropriate intervention quickly (e.g., offers a food source containing glucose) (Ferrario, 2004). Considering the context of the situation enhances the nurse's analytic skills (Ironside, 2005) and results in a more accurate diagnosis.

Part of diagnostic reasoning is **clinical inference**: the process of drawing conclusions from related pieces of evidence (Smith Higuchi & Donald, 2002). An inference involves forming patterns of information from data before making a diagnosis. Seeing that a client has lost his appetite and experienced a loss of weight over the past month, the nurse infers that the client has a nutritional problem. An example of diagnostic reasoning is forming a nursing diagnosis such as *imbalanced nutrition, less than body requirements* (see Chapter 43).

Often you cannot make a precise nursing diagnosis during your first meeting with a client. You will sometimes sense that a problem or health concern exists, but you do not have sufficient data to make a specific diagnosis. Some clients' physical conditions limit their ability to tell you about symptoms. Other clients may choose not to share sensitive and important information during your initial assessment. Clients' behaviours and physical responses may become observable only under certain conditions not present during your initial assessment. When you are uncertain of a diagnosis, continue data collection, which may include consulting with expert nurses or other health care professionals. As a nurse, you have to critically analyze changing clinical situations until you are able to determine the client's unique situation. Diagnostic reasoning is a continuous behaviour in nursing practice.

In diagnostic reasoning, use client data that you gather to logically explain a clinical judgement. For example, after turning a client over in bed, you see an area of redness on his right hip. You palpate the area and note that it is warm to the touch, and the client complains of tenderness there. You push on the area with your finger, and, after you release pressure, the area does not blanch or turn white. You think about what you know about normal skin integrity and the effects of pressure. You form the conclusion the client has a pressure ulcer. As a new student, confirm your judgement with experienced nurses. At times, your clinical judgement may be incorrect; however, nurse experts will give you feedback to build on in future clinical situations.

Nurses do not make medical diagnoses, but they do assess and monitor clients closely and compare the client's signs and symptoms with those that are common to a medical diagnosis. This type of diagnostic reasoning helps nurses and other health care professionals pinpoint the nature of a problem more quickly and select proper interventions. Similarities and differences between medical and nursing diagnoses are described in more detail in Chapter 13.

Clinical Decision Making. Clinical decision making is a problem-solving activity that focuses on defining client problems and selecting appropriate treatments (Smith Higuchi & Donald, 2002). Nurses are responsible for making accurate and appropriate clinical decisions. Clinical decision making distinguishes professional nurses from technical personnel. It is the professional nurse, for example, who takes immediate action when a client's clinical condition deteriorates, decides whether a client is experiencing complications that call for notification of a physician, or decides whether a teaching plan for a client is ineffective and necessitates revision. Benner (1984) described clinical decision making as judgement that includes critical and reflective thinking and action and the application of scientific and practical knowledge.

Clinical judgement requires that you recognize the salient aspects of a clinical situation, interpret their meanings, and respond appopriately. It includes four components: noticing or grasping the situation; interpreting or developing a sufficient understanding of the situation to respond; responding or deciding on a course of action; and reflecting on or reviewing the actions taken and their outcomes. In making a clinical judgement, you consider the context of the situation and rely on analytic processes, intuition, and narrative thinking (i.e., thinking that occurs as a result of telling and interpreting stories). As you reflect on actions taken, you acquire clinical learning, which contributes to future clinical judgements (Tanner, 2006).

Most clients have health concerns for which no clear textbook solutions exist. Each client's problems are unique and products of many factors, including the client's physical health, lifestyle, culture, relationship with family and friends, living environment, and experiences. As a nurse, you do not always have a clear picture of the client's needs and the appropriate actions to take when you first meet a client. Instead, you must learn to question and explore different perspectives and interpretations in order to find a solution that benefits the client.

When you approach a clinical problem, such as a client who is experiencing difficulty walking, you make a decision that identifies the problem (e.g., right-sided weakness) and choose nursing interventions (e.g., teaching the use of appropriate assistive devices) for that client. Nurses constantly make clinical decisions to improve a client's health or maintain wellness. Clinical decision making requires careful reasoning so that you choose the options for the best client outcomes on the basis of the client's condition and the priority of the problem or health concern.

You improve your clinical decision making by knowing your clients. Nurse researchers found that expert nurses develop a level of knowing that leads to pattern recognition of client's symptoms and responses (White, 2003). For example, an expert nurse who has worked on a general surgery unit for many years is more likely to detect signs of internal hemorrhage (e.g., fall in blood pressure, rapid pulse, change in consciousness) than is a new nurse. Over time, a combination of knowledge, experience, time spent in a specific clinical area, and the quality of relationships formed with clients allow expert nurses to know clinical situations and quickly anticipate and select the right course of action (Tanner et al., 1993). Spending more time during initial client assessments to both observe client behaviour and measure physical findings is a way to improve knowing your clients. Also, consistently monitoring clients as problems occur helps you see how clinical changes develop over time. The selection of nursing actions is built on both clinical knowledge and client data, including the following:

- The identified status and situation of the client.
- Knowledge about the clinical variables (e.g., client's age, seriousness of the problem, pathological process of the problem, client's pre-existing disease conditions) involved in the situation and how the variables are linked together.
- Knowledge about the usual patterns of any diagnosed problem or prognosis and a judgement about the likely course of events and outcomes of the diagnosed problem, in view of any health risks the client also has.
- Any additional relevant information about requirements in the client's daily living situation, functional capacity, and social resources.

- Knowledge about the nursing interventions available and the way in which specific actions will predictably affect the client's situation.

Making an accurate clinical decision allows you to set priorities for nursing action (see Chapter 13). Because each situation involves different clients and different variables, a certain activity is sometimes more of a priority in one situation and less of a priority in another. For example, if a home care client is physically dependent, unable to eat, and incontinent of urine, skin integrity is of higher priority than if the client were immobile but continent of urine and able to eat a normal diet. Do not assume that certain health situations produce automatic priorities. For example, an adolescent who has embarked on a smoking cessation program is expected to experience some withdrawal symptoms, which often become a priority of care. However, if the client is experiencing anxiety about potential weight gain that decreases her ability to participate fully in the program, it becomes necessary for you to focus on ways to relieve the anxiety before the smoking cessation measures will be effective.

After determining a client's nursing care priorities, you select actions most likely to relieve each problem or to promote health, wellness, and quality of life. A wide range of choices is often available, from nurse-administered to client self-care strategies. You collaborate with the client and then select, test, and evaluate the chosen approaches.

Nurses make decisions about individual clients and about groups of clients. You use criteria such as the clinical condition of the clients, Maslow's hierarchy of needs, risks involved in treatment delays, and clients' expectations of care to determine which clients have the most urgent priorities for care. For example, a client in a community care centre who is experiencing a sudden drop in blood pressure along with a change in consciousness requires your attention immediately, as opposed to a small child who requires a routine immunization or a group of expectant parents attending a prenatal class. In order for you to manage the wide variety of problems associated with groups of clients, skillful, prioritized decision making is crucial (Box 12–2).

Nursing Process as a Critical Thinking Competency

Nurses apply the **nursing process** as a critical thinking competency when delivering client care (Kataoka-Yahiro & Saylor, 1994). The nursing process is a five-step clinical decision-making approach that

---

> **BOX 12-2** **Clinical Decision Making for Groups of Clients**

- Identify the nursing diagnosis and collaborative problems of each client (see Chapter 13).
- Analyze clients' diagnoses or problems and decide which are most urgent on the bases of basic needs, the clients' changing or unstable status, and problem complexity (see Chapter 13).
- Consider the resources available for managing each problem, including unregulated care providers assigned to work with you, as well as clients' family members.
- Consider how to involve the clients as decision makers and participants in care.
- Decide how to combine activities to resolve more than one client problem at a time.
- Decide what, if any, nursing care procedures to delegate to unregulated care providers so that you are able to spend your time on activities requiring professional nursing knowledge.

consists of assessment, diagnosis, planning, implementation, and evaluation (see Chapters 13 to 15). The purpose of the nursing process is to assist nurses in identifying and treating clients' health concerns. Use of the nursing process allows nurses to help clients meet agreed-upon outcomes for better health (Figure 12–2). The nursing process incorporates general (e.g., scientific method, problem solving, and decision making) and specific critical thinking competencies (e.g., diagnostic reasoning, inference, and clinical decision making), described earlier in this chapter, in a manner that focuses on a particular client's unique needs. The format of the nursing process is unique to the discipline of nursing and provides a common language and process for nurses to "think through" clients' clinical problems (Kataoka-Yahiro & Saylor, 1994). Chapter 13 describes the nursing process in more detail.

The nursing process is often called a *blueprint* or *plan for care*. It allows flexibility for use in all clinical settings. When you use the nursing process, you identify a client's health-related concerns, clearly define a nursing diagnosis or collaborative problem, determine priorities of care, and set goals and expected outcomes of care. Then you develop and communicate a plan of care, perform nursing interventions, and evaluate the effects of your care. Involving your client in each step of the nursing process helps ensure that care is client centered. When you become more competent in using the nursing process, you are able to focus not merely on a single client problem or diagnosis but on multiple problems or diagnoses and to move back and forth between steps when considering all of the information available to you about a client's concerns. With each step, you apply critical thinking to provide the very best professional care to your clients.

Qualities for Critical Thinking

The fourth component of the critical thinking model is qualities. An important part of critical thinking is interpreting, evaluating, and making judgements about the adequacy of various arguments and available data. Qualities define how a successful critical thinker approaches a problem or a situation that necessitates decision making. For example, when a client complains of anxiety before undergoing a diagnostic procedure, the curious nurse explores possible reasons for the client's concerns. The nurse also exhibits discipline and perseverance in taking responsibility to complete a thorough assessment to find the sources of the client's anxiety. The quality of inquiry involves an ability to recognize that problems exist and that you need evidence in support of what you suppose to be true (Watson & Glaser, 1980). Knowing when you need more information, knowing when information is misleading, and recognizing your own knowledge limits and personal biases are examples of how critical thinking qualities play a key role in decision making.

Standards for Critical Thinking

The fifth component of the critical thinking model includes intellectual and professional standards (Kataoka-Yahiro & Saylor, 1994).

Intellectual Standards. An intellectual standard is a guideline or principle for rational thought. You apply such standards when you conduct the nursing process. When you consider a client problem, apply intellectual standards such as thoroughness, preciseness, accuracy, and consistency to make sure that all clinical decisions are sound. Efficacious use of the intellectual standards in clinical practice ensures that you do not perform critical thinking haphazardly.

Professional Standards. Professional standards for critical thinking refer to ethical criteria for nursing judgements, evidence-informed criteria used for evaluation, and criteria for professional responsibility. Professional standards promote the highest level of

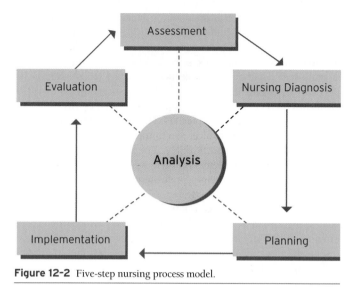

Figure 12-2 Five-step nursing process model.

quality nursing care for individuals and groups in institutional and community-based settings.

Ethical Criteria for Nursing Judgement. Client care requires more than just the memorization and application of scientific knowledge (Ironside, 2005). Efficacious nursing practice reflects sound ethical principles. Being able to focus on a client's values and beliefs helps you make clinical decisions that are just, faithful to the client's choices, and beneficial to the client's health and well-being. The *Code of Ethics for Registered Nurses* (Canadian Nurses Association, 2008) is based on core values that serve as a guide to ethical decision making in nursing practice. Among these values and ethical responsibilities are providing safe, compassionate, competent, and ethical care; promoting health and well-being; promoting and respecting informed decision making; preserving dignity; maintaining privacy and confidentiality; promoting justice; and being accountable. Critical thinkers maintain a sense of self-awareness through conscious awareness of their own values, beliefs, and feelings and of the multiple perspectives of clients, family members, staff, and peers in clinical situations. Chapter 8 summarizes ethical standards to use when you are faced with ethical dilemmas or problems.

One of the clients in a community health clinic is a young man who has signs and symptoms of chlamydia, a sexually transmitted disease. The client has had the symptoms for more than 3 weeks and voices concern about what it will mean to have the disease. Richard, a nurse, examines the young man and finds that the client has redness and itching on his penis, with a yellowish discharge. Richard checks further and asks whether the client has pain on urination. He also assesses the client for fever. Richard has limited knowledge about chlamydia, and so he consults with the clinic nurse practitioner, who explains the nature of the infection, the risks it poses to the client, the usual course of treatment, and some of the legal and ethical guidelines that govern nurses' actions when working with clients with sexually transmitted diseases. Richard returns to the client and speaks confidently with him about chlamydia, the reason for his symptoms, the need to tell sex partners about the infection, and the importance of wearing a condom.

Criteria for Evaluation. Nurses routinely use evidence-informed criteria to assess clients' conditions and to determine the efficacy of nursing interventions. For example, accurate assessment of symptoms such as pain or shortness of breath requires use of assessment criteria such as the duration, severity, location, aggravating or relieving factors, and effects on daily lifestyle (see Chapter 42). In this case, assessment criteria allow you to accurately determine the nature of a client's symptoms, select appropriate interventions, and later evaluate whether the interventions are effective. Another example is the determination of the stage of a pressure ulcer on the basis of scientific criteria, including temperature, tissue consistency, and depth of the wound (see Chapter 47). The criteria allow you to identify the stage of a pressure ulcer and to track how quickly it heals.

Professional Responsibility. The standards of professional responsibility that a nurse strives to achieve are the standards cited in institutional practice guidelines, professional organizations' standards of practice, and nursing practice acts. To view the nursing practice standards practice that govern nurses' actions in your jurisdiction, visit the Web site of the professional nursing association in the province or territory in which you reside. These standards outline the responsibilities and accountabilities that a nurse assumes in guaranteeing high-quality health care to the public.

Developing Critical Thinking Skills

To develop critical thinking skills, it is important to learn how to connect knowledge and theory in practice (Box 12–3). Making sense of what you learn in the classroom, from reading, or from dialogue with other students and then applying it during client care are always challenging. Learning approaches will assist you in developing and improving your critical thinking skills.

Reflective Journal Writing

How often do you think back on a situation to consider why it occurred? How did you act? What could you have done differently? What knowledge could you have used? **Reflection** is the process of purposefully thinking back or recalling a situation to discover its purpose or meaning. Reflection is necessary for self-evaluation and improvement of nursing practice.

Reflective journal writing is a tool for developing critical thought and reflection through clarifying concepts (Bilinski, 2002). Reflective writing gives you the opportunity to define and express a clinical experience in your own words (Di Vito-Thomas, 2005). By keeping a reflective journal of each of your clinical experiences, you are able to explore personal perceptions or understanding of the experience and develop the ability to apply theory in practice. The use of a journal improves your observation and descriptive skills.

The "Circle of Meaning" model, which was adapted to nursing practice, encourages reflection, concept clarification, and a search for meaning in nursing practice (Bilinski, 2002). The model features a series of questions that enable nurses to journey through the clinical experience and find meaning and connections. The questions include the following:

- What experience or situation in your clinical practice seems confusing, difficult, or interesting?
- What is the meaning of the experience? What feelings did you have about it? What feelings did your client have? What influenced the experience?
- Do your responses to the preceding questions remind you of any experience from the past or present, or something that you think is desirable future experience? How does it relate? What are the implications or significance?
- What are the connections between what is being described and the things you have learned about nursing science, research, and

theory? What are some possible solutions? What approach or solution would you choose, and why would you choose it? What is the effectiveness of this approach?

Keeping a journal of your client care experiences will help you become aware of how you use clinical decision making skills (Kessler & Lund, 2004). Begin by recording notes after a clinical experience. Telling a story and drawing a picture are two additional ways to identify the experience you wish to reflect on. Describe in detail what you felt, thought, and did. Analyze your experience by considering thoughts, feelings, and possible meanings for you and the client. Challenge any preconceived ideas you have when you look at actual clinical situations. Describe the significance of the experience. Refer to your journal often when you care for clients in similar circumstances. Reflecting on your experiences is an important component of monitoring your competence in nursing practice. It also promotes knowledge transfer by enabling you to identify how previously acquired knowledge can be applied in a current or future situation (Nielsen et al., 2007).

Concept Mapping

As a nurse, you care for clients who have multiple nursing diagnoses or collaborative problems. A **concept map** is a visual representation of client problems and interventions that depicts their relationships to one another (Schuster, 2003). The primary purpose of concept

---

✳ BOX 12-3   RESEARCH HIGHLIGHT

How to "Think Like a Nurse"

Research Focus

Faculty members use a variety of teaching and learning strategies to aid students in developing critical thinking. Di Vito-Thomas (2005) invited junior and senior nursing students from four schools of nursing to answer two questions: (1) "How would you describe how you think when making clinical judgements?" and (2) "What were the most important teaching/learning strategies in the development of your clinical judgement?"

Research Abstract

Students described their thinking as a process that developed through experience in practice. Education and practice are combined so that knowledge gained in the classroom becomes second nature in practice. Students noted that they learned to think through different options and then to weigh those options determine what to do first to improve client outcomes. Clinical experience was the most important strategy in developing clinical judgement. Concept maps showing the interrelatedness of all aspects of client care were also useful. Case studies allowed students to focus on, think critically about, and understand the relationships between those aspects.

Evidence-Informed Practice

Teaching and learning strategies that help develop clinical judgement include the following:
- Scrutinizing case studies displayed on concept maps
- Having in-depth discussion with instructors while observing clinical changes in clients
- Making joint decisions with peers and instructors on client care

References: Di Vito-Thomas, P. (2005). Nursing student stories on learning how to think like a nurse. *Nurse Education, 30*(3), 133.

mapping is to synthesize relevant data about a client, including assessment data, nursing diagnoses, health needs, nursing interventions, and evaluation measures (Hill, 2006). Through drawing a concept map, you learn to organize or link information in a unique way so that the diverse information you have about a client begins to connect to form meaningful patterns and concepts. When you see the relationship between the various client diagnoses and the data that support them, you gain a better understanding of a client's clinical situation. Over time, concept maps become more detailed, integrated, and comprehensive as you learn more about the care of a client and as you care for similar clients (Ferrario, 2004). You will see similarities and differences between clients, which helps you hone decision-making skills.

Concept maps take many visual forms. Several examples of concept maps are included in Chapters 31 to 49 of this textbook. Additional resources are also found in the reference list at the end of this chapter. Most students follow a model that makes the concept map a working document. As a student, you develop the map during your care for the client. You begin by obtaining client data from a variety of sources (e.g., the medical record, pertinent nursing literature, the client's history and physical examination, and other health care professionals). The client's major medical diagnosis and any comorbid conditions (unrelated medical conditions) usually form the center of the map. From there, you group patterns of assessment data along the edges of the map. As you identify the different nursing diagnoses, you draw dotted lines to connect the diagnoses that are related.

The links must be accurate in order to show true clinical relationships. On the map, you also list the nursing interventions chosen for the client. Once again, you see how any one intervention applies to more than one nursing diagnosis. While caring for a client, you write down the client's responses to your interventions and any clinical impressions you may have.

The final map gives you a broader and more complex understanding of your client's health care needs. Save the concept maps you create and use them as a reference as you care for other clients with similar health concerns.

Critical Thinking Synthesis

Critical thinking is a reasoning process by which you reflect on and analyze your own thoughts, knowledge, and actions (Figure 12–3). To be think critically requires dedication and a desire to grow intellectually. For novice nurses, it is important to learn the steps of the nursing process and to incorporate the elements of the critical thinking model in your practice. The two processes are intertwined in making quality decisions about client care. The key components of critical thinking are integrated into Chapters 31 to 49 of this text to help you better understand its relationship to the nursing process and to making quality judgements and decisions about client care.

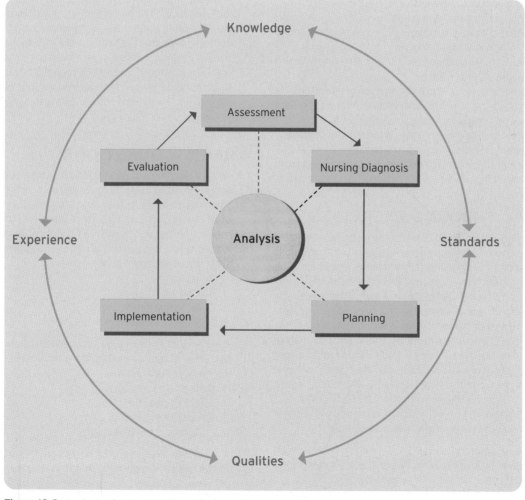

Figure 12-3 Synthesis of critical thinking with the nursing process competency.

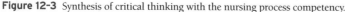

✱ KEY CONCEPTS

- Critical thinking is a process acquired through experience and an active curiosity about learning.
- Nurses who apply critical thinking in their work focus on options for solving problems and making decisions, rather than rapidly and carelessly quickly adopting simple solutions.
- Following a procedure step by step without adjusting to a client's unique needs is an example of basic critical thinking.
- In complex critical thinking, a nurse learns that alternative, and perhaps conflicting, solutions to problems exist.
- The critical thinking model combines a nurse's knowledge base, experience, competence in nursing process, qualities, and standards to explain how nurses make clinical judgements that are necessary for safe, effective nursing care.
- In diagnostic reasoning, you collect client data and then logically develop a clinical judgement, such as a nursing diagnosis.
- When you face a clinical problem or situation and choose a course of action from several options, you are making a clinical decision.
- Clinical learning experiences are necessary for you to acquire clinical decision-making skills.
- You improve your clinical decision making by knowing your clients.
- Clinical decision making involves judgement that includes critical and reflective thinking and the action and application of scientific and practical knowledge.
- The nursing process is a blueprint for client care that involves both general and specific critical thinking competencies in a way that focuses on the client's unique needs.
- Critical thinking qualities help a nurse to know when more information is needed, to know when information is misleading, and to recognize personal knowledge limits.
- The use of intellectual standards during assessment ensures a complete database of information.
- Professional standards for critical thinking refer to ethical criteria for nursing judgements, scientific and practice criteria to be used for evaluation, and criteria for professional responsibility.
- Reflective journal writing gives you the opportunity to define and express clinical experiences in your own words.
- Drawing a concept map enables you to gain a broader and more complex understanding of your client's complex health care needs.

✱ CRITICAL THINKING EXERCISES

1. You are meeting with an obese client for the first time. She states that she been successful in losing weight on several occasions but is frustrated by her inability to maintain her weight loss. She reports having tried "virtually every fad diet" and "multiple exercise programs." She admits that as her weight increases, she tends to be become less active. She has become increasingly reluctant to leave her home because of the negative reactions of other people. In listening to her story, you attempt to imagine what it would be like to be in her situation and to examine your biases and assumptions about people who are obese. Your goal is to begin to discuss potential options with her for dealing with her situation. Describe the level of critical thinking that is necessary in this scenario. How will your actions potentially assist in helping this client develop an effective plan of action?

2. Consider the following statements, and describe whether each is an example of problem solving, inference, or diagnostic reasoning. Support your answer with a rationale.

   a. As the nurse enters a client's room, she observes that the intravenous line is not infusing at the ordered rate. The nurse checks the flow regulator on the tubing, looks to see whether the client is lying on the tubing, checks the connection between the tubing and the intravenous catheter, and then checks the condition of the site where the intravenous catheter enters the client's skin. She readjusts the flow rate, and the infusion begins at the correct rate.

   b. The nurse sits down to talk with her client, who lost her sister 2 weeks ago. The client reports that she is unable to sleep, feels very fatigued during the day, and is having trouble at work. The nurse asks her clarify the type of trouble, and the client explains that she cannot concentrate or even solve simple problems. The nurse records the results of her assessment, describing the client's problem as ineffective coping.

   c. In observing a new mother breastfeeding her baby, the public health nurse observes that the baby is fussy and is not sucking effectively. The nurse reviews the baby's record and finds that he has lost a considerable amount of weight since birth. The nurse conducts an assessment and notes that the baby has poor skin turgor. The mother reports that he urinates infrequently and sleeps only for very short periods of time between feedings. The nurse concludes that the baby is dehydrated and is at risk of becoming malnourished.

3. Mr. Yousif is a terminally ill client receiving home care. His wife and son are asking you about his pain control. Mrs. Yousif is requesting that her husband's medication be increased, even if it means he will not be responsive. She does not want her husband to suffer. The son is vehemently opposed to too much narcotic and feels that his father is still able to make decisions for himself. Mr. Yousif remains alert much of the time and is able to talk with you about his feelings regarding death and his desire to die at home. He seems to appreciate your availability in talking with him. How might you use critical thinking to help the family resolve this complex problem?

✱ REVIEW QUESTIONS

1. You are teaching a 12-year-old boy how to self-administer insulin. After discussing the techniques and demonstrating an injection, you ask him to try it. After two attempts, it is obvious that he does not understand how to prepare the correct dose. You review your approach with the client carefully and ask a colleague for her suggestions about how to improve your teaching skills. This is an example of
   1. Reflection
   2. Risk taking
   3. Client assessment
   4. Care plan evaluation

2. A nurse uses an institution's procedure manual to confirm how to change a client's nasogastric tubing. The level of critical thinking the nurse is using is
   1. Commitment
   2. Scientific method
   3. Basic critical thinking
   4. Complex critical thinking

3. A client had hip surgery 24 hours ago. The nurse refers to the written plan of care, noting that the client has a device collecting wound drainage. The physician is to be notified when the

accumulation in the device exceeds 100 mL for the day. When the nurse enters the room, the nurse looks at the device and carefully notes the amount of drainage currently in the device. This is an example of

1. Planning
2. Evaluation
3. Intervention
4. Assessment

4. The nurse asks a client how she feels about her impending surgery for breast cancer. Before the discussion, the nurse reviewed the description in his textbook of loss and grief in addition to therapeutic communication principles. The critical thinking component involved in the nurse's review of the literature is

1. Experience
2. Problem solving
3. Knowledge application
4. Clinical decision making

✱ RECOMMENDED WEB SITES

Canadian Nurses Association: http://www.cna-nurses.ca
A wide range of valuable resources, including the *Code of Ethics for Registered Nurses* (CNA, 2008), can be found on the Web site of the Canadian Nurses Association. This Web site also links to the Web sites of each of the provincial and territorial professional nursing associations in Canada. Visit these Web sites and become familiar with the kinds of resources that are available to you. The position papers and other documents found on these Web sites demonstrate how Canadian nurse leaders have used critical thinking to explore important issues in nursing and nursing practice.

IHMC CMap Tools: A Modelling Kit: http://cmap.ihmc.us
This Web site not only provides an example of a concept map but also provides instruction about how to create one. It illustrates components of a concept map and their relationship to each other.

Insight Assessment/California Academic Press: http://www.insightassessment.com/articles.html
A wide array of articles and case studies related to critical thinking, tools to measure your critical thinking skills, and other valuable resources can be found on this Web site. Many of these resources can be downloaded for free; others are available for purchase.

The Critical Thinking Community: http://www.criticalthinking.org
The section of this Web site titled "The Thinker's Guide Series" includes links to a number of short booklets that explore subjects such as critical thinking concepts and tools, improving your reading, writing and study skills, and ethical reasoning.

Critical Thinking on the Web: A Directory of Quality Online Resources: http://www.austhink.org/critical/index.htm
This Web site links to a wide range of articles in which critical thinking is examined from a variety of perspectives, including nursing. It also contains links to a variety of tutorials that you can use to improve your critical thinking skills.

Critical Thinking Strategies: Concept Mapping: http://cord.org/txcollabnursing/onsite_conceptmap.htm
This Web site provides examples of the use of concept maps in nursing practice.

Student Resources: Critical Thinking Skills: http://distance.uvic.ca/courses/critical/index.htm
This online tutorial assists students in exploring the importance of critical thinking in reading, writing, reasoning, and making judgements.

13

Nursing Assessment and Diagnosis

Original chapter by Patricia A. Potter, RN, MSN, PhD, GMAC, FAAN

Canadian content written by Marilynn J. Wood, RN, BSN, MPH, DrPH,

and Janet C. Ross-Kerr, RN, BScN, MS, PhD

media resources

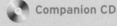 **Web Site**

- Audio Chapter Summaries
- Glossary
- Multiple-Choice Review Questions
- Student Learning Activities
- Weblinks

Companion CD

- Glossary
- Interactive Learning Activities
- Fluids and Electrolytes Tutorial
- Test-Taking Skills

The **nursing process** is a problem-solving approach to identifying, diagnosing, and treating the health issues of clients. It is fundamental to how nurses practice. As a nursing student, you will learn the five steps of the nursing process—assessment, diagnosis, planning, implementation, and evaluation—as if they were a linear process (Figure 13–1). However, the nursing process is, in fact, continuous, and in practice, you will learn to move back and forth between the various steps (Potter et al., 2005).

Consider the following scenario:

Lisa, a registered nurse on an orthopedic nursing unit, enters Ms. Devine's room for the first time at 0700 when her shift begins. Ms Devine is a 52-year-old woman who sustained an injury, a ruptured lumbar disc, in a fall 2 months ago. She is scheduled for a lumbar laminectomy this afternoon. When Lisa first observes Ms. Devine, she notes the client is moving in bed awkwardly and is grimacing when she turns. Ms. Devine looks up and states, "Oh, I am so glad you are here. [Sighs] The pain in my back seems worse, and I cannot get comfortable. I cannot sit at all, so I will stay in bed for now. I just dread having this surgery, I will be so glad when this is all over [looks away and avoids eye contact]." Lisa observes Ms. Devine's facial grimace and notes her sighing. She responds, "Ms. Devine, you obviously look uncomfortable and a bit upset. Let me ask you a few questions: Show me where the pain is. On a scale of 0 to 10, with 10 the worst pain ever and 0 no pain, how would you rate your pain? Does it become worse when you turn?" As Ms. Devine responds to the questions, Lisa analyzes the data and considers other relevant information, such as the client's medical diagnosis (ruptured lumbar disc) and knowledge of the alterations that the condition typically causes (e.g., sciatic pain and change in sensation of the lower extremities). Lisa decides that Ms. Devine has acute pain related to pressure on the spinal nerves. Lisa explains to Ms. Devine a plan to help relieve the discomfort. She then administers an ordered analgesic, repositions Ms. Devine, and discusses how Ms. Devine can practice relaxation exercises. Forty minutes later, Lisa returns to Ms. Devine's room to determine whether the pain is relieved and whether she wants to try the relaxation exercises.

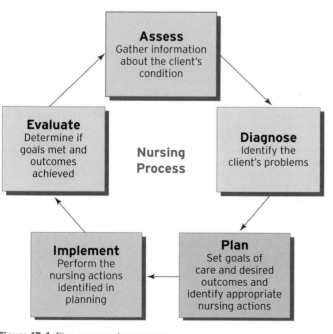

Figure 13-1 Five-step nursing process.

Lisa applied the nursing process while caring for Ms. Devine. Each time you meet a client, you will apply the nursing process to provide appropriate and effective nursing care. The process begins with the first step, **assessment**, the gathering and analysis of information about the client's health status. In the next step, **diagnosis**, you then make clinical judgements about the client's response to health problems in the form of nursing *diagnoses*. Once you establish appropriate nursing diagnoses, you create a plan of care. **Planning** includes interventions individualized to each of the client's nursing diagnoses. The next step, **implementation**, involves the actual performance of planned interventions. After administering interventions, you conduct an **evaluation** of the client's response and whether the interventions were effective. The nursing process is central to your ability to provide timely and appropriate care to your clients.

The nursing process is a variation of scientific reasoning that allows you to organize and systematize nursing practice. You learn to make inferences about the meaning of a client's response to a health problem or generalize about the client's functional state of health. A pattern begins to form. For example, if Ms. Devine is having acute back pain, the data allow Lisa to infer that the client's mobility is limited. Lisa gathers more information (e.g., noting how the client moves and whether the client is able to walk, stand, and sit normally) until the client's problem is classified accurately: for example, as the nursing diagnosis *impaired physical mobility related to acute back pain*. The clear definition of the client's problems provides the basis for planning and implementing nursing interventions and evaluating the outcomes of care.

Critical Thinking Approach to Assessment

Assessment is the deliberate and systematic collection of data to determine a client's current and past health status and functional status and to determine the client's present and past coping patterns (Carpenito-Moyet, 2005). Nursing assessment consists of two steps:

- Collection and verification of data from a primary source (the client) and secondary sources (e.g., family, health professionals, and patient record).
- The analysis of all data as a basis for developing nursing diagnoses, identifying collaborative problems, and developing a plan of individualized care.

The purpose of assessment is to establish a **database** about the client's perceived needs, health problems, and responses to these problems. In addition, the data reveal related experiences, health practices, goals, values, and expectations about the health care system.

When a plumber comes to your home to repair a problem you describe as a "leaking faucet," the plumber checks the faucet, its attachments to the water line, and the water pressure in the system to determine the actual malfunction. Similarly, you see clients who will present an initial health problem to you. You then proceed to observe each client's behaviour, ask questions about the nature of the problem, listen to the cues the client provides, and conduct a physical examination (see Chapter 32). Sometimes you also interview family members who are familiar with the client's health problem, and you review any existing medical record data. All of the data you collect form different sets or patterns of information that point to a diagnostic conclusion. Once a plumber knows the source of the faucet leak, he or she is able to repair the faucet. Similarly, once you know the nature and source of a client's health problems, you are able to provide interventions that will restore, maintain, or improve the client's health.

Critical thinking is important to good assessment (see Chapter 12). Critical thinking allows you to see the big picture when you form conclusions or make decisions about a client's health condition. While gathering data about a client, you synthesize relevant knowledge, recall prior clinical experiences, apply critical thinking **standards** and available evidence, and use standards of practice to direct your assessment in a meaningful and purposeful way (Figure 13–2). Your knowledge of the physical, biological, and social sciences enables you to ask relevant questions and collect history and physical assessment data relevant to the client's presenting health care needs. For example, by knowing that a client has a history of a ruptured lumbar disc, you know to ask whether the client has sciatic pain (characteristic pain that radiates or spreads from the buttocks down the leg) and to question how the discomfort affects the client's ability to walk or sit, inasmuch as these are common symptoms of disc disease. By using good communication skills and critical thinking intellectual standards, you can collect complete, accurate, and relevant data.

Prior clinical experience contributes to the skills of assessment. For example, if you have cared for a client with back pain, you know the pain is sometimes disabling and limits the client's normal motion. Thus, you thoroughly assess the extent to which the pain affects the current client's ability to walk normally and to perform daily living activities. By validating abnormal assessment findings and personally observing assessments performed by skilled professionals, you become competent in assessment. You also learn to apply standards of practice and accepted standards of "normal" for physical assessment data when assessing clients. Use of critical thinking qualities such as creativity, perseverance, and confidence ensure that you compile a comprehensive database.

Data Collection

As you begin a client assessment, think critically about what to assess. On the basis of your clinical knowledge and experience and your client's health history and responses, determine what questions or measurements are appropriate. When you first meet a client, make a quick observational overview or screening. Usually an overview is based on a treatment situation. For example, a community health nurse assesses the neighbourhood and the community of the client; an emergency room nurse uses the airway-breathing-circulation (ABC) approach; and an oncology nurse focuses on the client's symptoms from disease and from treatment and grief response. In the case of Ms. Devine, Lisa first focuses on the nature and severity of her client's pain, the risk of limited mobility, and the extent of the client's anxiety. She will later expand her assessment to determine whether Ms. Devine has been psychologically prepared for her upcoming surgery.

You learn to differentiate important data from the total data collected. A **cue** is information that you obtain through use of the senses. An **inference** is your judgement or interpretation of those cues. For example, a client's crying is a cue that possibly implies fear or sadness. You ask the client about any concerns and make known any nonverbal expressions you notice in an effort to direct the client to share his or her feelings. It is possible to miss important cues when you conduct an initial overview. However, always try to interpret cues from the client to know how in-depth to make your assessment. Remember that thinking is human and imperfect. You will acquire appropriate thinking processes in the conduct of assessment, but expect to make mistakes in missing important cues (Lunney, 2006).

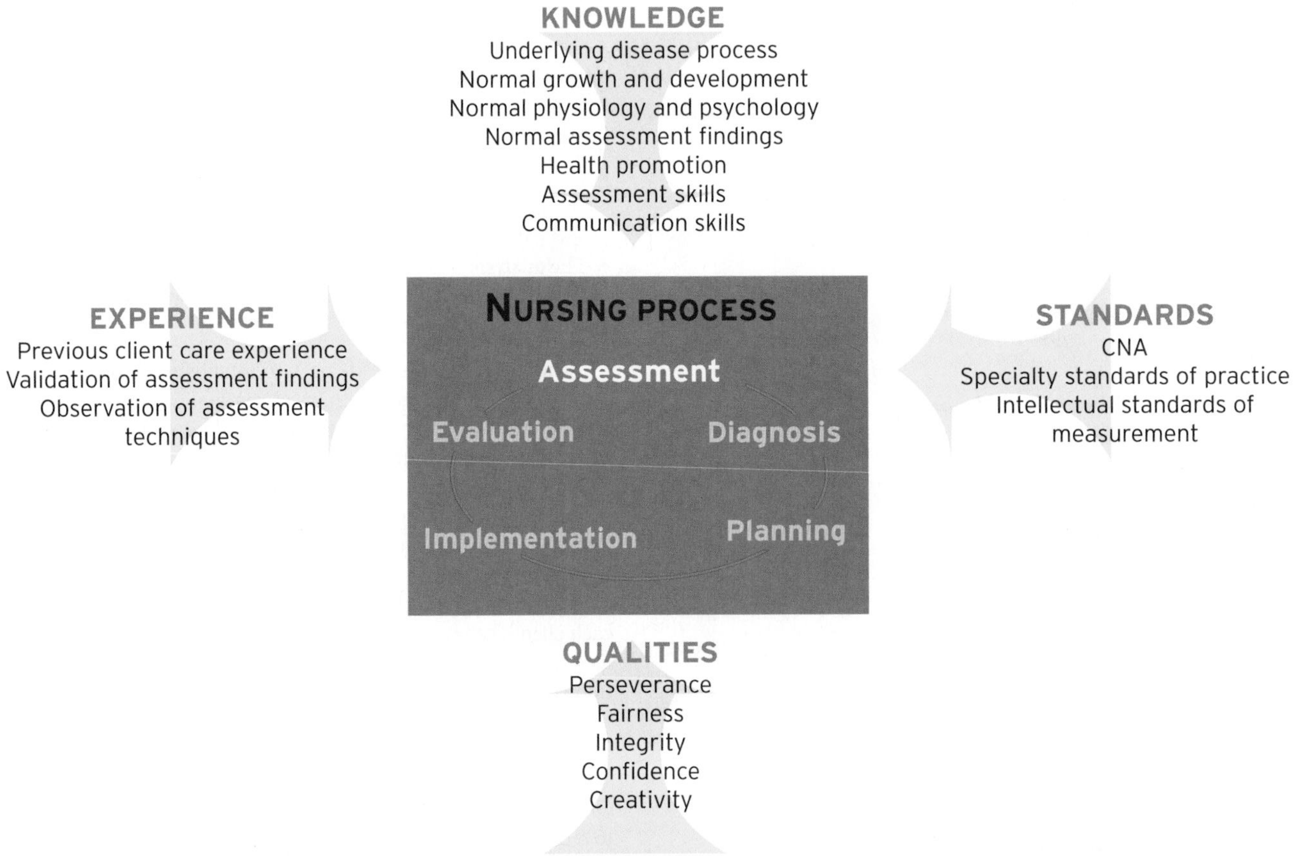

KNOWLEDGE
Underlying disease process
Normal growth and development
Normal physiology and psychology
Normal assessment findings
Health promotion
Assessment skills
Communication skills

EXPERIENCE
Previous client care experience
Validation of assessment findings
Observation of assessment techniques

NURSING PROCESS

Assessment

Evaluation   Diagnosis

Implementation   Planning

STANDARDS
CNA
Specialty standards of practice
Intellectual standards of measurement

QUALITIES
Perseverance
Fairness
Integrity
Confidence
Creativity

Figure 13-2 Critical thinking and the assessment process.

Assessment is dynamic and allows you to freely explore relevant client problems as you discover them.

Begin your assessment by documenting a comprehensive **nursing health history**, a detailed database that allows you to plan and carry out nursing care to meet the client's needs. Box 13–1 presents guidelines for documenting a comprehensive history. This approach encourages you to focus on your client's strengths and available supports, as well as on the presenting problem.

As you collect data, you begin to categorize cues, make inferences, and identify emerging patterns, potential problem areas, and

---

➤ BOX 13-1   **Guidelines for Documenting a Comprehensive Nursing Health History**

A. Identifying Data
Name, age, sex, date, and place of birth.

B. Reason for Health History Interview
Explain why you are interviewing the client at the present time (e.g., the client has just been admitted to an inpatient unit or clinic).

C. Current State of Health
General state of health and health goals. If an illness is present, gather data about the nature of the illness by conducting a symptom analysis (see Chapter 32).

D. Developmental Variables
- Marital status: single, married, separated, widowed, divorced.
- Number of children.
- Developmental stage (see Chapter 22).
- Current occupation.
- Significant life experiences (e.g., education, previous occupations, financial situations, retirement, coping or stress tolerance, and measures normally used to reduce stress).
- Safety hazards (e.g., biological, chemical, ergonomic, physical, psychosocial, reproductive).
- Housing, environmental hazards (e.g., type of housing, location, living arrangements; specific hazards in the home or community).
- Safety measures (e.g., use of seat belts, presence of smoke detectors and fire extinguishers, and other measures related to specific hazards of work, community, and home).

E. Psychological Variables
Mental processes, relationships, support systems, statements regarding client's feelings about self.

F. Spiritual Variables
Rituals, religious practices, beliefs about life, clients' source of guidance in acting on beliefs, and the relationship with family in exercising faith.

G. Sociocultural Variables
- Culture: beliefs and practices related to health and illness (see Chapter 10).
- Primary language and other languages spoken.
- Recreation (exercise, hobbies, socializing, use of leisure time).
- Family and significant others. Include family composition, relationships, special problems experienced by family, client's and family's response to stress, roles, and support systems. The family history provides information about family structure, interaction, and function that may be useful in planning care. For example, a cohesive, supportive family can help a client adjust to an illness or disability and should be incorporated into the plan of care. However, if the client's family members are not supportive, it may be better not to involve them in care. Outline a family tree (genogram; see Chapter 20) to determine whether the client is at risk for genetic illnesses and to identify areas of health promotion and illness prevention.

H. Physiological Variables (Body Structure and Function)
History of Past Illnesses and Injuries
Including dates.

Current Medications
Prescribed, over-the-counter, or illicit drugs. Include name, dosage, schedule, duration of and reason for use, and expected effects and side effects; if illicit drug, include type, amount, response, adverse reaction, drug-related accidents or arrests, attempts to quit.

Review of Systems
The **review of systems** is a systematic method for collecting data on all body systems. Not all questions in each system may be covered in every history. Nevertheless, some questions about each system are included, particularly when a client mentions a symptom or sign. The nurse begins with questions about the usual functioning of each body system and any noted changes and follows with specific questions such as the ones noted as follows for each system. Nurses also focus on measures taken by the client to promote and maintain health and those to prevent illness or injury. The following are included in the review of systems:
- *General manifestation of symptoms:* fever, chills, malaise, pain, sleep patterns and disturbances, fatigue, recent alterations in weight.
- *Integumentary:* itching, colour or texture change, lesions, dryness and use of creams or lotions, changes in hair or nails.
- *Ocular:* visual acuity, blurring, eye pain, recent change in vision, discharge, excessive tearing, date of last examination.
- *Auditory:* hearing loss, pain, discharge, dizziness, perception of ringing in ears, wax.
- *Upper respiratory:* nosebleeds, nasal discharge, nasal allergies, sinus problems, frequency of colds and usual method of treatment, sore throat and usual type of home remedy, hoarseness or voice changes.
- *Lower respiratory:* use of tobacco (amount and number of years of smoking; exposure to tobacco smoke; if smoker, attempts to stop smoking), exposure to airborne pollutants, cough, sputum, wheezing, shortness of breath, tuberculosis test and results, date of last chest X-ray examination.
- *Breasts and axillae:* rashes, lumps, discharge, pain, breast self-examination practices.
- *Lymphatic:* pain, swelling.
- *Cardiovascular:* chest pain or distress, precipitating causes, timing and duration, relieving factors, dyspnea, orthopnea, edema, hypertension, exercise tolerance, circulatory problems, varicose veins.
- *Gastrointestinal:* appetite, digestion, food intolerance, dysphagia, heartburn, abdominal pain, nausea or vomiting, bowel regularity, use of laxatives, change in stool colour or contents, constipation or diarrhea, flatulence, hemorrhoids, rectal examinations.
  a. Dietary pattern: calculate number of servings per day of each of the food groups, using *Canada's Food Guide to Healthy Eating* (http://www.nms.on.ca/Elementary/canada.htm) for serving size (see Chapter 43); restrictions to food choice; special diets; use of salt; calculate adequacy of fluid intake (should be 30 to 40 mL of fluid per kilogram of body weight); indicate sources of calcium and

Continued

➤ **BOX 13-1** **Guidelines for a Comprehensive Nursing Health History** *continued*

amounts per day, alcohol use (average number of ounces per week, recent changes in pattern of consumption).
- *Urinary:* painful urination; blood, stones, or pus in urine; bladder or kidney infections; difficulty stopping urinary stream; dribbling or hesitancy; sudden feeling of need to urinate; frequent urination; nocturia (having to get up to void during the night); incontinence (see Chapter 44).
- *Genital and reproductive:*
  a. Male: puberty onset, difficulty with erections, emissions, testicular pain, libido, infertility, urethral discharge, genital lesions, exposure to and history of sexually transmitted infections, testicular self-examinations, testicular lump or pain, hernias, sexual preference, birth control method, and safer sex practices used.
  b. Female: menses (onset, duration, regularity, flow, discomfort, date of most recent menstrual period), age at menopause (occurrence of hot flashes, night sweats, vaginal discharge), date of last Pap smear, pregnancies (number, miscarriages, abortions), exposure to and history of sexually transmitted infections, sexual preference, birth control method, and safer sex practices used.

- *Musculoskeletal:* pain, joint stiffness or swelling, restricted motion, muscle wasting, weakness, general mobility.
- *Neurological:* injury, headaches, dizziness, fainting, abnormalities of sensation or coordination, tremors, seizures.
- *Endocrine:* excessive sweating, thirst, hunger, or urination; intolerance of heat or cold; changes in distribution of facial hair; thyroid enlargement or tenderness; unexplained weight change; change in glove or shoe size.
- *Hematological:* anemia; bruise or bleed easily; transfusions.
- *Psychiatric:* depression, mood changes, difficulty concentrating, nervousness, anxiety, suicidal thoughts, irritability.
- *Immunological:* communicable diseases (indicate disease and age at or year of onset), immunization status (indicate year of most recent immunization), allergies (known allergens and reactions; MedicAlert identification worn).

Adapted from Skillen, D. L., & Day, R. A. (2004). *A syllabus for adult health assessment.* Edmonton, AB: University of Alberta, Faculty of Nursing.

solutions. To do this well, you critically anticipate patterns, problems, and solutions, which means you try to stay a step ahead of the assessment. Before you make an inference, remember to document cues that support the inference. Your inferences will direct you to further questions. Once you ask a question of a client or make an observation, the information "branches" to an additional series of questions or observations (Figure 13–3). If you do not anticipate assessment questions, your assessment may be incomplete, or you may fail to recognize cues and dismiss relevant problem areas. Knowing how to probe and frame questions is a skill that you hone with experience. You learn to decide which questions are relevant to a situation and to interpret the data accurately.

Types of Data

Data can be obtained from two primary sources: subjective and objective. **Subjective data** are your clients' verbal descriptions of their health problems. Only clients provide subjective data. For example, Ms. Devine's report of back pain and her expression of dread over anticipating surgery are subjective findings. Subjective data usually include feelings, perceptions, and self-report of symptoms. Although only clients provide subjective data relevant to their health condition, be aware that the data sometimes reflect physiological changes, which you further explore through objective data collection.

Objective data are observations or measurements of a client's health status. Inspection of the condition of a wound, a description of an observed behaviour, and the measurement of blood pressure are examples of objective data. The measurement of objective data is based on an accepted standard, such as the Fahrenheit or Celsius measure on a thermometer, centimetres on a measuring tape, or known characteristics of behaviours (e.g., anxiety or fear). When you collect objective data, apply critical thinking intellectual standards (e.g., whether the data are clear, precise, and consistent) so that you can correctly interpret your findings.

Sources of Data

As a nurse, you obtain data from a variety of sources. Each source of data provides information about the client's level of wellness, strengths, anticipated prognosis, risk factors, health practices and goals, and patterns of health and illness.

Client. A client is usually your best source of information. Clients who are conscious, alert, and able to answer questions correctly provide the most accurate information about their health care needs, lifestyle patterns, current and past illnesses, perception of symptoms, and changes in activities of daily living. Always consider the setting for your assessment. A client experiencing acute symptoms in an emergency department will not offer as much information as one who comes to an outpatient clinic for a routine checkup. Always be attentive, and show a caring presence with the client (see Chapter 19). Let the client know you are interested in what he or she has to say. Clients are less likely to reveal the nature of their health care problems fully when nurses show little interest or are easily distracted by activities around them.

Family and Significant Others. Family members and significant others are primary sources of information for infants or children, critically ill adults, and mentally handicapped, disoriented, or unconscious clients. In cases of severe illness or emergency situations, families are sometimes the only available sources of information for nurses and clients' health care professionals. The family and significant others are also important secondary sources of information. They confirm findings that a client provides (e.g., whether a client takes medications regularly at home or how well the client sleeps or eats). Include interviewing the family when appropriate. Remember also that a client does not always wish you to question the family.

Spouses or close friends often sit in during an assessment and provide their view of the client's health problems or needs. They not only supply information about the client's current health status but also are able to tell when changes in the client's status occurred. Family members are often very well informed because of their experiences living with the client and observing how health problems affect daily living activities. Family and friends make important observations about the client's needs that can affect the way care is delivered (e.g., how a client eats a meal or how a client makes choices).

Health Care Team. You frequently communicate with other health care team members in gathering information about clients. In the acute care setting, the change-of-shift report is the way for nurses from one shift to communicate information to nurses on the next

Client Data	Branching Questions	Client Patterns
Facial grimacing	Are you having pain?	Pain (Acute or Chronic?)
Client acknowledges "yes"	Tell me how long it has been bothering you.	Acute pain can affect client's normal lifestyle
Client reports 2 months' duration	Show me where the pain is located.	
Client moves hand to lower back	Are you able to bend over?	Mobility problem?
Client has limited range of motion in back	Take a few steps across the room so I can see you walk.	
Client walks with slow, exaggerated gait	What do you do to relieve the pain at home?	
Client uses ice and ibuprofen	Do the ice and medication help?	Health care management?
Treatments do not eliminate pain	Have you missed work because of the pain?	
Client has missed several days over last 2 months	What is it that you do at work that is affected by your pain?	Employment?
Client works in business office; cannot sit for long periods		

Figure 13-3 Example of branching logic for selecting assessment questions.

shift (see Chapter 16). When nurses, physicians, physical therapists, social workers, or other staff consult about a client's condition, they typically have information about the client. This information includes how the client is interacting within the health care environment, the client's physical or emotional reactions to treatment, the result of diagnostic procedures or therapies, and how the client responds to visitors. Every member of the team is a source of information for identifying and verifying information about the client.

Medical Records. The medical record is a source of the client's medical history, laboratory and diagnostic test results, current physical findings, and the medical treatment plan. Data in the records offer baseline and ongoing information about the client's response to illness and progress to date. Information in a client's record is confidential. The medical record is a valuable tool for checking the consistency and similarities of personal observations.

Literature. You complete your assessment database by reviewing nursing, medical, and pharmacological literature about a client's illness. This review increases your knowledge about the client's diagnosed problems, expected symptoms, treatment, prognosis, and established standards of therapeutic practice. A knowledgeable nurse obtains relevant, accurate, and complete information for the assessment database.

Nurse's Experience. Benner and Wrubel (1989) noted that through experience, a nurse learns to ask the right questions, choosing only the questions that will elicit the most useful information. A nurse's expertise develops after testing and refining propositions, questions, and principle- or standard-based expectations. For example, after Lisa has cared for Ms. Devine, she has learned some lessons. Lisa will more quickly recognize the behaviour the client showed while in acute pain when she cares for the next client with similar health problems. Lisa will also note how positioning techniques helped Ms. Devine relax and ameliorated her discomfort. Practical experience and the opportunity to make clinical decisions strengthen your critical thinking.

Methods of Data Collection

As a nurse, you use the client interview, nursing health history, physical examination findings, and results of laboratory and diagnostic tests to establish a client's assessment database.

Interview. The first step in establishing a database is to collect subjective information by interviewing the client. An **interview** is an organized conversation with the client. The initial formal interview involves obtaining the client's health history and information about the current illness. During the initial interview, you have the opportunity to do the following:

- Introduce yourself to the client, explain your role, and explain the role of other health care professionals during care.
- Establish a caring therapeutic relationship with the client.
- Obtain insight about the client's concerns and worries.
- Determine the client's goals and expectations of the health care system.
- Obtain cues about which parts of the data collection phase necessitate further in-depth investigation.

You and the client become partners during the interview, rather than your controlling the interview. An interview consists of three phases, similar to that of a therapeutic relationship: orientation, working, and termination.

A successful interview requires preparation. Collect any available information about the client, and then create a favourable environment for the interview. An environment in which the client is comfortable and relaxed helps you conduct a good interview. Some clients interviewed at home prefer that the interview take place in a bedroom, away from other family members, or in the living room, with a spouse present. Remember to let a client decide whether to involve the family. Finally, select a place private enough to allow the client to be comfortable when providing personal information.

Orientation Phase. During the orientation phase of the interview, you introduce yourself, describe your position, and explain the purpose of the interview. Explain to clients why you are collecting data (e.g., for a nursing history or for a focused assessment) and assure them that any information obtained will remain confidential and will be used only by health care professionals who provide their care.

After making Ms. Devine more comfortable, Lisa decides that it is time to get to know her client better. Lisa reviews the interview process and its objectives, confidentiality, and length. "I want to spend some time better understanding your back pain and then what you know about your surgery. If you are comfortable, I would like to spend about 10 minutes discussing this with you. Everything you share will be confidential." Lisa and Ms. Devine agree mutually on the interview time.

LISA: Now, I want to ask you some questions about your health so we can plan your care together. Before we get started, do you have any questions for me?

MS. DEVINE: Yes. I know they plan to remove the disc in my back. It has been hurting so bad. I can't even bend over. Is there a chance I could be paralyzed?

LISA: Tell me what your doctor has explained about surgery.

MS. DEVINE: She has told me that I have a, what was it called, a herniated disc. She said it is pinching nerves in my back. Well, if it pinches nerves, could I not become paralyzed? She did tell me that she has done this procedure many times before.

LISA: A herniated disc is serious. The disc is normally situated between two vertebrae, but in your case it is now pinching on your spinal nerves. That is why you have so much discomfort. Your surgery is aimed at removing pressure on your nerves. I would suggest you talk with your doctor about your concerns before going into surgery.

MS. DEVINE: Okay, that makes me feel a little better. I have some important things going on at my work. My husband and I own our own business. I just want this to be over.

LISA: Tell me more about your pain.

Working Phase. In the working phase of the interview, you gather information about the client's health status. Remember to stay focused, orderly, and unhurried. Use a variety of communication strategies such as active listening, paraphrasing, and summarizing to promote a clear interaction (see Chapter 18). The use of open-ended questions encourages clients to describe their health histories in detail.

During the working phase, obtain a nursing health history by exploring the client's current illness, health history, and expectations of care. The objective for collecting a health history is to identify patterns of health and illness, risk factors for physical and behavioural health problems, changes from normal function, and available resources for adaptation. The initial interview is normally the most extensive. Ongoing interviews, which occur each time you interact with your client, do not need to be as extensive; their purpose is to update the client's status and focus more on changes in previously identified ongoing and new problems. An example of Lisa's interview techniques is as follows:

LISA: Tell me, Ms. Devine, about your back pain. [Open-ended question]

MS. DEVINE: Sometimes it is really sharp, especially when I stand and try to walk.

LISA: On a scale of 0 to 10, with 0 being no pain and 10 being the worst imaginable, how would you rate your pain when it becomes sharp? [Close-ended question]

MS. DEVINE: Oh, it can be bad; I would rate it an 8 or 9.

LISA: Point to where you notice the pain. [Asking for specificity]

MS. DEVINE: [points to her lower sacral area] It hurts here, and I also get a deep burning pain in my right buttock.

LISA: Can you tell me if anything else aggravates the pain?

MS. DEVINE: This morning I sneezed and thought I was going to faint. Then I could feel the pain go down my right leg.

LISA: Does anything else worsen the pain? [Probes for completeness]

MS. DEVINE: Well, just about any way I move tends to make my back hurt.

LISA: Any way? [Clarification]

MS. DEVINE: It hurts when I turn or twist. If I lie flat, it does not bother me.

LISA: In what way has it limited you in your usual activities? [Open-ended question]

MS. DEVINE: Well, I have not been able to work. I went back about a month ago, but I was miserable when I tried to sit down. I could not tolerate the discomfort.

Termination Phase. As in the other phases of the interview, termination requires skill on the part of the interviewer. Give your client a clue that the interview is coming to an end. For example, say, "I want to ask just two more questions" or "We'll be finished in about 2 minutes." This helps the client maintain direct attention without being distracted by wondering when the interview will end. This approach also gives the client an opportunity to ask questions. When concluding an interview, summarize the important points and ask the client whether the summary was accurate. End the interview in a friendly manner, telling the client when you will return to provide care; for example:

"Thank you, Ms. Devine. You have given me a good picture of your back problem and what you have been told about surgery. I think pain control will be a priority before and after your surgery. Because this is your first time in the hospital, I want to be sure I explain whatever you would like to know. I am going to return in about an hour and talk with you about the surgery and what to expect. Can I do anything for you now?"

A skillful interviewer adapts interview strategies on the basis of the client's responses. You successfully gather relevant health data when you are prepared for the interview, and you are able to carry out each interview phase with minimal interruption.

Cultural Considerations in Assessment

As a professional nurse, it is important to conduct any assessment with cultural competence (see Chapter 10). This involves a conscientious understanding of your client's culture so that you can offer better care within differing value systems and act with respect and understanding without imposition of your own attitudes and beliefs (Seidel et al., 2003). Good communication techniques are important when assessing a client whose culture is different from your own. Communication and culture are interrelated in the way feelings are expressed verbally and nonverbally. If you can learn the variations in how people of different cultures communicate, you will probably be able to gather more accurate information from clients. For example, the Spanish and French use firm eye contact when speaking. However, this is considered rude or immodest by certain Asian or Middle Eastern cultures. North Americans often tend to let the eyes wander (Seidel et al., 2003). By using the right approach with eye contact, you show respect for your client, and the client is probably encouraged to share more information.

When you interact to assess any specific client, first know your own cultural self. You need to avoid forming a sense of the client on the basis of prior information about the client's culture. Instead, draw upon your knowledge and then ask questions in a constructive and probing way to allow you to truly understand the client.

Use **open-ended questions** whenever you are not sure what the answer will be and when you want description in the client's own words (Box 13–2). Remember that **closed-ended questions** can all be answered by "yes" or "no" (or a choice of answers that you provide), and limit these to issues in which you do not need additional information from the client.

> **BOX 13-2**   **Examples of Open- and Closed-Ended Questions**

Open-Ended Questions
Tell me how you are feeling.
Your discomfort affects your ability to get around in what way?
Describe how your wife has been helping you.
Give me an example of how you get relief from your pain at home.

Closed-Ended Questions
Do you feel as if the medication is helping you?
Who is the person who helps you at home?
Do you understand why you are having the X-ray examination?
Has the warm compress given you relief from your back pain?
Are you having pain now?
On a scale of 0 to 10, how would you rate your pain?

Nursing Health History

You document a nursing health history during either your initial contact or an early contact with a client. The history is a major component of assessment. Although many health history forms are structured, you learn to use the questions as starting points. A good assessor learns to refine and broaden questions as needed in order to correctly assess the client's unique needs. Time and client priorities determine how complete a history is. Identify patterns of information about a client's health and illness by collecting data about all health dimensions (see Box 13–1). Incorporating data from all dimensions allows you to develop a complete plan of care.

Family History

The purpose of documenting the family history is to obtain data about immediate and blood relatives. The objectives are to determine whether the client is at risk for illnesses of a genetic or familial nature and to identify areas of health promotion and illness prevention (see Chapter 21). The family history also provides information about family structure, interaction, and function that is often useful in planning care (see Chapter 20). For example, a close, supportive family will help a client adjust to an illness or disability, and so you incorporate information from the family into the plan of care. If the client's family is not supportive, however, it is better to not involve family members in care. Stressful family relationships are sometimes a significant barrier when you try to help clients with problems involving loss, self-concept, spiritual health, and personal relationships.

Documentation of History Findings

As you conduct the nursing health history, record your assessment in a clear, concise manner, using appropriate terminology. Standardized forms make it easy to enter data as the client responds to questions. In settings that have computerized documentation, entry of assessment data is very easy. A clear, concise record is necessary for use by other health care professionals (see Chapter 16). Regardless of the model used in a documentation system, you want a thorough database that provides historical and current information about the client's health. This information then becomes the baseline against which you evaluate any future changes.

Physical Examination

A physical examination is an investigation of the body to determine its state of health. A physical examination involves use of the techniques of inspection, palpation, percussion, auscultation, and smell (see

Chapter 32). A complete examination includes measurements of a client's height, weight, and vital signs and a head-to-toe examination of all body systems. By performing actual hands-on physical assessment, you gather valuable objective information that helps in forming accurate diagnostic conclusions. Always conduct an examination with sensitivity and competence to prevent your client from becoming anxious.

Observation of Client Behaviour. Throughout an interview and physical examination, it is important for you to observe a client's verbal and nonverbal behaviours closely. The information enhances your objective database. You learn to determine whether data obtained by observation matches what the client verbally communicates. For example, if a client expresses no concern about an upcoming diagnostic test but shows poor eye contact, shakiness, and restlessness, all suggestive of anxiety, then verbal and nonverbal data conflict. Observations direct you to gather additional objective information to form accurate conclusions about the client's condition. An important aspect of observation includes a client's level of function: the physical, developmental, psychological, and social aspects of everyday living. Observation of the level of function differs from observations you make during an interview. Observation of level of function involves watching what a client does, such as eating or making a decision about preparing a medication, rather than what the client tells you he or she can do. Observation of function can occur in the home or in a health care setting during a return visit.

Diagnostic and Laboratory Data. The results of diagnostic and laboratory tests reveal or clarify alterations questioned or identified during the nursing health history and physical examination. For example, during the history documentation, the client reports having a bad cold for 6 days and at present has a productive cough with brown sputum and mild shortness of breath. On physical examination, you notice an elevated temperature, increased respirations, and decreased breath sounds in the right lower lobe. You review the results of a complete blood cell count and note that the white blood cell count is elevated (indicating an infection). In addition, the radiologist's report of a chest X-ray examination shows the presence of a right lower lobe infiltrate. Such findings combined are suggestive of the medical diagnosis of pneumonia and the associated nursing diagnosis of *impaired gas exchange*.

Some clients collect and monitor laboratory data in the home. For example, clients with diabetes mellitus often perform daily blood glucose monitoring. Ask clients about their routine results to determine their responses to illness and elicit information about the effects of treatment measures. Compare laboratory data with the established norms for a particular test result, age group, and gender.

Interpreting Assessment Data and Making Nursing Judgements. The successful analysis and interpretation of assessment data requires critical thinking. When you correctly analyze data, you recognize patterns that lead you to make necessary clinical decisions about your client's care. These decisions are in the form of either nursing diagnoses or collaborative problems that require treatment from several disciplines (Carpenito-Moyet, 2005). When you critically think about interpreting assessment information, you determine the presence of abnormal findings, what further observations you need to clarify information, and the client's health problems.

Data Validation. Before you begin analyzing and interpreting data, validate the collected information you have, in order to avoid making incorrect inferences (Carpenito-Moyet, 2005). **Validation** of assessment data is the comparison of data with another source to determine data accuracy. For example, you observe a client crying and logically infer it is related to hospitalization or a medical diagnosis. Making such an initial inference is not wrong, but problems result if you do not validate the inference with the client. Instead, say, "I notice that you have been crying. Can you tell me about it?" By questioning the client, you will discover the real reason for the crying behaviour. Ask your client to validate the information obtained during the interview and history. Validate findings from the physical examination and observation of client behaviour by comparing data in the medical record and by consulting with other nurses or health care team members. Often family or friends are able to validate your assessment information. Validation opens the door for gathering more assessment data because it involves clarifying vague or unclear data. On occasion, you need to reassess previously covered areas of the nursing history or gather further physical examination data. Continually analyze and think about a client's database to make concise, accurate, and meaningful interpretations. Critical thinking applied to assessment enables you to fully understand the client's problems, to judge the extent of the problems carefully, and to discover possible relationships between the problems.

Lisa gathered initial data about the character of Ms. Devine's back pain. She applied critical thinking in her assessment as she considered what she knew about ruptured lumbar discs and the anticipated type of symptoms that clients experience. As she assessed Ms. Devine, she applied intellectual standards, obtaining information that was precise (location of pain), consistent and accurate (use of pain rating scale), and complete (probing for factors that worsen pain). Lisa learned additional information about Ms. Devine's concerns about surgery. Ms. Devine tells Lisa, "I hope the surgery goes well. You know, I have a friend who had back surgery, and she took a long time to recover. I want to get back to work without a long absence. If this had just not happened—why did I have to fall?" Lisa could make several inferences from this information, but she applies the critical thinking attitude of discipline and stays focused to ensure her assessment is accurate and comprehensive. She validates her inferences with Ms. Devine, "You sound anxious about having surgery. You know of others who have had difficult outcomes after surgery. Do you think you are uncertain about what to expect?" Ms. Devine confirms Lisa's assessment, "Yes, I am worried. I have never been in a hospital, as you know, and I feel I do not know what that involves. I am a person who likes to have information, so I can make the right decisions and know what to do."

Analysis and Interpretation. After you collect extensive information about a client, you analyze and interpret the data. You begin analysis by organizing the information into meaningful and usable clusters, keeping in mind your client's response to illness. A data cluster is a set of signs or symptoms that you group together in a logical way. During data clustering, organize data and focus attention on client functions for which support or assistance for recovery is needed. **Data analysis** involves recognizing patterns or trends in the clustered data, comparing them with standards, and then establishing a reasoned conclusion about the client's responses to a health problem (Box 13–3). Patterns of meaning begin to form, enabling you to make inferences about client problems. Through reasoning and judgement, you decide what information explains the client's health status. At times, you need to gather additional information to clarify your interpretation. For example, Ms. Devine told Lisa that she had not been in a hospital and did not know what that involved. Lisa inferred or guessed that Ms. Devine had limited knowledge about the laminectomy and the associated nursing care. Instead of making that conclusion, Lisa sought further information by asking, "Tell me what your doctor has told you about your surgery." Ms. Devine related,

"Well I know the doctor is going to remove something between my vertebrae. She said I will be in the hospital about 2 or 3 days." Lisa asked, "Has anyone talked with you about your care after surgery?" Ms. Devine replied, "No, not really. I have several questions I would like to ask about it." Lisa listened to the additional information provided by Ms. Devine. In looking for patterns of data, Lisa decided that Ms. Devine had a knowledge deficiency because of her limited preparation for the surgery but was interested in learning. If you are successful in clustering data well in your analysis, you will become proficient in identifying individualized nursing diagnoses and in identifying collaborative problems (see Figure 13–6).

During clustering, a cue or an individual sign, symptom, or finding will alert you more than others do. Such cues are especially helpful in identifying nursing diagnoses. In time, you will become experienced in recognizing clusters that indicate problems such as pain, anxiety, or immobility. Clustering also helps make documentation more concise and focused.

Data Documentation

Data documentation is the last part of a complete assessment. The timely, thorough, and accurate documentation of facts is necessary when client data are recorded. If you do not record an assessment finding or problem interpretation, that information is lost and unavailable to anyone else caring for the client. If specific information is lacking, the person reading the report is left with only general impressions. Observation and recording of client status is a legal and professional responsibility. Recording factual information is easy after it becomes a habit. The basic rule is to record all observations. When you record data, pay attention to facts, and make an effort to be as descriptive as possible. Anything heard, seen, felt, or smelled should be reported exactly. Record objective information in accurate terminology (e.g., "weighs 170 lbs," "abdomen is soft and nontender to palpation"). Record subjective information from a client in quotation marks. When entering data, do not generalize or form judgements through written communication. Conclusions about such data become nursing diagnoses and thus must be accurate. As you gain experience and become familiar with clusters and patterns of signs and symptoms, you will conclude the existence of the correct problem. (Review Chapter 16 for details on documentation.)

Concept Mapping. Most of the clients you care for have more than one health problem. A concept map is a visual representation that allows you to graphically show the connections between a client's many health problems. Hinck et al. (2006) showed that concept mapping is an effective learning strategy to understand the relationships that exist between client problems. Your first step in concept mapping is to organize the assessment data you collect for your client. Placing all of the cues together into clusters that form patterns will

---

▶ **BOX 13-3** **Steps of Data Analysis**

1. Recognize a pattern or trend by cues:
   Turns slowly
   Is unable to bend over
   Walks with hesitation
2. Compare with normal standards:
   Has normal range of motion
   Initiates movement without hesitation
3. Make a reasoned conclusion:
   Has limited mobility
   Has reduced activity level

lead you to the next step of the nursing process: nursing diagnosis. Through concept mapping, you obtain a holistic perspective of your client's health care needs, which ultimately leads you to make better clinical decisions (King & Shell, 2002). Figure 13–4 shows the first step in a concept map that Lisa will develop for Ms. Devine as a result of her nursing assessment.

Nursing Diagnosis

After you assess a client thoroughly to compile a database, the next step of the nursing process is to form diagnostic conclusions that determine the nursing care that a client receives (Figure 13–5). Some of the conclusions lead to nursing diagnoses, whereas others do not. Diagnostic conclusions include problems treated primarily by nurses (nursing diagnoses) and problems necessitating treatment by several disciplines (collaborative problems). Together, nursing diagnoses and collaborative problems represent the range of client conditions that necessitate nursing care (Carpenito-Moyet, 2005).

When physicians refer to commonly accepted medical diagnoses, such as myocardial infarction, diabetes mellitus, or osteoarthritis, they all know the meaning of the diagnoses and the standard approaches to treatment. A **medical diagnosis** is the identification of a disease condition on the basis of a specific evaluation of physical signs, symptoms, the client's medical history, and the results of diagnostic tests and procedures. Physicians are licensed to treat diseases or pathological processes described in medical diagnostic statements. Nurses have a similar diagnostic language. **Nursing diagnosis**, the second step of the nursing process, determines health problems within the domain of nursing. The process of diagnosing is the result of your analysis of data and your resultant identification of specific client responses to health care problems. The term *diagnose* means "distinguish" or "know." A nursing diagnosis is a clinical judgement about individual, family, or community responses to actual and potential health problems or life processes that is within the domain of nursing (NANDA International, 2007).

A **collaborative problem** is an actual or potential physiological complication that nurses monitor to detect the onset of changes in a client's status (Carpenito-Moyet, 2005). When collaborative problems develop, nurses intervene in collaboration with personnel from other health care disciplines. Nurses manage collaborative problems such as hemorrhage, infection, and cardiac arrhythmia by using both physician-prescribed and nursing-prescribed interventions to minimize complications. For example, a client who has a surgical wound is at risk for developing an infection, and so a physician prescribes antibiotics. The nurse monitors the client for fever and other signs of infection and implements appropriate wound care measures.

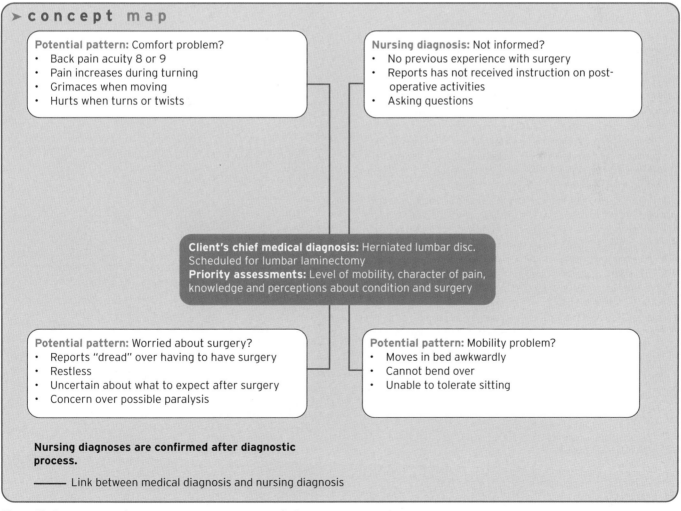

Figure 13-4 Concept map for Ms. Devine's nursing assessment findings.

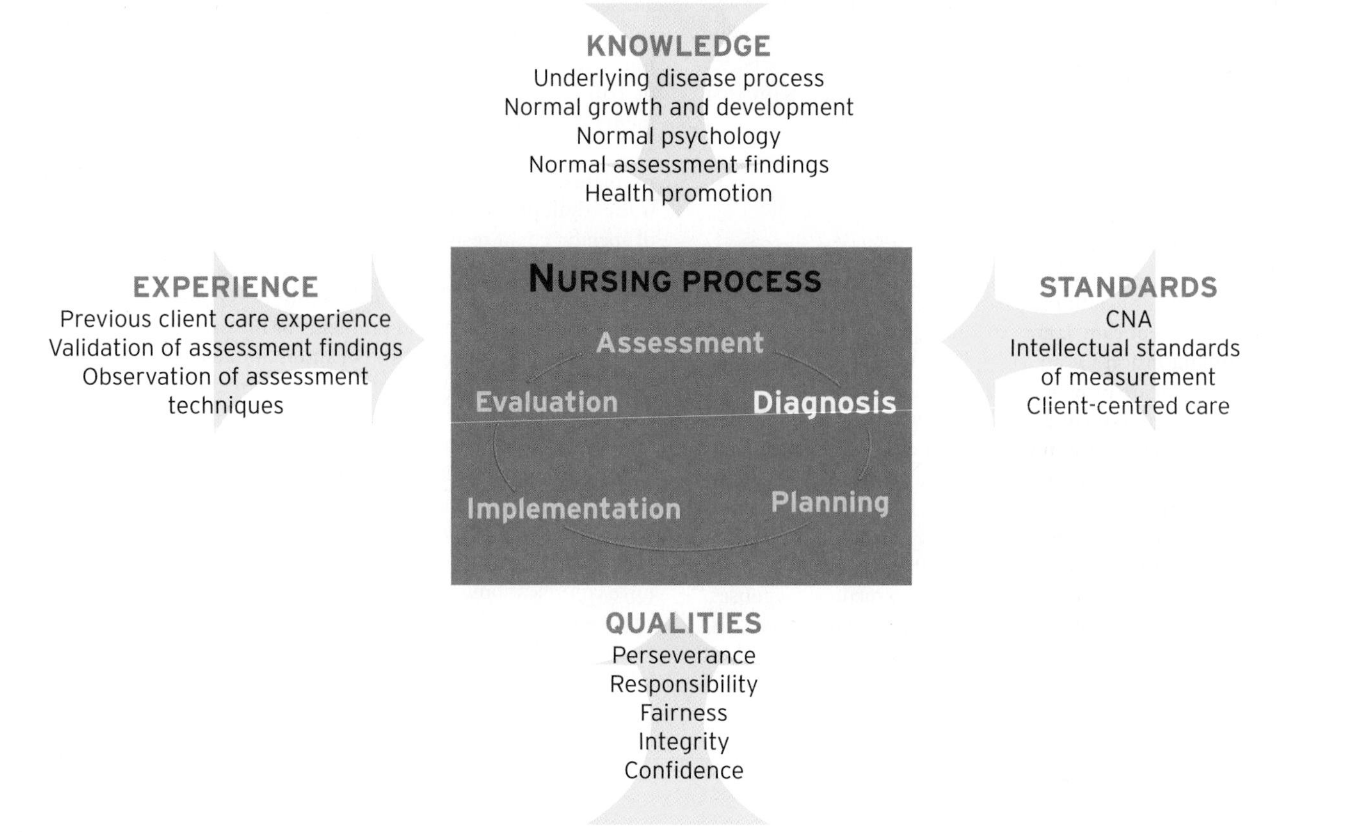

KNOWLEDGE
Underlying disease process
Normal growth and development
Normal psychology
Normal assessment findings
Health promotion

EXPERIENCE
Previous client care experience
Validation of assessment findings
Observation of assessment
techniques

NURSING PROCESS

Assessment

Evaluation | Diagnosis

Implementation | Planning

STANDARDS
CNA
Intellectual standards
of measurement
Client-centred care

QUALITIES
Perseverance
Responsibility
Fairness
Integrity
Confidence

Figure 13-5 Critical thinking and the nursing diagnostic process.

Ms. Devine is scheduled to undergo a lumbar laminectomy for a herniated lumbar disc (her medical diagnosis). Lisa has conducted an assessment of Ms. Devine's health status and needs and has collected information in four different problem areas. Lisa then reviews the clusters and patterns of data she collected to correctly identify the nursing diagnoses that apply to Ms. Devine's situation. One cluster of data includes information about Ms. Devine's inexperience with surgery and her statement that she has not received information about postoperative activities. Lisa decides that the data include defining characteristics for the nursing diagnosis deficient knowledge regarding postoperative routines related to inexperience. Lisa has been assigned to care for the client on the day after surgery. Lisa knows from experience that common postoperative collaborative problems include wound infection and acute urinary retention. Lisa will work closely with the physician and other members of the nursing team in an effort to prevent or minimize these problems. Ms. Devine's health care plan will include a combination of interventions directed to resolve or manage nursing and medical diagnoses and any related collaborative problems.

Nursing diagnoses provide the basis for selection of nursing interventions to achieve outcomes for which you, as a nurse, are accountable (NANDA International, 2007). A nursing diagnosis focuses on a client's actual or potential response to a health problem rather than on the physiological event, complication, or disease. In the case of the diagnosis *deficient knowledge regarding postoperative routines,* Lisa will offer instruction to improve Ms. Devine's knowledge of what to expect after surgery and how she is able to participate in her postoperative care. A nurse cannot independently treat a medical diagnosis such as a herniated

disc. However, Lisa will manage Ms. Devine's postoperative care, monitoring her postoperative progress and managing wound care, fluid administration, and medication therapy to prevent collaborative problems from developing. Collaborative problems occur or probably will occur in association with a specific disease, trauma, or treatment (Carpenito-Moyet, 2005). You will need expert nursing knowledge to assess a client's specific risk for these problems, to identify the problems early, and then to take preventive action (Figure 13–6). Critical thinking is necessary in identifying nursing diagnoses and collaborative problems so that you individualize care appropriately for your clients.

Nursing diagnosis is recognized in Canada and the United States as an innovative means of translating nursing observations and assessments into standard conclusions in a common nomenclature. Although nursing diagnosis is part of basic nursing preparation in Canada, it has not yet been incorporated into provincial and territorial nursing practice standards or legislation. The exceptions are in Ontario and Saskatchewan, where practice standards require the formulation and documentation of nursing diagnoses. However, the Canadian Nurses Association (2008) described the competencies required of registered nurses in the area of assessment and diagnosis in the following statements taken from the list of competencies required of nurses for professional practice:

The registered nurse:

• Uses data collection techniques pertinent to the person and the situation (e.g., community assessment, selected screening tests, risk assessment scales, measuring and monitoring).
• Identifies determinants of health that are pertinent to the person and the situation (e.g., income, social status, education, employment, work conditions).

- Identifies actual or potential health problems/risk factors (e.g., hypertension, diabetes, obesity).
- Identifies actual or potential safety risks to the person (e.g., incidents and accidents, environmental pollution, mechanical equipment).
- Identifies actual or potential risks of abuse (e.g., domestic violence, elder abuse, bullying).
- Uses a holistic approach in collecting relevant data (e.g., biological, psychological, sociological, cultural, spiritual).
- Collects data from a range of appropriate sources (e.g., the person, previous and current health records/nursing care plans/collaborative plans of care, family members/significant persons/substitute decision maker, census data, and epidemiological data, other health care providers).
- Uses appropriate assessment techniques for data collection (e.g., observation, inspection, auscultation, palpation, percussion, selected screening tests, interview, consultation, focus group, measuring and monitoring).
- Assesses psychological and psychosocial adaptation (e.g., recognizes depression and uses resources to assess depression).
- Individualizes the assessment to the person (e.g., growth and development stage, culture, physical and mental challenges).
- Validates data collected with the person and appropriate sources.
- Analyses data to establish relationships among the various data collected (e.g., determines relationship between health assessment and laboratory values).
- Integrates nursing knowledge with knowledge from the arts, humanities, and medical and social sciences to interpret data.
- Identifies actual and potential health problems or issues.

It is clear from these statements regarding nursing competencies that nursing diagnosis is intrinsic to professional practice in Canada. The use of standard formal nursing diagnostic statements (Box 13–4) serves several purposes:

1. They provide a precise definition that gives all members of the health care team a common language for understanding the client's needs.
2. They allow nurses to communicate their actions among themselves, to other health care professionals, and to the public.
3. They distinguish the nurse's role from that of the physician or other health care professionals.
4. They help nurses focus on the scope of nursing practice.
5. They foster the development of nursing knowledge.

Critical Thinking and the Nursing Diagnostic Process

Diagnostic reasoning is a process of using assessment data about a client to logically explain a clinical judgement: in this case, a nursing diagnosis. The diagnostic process flows from the assessment process and includes decision-making steps. These steps include data clustering, identifying client needs, and formulating the diagnosis or problem.

Clusters and patterns of data often contain **defining characteristics**, the clinical criteria or assessment findings that help confirm an actual nursing diagnosis. **Clinical criteria** are objective or subjective signs and symptoms, clusters of signs and symptoms, or risk factors

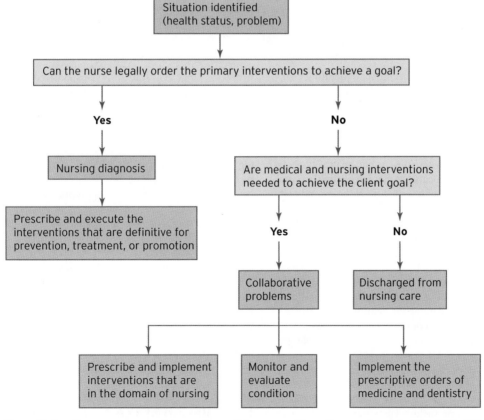

Figure 13-6 Differentiating nursing diagnoses from collaborative problems. **Source:** Copyright 1990, 1988, 1985 by Lynda Juall Carpenito. Redrawn from Carpenito, L. J. (1995). *Nursing diagnosis: Application to clinical practice* (6th ed.). Philadelphia, PA: J. B. Lippincott.

> **BOX 13-4**   **Examples of NANDA International Nursing Diagnoses**

Activity intolerance

Risk for *activity* intolerance

Ineffective *airway* clearance

Latex *allergy* response

Risk for latex *allergy* response

Anxiety

Death *anxiety*

Risk for *aspiration*

Risk for impaired parent–child *attachment*

Autonomic dysreflexia

Risk for *autonomic* dysreflexia

Risk-prone health *behaviour*

Disturbed *body* image

Risk for imbalanced *body* temperature

Bowel incontinence

Effective *breastfeeding*

Ineffective *breastfeeding*

Interrupted *breastfeeding*

Ineffective *breathing* pattern

Decreased *cardiac* output

Caregiver role strain

Risk for *caregiver* role strain

Readiness for enhanced *comfort*

Impaired verbal *communication*

Readiness for enhanced *communication*

Decisional *conflict*

Parental role *conflict*

Acute *confusion*

Chronic *confusion*

Risk for acute *confusion*

Constipation

Perceived *constipation*

Risk for *constipation*

Contamination

Risk for *contamination*

Compromised family *coping*

Defensive *coping*

Disabled family *coping*

Ineffective *coping*

Ineffective community *coping*

Readiness for enhanced *coping*

Readiness for enhanced community *coping*

Readiness for enhanced family *coping*

Risk for sudden infant *death* syndrome

Readiness for enhanced *decision making*

Ineffective *denial*

Impaired *dentition*

Risk for delayed *development*

Diarrhea

Risk for compromised human *dignity*

Moral *distress*

Risk for *disuse* syndrome

Deficient *diversional* activity

Disturbed *energy* field

Impaired *environmental* interpretation syndrome

Adult *failure* to thrive

Risk for *falls*

Dysfunctional *family* processes: alcoholism

Interrupted *family* processes

From NANDA International. (2007). *NANDA-I nursing diagnoses: Definitions and classification, 2007–2008*. Philadelphia, PA: Author. Reprinted with permission.

that lead to a diagnostic conclusion. A specific set of defining characteristics helps confirm identification of each **NANDA International**–approved nursing diagnosis (NANDA International, 2007). As a nurse, you learn to recognize patterns of defining characteristics and then readily select the corresponding diagnosis.

Table 13–1 shows two examples of approved nursing diagnoses and their associated defining characteristics. As you analyze clusters of data, begin to consider various diagnoses that might apply to your client. For example, the diagnoses of *impaired gas exchange* and *ineffective breathing pattern* have similar defining characteristics, including dyspnea, abnormal respiratory rate, and abnormal depth of breathing. When you determine a diagnosis, however, remember that the absence of certain defining characteristics suggests that you reject a diagnosis under consideration. Thus, in the same example, if a client uses accessory muscles to breathe and demonstrates pursed-lip breathing, the correct diagnosis is not *impaired gas exchange* but *ineffective breathing pattern*. Always examine the defining characteristics in your database carefully to confirm or eliminate a nursing diagnosis. To be more accurate, review all characteristics, eliminate irrelevant ones, and confirm the relevant ones.

While focusing on patterns of defining characteristics, you also compare a client's pattern of data with data that are consistent with normal, healthy patterns. Use accepted norms as the basis for comparison and judgement. These norms include laboratory and diagnostic test values, professional standards, and normal anatomical or physiological limits. When comparing patterns, judge whether the grouped signs and symptoms are normal for the client and whether they are within the range of healthy responses. Isolate any defining characteristics not within healthy norms in order to identify a problem.

Before finalizing a nursing diagnosis, review the client's general health care needs or problems. Identifying client needs allows you to individualize nursing diagnoses by considering all assessment data and focusing on the more relevant data. For example, after reviewing clusters of data from Ms. Devine's assessment, Lisa was able to recognize that the client had a knowledge deficiency. However, before Lisa was able to provide appropriate care, it was necessary to define Ms. Devine's problem more specifically. NANDA International (2007) has two nursing diagnoses that apply to knowledge: *deficient knowledge* and *readiness for enhanced knowledge*. A careful review of Ms. Devine's presenting behaviours and self-report of the problem led to the selection of *deficient knowledge* because the client had no previous knowledge of postoperative activities. Her problem was not a need for knowledge reinforcement but the absence of knowledge. It is crucial to select the correct diagnostic label for a client's need. Usually from assessment to diagnosis, the information that you gather progresses from general to specific. It helps to think of the problem identification phase in terms of the general health care problem and to think of the formulation of the nursing diagnosis in terms of the specific health problem.

Formulation of the Nursing Diagnosis

NANDA International (2007) identified four types of nursing diagnoses: actual diagnoses, risk diagnoses, health promotion diagnoses, and wellness diagnoses. An **actual nursing diagnosis**

> **TABLE 13-1**   Examples of NANDA International-Approved Nursing Diagnoses With Defining Characteristics

Diagnosis: Impaired Gas Exchange	**Diagnosis: Ineffective Breathing Pattern**
Defining Characteristics	
Dyspnea	Dyspnea
Abnormal rate, rhythm, depth of breathing	Bradypnea: in clients aged 14 years and older, ≤11 respirations/minute
Abnormal arterial pH	Decreased vital capacity
Abnormal skin colour (pale, dusky)	Orthopnea
Hypoxemia	Altered chest excursion
Hypercarbia	Use of accessory muscles to breathe
Hypoxia	Tachypnea: in clients aged 14 years and older, >24 respirations/minute
Confusion	Pursed-lip breathing
Related Factors	
Ventilation perfusion imbalance	Hyperventilation
Alveolar–capillary membrane changes	Pain
	Chest wall deformity
	Anxiety
	Musculoskeletal impairment
	Body position

Data from NANDA International. (2007). *NANDA-I nursing diagnoses: Definitions and classification, 2007–2008.* Philadelphia, PA: Author.

describes responses to health conditions or life processes that exist in an individual, family, or community. Defining characteristics (manifestations, signs, and symptoms) that cluster in patterns of related cues or inferences support this diagnostic judgement (NANDA International, 2007). The selection of an actual diagnosis indicates that sufficient assessment data are available to establish the nursing diagnosis. In the case of Ms. Devine, Lisa assessed the client to have back pain with a severity rated from 8 to 9 on a 10-point scale. The pain increased with movement. As a result of the pain, Ms. Devine has slept poorly. *Acute pain* is an actual nursing diagnosis.

A **risk nursing diagnosis** describes human responses to health conditions or life processes that will possibly develop in a vulnerable individual, family, or community (NANDA International, 2007). For example, after Ms. Devine undergoes the laminectomy, she has a surgical incision. The hospital environment poses a risk for infection. Thus, after Ms. Devine's surgery, Lisa chooses the nursing diagnosis *risk for infection.* The key assessment for this type of diagnosis is the presence of data that reveal risk factors (incision and hospital environment) that confirm Ms. Devine's vulnerability. Such data include physiological, psychosocial, familial, lifestyle, and environmental factors that increase the client's vulnerability to, or likelihood of developing, the condition.

A **health-promotion nursing diagnosis** is a clinical judgement of a person's, family's, or community's motivation and desire to increase well-being and actualize human health potential, as expressed in their readiness to enhance specific health behaviours, such as nutrition and exercise. Health-promotion diagnoses can be used in any health state; they do not reflect current levels of wellness (NANDA International, 2007).

A **wellness nursing diagnosis** describes levels of wellness in an individual, family, or community that can be enhanced (NANDA International, 2007). It is a clinical judgement about an individual, group, or community in transition from a specific level of wellness to a higher level of wellness. You select this type of diagnosis when the client wishes to or has achieved an optimal level of health. For example, *readiness for enhanced coping related to successful cancer treatment* is a wellness diagnosis, and the nurse and the family unit work together to adapt to the stressors associated with cancer

survivorship. In doing so, the nurse incorporates the client's strengths and resources into a plan of care, with the outcome directed at improving the level of coping.

Components of a Nursing Diagnosis

The nursing diagnosis results from the assessment and diagnostic process. Throughout this text, nursing diagnoses are in a two-part format: the diagnostic label followed by a statement of a related factor (Table 13–2). It is this two-part format that provides a diagnosis meaning and relevance for a particular client. In addition, all NANDA International–approved diagnoses have a definition. Risk factors are a component of all risk nursing diagnoses.

Diagnostic Label. The **diagnostic label** is the name of the nursing diagnosis as approved by NANDA International (2007) (see Table 13–1). It describes the essence of a client's response to health conditions in as few words as possible. Diagnostic labels include

> **TABLE 13-2**   NANDA International (2007) Nursing Diagnosis Format

Diagnostic Statement	Related Factors
Acute pain	Biological, chemical, physical, or psychological injury agents (e.g., inflammation, edema, burn)
Anxiety	Stress
	Unmet needs
	Interpersonal transmission
	Situational or maturational crises
	Fluid retention
	Impaired skin integrity
	Excessive secretions
	Immobilizations
	Altered circulation

descriptors used to give additional meaning to the diagnosis. For example, the diagnosis *impaired physical mobility* includes the descriptor *impaired* to describe the nature or change in mobility that best describes the client's response. Examples of other descriptors are *compromised, decreased, deficient, delayed, effective, imbalanced, impaired,* and *increased.*

Related Factors. The **related factor** is a condition or **etiology** identified from the client's assessment data. It is associated with the client's actual or potential response to the health problem and can be changed through the use of nursing interventions. For example, in the case of Ms. Devine, Lisa assessed that Ms. Devine had not received instruction on postoperative activities and that Ms. Devine was asking questions. Lisa also learned that Ms. Devine had not undergone surgery before. The nursing diagnostic statement for Ms. Devine will include the diagnostic label (e.g., *deficient knowledge regarding postoperative routines*) and the related factor (e.g., *related to lack of exposure to instruction*) (Figure 13–7). Because of the related factor *lack of exposure to instruction,* Lisa will implement client instruction on postoperative activities. The "related to" phrase is not a cause-and-effect statement; rather, it indicates that the etiology contributes to or is associated with the client's diagnosis (Figure 13–8). The inclusion of the "related to" phrase requires you to use critical thinking skills to individualize the nursing diagnosis and then select nursing interventions (Table 13–3). The origin or cause of the nursing diagnosis is always within the domain of nursing practice and a condition that responds to nursing interventions.

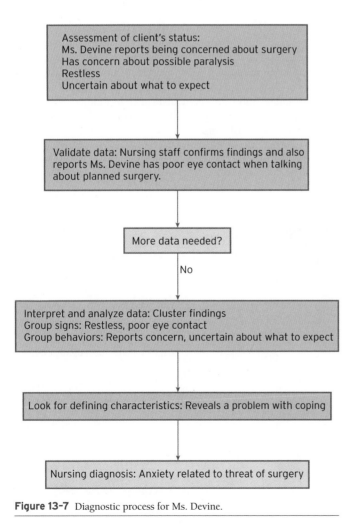

Figure 13-7 Diagnostic process for Ms. Devine.

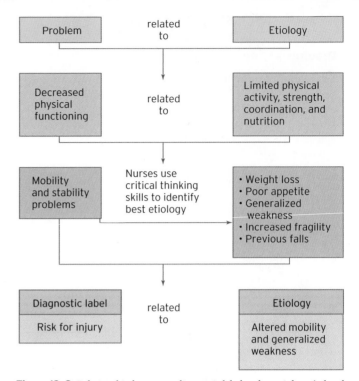

Figure 13-8 Relationship between a diagnostic label and an etiology (related factor). **Source:** Redrawn from Hickey, P. (1990). *Nursing process handbook.* St. Louis, MO: Mosby.

Sometimes health care professionals record medical diagnoses as the etiology in the nursing diagnosis. This is incorrect. Nursing interventions do not change a medical diagnosis. However, you direct nursing interventions at behaviours or conditions that you are able to treat or manage. For example, the nursing diagnosis *acute pain related to herniated disc* is incorrect; nursing actions do not affect the medical diagnosis of a herniated disc. Instead, a diagnosis of *acute pain related to pressure on spinal nerves* results in nursing interventions directed at reducing stress on the vertebrae, improving body alignment, and offering nonpharmacological comfort measures.

Table 13–4 demonstrates the association between a nurse's assessment of a client, the clustering of defining characteristics, and formulation of nursing diagnoses. The diagnostic process results in the formation of a total diagnostic label that enables a nurse to develop an appropriate, **client-centred plan of care.** The defining characteristics and relevant etiologies are from NANDA International (2007).

Definition. NANDA International (2007) approved a definition for each diagnosis that follows clinical use and testing. The definition describes the characteristics of the human response identified. For example, the definition of the diagnostic label *impaired physical mobility* is the "limitation in independent, purposeful physical movement of the body or of one or more extremities" (NANDA International, 2007). You will refer to definitions of nursing diagnoses to assist in identifying a client's correct diagnosis.

Risk Factors. Risk factors are environmental, physiological, psychological, genetic, or chemical elements that increase the vulnerability of an individual, family, or community to an unhealthful event (NANDA International, 2007). They are a component of all risk nursing diagnoses. The risk factors are cues to indicate that a risk nursing diagnosis is applicable to a client's condition. Examples of risk factors for the nursing diagnosis *risk for infection* include

> **TABLE 13-3**   **Comparison of Interventions for Nursing Diagnoses with Different Etiologies**

Nursing Diagnoses	Interventions
Client A	
Anxiety related to uncertainty over surgery	Provide detailed instructions about the surgical procedure, recovery process, and postoperative care activities Plan formal time for client to ask questions
Impaired physical mobility related to acute pain	Administer analgesics 30 minutes before planned exercise Instruct client in technique to splint painful site during activity
Client B	
Anxiety related to loss of job	Consult with social work to arrange for job consulting Encourage client to continue health promotion activities (e.g., exercise, routine social activities)
Impaired physical mobility related to musculoskeletal injury	Have client perform active range-of-motion exercises to affected extremity every 2 hours Instruct client on use of three-point crutch gait

invasive procedures, trauma, malnutrition, immunosuppression, and insufficient knowledge to avoid exposure to pathogens. The risk factors help you select the correct risk diagnosis, similar to the manner in which defining characteristics help you formulate actual nursing diagnoses. In addition, risk factors are valuable when you plan preventive nursing interventions.

Support of the Diagnostic Statement. Nursing assessment data must support the diagnostic label, and the related factors need must be included in these data. To collect complete, relevant, and correct assessment data, it helps to identify assessment activities that produce specific kinds of data. For example, asking the client about the quality and perception of pain elicits subjective data. However, if palpating an area elicits a facial grimace, that grimace is objective information. Likewise, asking a client to describe the perception of an irregular heartbeat elicits subjective information, and using auscultation to obtain a pulse elicits an objective measurement of heart rate and rhythm. When you review assessment data to look for clusters of defining characteristics, consider whether you have probed and assessed the client accurately and thoroughly to gather a complete database.

Concept Mapping for Nursing Diagnoses

When caring for a client or groups of clients, you need to think critically about client needs and how to prevent problems from developing. Your holistic view of a client heightens the challenge of thinking about all client needs and problems. Few clients have single problems. Nurses often care for clients with multiple nursing diagnoses. Therefore, a "picture" of each client usually consists of several interconnections between sets of data all associated with identified client problems (Mueller et al., 2002). Concept mapping is one way to graphically represent the connections between concepts and ideas that are related to a central subject (e.g., the client's health problems).

Hsu and Hsieh (2005) described a concept map as a scheme that displays visual knowledge in the form of a hierarchical graphic network. In a concept map, assessment data are depicted as the relationships of a client's problems to one another (Schuster, 2003). As you proceed in applying each step of the nursing process, your concept map expands with more detail about planned interventions. A concept map promotes critical thinking by causing you to identify,

> **TABLE 13-4**   **Defining Characteristics and Etiologies to Confirm Nursing Diagnoses**

Assessment Activities	Defining Characteristics (Clustering Cues)	Nursing Diagnoses	Etiologies ("Related to")
Ask client to rate severity of pain on a scale from 0 to 10 Observe client's positioning in bed	Client verbally reports pain at a level of 8 or 9 when it becomes sharp Client bends knees while on back to lessen pain	Acute pain	Physical pressure on spinal nerves
Ask whether client has difficulty falling asleep or awakens during night from pain Observe for any nonverbal signs of discomfort	Client reports feeling tired, awakens easily Client moans and sighs when attempting to find comfortable position in bed	Acute pain	Physical pressure on spinal nerves
Observe client's eye contact when client is talking Observe client's body language Ask client to describe feelings about surgery	Client has poor eye contact when discussing surgery Client is restless Client is uncertain about what to expect after surgery and the outcome of surgery	Anxiety	Threat to health status as a result of surgery
Give instruction in topic of interest, and return in 15 minutes to measure retention	Client forgets details of explanation	Anxiety	Threat to health status as a result of surgery

graphically display, and link key concepts by organizing and analyzing information (Hsu & Hsieh, 2005).

Figure 13–9 shows the development of Lisa's concept map for Ms. Devine. Lisa began during the assessment step of the nursing process to gather a database for Ms. Devine. Her assessment included Ms. Devine's perspective of her health problems, as well as the objective and subjective data Lisa collected through observation and examination. Lisa validated findings and added to the database as she learned new information. Data sources include physical, psychological, and sociocultural domains.

Lisa applies clinical reasoning and intuition that reflects her own basic nursing knowledge, her past experiences with clients, patterns that she observed in similar situations, and reference to institutional standards and procedures (e.g., pain management policies or postoperative teaching protocols) (Ferrario, 2004). As Lisa begins to observe patterns of defining characteristics, she places labels to identify the four nursing diagnoses that apply to Ms. Devine. She is also able to see the relationship between the diagnoses and connects them on the care map graphic. If Ms. Devine continues to be anxious, Lisa knows from her experience in caring for clients with pain that Ms. Devine's pain will increase. Likewise, increased pain will heighten anxiety. Anxiety also

influences how well Ms. Devine will attend to any instructions, but until she understands what to expect, her anxiety will not diminish. Ms. Devine's pain, if unrelieved, will likely worsen her immobility.

Concept mapping organizes and links information to allow you to see new wholes and appreciate the complexity of client care (Ferrario, 2004). Lisa's next step on the care map will be to identify the nursing interventions appropriate for Ms. Devine's care.

The advantage of a concept map is its central focus on the client rather than on the client's disease or health alteration. This focus encourages students of nursing to concentrate on clients' specific health concerns and nursing diagnoses (Mueller et al., 2002). It also promotes client participation with the eventual plan of care.

Sources of Diagnostic Errors

Errors occur in the nursing diagnostic process during data collection, interpretation and analysis, clustering, and in statement of the diagnosis. As a nurse, you need to apply methodical critical thinking so that the nursing diagnostic process is accurate.

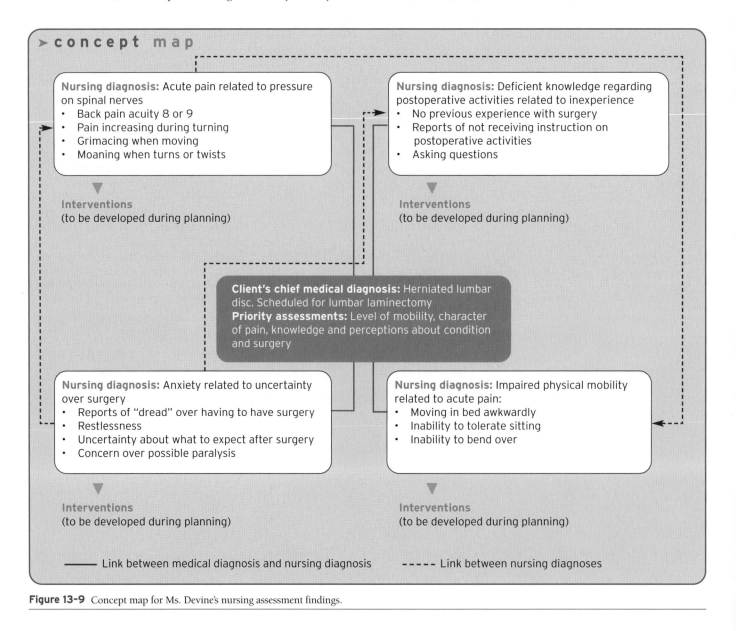

Figure 13-9 Concept map for Ms. Devine's nursing assessment findings.

Errors in Data Collection

To avoid errors in data collection, you should be knowledgeable and skilled in all assessment techniques (Box 13–5). Check for inaccurate or missing data, and collect data in an organized way. The following practice tips are essential to avoid data collection errors:

- Review your level of comfort and competence with interview and physical assessment skills before you begin data collection.
- Approach assessment in steps. Focus on completing a client interview before starting a physical examination. Perhaps focus on only one body system to learn how to gather a complete assessment. Then move to a more complex head-to-toe examination.
- Review your clinical assessments in clinical or classroom settings. They will provide you with a constructive learning opportunity to determine how to revise an assessment or to gather additional information.
- Determine the accuracy of your data. When you auscultate abnormal lung sounds for the first time, be sure of what you hear through the stethoscope. If assessment data are inaccurate, you will misinterpret data from clients, select inappropriate interventions, compromise the quality of care, and possibly endanger the client (Lunney, 1998). To minimize the risk of inaccuracy, have a more experienced coworker validate your findings or explain why they are incorrect.
- Be organized in any examination. Have the appropriate forms and examination equipment ready to use. Be sure the environment is private, quiet, and comfortable for the client.

Errors in Interpretation and Analysis of Data

After data collection, review your database to decide whether it is accurate and complete. Review data to confirm that measurable, objective physical findings support subjective data. For example, when a client reports "difficulty breathing," you should also listen to lung sounds, assess respiratory rate, and measure the client's chest excursion. When you are not able to validate data, the correspondence between clinical cues and the nursing diagnosis is inaccurate (Lunney, 1998). Begin interpretation by identifying and organizing relevant assessment patterns to confirm the presence of client problems. Be careful to consider any conflicting cues or to decide whether cues are insufficient for forming a diagnosis. Also, it is very important to consider a client's cultural background or developmental stage when you interpret the meaning of cues. For example, clients from the Middle East may express pain very differently than do Asian clients. Misinterpreting clients' expressions of pain will easily lead to an inaccurate diagnosis.

Errors in Data Clustering

Errors in data clustering occur when data are clustered prematurely or incorrectly or are not clustered at all. Premature closure of clustering occurs when you make the nursing diagnosis before grouping all data. For example, you learn that a client has had urinary incontinence and complains of urgency and nocturia. You cluster the available data and consider that *impaired urinary elimination* is a probable diagnosis. However, incorrect clustering occurs when you try to make the nursing diagnosis fit the signs and symptoms obtained. In this example, further assessment reveals the client has bladder distension and dribbling, and the condition is probably overflow incontinence. As a result of these findings, you are able to make a more accurate diagnosis: *urinary retention*. Always identify the nursing diagnosis from the data, not the reverse. An incorrect nursing diagnosis affects quality of client care.

> **► BOX 13-5**   **Sources of Diagnostic Error**

Collecting
Lack of knowledge or skill
Inaccurate data
Missing data
Disorganization

Interpreting
Inaccurate interpretation of cues
Failure to consider conflicting cues
Using an insufficient number of cues
Using unreliable or invalid cues
Failure to consider cultural influences or developmental stage

Clustering
Insufficient clustering of cues
Premature or early closure of clustering
Incorrect clustering

Labelling
Wrong diagnostic label selected
Existence of evidence that another diagnosis is more likely
Condition incorrectly overlooked as a collaborative problem
Failure to validate nursing diagnosis with client
Failure to seek guidance

Errors in the Diagnostic Statement

The correct selection of a diagnostic statement is more likely to result in the selection of appropriate nursing interventions and outcomes (Dochterman & Jones, 2003). To reduce errors, word the diagnostic statement in appropriate, concise, and precise language. Use correct terminology reflecting the client's response to the illness or condition. Use of standardized nursing language from NANDA International (2007) helps ensure accuracy. A diagnostic statement such as "unhappy and worried about health" is not a scientifically based diagnosis, and it will lead to errors. The language needs to be more precise and appropriate, such as *ineffective coping related to fear of medical diagnosis*. Also, the problem and etiological portions of the diagnostic statement need to be within the scope of nursing in order to be diagnosed and treated.

Documentation

Once you identify a client's nursing diagnoses, list them on the written plan of care. In the clinical facility, list nursing diagnoses chronologically as you identify them. When you initiate the original care plan, always list the highest priority nursing diagnoses first.

Thereafter, add additional nursing diagnoses to the list. Date a nursing diagnosis at the time of entry. When you care for a client, always review the list and identify the nursing diagnoses with the highest priority, regardless of chronological order.

Nursing Diagnoses: Application to Care Planning

Nursing diagnosis is a mechanism for identifying the nursing care necessary for clients. Diagnoses provide direction for the planning process and the selection of nursing interventions to achieve desired outcomes for clients. Just as the medical diagnosis of diabetes guides a physician to prescribe a low-carbohydrate diet and medication for blood glucose control, the nursing diagnosis of *impaired skin integrity* directs a nurse to apply certain support surfaces to a client's bed and to initiate a turning schedule. In Chapter 14, you learn how unifying the language of NANDA International, along with the Nursing Interventions Classification (NIC), and Nursing Outcomes Classification (NOC), facilitate the process of matching nursing diagnoses with accurate and appropriate interventions and outcomes (Dochterman & Jones, 2003). The care plan is a map for nursing care and demonstrates your accountability for client care. By learning to make accurate nursing diagnoses, your subsequent care plan will assist in communicating to other professionals the client's health care problems and ensure that you select relevant and appropriate nursing interventions.

✳ KEY CONCEPTS

- The nursing process employs critical thinking to identify, diagnose, and treat clients' responses to health and illness.
- Nursing assessment involves the collection and verification of data and the analysis of all data to establish a database about a client's perceived needs, health problems, and responses to those problems.
- By interpreting the meaning of cues, you form an inference, which then enables you to identify meaningful clusters of information.
- To conduct a comprehensive assessment, you use a structured database format or a problem-oriented approach.
- The interview is an organized conversation with a client that begins by establishing a therapeutic relationship with the client and that aids in the investigation and discussion of the client's health care needs.
- Open-ended questions encourage clients to describe their health histories in detail, whereas closed-ended questions present a list of possible choices for the client.
- An interview includes three phases: orientation, working, and termination.
- Once a client provides subjective data, you consider exploring the findings further by collecting objective data.
- During assessment, you critically anticipate and use an appropriate branching set of questions or observations to collect data, and cues of assessment information are clustered to identify emerging patterns and problems.
- Written data statements are descriptive, to the point, and complete and do not include inferences or interpretative statements.
- Family members and friends sometimes offer observations about the client's needs; these observations will affect the way you deliver care.
- During assessment, you encourage clients to describe their histories of illnesses or health care problems.
- To form a nursing judgement, you critically assess a client, validate the data, interpret the information gathered, and look for diagnostic cues that will lead you to identify the client's problems.
- NANDA International has developed a common language that enables all members of the health care team to understand a client's needs.
- The analysis and interpretation of data requires you to validate data, recognize patterns or trends, compare data with healthful standards, and then form diagnostic conclusions.
- The absence of defining characteristics suggests that you reject a proposed diagnosis.
- Three types of nursing diagnoses exist: actual, at risk, and wellness diagnoses.
- A nursing diagnosis is written in a two-part format, including a diagnostic label and an etiological or related factor.

- The "related to" factor of the diagnostic statement assists you in individualizing a client's nursing diagnoses and provides direction for your selection of appropriate interventions.
- Risk factors serve as cues to indicate that a risk nursing diagnosis applies to a client's condition.
- Concept mapping is a visual representation of a client's nursing diagnoses and their relationship with one another.
- Nursing diagnostic errors occur through errors in data collection, in interpretation and analysis of data, in clustering of data, or in the diagnostic statement.
- Nursing diagnoses improve communication between nurses and other health professionals.

✳ CRITICAL THINKING EXERCISES

1. Mrs. Lewis comes to the well-baby clinic for her infant's 1-month examination. She tells her nurse, Ethan, that the baby has not been sleeping well during the night. In addition, Mrs. Lewis has noted a rash on the baby's abdomen. Write three questions that Ethan might ask to assess the two potential problems Mrs. Lewis has presented. What assessment technique might the nurse apply to assess the rash that would not be used to assess the baby's sleep pattern?

2. Mrs. Spezio has a pressure ulcer over the coccyx that is 5 cm in diameter and approximately 1 cm deep. The tissue surrounding the ulcer is inflamed and tender to touch. Mrs. Spezio is transferring from a long-term care facility where she had resided for 6 months after a massive stroke. She is unable to move independently in bed and does not sense pressure or discomfort over her coccyx or hips. In view of this clinical situation, identify the defining characteristics and related factors for the nursing diagnosis *impaired skin integrity*.

✳ REVIEW QUESTIONS

1. The purpose of assessment is to
   1. Make a diagnostic conclusion
   2. Delegate nursing responsibility
   3. Teach the client about his or her health
   4. Establish a database concerning the client

2. Assessment data must be descriptive, concise, and complete. An assessment should *not* include
   1. Subjective data from the client
   2. A detailed physical examination
   3. The use of interpersonal and cognitive skills
   4. Inferences or interpretative statements not supported by data

3. During data clustering, a nurse
   1. Provides documentation of nursing care
   2. Reviews data with other health care professionals
   3. Makes inferences about patterns of information
   4. Organizes cues into patterns that enable the nurse to identify nursing diagnoses

4. You gather the following assessment data. Which of the following cues form a pattern? (Choose all that apply.)
   1. The client is restless.
   2. Fluid intake for 8 hours is 800 mL.
   3. The client complains of feeling short of breath.
   4. The client has drainage from surgical wound.
   5. Respirations are 24 per minute and irregular.
   6. Client reports loss of appetite for more than two weeks.

5. A nursing diagnosis is
   1. The diagnosis and treatment of human responses to health and illness
   2. The advancement of the development, testing, and refinement of a common nursing language
   3. A clinical judgement about individual, family, or community responses to actual and potential health problems or life processes
   4. The identification of a disease condition on the basis of a specific evaluation of physical signs, symptoms, the client's medical history, and the results of diagnostic tests

6. Lisa reviews data that she has collected regarding Ms. Devine's pain symptoms. She compares the defining characteristics for *acute pain* with those for *chronic pain*. In the end, she selects *acute pain* as the correct diagnosis. This is an example of how Lisa avoids an error in
   1. Data collection
   2. Data clustering
   3. Data interpretation
   4. Making a diagnostic statement

7. One of the purposes of the use of standard formal nursing diagnostic statements is to
   1. Evaluate nursing care
   2. Gather information on client data
   3. Help nurses to focus on the role of nursing in client care
   4. Facilitate understanding of client problems among health care professionals

8. The nursing diagnosis *readiness for enhanced communication* is an example of
   1. A risk nursing diagnosis
   2. An actual nursing diagnosis
   3. A potential nursing diagnosis
   4. A wellness nursing diagnosis

9. The nursing diagnosis *hypothermia* is an example of
   1. A risk nursing diagnosis
   2. An actual nursing diagnosis
   3. A potential nursing diagnosis
   4. A wellness nursing diagnosis

10. The word *impaired* in the diagnosis *impaired physical mobility* is an example of a
    1. Descriptor
    2. Risk factor
    3. Related factor
    4. Nursing diagnosis

11. In the following examples, which nurse is acting to avoid a data collection error?
    1. The nurse asks a colleague to chart his or her assessment data.
    2. The nurse considers conflicting cues in deciding the correct nursing diagnosis.

3. The nurse assessing the edema in a client's lower leg is unsure of its severity and asks a coworker to check it with him or her.
    4. After performing an assessment, the nurse critically reviews his or her level of comfort and competence with interview and physical assessment skills.

12. Casey is reviewing a client's list of nursing diagnoses in the medical record. The most recent nursing diagnosis is *diarrhea related to intestinal colitis*. This is an incorrectly stated diagnostic statement, best described as
    1. Identifying the clinical sign instead of an etiology
    2. Identifying a diagnosis on the basis of prejudicial judgement
    3. Identifying the diagnostic study rather than a problem caused by the diagnostic study
    4. Identifying the medical diagnosis instead of the client's response to the diagnosis

13. Which of the following are defining characteristics for the nursing diagnosis *impaired urinary elimination?* (Choose all that apply.)
    1. Nocturia
    2. Frequency
    3. Urine retention
    4. Inadequate urinary output
    5. Treatment with intravenous fluids
    6. Sensation of bladder fullness

✳ RECOMMENDED WEB SITES

Center for Nursing Classification & Clinical Effectiveness: www.nursing.uiowa.edu/excellence/nursing_knowledge/clinical_effectiveness/index.htm
The University of Iowa's Center for Nursing Classification & Clinical Effectiveness was established to facilitate ongoing research of the Nursing Interventions Classification (NIC) and Nursing Outcomes Classification (NOC). This site provides an overview of the NIC and NOC and offers information about new classification material and publications.

NANDA International: http://www.nanda.org/
Through this Web site, NANDA International (formerly the North American Nursing Diagnosis Association) provides current information on nursing diagnosis research, publications, links, and Internet resources.

Registered Nurses Association of Ontario (RNAO): Nursing Best Practices Guidelines: http://www.rnao.org/bestpractices/
The RNAO has developed an extensive process to develop best practices guidelines in a variety of areas of clinical nursing. They have received federal as well as provincial funding for this process, and their work has been made available to all Canadian nurses through this Web site, which lists all current guidelines that have been developed.

14

Planning and Implementing Nursing Care

Original chapter by Patricia A. Potter, RN, MSN, PhD, GMAC, FAAN

Canadian content written by Janet C. Ross-Kerr RN, BScN, MS, PhD, and Marilynn J. Wood, RN, BSN, MPH, DrPH

objectives

Mastery of content in this chapter will enable you to:

- Define the key terms listed.
- Explain the relationship between planning and nursing assessment and diagnosis.
- Discuss the criteria used in priority setting.
- Describe goal setting.
- Discuss the difference between a goal and an expected outcome.
- List the seven guidelines for writing an outcome statement.
- Develop a plan of care from a nursing assessment.
- Discuss the differences between nurse-initiated, physician-initiated, and collaborative interventions.
- Discuss the process of selecting nursing interventions.
- Describe the purposes of a written nursing care plan.
- Describe the elements of a concept map.
- Describe the consultation process.
- Explain the relationship of implementation to the nursing diagnostic process.
- Discuss the differences between protocols and medical directives or standing orders.
- Describe the association between critical thinking and selecting nursing interventions.
- Identify preparatory activities to perform before implementation.
- Discuss steps taken to revise a plan of care before performing implementation.
- Define the three implementation skills.
- Describe and compare direct and indirect nursing interventions.
- Select appropriate interventions for an assigned client.

key terms

Activities of daily living, p. 194
Adverse reaction, p. 195
Client-centred goal, p. 180
Collaborative interventions, p. 183
Consultation, p. 190
Counselling, p. 195
Critical pathways, p. 187
Dependent nursing intervention, p. 183
Direct care, p. 190
Expected outcome, p. 180
Goal, p. 180
Independent nursing interventions, p. 183
Instrumental activities of daily living, p. 195

Kardex, p. 187
Lifesaving measure, p. 195
Long-term goal, p. 180
Medical directive, p. 192
Nursing care plan, p. 187
Nursing intervention, p. 190
Nursing-sensitive client outcome, p. 182
Planning, p. 179
Preventive nursing actions, p. 195
Priority setting, p. 179
Scientific rationale, p. 184
Short-term goal, p. 180
Standing order, p. 192

media resources

evolve Web Site
- Audio Chapter Summaries
- Glossary
- Multiple-Choice Review Questions
- Student Learning Activities
- Weblinks

Companion CD
- Glossary
- Interactive Learning Activities
- Fluids and Electrolytes Tutorial
- Test-Taking Skills

Planning Nursing Care

Lisa is beginning to plan the nursing care for Ms. Devine. In the diagnostic step of the nursing process (see Chapter 13), Lisa identified four nursing diagnoses relevant to Ms. Devine's case: acute pain, anxiety, deficient knowledge, and impaired physical mobility. Lisa is responsible for planning Ms. Devine's care from this morning until the time Ms. Devine leaves for surgery. Lisa will have left work on the unit by the time Ms. Devine returns from surgery, but as her primary nurse, Lisa will provide direction for the staff who assume Ms. Devine's care. Careful planning involves seeing a relationship between a client's problems, recognizing that certain problems take precedence over others, and proceeding with a safe and efficient approach to care. For each of the diagnoses, Lisa identifies the goals and expected outcomes that she and the client hope to achieve. The goals and outcomes direct Lisa in selecting appropriate therapeutic interventions. Ms. Devine is a client who will partner well with Lisa in selecting interventions suited to her own needs, strengths, and limitations. Lisa knows she needs to develop a plan quickly, because Ms. Devine is to go to the operating room by noontime.

After you identify a client's nursing diagnoses and strengths, you begin planning nursing care. **Planning** is a category of nursing behaviour in which a nurse sets client-centred goals, outlines expected outcomes, plans nursing interventions, and selects interventions that will resolve the client's problems and achieve the goals and outcomes. Planning requires critical thinking, applied through deliberate decision making and problem solving. Another aspect of planning is to set priorities for a client. Many clients have multiple diagnoses and a number of health problems. Successful planning requires that you collaborate with the client and family, consult with other members of the health care team, and review related literature. This literature includes available evidence concerning the client's health care problems. A plan of care is dynamic and will change as you meet the client's needs or identify new needs.

Establishing Priorities

Priority setting is the ordering of nursing diagnoses or client problems, through the use of principles such as urgency or importance, to establish a preferential order for nursing actions (Hendry & Walker, 2004; Figure 14–1). By ranking nursing diagnoses in order of importance, you attend to the client's most important needs first. Priorities help you to anticipate and sequence nursing interventions for a client who has multiple nursing diagnoses and health problems. You and your clients select mutually agreed-on priorities on the bases of the urgency of the problems, safety, the nature of the treatment indicated, and the relationship among the diagnoses.

Establishing priorities is not merely a matter of numbering the nursing diagnoses on the basis of severity or physiological importance. Fontana (1993) suggested that nurses establish priorities in relation to importance and time. Nursing diagnoses of conditions that, if untreated, result in harm to the client or others have the highest priorities. For example, *risk for other-directed violence, impaired gas exchange,* and *decreased cardiac output* are typically high-priority nursing diagnoses that raise issues of safety, adequate oxygenation, and adequate circulation. High priorities are sometimes both physiological and psychological and may address other basic human needs. Consider Ms. Devine's case. Among Ms. Devine's nursing diagnoses,

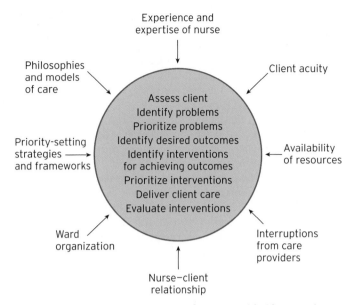

Figure 14-1 A model for priority setting. **Source:** Modified from Hendry, C., & Walker, A. (2004). Priority setting in clinical nursing practice. *Journal of Advanced Nursing, 47,* 427–436.

acute pain and *anxiety* are of the highest priority. Lisa knows that she needs to relieve Ms. Devine's acute pain and lessen the client's anxiety so that the client will approach surgery in less distress.

Intermediate priority nursing diagnoses involve the non-emergency, non–life-threatening needs of the client. In Ms. Devine's case, *deficient knowledge* is an intermediate diagnosis. It is very important that Lisa properly prepare Ms. Devine for surgery. Focused and individualized instruction will help Ms. Devine understand what to expect during her preoperative preparation and how to participate in postoperative care activities. Attending to the diagnosis of *deficient knowledge* will help minimize postoperative complications. Once Lisa addresses the higher priority nursing diagnoses of pain and anxiety, Ms. Devine will probably be more able to learn postoperative care. Also, greater understanding of the surgical procedure may help relieve Ms. Devine's anxiety.

Low-priority nursing diagnoses are not always directly related to a specific illness or prognosis but affect the client's future well-being. Many low-priority diagnoses focus on the client's long-term health care needs. In Ms. Devine's situation, *impaired physical mobility* is caused in part by her pain but also by her medical condition: a herniated disc. Lisa will monitor this diagnosis carefully, especially postoperatively. For now, Lisa will try to make Ms. Devine as comfortable as possible, which may improve Ms. Devine's ability to turn and position herself. After the surgery, Lisa will reassess her client. If *impaired physical mobility* remains a problem, the diagnosis is a higher priority because it is essential for Ms. Devine to achieve more normal mobility for a full recovery and to prevent postoperative complications.

The order of priorities changes as a client's condition changes, sometimes within a matter of minutes. Ongoing client assessment is crucial for determining the status of your client's nursing diagnoses.

In considering time as a factor in setting priorities, White (2003) explained that the planning of nursing care occurs in three phases: initial, ongoing, and discharge. Initial planning involves development of a preliminary plan of care after admission assessment and initial selection of nursing diagnoses. Because of progressively shorter lengths of hospitalization, initial planning is important in addressing nursing diagnoses and collaborative problems in order to hasten problem resolution. Ongoing planning involves continuous updating of the client's plan of care. As the client's condition changes, you assess new information about the client and evaluate the client's status. Discharge planning involves the critical anticipation and preparation for meeting the client's needs after discharge. This is a crucial phase of planning that should begin upon admission or when care begins. It continues throughout the period of care.

Lisa is now involved with the initial planning of Ms. Devine's care. Lisa needs to initiate interventions to manage each of Ms. Devine's nursing diagnoses before surgery. Once Ms. Devine returns from the operating room, Lisa, or another nurse, will conduct ongoing planning by further assessing Ms. Devine's status and then redefining nursing diagnoses that apply postoperatively. As Ms. Devine recovers from surgery, Lisa and her colleagues will work together in developing a discharge plan that will assist Ms. Devine in returning home in as healthy a condition as possible.

Priority setting begins at a holistic level when you identify and prioritize a client's main diagnoses or problems (Hendry & Walker, 2004). However, you also need to prioritize the specific interventions or strategies that you will use to help a client achieve desired goals and outcomes. For example, as Lisa considers the high-priority diagnosis of *acute pain* for Ms. Devine, she decides which intervention, among the interventions of administering an analgesic, repositioning, and teaching relaxation exercises, to perform first. Lisa knows that a certain degree of pain relief is necessary before a client can attend to relaxation exercises. She may decide to turn and reposition Ms. Devine and then give her an analgesic. However, if Ms. Devine is too uncomfortable to turn, Lisa will select administering the analgesic as her first priority. It is important to involve the client in priority setting whenever possible; in some situations, you and your client have different priorities.

Critical Thinking in Establishing Goals and Expected Outcomes

Once you identify a nursing diagnosis, you must identify the best approach to address and resolve the problem. What do you plan to achieve? **Goals** and **expected outcomes** are specific client behaviour or physiological responses that you set to achieve through nursing diagnosis or collaborative problem resolution. They provide a clear focus for the type of interventions necessary to care for your client.

For example, in the case of Ms. Devine, who has a diagnosis of *acute pain related to pressure on spinal nerves*, a goal of care includes "Client achieves improved pain control before surgery." To monitor Ms. Devine's progress, Lisa must use expected outcomes or measurable criteria to evaluate goal achievement. Measurable outcomes for the goal of pain relief include "Client's self-report of pain will be 3 or less on a scale of 0 to 10," and "Client will be able to turn without reported discomfort." The outcomes will reflect Lisa's success in selecting interventions for Ms. Devine's pain relief. After administering an analgesic and repositioning the client a few minutes later, Lisa will return to Ms. Devine's room in 30 minutes and ask the client to rate her pain and to report on her comfort level. If Ms. Devine rates her pain at a 3 or less and similarly reports minimal discomfort when turning, her goals will have been met. Lisa will follow her plan until Ms. Devine goes to the operating room. Goals and expected outcomes serve two purposes: to provide clear direction for the selection and use of nursing interventions and to provide focus for evaluating the effectiveness of the interventions.

Planning nursing care requires critical thinking (Figure 14–2). You need to carefully evaluate the identified nursing diagnoses, the urgency of the problems, and the resources of the client and the health care delivery system. You apply knowledge from the medical, sociobehavioural, and nursing sciences to plan client care. To select goals, expected outcomes, and interventions, you must consider your previous experience with similar client problems, as well as any established standards for clinical problem management. Goals and outcomes need to be relevant to client needs and to be specific, observable, measurable, and time-limited; they must also have the greatest likelihood of success.

For example, in choosing a plan for managing the client's acute pain, Lisa creatively selects a comfort measure that Ms. Devine practises at home. The diagram in Figure 14–3 graphically illustrates the relationships between nursing diagnoses, goals, expected outcomes, and nursing interventions.

Goals of Care

A **client-centred goal** is a specific and measurable behavioural response that reflects a client's highest possible level of wellness and independence in function. Examples are "Client will perform self-care hygiene independently" and "Client will remain free of infection." A goal is realistic and based on client needs and resources. A client-centred goal represents predicted resolution of a diagnosis or problem, evidence of progress toward resolution, progress toward improved health status, or continued maintenance of good health or function (Carpenito-Moyet, 2005). A goal involves only one behaviour or response. The example of "Client will administer a self-injection and demonstrate infection control measures" is incorrect because the statement includes two different behaviours: "administer" and "demonstrate." Instead, the goal should be worded as follows: "Client will administer a self-injection." The specific criteria you use to measure success of the goal are the expected outcomes: for example, "Client will prepare medication dose correctly" and "Client uses medical asepsis when preparing injection site." Each goal is time-limited so that the health care team has a common time frame for problem resolution. The time frame depends on the nature of the problem, etiology, overall condition of the client, and treatment setting.

A **short-term goal** is an objective behaviour or response that you expect a client to achieve in a short time, usually less than a week. In an acute care setting, you set goals for over a course of just a few hours. Such was the case when Lisa set for Ms. Devine the goal "Client's level of comfort will improve before surgery." A **long-term goal** is an objective behaviour or response that you expect a client to achieve over a longer period, usually over several days, weeks, or months: for example, "Client will be tobacco free within 60 days." Goal setting establishes the framework for the nursing care plan. Table 14–1 outlines the progression from nursing diagnoses to goals and expected outcomes, which Lisa individualizes to meet Ms. Devine's needs.

Role of the Client in Goal Setting. It is important to work closely with clients in setting goals. Mutual goal setting is an activity that includes clients and families in prioritizing goals of care and in developing plans for action (Bulechek et al., 2008). Clients need to be able to engage in problem solving and decision making in order to participate effectively in goal-setting. Unless you set goals mutually and make a clear plan for action, clients will not follow the care plan. For example, Lisa and Ms. Devine set the goal "Client will report greater comfort." They agreed that this would be demonstrated by pain acuity rated less than 3 on a scale of 0 to 10, a level that Ms. Devine reports is tolerable for her.

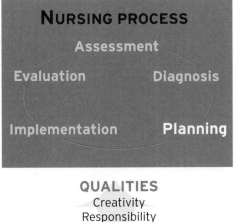

KNOWLEDGE
Client's database and selected nursing diagnoses
Anatomy and physiology
Pathophysiology
Normal growth and development
Evidence-informed nursing interventions
Role of other health care disciplines
Community resources
Family dynamics
Teaching and learning process
Delegation principles
Priority-setting principles

EXPERIENCE
Previous client care experience
Personal experience in
organizing activities

NURSING PROCESS
Assessment
Evaluation   Diagnosis
Implementation   Planning

STANDARDS
CNA
Specialty standards of practice
Client-centred goals and outcomes
Intellectual standards

QUALITIES
Creativity
Responsibility
Perseverance
Discipline

Figure 14-2 Critical thinking and the process of planning care. *CNA*, Canadian Nurses Association.

Expected Outcomes

An expected outcome is a specific measurable change in a client's status that you expect in response to nursing care. Expected outcomes provide a focus or direction for nursing care because they are the desired physiological, psychological, social, developmental, or spiritual responses that indicate resolution of clients' health problems. Derived from both short- and long-term goals, outcomes determine when a specific client-centred goal has been met.

Usually you list several expected outcomes for each nursing diagnosis and goal. The reason for the multiple expected outcomes is that sometimes one nursing action is not enough to resolve a specific problem. In addition, the listing of the step-by-step expected outcomes assists in planning interventions. Write expected outcomes sequentially, specifying time frames for each (see Table 14–1). Time frames provide progressive steps to recovery and assist in ordering nursing interventions. In addition, time frames set limits for problem resolution. In the case of Ms. Devine, Lisa plans to relieve the client's pain enough so that she is able to turn comfortably in bed within the next two hours and to successfully reduce pain severity before surgery.

Write expected outcome statements in measurable terms. This enables you to note the specific behaviour or physiological response expected for resolution of the problem. For example, "Client will have less pain" is an inaccurate outcome statement because the phrase "less pain" is nonspecific. The statement "Client will report pain acuity of less than 3 on a scale of 0 to 10" is accurate.

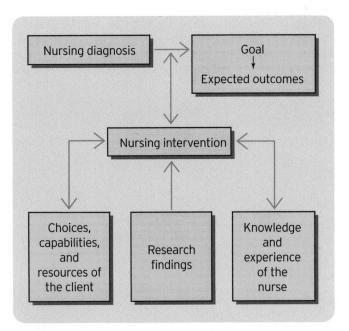

Figure 14-3 From diagnosis to outcome. **Source:** Revised and redrawn from Gordon, M. (1994). *Nursing diagnosis: Process and application* (3rd ed.). St. Louis, MO: Mosby.

> **TABLE 14-1**   **Examples of Goal Setting with Expected Outcomes for Ms. Devine**

Nursing Diagnoses	Goals	Expected Outcomes
Acute pain related to pressure on spinal nerves	Ms. Devine's level of comfort will improve before surgery	Client will be able to turn without reported discomfort in two hours Client's self-report of pain will be 3 or less on a scale of 0 to 10 by the time of scheduled surgery
Anxiety related to uncertainty over surgery	Ms. Devine will accept plan for surgical care before scheduled surgery	Client will express less uneasiness about surgical experience in next four hours
Deficient knowledge regarding postoperative activities related to inexperience	Ms. Devine will understand treatment procedures planned postoperatively within four hours	Client will exhibit less facial tension before scheduled surgery Client will describe purpose of postoperative exercises before scheduled surgery Client will demonstrate use of incentive spirometer and coughing before scheduled surgery Client will explain purpose of postoperative monitoring activities before scheduled surgery
Impaired physical mobility related to acute back pain	Ms. Devine will move independently in bed before surgery	Client will initiate turning without discomfort within 2 hours. Client will position self for care procedures within 2 hours

Nursing Outcomes Classification. The current health care environment pays considerable attention to measuring outcomes sensitive to nursing interventions. Many health care administrators focus on outcomes in determining staffing and other resources in health care settings. The Iowa Intervention Project published the Nursing Outcomes Classification (NOC) and has linked the outcomes to NANDA International (2007) nursing diagnoses (University of Iowa College of Nursing, 2008). The Iowa researchers defined a **nursing-sensitive client outcome** as an individual, family, or community state, behaviour, or perception that is measurable along a continuum in response to a nursing intervention. For any given NANDA International nursing diagnosis, multiple outcomes are suggested in NOC. These outcomes provide descriptions of the focus of nursing care and include indicators for measuring success with interventions (Table 14–2).

Combining Goals and Outcome Statements
Many schools of nursing and health care institutions combine goal and outcome statements. Staff members within health care settings often refer to the terms *goals* and *outcomes* interchangeably. This is acceptable

as long as the criteria for writing goals and outcomes are met. For example, the statement "Client will achieve pain control as evidenced by reporting pain acuity of less than 3 on a scale of 0 to 10 within 24 hours" is an acceptable statement. The goal portion of the statement broadly describes the desired client status ("achieve pain control"), and the outcome portion of the statement contains the observable criterion ("3 on a [pain] scale") needed to measure success.

Guidelines for Writing Goals and Expected Outcomes
There are seven guidelines for writing goals and expected outcomes: client-centred, singular, observable, measurable, time-limited, mutual, and realistic.

Client-Centred Goal or Outcome. Outcomes and goals reflect client responses that are expected after nursing interventions. Write a goal to reflect client behaviour, not to reflect your goals or interventions. A correct outcome statement is "Client will ambulate in the hall three times a day." A common error is to write "Ambulate client in the hall three times a day."

> **TABLE 14-2**   **Examples of NANDA International Nursing Diagnoses and Suggested NOC Linkages**

Nursing Diagnosis	Suggested NOC-Based Outcomes (Examples)	Outcome Indicators (Examples)
Deficient knowledge	Knowledge: treatment procedures	Description of treatment procedure Description of steps in procedure
	Client satisfaction: teaching	Explanations provided in understandable terms Explanation of activity restrictions
Activity intolerance	Activity tolerance	Oxygen saturation with activity Pulse rate with activity Respiratory rate with activity
	Self-care status	Bathes self Dresses self Prepares food and fluid for eating

Source: Moorhead, S., Johnson, M., & Maas, M. (2008). *Nursing Outcomes Classification* (4th ed.). St. Louis, MO: Mosby.
NOC, Nursing Outcomes Classification.

Singular Goal or Outcome. Be precise in evaluating a client response to a nursing action. Each goal and outcome addresses only one behaviour or response.

Observable Goal or Outcome. You need to be able to observe whether change in a client's status occurs. Changes in physiological findings and in the client's knowledge, perceptions, and behaviour are observable. You observe outcomes by directly asking clients about their condition and by using assessment skills. For the outcome "Lungs will be clear on auscultation by 8/31," you auscultate the client's lungs routinely after therapy. The outcome statement "Client will appear less anxious" is not a correct statement because no specific behaviour for "will appear" is observable.

Measurable Goal or Outcome. You will learn to write goals and expected outcomes that set standards against which to measure the client's response to nursing care. Examples such as "Body temperature will remain 98.6°F" and "Apical pulse will remain between 60 and 100 beats per minute" enable you to objectively measure changes in the client's status.

Time-Limited Goal or Outcome. The time frame for each goal and expected outcome indicates when you expect the response to occur. Time frames assist in determining progress toward goals and outcomes.

Mutual Goal or Outcomes. Mutually set goals and expected outcomes ensure that client and nurse agree on the direction and time limits of care. Mutual goal setting increases clients' motivation and cooperation.

Realistic Goal or Outcome. Set goals and expected outcomes that are reachable. This provides clients with a sense of hope that increases motivation and cooperation. In order to establish realistic goals, you need to assess the resources of the health care facility, the family, and the client. You also need to be aware of the client's physiological, emotional, cognitive, and sociocultural potential and the economic cost and resources available to reach expected outcomes in a timely manner.

Types of Interventions

Nursing interventions belong to three categories: nurse-initiated, physician-initiated, and collaborative. Interventions are based on client needs. Some clients require all three categories of interventions, whereas others need only nurse- and physician-initiated interventions.

Nurse-initiated interventions are **independent nursing interventions.** These do not require direction or orders from other health care professionals. As a nurse, you act independently for clients. Nurse-initiated interventions are informed by the best available evidence. Examples include elevating an edematous extremity, instructing clients in side effects of medications, or directing a client to splint an incision during coughing.

Physician-initiated interventions are **dependent nursing interventions,** or actions that require orders or directions from physicians or other health professionals. The interventions are directed toward treating or managing a medical diagnosis. Nurse practitioners working under collaborative agreements with physicians or who are licensed through provincial or territorial nursing legislation are also able to provide such orders or directions for care. As the nurse, you intervene by carrying out these written or verbal orders. Administering a medication and changing a dressing are examples of physician-initiated interventions.

Each physician-initiated intervention requires specific nursing responsibilities that are based on nursing knowledge. For example, when administering medications, you are responsible for knowing the classification of the drug, its physiological action, the normal dosage, side effects, and nursing interventions related to its action or side effects (see Chapter 34).

Interdependent nursing interventions, or **collaborative interventions,** are therapies that require the combined knowledge, skill, and expertise of a number of health care professionals. Typically, when you plan care for a client, you review the necessary interventions and determine whether the collaboration is necessary. An interdisciplinary health care team conference about a client's care is useful in determining interdependent nursing interventions.

In the case study involving Lisa and Ms. Devine, Lisa will initiate independent interventions to help calm Ms. Devine's anxiety and to begin teaching her about postoperative care. In addition, Lisa independently positions Ms. Devine to minimize her discomfort and promote more normal mobility. Among the dependent interventions Lisa plans to implement are administering an analgesic and completing any necessary preoperative diagnostic tests. Lisa decides that consultation with the unit social worker is another way to help Ms. Devine with her anxiety over surgery.

Every nurse faces an inappropriate or incorrect order at some time (Table 14–3). The nurse with a strong knowledge base recognizes and questions errors. The ability to recognize incorrect therapies is particularly important in administering medications or implementing procedures. Errors may occur in writing or transcribing orders. Clarifying an order is competent nursing practice and protects clients from harm. When you carry out an incorrect or inappropriate intervention, you are responsible for an error in judgement and are legally responsible for any complications resulting from the error (see Chapter 9).

Selection of Interventions

Interventions are not selected randomly. Clients with the diagnosis of *anxiety,* for example, may require a variety of interventions. You treat anxiety related to the uncertainty of impending surgery very differently than anxiety related to a possible loss of family role function. When choosing interventions, consider six factors: (1) the nursing diagnosis, (2) goals and expected outcomes, (3) the evidence base (e.g., research or proven practice guidelines), (4) feasibility, (5) acceptability to the client, and (6) your own competence (Bulechek et al., 2008) (Box 14–1). During deliberation, review resources such as the nursing literature, standard protocols or guidelines, the Nursing Interventions Classification (NIC), critical pathways, policy or procedure manuals, and textbooks. As you select interventions, collaborate with other professionals, review your clients' needs and priorities, and review your previous experiences to select interventions that have the best potential for achieving the expected outcomes.

Nursing Interventions Classification

The Iowa Intervention Project (1993) developed a set of nursing interventions that provides a level of standardization, which enhances communication of nursing care across all health care settings and enables health care professionals to compare outcomes (Bulecheck et al., 2008; McCloskey & Bulechek, 2004). The NIC model includes three levels: domains, classes, and interventions for

> **TABLE 14-3**   **Frequent Errors in Writing Nursing Interventions**

Type of Error	Incorrectly Stated Nursing Intervention	Correctly Stated Nursing Intervention
Failure to precisely or completely indicate nursing actions	Turn client every two hours	Turn client every two hours, using the following schedule: 8 A.M.: supine 10 A.M.: left side Noon: prone 2 P.M.: right side (repeat this routine beginning at 4 P.M. and midnight)
Failure to indicate frequency	Perform blood glucose measurements	Measure blood glucose before each meal: 7 A.M., 11 A.M., and 5 P.M.
Failure to indicate quantity	Irrigate wound once a shift: 6 A.M., 11 A.M., and 5 P.M.	Irrigate wound with 100 mL normal saline until clear: 6 A.M., 11 A.M., and 5 P.M.
Failure to indicate method	Change client's dressing once a shift: 6 A.M., 2 P.M., and 10 P.M.	Replace client's dressing with Neosporin ointment to wound and two dry 4×4 dressings secured with hypoallergenic tape, once a shift: 6 A.M., 2 P.M., and 10 P.M.

ease of use. The domains are the highest level (Level 1) of the model, worded in broad terms (e.g., "safety" and "physiological: basic") to organize the more specific classes and interventions (Table 14–4). The second level of the model includes 30 classes, which offer useful clinical categories for reference in selecting interventions. The third level of the model includes the 514 interventions, defined as any treatment based on clinical judgement and knowledge, that a nurse performs to enhance the condition of a client who presents an alteration within the class (Bulechek et al.,

2008) (Box 14–2). Each intervention can be performed with a variety of nursing activities (Box 14–3). Nursing activities are those commonly used in a plan of care. NIC-based interventions are also linked with NANDA International (2007) nursing diagnoses for ease of use. For example, if a client has a nursing diagnosis of *acute pain*, 21 recommended interventions, including pain management, cutaneous stimulation, and anxiety reduction, may be used. A variety of nursing care activities are presented with each of the recommended interventions.

> **BOX 14-1**   **Choosing Nursing Interventions**

Characteristics of the Nursing Diagnosis
Interventions should alter the etiological ("related to") factor or signs and symptoms associated with the diagnostic label.
- When an etiological factor cannot change, direct the interventions toward treating the signs and symptoms (e.g., NANDA International [2007] defining characteristics).
- For potential or high-risk diagnoses, direct interventions at altering or eliminating risk factors for the diagnosis.

Expected Outcomes
Because nurses state outcomes in terms used to evaluate the effect of an intervention, this language assists in selecting the intervention.
NIC is designed to show the link to NOC (University of Iowa College of Nursing, 2008).

Evidence Base
Research evidence in support of a nursing intervention indicates the effectiveness of the intervention in certain types of clients.
- Refer to the evidence (e.g., research articles or evidence-informed practice protocols that describe the use of the evidence in similar clinical situations and settings.
- When research is not available, use scientific principles (e.g., infection control) or consult a clinical expert about your client population.

Feasibility
A specific intervention has the potential for interacting with other interventions.
- Be knowledgeable about the total plan of care.
- Consider cost: Is the intervention clinically effective and cost efficient?
- Consider time: Are time and personnel resources available?

Acceptability to the Client
A treatment plan needs to be acceptable to the client and family and must match the client's goals, health care values, and culture.
- Promote informed choice; help a client know how to participate in and anticipate the effect of interventions.

Capability of the Nurse
The nurse needs to have up-to-date knowledge of the intervention, its scientific basis, and considerations for implementation.
- Be prepared to carry out the intervention.
- Know the **scientific rationale** for the intervention.
- Have the necessary psychosocial and psychomotor skills to complete the intervention.
- Be able to function within the specific setting and to use health care resources effectively and efficiently.

Modified from Dochterman, J. M., & Bulechek, G. M. (2004). *Nursing Interventions Classification (NIC)* (4th ed.). St. Louis, MO: Mosby.

► **TABLE 14-4** **Nursing Interventions Classifications (NIC) Taxonomy**

Domain 1	Domain 2	Domain 3	Domain 4	Domain 5	Domain 6	Domain 7
Level 1 Domains						
1. Physiological: Basic Care that supports physical functioning	2. Physiological: Complex Care that supports homeostatic regulation	3. Behavioural Care that supports psychosocial functioning and facilitates lifestyle changes	4. Safety Care that supports protection against harm	5. Family Care that supports the family	6. Health System Care that supports effective use of the health care delivery system	7. Community Care that supports the health of the community
Level 2 Classes						
A. *Activity and Exercise Management:* Interventions to organize or assist with physical activity and energy conservation and expenditure	G. *Electrolyte and Acid–Base Management:* Interventions to regulate electrolyte/acid–base balance and prevent complications	O. *Behaviour Therapy:* Interventions to reinforce or promote desirable behaviours or alter undesirable behaviours	U. *Crisis Management:* Interventions to provide immediate short-term help in both psychological and physiological crises	W. *Childbearing Care:* Interventions to assist in understanding and coping with the psychological and physiological changes during the childbearing period	Y. *Health System Mediation:* Interventions to facilitate the interface between patient/family and the health care system	c. *Community Health Promotion:* Interventions that promote the health of the whole community
B. *Elimination Management:* Interventions to establish and maintain regular bowel and urinary elimination patterns and manage complications due to altered patterns	H. *Drug Management:* Interventions to facilitate desired effects of pharmacological agents	P. *Cognitive Therapy* Interventions to reinforce or promote desirable cognitive functioning or alter undesirable cognitive functioning	V. *Risk Management:* Interventions to initiate risk-reduction activities and continue monitoring risks over time	Z. *Childrearing Care:* Interventions to assist in rearing children	a. *Health System Management:* Interventions to provide and enhance support services for the delivery of care	d. *Community Risk Management:* Interventions that assist in detecting or preventing health risks to the whole community
C. *Immobility Management:* Interventions to manage restricted body movement and the sequelae	I. *Neurologic Management:* Interventions to optimize neurologic functions	Q. *Communication Enhancement:* Interventions to facilitate delivering and receiving verbal and nonverbal messages		X. *Lifespan Care:* Interventions to facilitate family unit functioning and promote the health and welfare of family members throughout the lifespan	b. *Information Management:* Interventions to facilitate communication among health care providers	

Continued

▶ TABLE 14-4   Nursing Interventions Classifications (NIC) Taxonomy   *continued*

Domain 1	Domain 2	Domain 3	Domain 4	Domain 5	Domain 6	Domain 7
Level 2 Classes						
D. *Nutrition Support:* Interventions to modify or maintain nutritional status	J. *Perioperative Care:* Interventions to provide care before, during, and after surgery	R. *Coping Assistance:* Interventions to assist another to build on own strength, to adapt to a change in function, or to achieve a higher level of function				
E. *Physical Comfort Promotion:* Interventions to promote comfort using physical techniques	K. *Respiratory Management:* Interventions to provide care before, during, and immediately after surgery	S. *Patient Education:* Interventions to facilitate learning				
F. *Self-Care Facilitation:* Interventions to provide or assist with routine activities of daily living	L. *Skin/Wound Management:* Interventions to maintain or restore tissue integrity	T. *Psychological Comfort Promotion:* Interventions to promote comfort using psychological techniques				
	M. *Thermoregulation:* Interventions to maintain body temperature within a normal range					
	N. *Tissue Perfusion Management:* Interventions to optimize circulations of blood and fluids to the tissue					

From Bulechek, G. M., Butcher, H. K., & Dochterman, J. M. (2008). *Nursing Interventions Classification (NIC)* (5th ed.). St. Louis, MO: Mosby.

> **BOX 14-2** **Example of Interventions for Physical Comfort Promotion**

Class: Physical Comfort Promotion
Interventions to promote comfort [by] using physical techniques

Interventions (Examples)
Acupressure
Aromatherapy
Cutaneous stimulation
Environmental management
Heat/cold application
Nausea management
Pain management
Progressive muscle relaxation
Simple massage

Examples of Linked Nursing Diagnoses
Acute pain
Chronic pain

From Dochterman, J. M., & Bulechek, G. M. (2004). *Nursing Interventions Classification (NIC)* (4th ed.). St. Louis, MO: Mosby.

> **BOX 14-3** **Example of Interventions and Associated Nursing Activities**

Class: Physical Comfort Promotion Intervention–Environmental Management

Examples of Activities
Create a safe environment for client
Provide a clean, comfortable bed and environment
Avoid unnecessary exposure, drafts, overheating, or chilling
Provide music of choice
Limit visitors
Manipulate lighting for therapeutic benefit
Bring familiar objects from home
Allow family/significant other to stay with client

From Dochterman, J. M., & Bulechek, G. M. (2004). *Nursing Interventions Classification (NIC)* (4th ed.). St. Louis, MO: Mosby.

Planning Nursing Care

In any health care setting, a nurse is responsible for developing a written plan of care for clients. The plan of care sometimes takes several forms (e.g., a nursing card-filing system, standardized care plans, and computerized plans). In general, a written **nursing care plan** includes nursing diagnoses; goals, expected outcomes, or both; and specific nursing interventions, so that any nurse is able to quickly identify a client's clinical needs and situation. In hospitals and community-based settings, the client often receives care from more than one nurse, physician, or allied health professional. A written nursing care plan makes possible continuity and coordination of nursing care and consultation by a number of health professionals.

Written care plans organize information exchanged by nurses in change-of-shift reports (see Chapter 16). You will learn to focus your reports on the nursing care, treatments, and expected outcomes documented in your care plans, and the end-of-shift report allows for discussion of care plans and the overall progress with the next caregiver. The nursing care plan (Box 14–4) on p. 188 provides an example of a care plan for Ms. Devine.

When developing an individualized care plan, involve the family and client. The family is a resource for helping the client meet health care goals. In addition, meeting some of the family's needs may improve the client's level of wellness.

Institutional Care Plans

Institutional care plans become part of a client's legal medical record. Many hospitals still use a written Kardex nursing care plan. The **Kardex** card-filing system allows quick reference to the needs of the client for certain aspects of nursing care (see Chapter 16). The care plan section of a Kardex system varies by agency and focuses on planned interventions to meet the needs of the client and family and to prepare the client for discharge from the hospital. The focus of a nursing care plan differs by setting and the evolving client situation. For example, nursing care plans developed for clients returning home are usually based solely on long-term health needs. Nursing care plans for same-day surgeries are usually focused on clients' short-term

needs (e.g., immediate recovery from surgery and instructions for self-care at home). In a long-term care facility, plans of care focus on clients' long-term rehabilitation needs.

Computerized Care Plans. A majority of health care facilities now have some type of electronic health record (EHR) and documentation system (Moody et al., 2004). Software programs are available for nursing care plans. In many facilities, the format is for standardized plans that are based on nursing diagnoses or select problem areas, which nurses are able to individualize for a specific client. Even if a standardized care plan is generally appropriate for a client, you need to add or delete information on the standardized form to individualize it for a client's needs. For example, you select a nursing diagnosis and then individualize the standard care plan by making selections from menus. Each care plan lists generalized nursing diagnoses, goals, outcome criteria, and interventions for specific clients. Computerized and standardized nursing care plans organize and enhance care planning. Their design incorporates current evidence-informed practice guidelines to achieve the desired client outcomes for a specific group of clients.

Care Plans for Community-Based Settings. Planning care for clients in community-based settings—for example, clinics, community centres, or clients' homes—involves using the same principles of nursing practice. In these settings, however, you need to complete a more comprehensive community, home, and family assessment. Ultimately, the client or family unit must be able to provide the majority of health care independently.

Critical Pathways. **Critical pathways** are multidisciplinary treatment plans that outline treatments or interventions that clients may require for treatment of a condition. Most pathways are based on medical rather than nursing diagnoses, but they incorporate related nursing diagnoses and associated nursing interventions. A critical pathway maps out, day to day or even hour to hour, the recommended interventions and expected outcomes. For example, a pathway for a surgical procedure such as a bowel resection will recommend on a day-by-day basis the client's activities, procedures, and discharge planning activities. A critical pathway ensures better continuity of care because it clearly maps out the responsibility of each health discipline. Well-developed pathways incorporate current evidence in caring for clients with a specific condition. Nurses

➤ BOX 14-4   NURSING CARE PLAN

Acute Pain

Assessment

Ms. Devine is a 52-year-old woman who was injured in a fall two months ago that caused rupture of a lumbar disc. She is scheduled for a lumbar laminectomy this afternoon. Ms. Devine is the office manager for a realty business she runs with her husband. She was not able to work regularly over the first month after the injury. She has sciatic pain that is sharp and burning, radiating down from her right hip to her right foot. The pain worsens when she sits. Her vital signs are as follows: temperature, 99.2°F; blood pressure, 138/82 mm Hg; pulse, 84 beats per minute; and respirations, 24 breaths per minute.

Assessment Activities	Findings and Defining Characteristics*
Observe client's body movements	Client limps **slightly with right leg. Turns** in bed **slowly.**
Observe client's facial expression	Client **grimaces** when she attempts to sit down.
Ask client to rate pain at its worst	Client **rates pain on a scale of 0 to 10 at an 8 or 9 at its worst.**

*Defining characteristics are in boldface type.

Nursing Diagnosis: Acute pain related to pressure on spinal nerves

Planning

Goal (Nursing Outcomes Classification)†	Expected Outcomes†
Pain Control	**Knowledge of Treatment Procedures**
Client will achieve improved pain control before surgery.	Client's self-report of pain will be 3 or less on a scale of 0 to 10
	Client's facial expressions reveal less discomfort when turning and repositioning.

†Outcomes classification labels from Moorhead S, Johnson, M., & Maas, M. (2008). *Nursing Outcomes Classification (NOC)* (3rd ed). St. Louis, MO: Mosby.

Interventions (Nursing Interventions Classification)‡	Rationale
Analgesic Administration	
Set positive expectations regarding effectiveness of analgesics.	Optimizes client's response to medication (Bulechek et al., 2008).
Give analgesic 30 minutes before turning or positioning client and before pain increases in severity.	Medication will exert peak effect when client attempts to increase movement.
Pain Management	
Reduce environmental factors in client's room (e.g., noise, lighting, temperature extremes).	Pleasurable sensory stimuli reduce pain perception.
Offer client information about any procedures and efforts at reducing discomfort.	Information satisfies client's interests and enables client to evaluate and communicate pain (McCaffery & Pasero, 1999).
Progressive Muscle Relaxation	
Direct client through progressive muscle relaxation exercise.	Relaxation techniques enable self-control when pain develops, reversing
Coach client through exercise.	the cognitive and affective–motivational component of pain perception.

‡Intervention classification labels from Bulechek, G. M., Butcher, H. K., & Dochterman, J. M. (2008). *Nursing Interventions Classification (NIC)* (4th ed.). St. Louis, MO: Mosby.

Evaluation

Nursing Actions	Client Response and Finding	Achievement of Outcome
Ask client to report severity of pain 30 minutes after analgesic administration.	Ms. Devine reports pain at a level of 5 on a scale of 0 to 10.	Pain is reduced, necessitates further nonpharmacological intervention to achieve outcome.
Observe client's facial expressions.	Ms. Devine is observed to have a relaxed facial expression.	Client's level of comfort is improving.

and other health care team members use these to monitor a client's progress. When critical pathways are used to plan care, some forms of documentation are eliminated (e.g., the nursing care plan, flow sheets, and nurses' notes) because all of the pertinent components are included in the pathway.

Concept Maps

Concept maps and their use in care planning are described in Chapter 13. Because you care for clients with multiple health problems and related nursing diagnoses, concept maps are useful in that they incorporate a visual representation of client problems and interventions and of their relationships to one another (Schuster, 2003). The concept map groups and categorizes nursing concepts to give you a holistic view of your client's health care needs and to help you make better clinical decisions in planning care (King & Shell, 2002). There are different approaches to writing concept maps. Schuster (2003) suggested some simple steps in preparing for concept mapping and in developing a clinical plan of care:

1. First, retrieve the clinical assessment database from the medical record, including health history, physical assessment data, laboratory and diagnostic data, medication history, and treatment plan.
2. Review all information concerning health problems, treatments, and medications in the literature, course textbooks, pharmacology texts, and other resources.
3. On the nursing unit, review standardized nursing care plans, critical pathways, clinical protocols, or client education materials.
4. Develop a preliminary diagram of the client's chief medical diagnosis and the patterns of assessment data that you have gathered. Write the client's major medical diagnoses in the middle of the map, and then add the assessment patterns like spokes on a wheel (see Chapter 13). Identify and group the related patterns of clinical assessment and medical history data. Remember that sometimes symptoms apply to more than one nursing diagnosis. Repeat symptoms under different categories when appropriate: for example, when pain is a symptom of both a problem with comfort and a problem with mobility.
5. Next, review your assessment patterns and attempt to identify the nursing diagnoses (see Chapter 13). Do not worry if you have difficulty developing nursing diagnoses at first. It is important to recognize the major nursing care focus for the client. Add diagnostic statements later if necessary.
6. Analyze relationships among nursing diagnoses, and draw dotted lines between them to indicate relationships (Figure 14–4). It is important for you to make meaningful associations between concepts because the links need to be accurate, meaningful, and complete. You need to be able to explain why nursing diagnoses are related. For example, in the case of Ms. Devine, anxiety and acute pain are interrelated, and pain is a cause of her reduced mobility.
7. List nursing interventions to attain the outcomes for each nursing diagnosis (see Figure 14–4). This step corresponds to the planning phase of the nursing process.
8. While caring for the client, use the map to write down the client's responses to each nursing activity. Also, note your clinical impressions and inferences about effectiveness of interventions and progress toward meeting expected outcomes.
9. Keep the concept map with you throughout the clinical day. As you revise the plan, take notes and add or delete nursing

interventions. Use the information recorded on the map for your documentation of client care.

Concept maps help nurses link concepts such as nursing diagnoses and to identify relationships between them to organize and understand information.

Consulting Other Health Care Professionals

Planning involves **consultation** with members of the health team. Although consultation can occur at any step in the nursing process, it occurs most often during planning and implementation, when problems necessitating additional knowledge, skills, or resources arise. Consulting involves seeking the expertise of a specialist, such as a nursing instructor, registered nurse, or clinical nurse specialist to identify ways of approaching and managing the planning and implementation of therapies.

Nurse consultants frequently offer advice about difficult clinical problems. For example, a nursing student will consult with the registered nurse assigned to the same client about ways to individualize interventions, with a clinical specialist for wound care techniques, or with an educator for useful teaching resources. Nurses are consulted for their clinical expertise, client education skills, or staff education skills. Nurses also consult with other members of the health care team, such as physical therapists, nutritionists, and social workers.

Implementing Nursing Care

Lisa enters Ms. Devine's room to administer morphine sulphate ordered for her severe back pain. The client is probably not going to the operating room for another four to six hours, and so Lisa aims to reduce the client's discomfort before then. Lisa administers the medication, using physical care principles to promote safety and prevent infection. She communicates with Ms. Devine in a calm and reassuring manner to allay anxiety. Lisa explains that she will return to Ms. Devine's room in about 30 minutes to help her turn and become comfortable and to offer basic instruction about anticipated postoperative routines. Lisa's interventions are designed to prepare Ms. Devine for her upcoming surgery.

Implementation. With a care plan based on clear and relevant nursing diagnoses, you initiate interventions that are most likely to achieve goals and expected outcomes needed to support or improve the client's health status. A **nursing intervention** is any treatment, based on clinical judgement and knowledge, to enhance client outcomes (Bulechek et al., 2008). Ideally, interventions are evidence informed (see Chapter 7), providing the most current, up-to-date, and effective approaches addressing client problems and include both direct and indirect care measures.

Direct care interventions are treatments performed through interactions with clients. For example, a client receives direct intervention in the form of medication administration, insertion of an intravenous infusion, or counselling during a time of grief. Indirect care interventions are treatments performed away from the client but on behalf of the client or group of clients (Bulechek et al., 2008). For example, indirect care measures include actions for managing the

➤ concept map

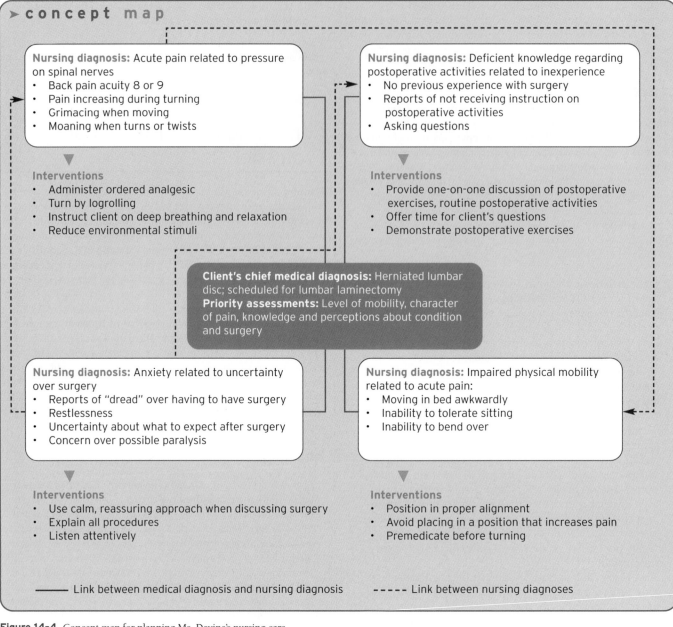

Nursing diagnosis: Acute pain related to pressure on spinal nerves
• Back pain acuity 8 or 9
• Pain increasing during turning
• Grimacing when moving
• Moaning when turns or twists

Interventions
• Administer ordered analgesic
• Turn by logrolling
• Instruct client on deep breathing and relaxation
• Reduce environmental stimuli

Nursing diagnosis: Deficient knowledge regarding postoperative activities related to inexperience
• No previous experience with surgery
• Reports of not receiving instruction on postoperative activities
• Asking questions

Interventions
• Provide one-on-one discussion of postoperative exercises, routine postoperative activities
• Offer time for client's questions
• Demonstrate postoperative exercises

Client's chief medical diagnosis: Herniated lumbar disc; scheduled for lumbar laminectomy
Priority assessments: Level of mobility, character of pain, knowledge and perceptions about condition and surgery

Nursing diagnosis: Anxiety related to uncertainty over surgery
• Reports of "dread" over having to have surgery
• Restlessness
• Uncertainty about what to expect after surgery
• Concern over possible paralysis

Interventions
• Use calm, reassuring approach when discussing surgery
• Explain all procedures
• Listen attentively

Nursing diagnosis: Impaired physical mobility related to acute pain:
• Moving in bed awkwardly
• Inability to tolerate sitting
• Inability to bend over

Interventions
• Position in proper alignment
• Avoid placing in a position that increases pain
• Premedicate before turning

——— Link between medical diagnosis and nursing diagnosis   - - - - Link between nursing diagnoses

Figure 14-4 Concept map for planning Ms. Devine's nursing care.

client's environment (e.g., safety and infection control), documentation, and interdisciplinary collaboration. Both direct and indirect care measures can be nurse-initiated, physician-initiated, and collaborative interventions. For example, client teaching is a direct, nurse-initiated intervention. The indirect intervention of consultation is a collaborative intervention.

Nursing is both an art and a science. Each intervention is rendered within the context of a client's unique situation. As you learn to intervene for a client, consider the context of the clinical situation. What is the client's particular situation? Why do you need to intervene in the clinical situation? How does the client perceive your proposed interventions? How can you support the client as you intervene? The answers to these questions enable you to deliver care compassionately and effectively with the best outcomes for your clients.

Critical Thinking in Implementation

The selection of nursing interventions involves complex decision making and is based on critical thinking to ensure that an intervention is correct and appropriate for the clinical situation. Even though you have planned a set of interventions for a client, good judgement, decision making, and reassessment are needed before each intervention is actually performed, inasmuch as clients' conditions sometimes change rapidly. Some points to consider when you work with clients to meet their needs are as follows:

• Review the set of all possible nursing interventions for the client's problem (e.g., for Ms. Devine's pain, Lisa considers analgesic administration, positioning, relaxation, and other nonpharmacological approaches).

- Review all possible consequences associated with each possible nursing action (e.g., Lisa considers that the analgesic may relieve pain, may have little or insufficient effect, or may cause an adverse reaction).
- Determine the probability of all possible consequences (e.g., if Ms. Devine's pain has decreased with analgesia and positioning in the past, it is unlikely adverse reactions will occur, and the intervention will probably be successful; however, if the client continues to remain highly anxious, her pain may not be relieved).
- Determine the effect of the intervention on the client (e.g., if the administration of an analgesic is effective, Ms. Devine will become less anxious and will be more responsive to preoperative instruction).

The selection and performance of nursing interventions for a client is part of clinical decision making. The critical thinking model described in Chapter 12 provides a framework for making decisions about nursing care. As you proceed with an intervention, you should consider the purpose of the intervention, the steps in performing the intervention correctly, and the medical condition of the client (Figure 14–5). It is essential to know the clinical standards of practice of each agency because procedures and standards of practice vary considerably. The standards of practice are guidelines for selection of interventions, their frequency, and information about whether they can be delegated.

Standard Nursing Interventions

To facilitate good care planning, systems of standard nursing interventions are available to help you. These are based on common health care problems for which standard interventions can serve as a reference point in determining what is necessary. Of more importance, if the standards are informed by evidence, interventions are more likely to improve client outcomes (see Chapter 7). Standard interventions, both nurse initiated and physician initiated, are available in the form of clinical guidelines or protocols, preprinted medical directives or standing orders, and NIC-based interventions.

Clinical Practice Guidelines and Protocols

A clinical guideline or protocol is a document that guides decisions and interventions for specific health care problems. The guideline or protocol is developed on the basis of an authoritative examination of current scientific evidence and assists nurses, physicians, and other health care professionals in making decisions about appropriate health care for specific clinical circumstances. Clinicians within a health care agency sometimes choose to review the scientific literature and their own standard of practice to develop guidelines and protocols in an effort to improve their standard of care. For example, a hospital develops a rapid assessment protocol to improve the identification and early treatment of clients

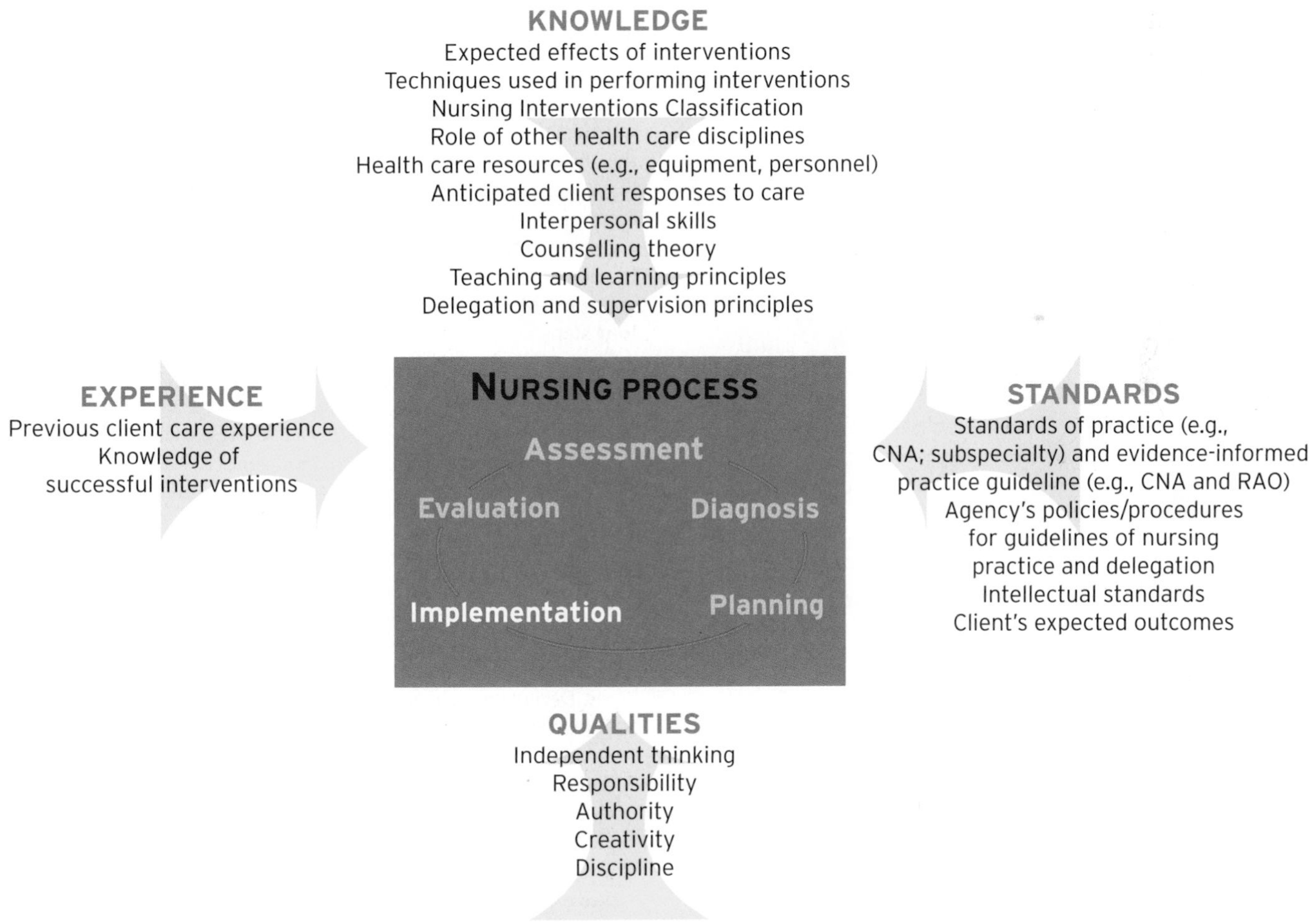

KNOWLEDGE
Expected effects of interventions
Techniques used in performing interventions
Nursing Interventions Classification
Role of other health care disciplines
Health care resources (e.g., equipment, personnel)
Anticipated client responses to care
Interpersonal skills
Counselling theory
Teaching and learning principles
Delegation and supervision principles

EXPERIENCE
Previous client care experience
Knowledge of
successful interventions

NURSING PROCESS

Assessment

Evaluation   Diagnosis

Implementation   Planning

STANDARDS
Standards of practice (e.g.,
CNA; subspecialty) and evidence-informed
practice guideline (e.g., CNA and RAO)
Agency's policies/procedures
for guidelines of nursing
practice and delegation
Intellectual standards
Client's expected outcomes

QUALITIES
Independent thinking
Responsibility
Authority
Creativity
Discipline

Figure 14-5 Critical thinking and the process of implementing care.

suspected of having a stroke. Clinical practice guidelines also assist you in providing the best possible care. The *Best Practice Guidelines* developed by the Registered Nurses Association of Ontario (2008) is an excellent example of these.

Medical Directives or Standing Orders

A **medical directive** or **standing order** is a statement of orders for the conduct of routine therapies, monitoring guidelines, or diagnostic procedures, or a combination of these, for specific clients with identified clinical problems. These statements direct client care in various clinical settings and must be approved and signed by the prescribing physician or health care professional. Medical directives or standing orders are common in critical care settings and other specialized practice settings in which clients' needs change rapidly and require immediate attention. Examples include those for preoperative blood tests, those for postoperative exercises and positioning, and those for certain medications (such as lidocaine or propranolol) for an irregular heart rhythm. When these statements are in place, the critical care nurse may administer the specified medication or conduct the specified action without first notifying the physician. Medical directives or standing orders are also common in community health settings in which physicians are not immediately available for contact. Medical directives, standing orders, and clinical protocols give the nurse legal protection to intervene appropriately in the client's best interest.

Nursing Intervention Classifications System

The NIC system developed at the University of Iowa helps differentiate nursing practice from the practice of other health care professionals (Box 14–5; see also Box 14–2). The NIC-based interventions are common interventions recommended for various NANDA International (2007) nursing diagnoses and care activities for NIC-based interventions. They define a level of standardization for nursing care across settings and for comparison of outcomes.

> **BOX 14-5** **Purposes of the Nursing Interventions Classification (NIC)**
>
> 1. Standardization of the nomenclature (e.g., labelling, describing) of nursing interventions. Standardizes the language nurses use to describe sets of actions in delivering client care.
> 2. Expansion of nursing knowledge about connections between nursing diagnoses, treatments, and outcomes. These connections will be determined through the study of actual client care through the use of a database that the classification will generate.
> 3. Development of nursing and health care information systems.
> 4. Teaching decision making to nursing students. Defining and classifying nursing interventions help teach beginning nurses how to determine a client's need for care and to respond appropriately.
> 5. Determination of the cost of services provided by nurses.
> 6. Planning for resources needed in all types of nursing practice settings.
> 7. Language to communicate the unique functions of nursing.
> 8. Link with the classification systems of other health care professionals.
>
> Modified from Dochterman, J. M., & Bulechek, G. M. (2004). *Nursing Interventions Classification (NIC)* (4th ed.). St. Louis, MO: Mosby.

Implementation Process

Preparation for implementation ensures efficient, safe, and effective nursing care. Preparatory activities include reassessing the client, reviewing and revising the existing nursing care plan, organizing resources and care delivery, anticipating and preventing complications, and implementing nursing interventions.

Reassessing the Client

Assessment is a continuous process that occurs each time you interact with a client. When you collect new data and identify a new client need, you modify the care plan. You also modify a plan when you resolve a client's health care need. During the initial phase of planning nursing care, assessment is partial and sometimes focuses on one dimension of the client, such as level of comfort, or on one system, such as the cardiovascular system. Reassessment helps you decide whether the proposed nursing action continues to be appropriate for the client's level of wellness. For example, Lisa plans to spend a few minutes talking further with Ms. Devine about her concerns relating to surgery. However, her reassessment reveals that Ms. Devine is still a bit uncomfortable and fatigued, and so Lisa must postpone her discussion. She decides to combine her discussion of Ms. Devine's concerns when she begins preoperative teaching in 30 minutes.

Reviewing and Revising the Existing Nursing Care Plan

After reassessing a client, review the care plan, compare assessment data in order to validate the nursing diagnoses, and determine whether the nursing interventions remain the most appropriate for the clinical situation. If the client's status has changed and the nursing diagnosis and related nursing interventions are no longer appropriate, modify the nursing care plan. An outdated or incorrect care plan compromises quality of nursing care. Review and modification enable you to provide timely and appropriate nursing interventions. Modification of the existing written care plan includes four steps:

1. Revise data in the assessment column to reflect current status. Date any new data to communicate the time of the change.
2. Revise the nursing diagnoses. Delete those that are no longer relevant, and add and date any new ones.
3. Revise specific interventions that correspond to the new nursing diagnoses and goals.
4. Determine the method of evaluation for any outcomes achieved.

It has been 45 minutes since Ms. Devine received an analgesic for her pain. She reports less discomfort, and so Lisa initiates preoperative instruction. After about 10 minutes of discussion, Lisa notes that Ms. Devine expresses less concern about surgery; Ms. Devine says, "I feel better now that I understand what surgery involves." Ms. Devine's movements are calmer and less restless. Lisa enters her new findings into the care plan. However, she decides not to delete the nursing diagnosis of anxiety just yet and adds an intervention to her plan: Encourage verbalization of client's remaining concerns about surgery *(see Figure 14–2). Seeing that Ms. Devine responded well to the analgesic, Lisa also adds more nonpharmacological interventions to her plan for pain management.*

Organizing Resources and Care Delivery

A facility's resources include equipment and skilled personnel. Organization of equipment and personnel makes timely, efficient, skilled client care possible. Preparation for giving care involves preparing the environment, as well as clients.

Equipment. Most nursing procedures require some equipment or supplies. Before you perform an intervention, you must identify which supplies are needed, determine whether they are available, and ensure that equipment is in working order to ensure safe use.

Personnel. You are responsible for determining whether to perform an intervention or to delegate it to another member of the nursing team. Your assessment of a client directs delegation decisions. For example, trained nursing assistants are able to competently measure a client's vital signs, but if you learned in the change-of-shift report that a particular client experienced cardiac irregularities during that shift, you must measure the client's vital signs yourself to evaluate cardiac status. Your judgement is important for determining health status and the need for intervention.

Environment. A care environment needs to be safe and conducive to the implementation of therapies. Client safety is your first concern. If the client has sensory deficits, a physical disability, or an alteration in level of consciousness, arrange the environment to prevent injury. Ensure privacy during procedures that may require some body exposure. Also, ensure that lighting is adequate for performing procedures correctly.

Client. Before you provide care, be sure the client is as physically and psychologically comfortable as possible. Ensure that clients are comfortable during interventions. Control environmental factors at the outset, taking care of physical needs (e.g., elimination), minimizing the potential for interruptions, and positioning the client correctly. Also, consider the client's strength and endurance, and plan only the level of activity that the client is able to tolerate comfortably. Awareness of the client's psychosocial needs helps you create a favourable emotional climate. Some clients feel reassured by having a significant other present for encouragement and moral support.

Anticipating and Preventing Complications

Risks to clients arise from both illness and treatment. Be alert for and recognize these risks, adapt your choice of interventions to the situation, evaluate the benefit of the treatment in relation to the risk, and, finally, initiate risk-prevention measures (Figure 14–6). Many conditions heighten the risk for complications. For example, the client with pre-existing left-sided paralysis that followed a stroke two years earlier is at risk for developing a pressure ulcer after orthopedic surgery because postoperative care entails traction and bed rest.

Your knowledge of pathophysiology and your experience with previous clients help you identify risk of complications. A thorough assessment reveals the level of the client's current risk. The **scientific rationale,** which concerns how certain interventions (e.g., pressure-relief devices, repositioning, or wound care) prevent or minimize complications, helps you select the most useful preventive measures. For example, if an obese client has uncontrolled postoperative pain, the risk for pressure ulcer development increases because the client may be unwilling or unable to change position frequently. The nurse anticipates when the client's pain will be aggravated, administers ordered analgesics, and then positions the client to remove pressure on the skin and underlying tissues. If the client continues to have difficulty turning or repositioning, the nurse may then select a pressure-relief device to place on the client's bed.

Identifying Areas of Assistance. Certain nursing situations require you to obtain assistance by seeking additional knowledge, nursing skills, unregulated care providers, or a combination of these. Before you begin care, review the plan to determine the need for assistance. Sometimes you need assistance in performing a procedure, comforting a client, or preparing the client for a diagnostic test. For example, when you care for an overweight, immobilized client, you may require additional personnel to help turn and position the client safely. Be sure to determine the number of additional personnel in advance. You can consult about this matter with other nurses or unregulated care providers.

You require additional knowledge and skills in situations with which you are less familiar or experienced. Because of the continual updating of health care technology, you may lack the skills to perform a procedure. In these situations, you need to prepare by seeking the necessary knowledge and requesting assistance from a more experienced nurse.

Implementation Skills

Nursing practice includes cognitive, interpersonal, and psychomotor (technical) skills. You need each type of skill to implement direct and indirect nursing interventions. You are responsible for knowing which skill is needed in a particular situation and for having the necessary knowledge and skill to perform each.

Cognitive Skills. Cognitive skills involve the application of critical thinking in the nursing process. To perform any intervention, always use good judgement and make sound clinical decisions. No nursing intervention is automatic or routine. You must continually think and anticipate so that you individualize care for clients. For example, Lisa knows the pathophysiological process of a ruptured disc, the anatomy of the spinal cord, and normal pain mechanisms. She considers each of these as she observes Ms. Devine, noting how the client's movement, posture, and position either aggravate or lessen her back pain. Lisa focuses on relieving Ms. Devine's acute pain with an analgesic but then considers the noninvasive interventions needed to minimize stress on the back so that the client will remain comfortable.

Interpersonal Skills. Interpersonal skills are essential for effective nursing action. The nurse develops a trusting relationship, expresses a caring attitude, and communicates clearly with the client and family (see Chapter 19). Good interpersonal communication is crucial for keeping clients informed, providing individualized client teaching, and effectively supporting clients with challenging emotional needs.

Psychomotor Skills. Psychomotor skills require the integration of cognitive and motor activities. For example, when giving an injection, you need to understand anatomy, physiology, and pharmacology (cognitive skills) and use good coordination and precision to administer the injection correctly (motor skills). You are responsible for acquiring necessary psychomotor skills, through your experience in the nursing laboratory, through the use of interactive instructional technology, or through actual hands-on care of clients. In the case of a new skill, always assess your level of competency and obtain the necessary resources to ensure that the client receives safe treatment.

➤ **concept map**

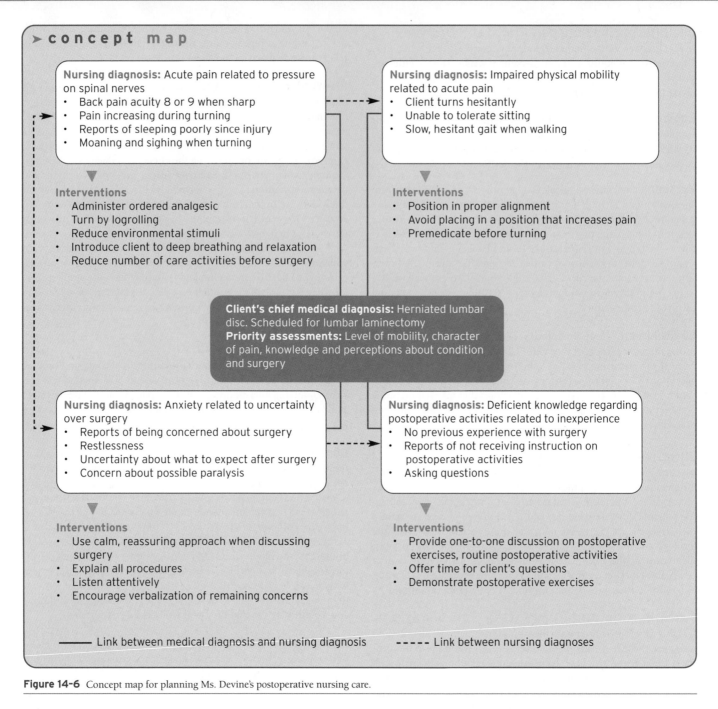

Nursing diagnosis: Acute pain related to pressure on spinal nerves
- Back pain acuity 8 or 9 when sharp
- Pain increasing during turning
- Reports of sleeping poorly since injury
- Moaning and sighing when turning

Interventions
- Administer ordered analgesic
- Turn by logrolling
- Reduce environmental stimuli
- Introduce client to deep breathing and relaxation
- Reduce number of care activities before surgery

Nursing diagnosis: Impaired physical mobility related to acute pain
- Client turns hesitantly
- Unable to tolerate sitting
- Slow, hesitant gait when walking

Interventions
- Position in proper alignment
- Avoid placing in a position that increases pain
- Premedicate before turning

Client's chief medical diagnosis: Herniated lumbar disc. Scheduled for lumbar laminectomy
Priority assessments: Level of mobility, character of pain, knowledge and perceptions about condition and surgery

Nursing diagnosis: Anxiety related to uncertainty over surgery
- Reports of being concerned about surgery
- Restlessness
- Uncertainty about what to expect after surgery
- Concern about possible paralysis

Interventions
- Use calm, reassuring approach when discussing surgery
- Explain all procedures
- Listen attentively
- Encourage verbalization of remaining concerns

Nursing diagnosis: Deficient knowledge regarding postoperative activities related to inexperience
- No previous experience with surgery
- Reports of not receiving instruction on postoperative activities
- Asking questions

Interventions
- Provide one-to-one discussion on postoperative exercises, routine postoperative activities
- Offer time for client's questions
- Demonstrate postoperative exercises

——— Link between medical diagnosis and nursing diagnosis   - - - - - Link between nursing diagnoses

Figure 14-6 Concept map for planning Ms. Devine's postoperative nursing care.

Direct Care

Nurses provide a wide variety of direct care measures. How a nurse interacts affects the success of any direct care activity, and a caring approach is essential. You need to be sensitive at all times to a client's clinical condition, values and beliefs, expectations, and cultural views. All direct care measures require safe and competent practice.

Activities of Daily Living

Activities of daily living (ADLs) are activities usually performed in the course of a normal day, including ambulation, eating, dressing, bathing, brushing the teeth, and grooming (see Chapter 38). A client's need for assistance with ADLs is temporary, permanent, or rehabilitative. A client with impaired mobility because of bilateral arm casts has a temporary need for assistance. A client with an irreversible injury to the cervical spinal cord is paralyzed and thus has a permanent need for assistance. Occupational and physical therapists play key roles in rehabilitation to restore ADL function.

When your assessment reveals that a client is experiencing fatigue, a limitation in mobility, confusion, and pain, the client probably needs assistance with ADLs. For example, a client who experiences shortness of breath avoids eating because of the associated fatigue. Assist the client by setting up meals, offering to cut up food, and planning for small and frequent meals to maintain nutrition. Determine the client's preferences when you assist with ADLs, and let the client participate as much as possible. Involving the client in planning the timing and types of interventions enhances the client's self-esteem and willingness to assume more independence.

Instrumental Activities of Daily Living

Illness or disability sometimes alters a client's ability to be independent in society. **Instrumental activities of daily living** (IADLs) include such skills as shopping, preparing meals, writing cheques, and taking medications. Nurses within the home care and community health care settings frequently assist clients in finding ways to accomplish IADLs. Often, family and friends are excellent resources for assisting clients. In acute care, it is important to anticipate how illness will affect the client's ability to perform IADLs and to involve other health professionals such as occupational therapists.

Physical Care Techniques

You routinely perform a variety of physical care techniques when caring for a client. Examples include turning and positioning, changing dressings, administering medications, and providing comfort measures. Considerations in providing physical care include protecting yourself and the client from injury, using proper infection control practices, staying organized, and following applicable practice guidelines. To carry out a procedure, you need to be knowledgeable about the procedure and how to perform it and about the expected outcomes.

Lifesaving Measures

A **lifesaving measure** is a physical care technique performed when a client's physiological or psychological state is threatened (see Chapter 39). The purpose of lifesaving measures is to restore physiological or psychological equilibrium. Such measures include administering emergency medications, instituting cardiopulmonary resuscitation, intervening to protect a confused or violent client, and obtaining immediate counselling from a crisis centre for an emotionally disturbed client. If an inexperienced nurse faces a situation necessitating emergency measures, the proper nursing action is to summon an experienced health professional.

Counselling

Counselling is a direct care method that helps the client use a problem-solving process to recognize and manage stress and to facilitate interpersonal relationships. Counselling involves emotional, intellectual, spiritual, and psychological support. A client and family who need nursing counselling may be upset or frustrated, but they are not necessarily disabled psychologically. Family caregivers need assistance in adjusting to the physical and emotional demands of caregiving. Likewise, the recipient of care also needs assistance in adjusting to the disability. Clients with psychiatric diagnoses require therapy provided by psychiatric nurses or by social workers, psychiatrists, or psychologists.

Many counselling techniques foster cognitive, behavioural, developmental, experiential, and emotional growth in clients. Most of the techniques listed in Box 14–3 require additional knowledge beyond the scope of this text. Counselling encourages individuals to examine available alternatives and decide which choices are useful and appropriate.

Teaching

Teaching is an important nursing responsibility and is related to counselling. Both involve using communication skills to create a change in the client. However, in counselling, the focus is on the development of new attitudes and feelings, whereas in teaching, the focus is on intellectual growth or the acquisition of new knowledge or psychomotor skills (Redman, 2005).

The purpose of health teaching is to help clients learn about their health status, ways of promoting health, and ways of caring for themselves. Some common examples of teaching by nurses are related to medication administration, activity restrictions, health promotion activities (e.g., diet and exercise), and knowledge about disease and related implications. Your role includes assessment of clients' learning needs and readiness to learn. It is important to know your client and to be aware of cultural and social factors that influence a client's willingness and ability to learn. It is also important to know the client's health literacy levels: that is, whether the client can read directions or make calculations that sometimes are necessary with self-care skills. The teaching–learning process is an interaction between you and the client in which you address specific learning objectives (see Chapter 21).

Controlling for Adverse Reactions

An **adverse reaction** is a harmful effect of a medication, diagnostic test, or therapeutic intervention. Because adverse reactions can follow any nursing intervention, it is important to know which ones might occur. Nursing actions that control for adverse reactions reduce or counteract the reaction. For example, when applying a moist heat compress, you must take steps to prevent burning the client's skin. First, assess the area where the compress is to be applied. Then, inspect the area every five minutes for any adverse reaction, such as excessive reddening of the skin from the heat or skin maceration from the moisture of the compress. When completing a physician-directed intervention, such as medication administration, you need to understand the known and potential side effects of the drug. After administration of the medication, you evaluate the client for any adverse effects. Also, be aware of drugs that counteract the side effects. For example, a client has a previously unknown hypersensitivity to penicillin, and hives develop after three doses. You record the reaction, stop further administration of the drug, and consult with the physician. You then administer an ordered dose of diphenhydramine (Benadryl), an antihistamine and antipruritic medication, to reduce the allergic response and to relieve the itching.

Preventive Measures

Preventive nursing actions promote health and prevent illness in order to avoid the need for acute or rehabilitative health care. Health promotion and illness prevention are very important. Prevention includes assessment and promotion of the client's health potential, carrying out prescribed measures (e.g., immunizations), health teaching, and identification of risk factors for illness, trauma, or both. Consider, for example, the case of Ms. Devine. Lisa learns that her client does not exercise regularly. Ms. Devine is 5 feet 6 inches tall and weighs 160 pounds. Because she is overweight and inactive, she is at risk when she performs activities that place stress on her back. If the client is able to lose some weight and start exercise therapy, she will be less likely to reinjure her back. Lisa plans to consult with the surgeon and physical therapist after surgery to design a plan to help Ms. Devine with weight loss and strengthening of back muscles.

Indirect Care

Indirect care measures are actions that support the effectiveness of direct care interventions (Bulechek et al., 2008). Many of the measures, such as emergency care maintenance and environmental and supply management, are managerial in nature (Box 14–6). Nurses spend a good amount of time in indirect and unit management activities. Communication of information about clients (e.g., change-of-shift report and consultation) is essential to ensure that direct care activities are planned, coordinated, and performed with the proper

> **BOX 14-6** **Examples of Indirect Care Activities**

- Documentation
- Delegation of care activities to unregulated care providers
- Medical order transcription
- Infection control (e.g., proper handling and storage of supplies, use of protective isolation)
- Environmental safety management (e.g., make client rooms safe, strategically assigning clients in a geographic proximity to a single nurse)
- Computer data entry
- Telephone consultations with physicians and other health care professionals
- Change-of-shift report
- Collecting, labelling, and transporting laboratory specimens
- Transporting patients to procedural areas and other nursing units

Modified from Dochterman, J. M., & Bulechek, G. M. (2004). *Nursing Interventions Classification (NIC)* (4th ed.). St. Louis, MO: Mosby.

resources. Delegation of care to unregulated care providers is another indirect care activity.

Communicating Nursing Interventions

Any intervention you provide for a client will be communicated in a written or oral format, or both. Written interventions are part of both the nursing care plan and the permanent medical record. In many institutions, staff develop interdisciplinary care plans, which are plans that represent the contributions of all disciplines involved in caring for a client. For example, when Ms. Devine begins recovering from back surgery, her nursing diagnosis of *impaired physical mobility* will prompt interventions by nurses (e.g., nonpharmacological pain control and positioning), the surgeon (e.g., activity guidelines and pharmacological pain control), and the physical therapist (e.g., ambulation training and exercises).

After completing nursing interventions, you document the treatment and client's response in the appropriate record (see Chapter 16). The entry usually includes a brief description of pertinent assessment findings, the specific procedure, the time and details of the procedure, and the client's response. You also communicate nursing interventions verbally to other health care professionals. Unless communication is clear, concise, accurate, and timely, caregivers can be uninformed, interventions may be needlessly duplicated, procedures may be delayed, or tasks may be left undone.

Delegating, Supervising, and Evaluating the Work of Other Staff Members

Depending on the staffing system, not all of the nursing interventions may be performed by the nurse who develops the care plan. Some activities are delegated to other members of the health care team.. Interventions such as skin care, ambulation, grooming, measuring vital signs in stable clients, and hygiene measures are examples of care activities that you may assign to unregulated care providers and licensed practice nurses who are competent to carry out these activities. When a nurse delegates aspects of a client's care to another staff member, the nurse assigning tasks is responsible for ensuring that each task is appropriately assigned and completed.

Achieving Client-Centred Goals

You implement nursing care to meet client-centred goals and outcomes. In most clinical situations, multiple interventions are necessary to achieve selected outcomes. Because clients' conditions may change rapidly, it is important to apply principles of care coordination, such as good time management, organizational skills, and appropriate use of resources, to ensure that you deliver interventions effectively and that clients achieve desired outcomes. Priority setting is also crucial in successful implementation because it helps you to anticipate and sequence nursing interventions when a client has multiple nursing diagnoses and collaborative problems. Another way to achieve client-centred goals is to encourage and assist clients to follow their treatment plan.

Effective discharge planning and teaching for clients and families require individualized care that is consistent with culture and health beliefs. The process should be initiated at the outset of care. Adequate and timely discharge planning and education of the client and family are the first steps in promoting a smooth transition from one health care setting to another or to home. To be effective with discharge planning and education, you individualize your care and take into consideration the various factors that influence a client's health beliefs. For example, to help Ms. Devine adopt better exercise habits when she returns home, Lisa needs to determine what knowledge and psychosocial factors may influence Ms. Devine to exercise when she returns home. Reinforcing successes with the treatment plan encourages clients to follow their care plans.

✳ KEY CONCEPTS

- During planning, you determine client-centred goals, set priorities, develop expected outcomes of nursing care, and develop a nursing care plan.
- Priority setting helps you anticipate and sequence nursing interventions when a client has multiple nursing diagnoses and collaborative problems.
- Multiple factors in the nursing care environment influence your ability to set priorities.
- Goals and expected outcomes provide clear direction for the selection and use of nursing interventions and provide focus for evaluation of the effectiveness of the interventions.
- In setting goals, the time frame depends on the nature of the problem, etiology, overall condition of the client, and treatment setting.
- A client-centred goal is singular, observable, measurable, time limited, mutual, and realistic.
- An expected outcome is an objective criterion for goal achievement.
- Care plans and critical pathways increase communication among nurses and facilitate the continuity of care from one nurse to another and from one health care setting to another.
- A concept map provides a visually graphic way to understand the relationship between a client's nursing diagnoses and interventions.
- The NIC taxonomy provides a standardization to assist you in selecting suitable interventions for clients' problems.
- Correctly written nursing interventions include actions, frequency, quantity, and method, and they specify the person to perform them.

- Consultation increases your knowledge about a client's problem and helps you learn skills and obtain the resources needed to solve the problem.
- Implementation is the step of the nursing process in which you provide direct and indirect nursing care interventions to clients.
- Clinical guidelines or protocols are evidence-informed documents that guide decisions and interventions for specific health care problems.
- During the initial phase of implementation, you reassess the client to determine whether the proposed nursing action is still appropriate for the client's level of wellness.
- To anticipate and prevent complications, you identify risks to the client, adapt interventions to the situation, evaluate the benefit of a treatment in relation to the risk, and initiate risk-prevention measures.
- Successful implementation of nursing interventions requires you to use appropriate cognitive, interpersonal, and psychomotor skills.
- Counselling is a direct care method that helps clients use problem solving to recognize and manage stress and to facilitate interpersonal relationships.
- Preventive nursing actions include assessment and promotion of the client's health potential, application of prescribed measures (e.g., immunizations), health teaching, and identification of risk factors for illness, trauma, or both.

✳ CRITICAL THINKING EXERCISES

Shawn, a nurse, has two different clients. Mr. Gordon is a 52-year-old client who was admitted to the hospital after a motor vehicle accident. He suffered rib fractures and has a laceration along his right thigh. Shawn has identified the following nursing diagnoses: *ineffective breathing pattern related to chest pain, acute pain related to musculoskeletal trauma,* and *risk for infection related to open wound.* Shawn's second client, Ms. Lawrence, is a 63-year-old woman who had surgery yesterday evening for repair of a foot fracture. Her foot is in a cast. Ms. Lawrence's nursing diagnoses include *acute pain related to tissue swelling, impaired mobility related to restricted movement from cast,* and *deficient knowledge regarding cast care related to inexperience.* Ms. Lawrence will probably be discharged in the morning. She lives alone. Shawn begins to plan care by establishing goals and outcomes for the nursing diagnoses.

1. Between the two clients, which diagnoses are high priority and which are intermediate priority?
2. Of the two clients, which one has higher priority regarding pain management?
3. For the nursing diagnosis *deficient knowledge regarding cast care related to inexperience,* write one goal and two expected outcomes.

Sue is a nursing student. She is to care for Mr. Nelson, a 63-year-old client who was admitted to the hospital with congestive heart failure and pneumonia. He is receiving medications to improve his heart failure and intravenous antibiotics to treat his pneumonia. He reports becoming fatigued easily during care activities and states, "I feel short of breath if I try to do too much." Sue notes he has 3+ edema in his lower extremities. Sue has identified nursing diagnoses of *decreased cardiac output* and *activity intolerance.* Sue must still perform hygiene measures, change the client's intravenous dressing, get him up into a chair, and measure noontime vital signs.

4. Before she begins to intervene, how can Sue make Mr. Nelson more comfortable?
5. What type of intervention is vital sign measurement?
6. Because Sue thinks that Mr. Nelson may be at risk of falling, she decides to get assistance from a colleague before trying to get him into a chair. This is an example of what type of implementation skill?
7. When changing Mr. Nelson's intravenous dressing, Sue cleans the insertion site in accordance with clinical practice guidelines and checks the site for signs of phlebitis. These steps are examples of what type of direct care measure?

✳ REVIEW QUESTIONS

1. Sheila, a nurse, is assigned to a client who has returned from the recovery room after surgery for a colorectal tumour. After an initial assessment, Sheila anticipates the need to monitor the client's abdominal dressing, intravenous infusion, and function of drainage tubes. The client is in pain and will not be able to eat or drink until intestinal function returns. Sheila will have to establish priorities of care in which of the following situations? (Choose all that apply.)
   1. The family comes to visit the client.
   2. The client expresses concern about pain control.
   3. The client's vital signs change, showing a drop in blood pressure.
   4. The charge nurse approaches Sheila and requests a report at end of shift.

2. Sheila's client signals with her call light. Sheila enters the room and finds that the drainage tube is disconnected, the intravenous line has 100 mL of fluid remaining, and the client has asked to be turned. Which of the following should Sheila perform first?
   1. Reconnect the drainage tubing.
   2. Inspect the condition of the intravenous dressing.
   3. Improve client's comfort, and turn her onto her side.
   4. Go to the medication room, and obtain the next intravenous fluid bag.

3. In her nursing care plan, Sheila writes expected outcomes for her client. Which of the following expected outcomes are written correctly? (Choose all that apply.)
   1. Client will remain afebrile until discharge.
   2. Intravenous site will be without phlebitis by the third postoperative day.
   3. Provide incentive spirometer for deep breathing every 2 hours.
   4. Client will report pain and turn more freely by the first postoperative day.

4. The nurse writes an expected outcome statement in measurable terms. An example is:
   1. Client will be pain free
   2. Client will have less pain
   3. Client will take pain medication every 4 hours
   4. Client will report pain acuity less than 4 on a scale of 0 to 10

5. Collaborative interventions are therapies that require:
   1. Nurse and client intervention
   2. Physician and nurse intervention
   3. Client and physician intervention
   4. Multiple health care professionals

6. When does implementation begin in the nursing process?
   1. During the assessment phase
   2. Immediately, in some critical situations
   3. After the care plan has been developed
   4. After mutual goal setting by the nurse and client

7. Mr. Switzer is a 34-year-old client who underwent surgical repair of an abdominal hernia this morning. At noon, the nurse records Mr. Switzer's vital sign measurements on the recovery room flow sheet. The recording of vital sign measurements is an example of:
   1. Psychomotor skill
   2. Indirect care measure
   3. Physical care technique
   4. Anticipating complications

8. Environmental factors heavily affect a client's care. Your first concern for the client includes which of the following?
   1. Safety
   2. Nurse staffing
   3. Confidentiality
   4. Adequate pain relief

9. An out-of-date care plan:
   1. Means the client was discharged
   2. Compromises the quality of care
   3. Ensures that the nursing care was delivered
   4. Identifies that the client response was successful

✳ RECOMMENDED WEB SITES

Center for Nursing Classification & Clinical Effectiveness: http://www.nursing.uiowa.edu/excellence/nursing_knowledge/ clinical_effectiveness/index.htm
The University of Iowa's Center for Nursing Classification and Clinical Effectiveness was established to facilitate ongoing research of the Nursing Interventions Classification (NIC) and Nursing Outcomes Classification (NOC). This Web site provides an overview of the NIC and NOC and offers information about new classification material and publications.

NANDA International: http://www.nanda.org/
Through this Web site, NANDA International provides current information on nursing diagnosis research, publications, and Internet resources.

Registered Nurses Association of Ontario: Best Practices Guidelines: http://www.rnao.org/bestpractices/
The Registered Nurses Association of Ontario has an extensive process for developing best practices guidelines in a variety of areas of clinical nursing. They have received federal and provincial funding for this process, and the results of their work have been made available to all Canadian nurses through this Web site, which lists all current guidelines that have been developed.

15

Evaluation of Nursing Care

Original chapter by Patricia A. Potter, RN, MSN, PhD, GMAC, FAAN

Canadian content written by Marilyn J. Wood, RN, BSN, MPH, DrPH,

and Janet C. Ross-Kerr, RN, BScN, MS, PhD

When a plumber comes to a home to fix a leaking faucet, he or she turns on the faucet to determine the problem, changes or adjusts parts to the faucet, and then turns on the faucet once again to determine whether the leak is fixed. Similarly, after a client with a diagnosis of pneumonia completes a five-day dose pack of antibiotics, the physician often has the client return to the office to have a chest X-ray examination to determine whether the pneumonia has cleared. When a nurse delivers an intervention such as applying a warm compress to a wound, several steps are involved. The nurse assesses the appearance of the wound, determines the severity of the wound, applies the appropriate form of compress, and then returns to determine whether the condition of the wound has improved. These three scenarios depict what ultimately occurs during the process of **evaluation**. The plumber rechecks the faucet, the physician orders a chest X-ray film, and the nurse inspects the wound.

Evaluation involves two components: an examination of a condition or situation and then a judgement as to whether change has occurred. Ideally, after an intervention takes place, evaluation will reveal an improvement.

Chapters 13 and 14 describe how you use critical thinking skills to gather client data, form nursing diagnoses, develop a plan of care, and implement the care plan. Evaluation, the final step of the nursing process, is crucial for determining whether, after application of the nursing process, the client's condition or well-being improves. You apply all that you know about a client and the client's condition, as well as experience with previous clients, to evaluate whether nursing care was effective. *You conduct evaluative measures to determine whether expected outcomes were attained, not whether nursing interventions were completed.* The expected outcomes are the standards against which you judge whether goals have been met and if care is successful.

In the continuing case study, Lisa is now making final preparations to send Ms. Devine to the operating room. Lisa evaluates the interventions she has implemented for the goals of achieving pain control, reducing anxiety, improving mobility, and improving Ms. Devine's knowledge of postoperative activities. Lisa had returned to Ms. Devine's room 30 minutes after administering an analgesic. At that time, the client reported having pain at a level of 4 on a scale of 1 (none) to 10 (worst). Lisa had documented the expected outcome of reduction of pain to a level of 3. Lisa then implemented further non-pharmacological interventions. It is now two hours later, and Lisa finds Ms. Devine lying in bed with her eyes closed. The client awakens as Lisa enters and says, "I just had my eyes closed; I am ready to get this over." Lisa asks, "Tell me how you are feeling." Ms. Devine responds, "Okay, really okay; I feel better, and I am a little less worried than when I first got here." Lisa asks, "On a scale of 0 to 10, tell me how you would rate your pain now." Ms. Devine, "I would say about a 4; it is still there but not as sharp." Lisa continues, "You said you were feeling less worried." Ms. Devine replies, "Yes, I think you have helped me feel less anxious. You know, surgery is nothing anyone wants to have, but I feel better knowing what to expect." Lisa observes that Ms. Devine is relaxed and does not grimace when she turns slightly to her side. Lisa asks, "Can you take just a moment to go over with me what we discussed about your care after surgery?" Ms. Devine responds, "Sure, that would be fine."

Critical Thinking and Evaluation

Evaluation is an ongoing process whenever you have contact with a client. Once you perform an intervention, you gather subjective and objective data from the client, family, and health care team members. You also review knowledge regarding the client's current condition,

treatment, resources available for recovery, and the expected outcomes. By referring to previous experiences caring for similar clients, you are in a better position to know how to evaluate your client's needs. Apply critical thinking qualities and standards to determine whether expected outcomes of care are achieved (Figure 15–1). If expected outcomes are achieved, the overall goals for the client also are met. Client behaviour and responses that you assessed before performing nursing interventions are compared with behaviour and responses that occur after you perform nursing care. Critical thinking directs you to analyze the findings from evaluation (Figure 15–2): Has the client's condition improved? Is the client able to improve, or do physical factors preventing recovery exist? To what degree does this client's motivation or willingness to pursue healthier behaviour influence response to therapies?

During evaluation, you make clinical decisions and continually redirect nursing care. For example, when Lisa evaluates Ms. Devine for a change in pain severity, she applies knowledge of the disease process, physiological responses to interventions (e.g., analgesics), and the correct procedure for pain severity measurement to interpret whether a change has occurred and whether the change is desirable. Lisa knows that the condition of the herniated disc will not change as a result of an analgesic, but the opioid medication she administered will alter the client's perception and reaction to pain (see Chapter 42). Use of the pain severity rating scale helps Lisa obtain an accurate measure of change in the client's pain perception. Evaluative findings determine Lisa's next course of action. In Ms. Devine's case, the pain score is a bit higher (4) than expected (3). However, the client is about to leave for surgery. Ms. Devine will probably receive a preoperative medication just before she goes to the preoperative holding area. The preoperative medication will include an analgesic, and so Lisa knows she cannot administer an additional analgesic at this time. She evaluates that Ms. Devine's pain has been reduced and decides to continue to use basic comfort measures to afford further pain relief.

Positive evaluations occur when you meet desired outcomes, and they lead you to conclude that the nursing intervention or interventions effectively met the client's goals. For example, in the case study, Lisa notes that Ms. Devine's pain rating fell from an 8 or 9 to a 4. With an expected outcome of a pain severity of 3, Lisa's interventions showed a successful reduction in pain severity, but

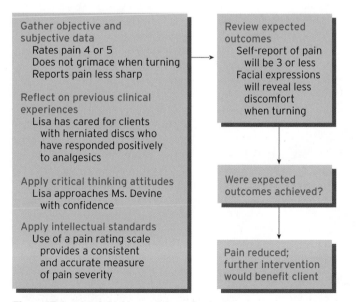

Figure 15-1 Critical thinking and the evaluation process.

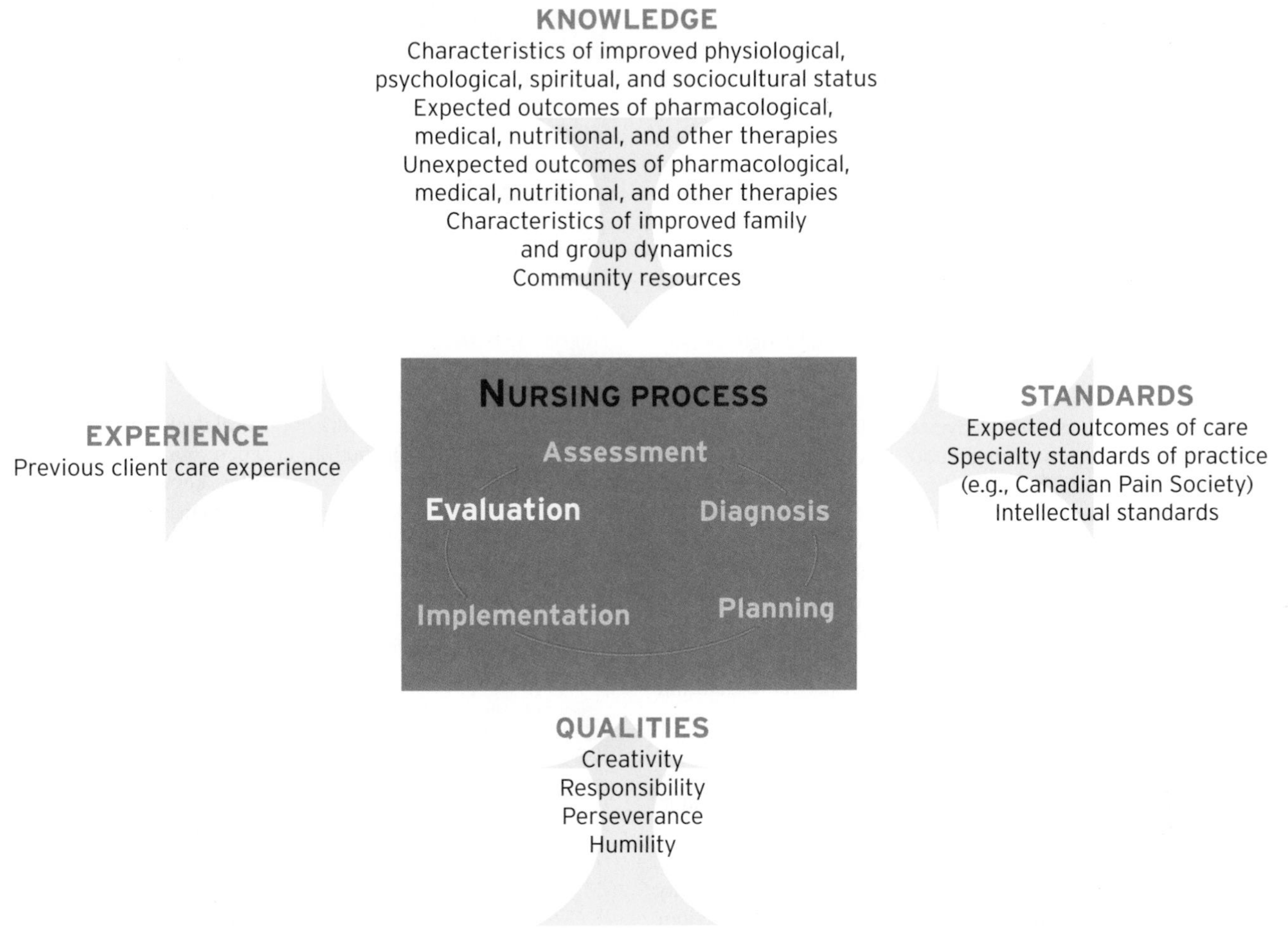

KNOWLEDGE
Characteristics of improved physiological,
psychological, spiritual, and sociocultural status
Expected outcomes of pharmacological,
medical, nutritional, and other therapies
Unexpected outcomes of pharmacological,
medical, nutritional, and other therapies
Characteristics of improved family
and group dynamics
Community resources

EXPERIENCE
Previous client care experience

NURSING PROCESS

Assessment

Evaluation   Diagnosis

Implementation   Planning

STANDARDS
Expected outcomes of care
Specialty standards of practice
(e.g., Canadian Pain Society)
Intellectual standards

QUALITIES
Creativity
Responsibility
Perseverance
Humility

Figure 15-2 Critical thinking and evaluation.

continuing intervention is necessary. Unmet or undesirable outcomes, such as the continuation of severe pain, indicate that interventions are not effective in minimizing or resolving the actual problem or avoiding the risk of a problem. Outcomes need to be realistic and adjusted on the basis of the client's prognosis and nursing diagnoses. An unmet outcome reveals the client has not responded to interventions as planned. As a result, the nurse changes the plan of care by trying different therapies or changing the frequency or approach of existing therapies.

This sequence of critically evaluating and revising therapies continues until you and the client successfully and appropriately resolve the problems, as defined by nursing diagnoses. Remember that evaluation is dynamic and ever changing, depending on the client's nursing diagnoses and condition. As problems change, so will expectations of outcomes. A client whose health status continuously changes requires more frequent evaluation. In addition, you will evaluate high-priority diagnoses first. For example, Lisa evaluates Ms. Devine's diagnosis of *acute pain* before evaluating the status of the diagnosis of *deficient knowledge*.

The Evaluation Process

The purpose of nursing care is to assist the client in resolving actual health problems, preventing the occurrence of potential problems, and maintaining a healthy state. The evaluation process, which determines the effectiveness of nursing care, consists of five ele-

ments: (1) identifying evaluative criteria and standards; (2) collecting data to determine whether the criteria or standards are met; (3) interpreting and summarizing findings; (4) documenting findings and any clinical judgement; and (5) terminating, continuing, or revising the care plan.

Identifying Criteria and Standards

You evaluate nursing care by knowing what to look for. A client's goals and expected outcomes are the objective criteria by which to judge a client's response to care.

Goals. A goal is the expected behaviour or response that indicates resolution of a nursing diagnosis or maintenance of a healthy state. It is a summary statement of what will be accomplished when the client has met all expected outcomes. In the case of Ms. Devine, Chapter 14 described Lisa's plan of care for *acute pain*. Lisa selected the goal "Client achieves improved pain control before surgery." Successful achievement of this goal depends on the success of Lisa's interventions, chosen from the Nursing Interventions Classification (NIC; Bulechek et al., 2008), for analgesic administration, pain management, and progressive muscle relaxation. Goals are also often based on standards of care or guidelines established for minimal safe practice. When a nurse cares for a client with a peripheral intravenous line, the goal "The intravenous site will remain free of phlebitis" is established on the basis of sound practice standards. (The Registered Nurses Association of Ontario's [2008] *Best Practice Guidelines* contains specific recommendations for care of peripheral intravenous lines).

Expected Outcomes. Outcomes have been broadly defined in the health care literature. Donabedian (1980) defined outcomes as favourable or adverse changes in clients' health states caused by prior or concurrent care. When nurses apply the nursing process, expected outcomes are the expected favourable and measurable results of nursing care. A nursing-sensitive client outcome is a measurable client or family state, behaviour, or perception largely influenced by and sensitive to nursing interventions (Moorhead et al., 2008). Examples of nursing-sensitive outcomes include reductions in pain severity, in incidence of pressure ulcers, and in incidence of falls (Box 15–1). In comparison, outcomes influenced largely by medical interventions include client mortality, hospital readmissions, and length of stay. **Outcomes** are statements of progressive, step-by-step responses or behaviours that must be achieved in order to accomplish the goals of care. An outcome defines the effectiveness, efficiency, and measurement of the results of nursing interventions. When you achieve outcomes, the related factors for a nursing diagnosis usually no longer exist. In Ms. Devine's case, the expected outcomes for the goal of achieving improved pain control are "Client's self-report of pain will be 3 or less on a scale of 0 to 10" and "Client's facial expressions reveal less discomfort when turning and repositioning." When Lisa evaluates Ms. Devine's pain at a level of 4 and notes an absence of facial grimacing during turning, she knows the client's pain has been reduced but that further pain relief is needed. However, the related factor for Ms. Devine's diagnosis of *acute pain* is pressure on spinal nerves, which will not be totally relieved until surgery. The analgesics and noninvasive nursing interventions are designed to reduce the perception of pain from pressure on the nerves, as well as to minimize additional pressure on nerves. It is important to understand that evaluation is not a description of the achievement of an intervention. Evaluation of Ms. Devine does *not* involve observation of her ability to turn correctly; it *does* involve observation of the client's behaviour (facial expression) during turning. During the planning phase of the nursing process (see Chapter 14), it is important for you to select an observable client state, behaviour, or self-reported perception that will reflect goal achievement.

One valuable resource is the Nursing Outcomes Classification (NOC; Moorhead et al., 2008), which provides a classification system of nursing sensitive outcomes. NOC is designed to provide the language for the evaluation step of the nursing process. The purposes of NOC are (1) to identify, label, validate, and classify nursing-sensitive client outcomes; (2) to field test and validate the classification; and (3) to define and test measurement procedures for the outcomes and indicators using clinical data. The NOC project complements the work of NANDA International (2007) and the NIC project. The NOC system offers nursing-sensitive outcomes for NANDA International nursing diagnoses (Table 15–1). For each outcome, the NOC system specifies recommended evaluation indicators: the client behaviours or responses that are measures of outcome achievement.

Collecting Evaluative Data

Proper evaluation enables you to determine the client's response to nursing care and whether the therapy was effective in improving the client's physical or emotional health. It is important to evaluate whether each client reaches a level of wellness or recovery that the health care team and client established in the goals of care. In addition, you must determine whether you met the client's expectations of care. You will ask clients questions about their perceptions of care, such as "Did you receive the type of pain relief you expected?" and "Did you receive enough information to care for your baby at home?" This level of evaluation is important for determining the client's satisfaction with care and for strengthening the partnering

---

✳ BOX 15-1   RESEARCH HIGHLIGHT

Nursing-Sensitive Outcomes

Evidence Summary

Although members of the general public recognize that oncology nurses aim to deliver high-quality care to people with cancer and to their families, nurses themselves struggle with ways to measure their influence on client outcomes. The Oncology Nursing Society (ONS) implemented a project to define and list nursing-sensitive patient outcomes (NSPOs) for the field of oncology. For each outcome, the ONS is working to provide references and links to best evidence in the literature, provide clinical guidelines, review existing knowledge, and discuss measurement of outcomes. Examples of NSPOs include control and management of symptoms (e.g., pain, fatigue, insomnia, nausea, constipation, breathlessness, diarrhea), functional status (activities of daily living, instrumental activities of daily living, role functioning, activity tolerance, nutritional status), psychological health status (anxiety, depression, spiritual distress, coping), and economic outcomes (home care visits, costs per day per episode of illness).

Application to Nursing Practice

- Establishing NSPOs for clients with cancer helps provide tools for you to use in measuring the impact of nursing care.
- Development of core measures linked to evidence-informed practice guidelines will improve nursing practice at the client's bedside.
- Use of NSPOs helps you clearly indicate to consumers the value nursing contributes to health care.

References: Given, B. A., & Sherwood, P. R. (2005). Nursing-sensitive patient outcomes—A white paper. *Oncology Nurses Forum, 32*, 773.

---

between you and the client. Always select appropriate evaluative measures to evaluate client response and expectations. Evaluating a client's response to nursing care requires the use of **evaluative measures,** which are simply assessment skills and techniques (e.g., auscultation of lung sounds, observation of a client's skill performance, discussion of the client's feelings, and inspection of the skin) (Figure 15–3). In fact, evaluative measures are the same as assessment measures, but you perform them when you make decisions about the client's status and progress.

The intent of assessment is to identify any problems that exist. The intent of evaluation is to determine whether the known problems have remained the same, improved, worsened, or otherwise changed. In many clinical situations, it is important to collect evaluative measures over a period of time to determine whether a pattern of improvement or change exists. A one-time observation of a pressure ulcer is insufficient to determine that the ulcer is healing. It is important to note a consistency in change. For example, over a period of two days, you can observe whether the pressure ulcer is gradually decreasing in size, whether the amount of drainage is declining, and whether the redness of inflammation is resolving. Recognizing a pattern of improvement or deterioration allows you to reason and decide whether the client's problems are resolved. The primary source of data for evaluation is the client. However, you also use input from the family and other caregivers. For example, if a client is at home, you can ask a family member to report on the amount of food the client eats during a meal or how well a client prepares to take medications. You will sometimes consult with a colleague about how a hospitalized client responded to pain medication during another shift.

In the case of Ms. Devine, Lisa's initial evaluation at the beginning of this chapter revealed the following: The client reported feeling better, rated pain at a level of 4, was lying in bed relaxed, felt less worried, and did not grimace when turning over.

When matching these actual behaviours and responses to expected outcomes, Lisa determines that Ms. Devine's pain and anxiety have lessened. Because the pain is less acute, Ms. Devine's mobility is less restricted. However, Lisa knows that the cause of Ms. Devine's pain has not been corrected. The surgery is still pending, and thus the client's anxiety will possibly increase. Lisa decides to continue the plan of care but makes revisions by adding additional basic comfort measures. The comfort measures help control both the pain and anxiety and help maintain the client's mobility. Lisa next evaluates whether Ms. Devine remembers the postoperative activities that they discussed earlier: "Ms. Devine, we talked about several things that you will be asked to do after surgery. I want to know whether you understand what we discussed. Tell me what to expect about your pain control and activity." Ms. Devine responds, "You said that I would have a device that lets me control how much pain medication I receive. I should not be afraid to use it. I know the doctors will get me up early to move around. You said if I can get control of the pain, it will be easier to get up and walk. What I do not remember is something you said about breathing." Lisa says, "Good, the device is a PCA. As for breathing, let's practise the incentive spirometer I showed you one more time." Lisa recognizes that Ms. Devine has learned about select postoperative activities but requires further instruction on the incentive spirometer. Deficient knowledge now becomes Lisa's priority until Ms. Devine leaves for surgery.

Careful monitoring and early detection of problems are a client's first line of defence. Always make clinical judgements of your observations of what is occurring with a specific client and not merely of what happens to clients in general. Frequently, changes are not obvious. Evaluations are client specific: based on a close familiarity with each client's behaviour, physical status, and reaction to caregivers. Critical thinking skills promote accurate evaluation, which enables appropriate revision of ineffective care plans and discontinuation of therapy that has successfully resolved a problem.

Discontinuing a Care Plan

After you determine that expected outcomes and goals have been met, you confirm this finding with the client when possible. If you and the client agree, then you discontinue that portion of the care plan. Documentation of a discontinued plan ensures that other nurses will not unnecessarily continue interventions for that portion of the plan of care. Continuity of care ensures that care provided to clients is relevant and timely. If you do not communicate achieved goals, you will waste much time.

Modifying a Care Plan

When goals are not met, you identify the factors that interfere with goal achievement. Change in the client's condition, needs, or abilities usually necessitates alteration of the care plan. For example, when teaching self-administration of insulin, you discover that the client has developed a new problem, a tremor associated with a side effect of a medication. The client is unable to draw medication from a syringe or inject the needle safely. As a result, the original outcomes "Client will correctly prepare insulin in a syringe" and "Client will administer insulin injection independently" cannot be met. You introduce new interventions (instructing a family member in insulin preparation and administration) and revise outcomes to meet the goal of care.

At times a lack of goal achievement results from an error in nursing judgement or failure to follow each step of the nursing process. Clients often have multiple and complex problems. Always remember the possibility of overlooking or misjudging something. When a goal is not achieved, no matter what the reason, repeat the entire nursing process sequence for that nursing diagnosis to discover which changes in the plan are needed. You then reassess the client, determine accuracy of the nursing diagnosis, establish new goals and expected outcomes, and select new interventions.

A complete reassessment of all client factors relating to the nursing diagnosis and etiology is necessary when you modify a plan. Reassessment requires critical thinking as you compare new data about the client's condition with previously assessed information.

Knowledge from previous experiences helps you direct the reassessment process. Caring for clients and families who have had similar health problems gives you a strong background of knowledge to use for anticipating client needs and knowing what to assess. Reassessment ensures that the database is accurate and current. It also reveals "missing links" (i.e., critical pieces of new information that were overlooked, which thus interfered with goal achievement). You sort, validate, and cluster all new data to analyze and interpret differences from the original database. You also document reassessment data to alert other nursing staff to the client's status. After reassessment, determine what nursing diagnoses are accurate for the situation. Ask whether you selected the correct diagnosis and whether it and the etiological factor are current. Then revise the problem list to reflect the client's changed status.

Sometimes you make a new diagnosis. You base your nursing care on an accurate list of nursing diagnoses. Accuracy is more important than the number of diagnoses selected. As the client's condition changes, the diagnoses also change. For example, you identified the nursing diagnosis *deficient knowledge related to inexperience* for a client with newly diagnosed diabetes. The original plan was to instruct the client in how to self-administer insulin. After finding that the client has difficulty self-administering insulin because of reduced visual acuity, you reassess the situation and find that a family member is available as a resource. To develop a plan designed to educate a caregiver about the administration of insulin, you then establish a new diagnosis: *ineffective health maintenance related to impaired dexterity.*

Goals and Expected Outcomes

When you revise care plans, review the goals and expected outcomes for needed changes. You even need to examine the appropriateness of goals for unchanged nursing diagnoses, because a change in one problem sometimes affects other problems. Determining that each goal and expected outcome is realistic for the problem, etiology, and time frame is particularly important. Unrealistic expected outcomes and time frames hamper goal achievement. Clearly document goals and expected outcomes for new or revised nursing diagnoses so that all team members are aware of the revised care plan. When the goal is still appropriate but has not yet been met, try changing the evaluation data to allow more time. You may also decide at this time to change interventions. For example, when a client's pressure ulcer does not show signs of healing, you choose to use a different support surface or a different type of wound cleanser. All goals and expected outcomes are client centred, with realistic expectations for client achievement.

Interventions

The evaluation of interventions concerns two factors: the appropriateness of the interventions selected and the correct application of the intervention. The appropriateness of an intervention is based on the standard of care for a client's health problem. A **standard of care** is the minimum level of care acceptable to ensure high quality of care. Standards of care define the types of therapies typically administered to clients with defined problems or needs. If a client who is receiving chemotherapy for leukemia has a specific nursing diagnosis, such as *nausea related to pharyngeal irritation*, the standard of care established by a nursing department for this problem includes pain control measures for pharyngeal irritation, mouth care guidelines, and diet therapy. The nurse reviews the standard of care to determine whether the right interventions have been chosen or whether additional ones are required. Increasing or decreasing the frequency of interventions is another approach for ensuring appropriate application of an intervention. You adjust interventions on the basis of the client's actual response to therapy, as well as previous experience with similar clients. For example, if a client continues to have congested lung sounds, you increase the frequency of the client's coughing and deep breathing exercises to remove secretions.

During evaluation, you find that some planned interventions are designed for an inappropriate level of nursing care. If you need to change the level of care, substitute a different action verb, such as *assist* in place of *provide* or *demonstrate* in place of *instruct*, in the revised care plan. For example, to assist a client to walk, a nurse must be at the client's side during ambulation, whereas providing an assistive device helps the client ambulate more independently. Also, demonstrating requires you to show a client how a skill is performed rather than simply telling the client how to perform it. Sometimes the level of care is appropriate but the interventions are unsuitable because of a change in the expected outcome. In this case, discontinue the interventions and plan new ones. Make any changes in the plan of care according to the nature of the client's unfavourable response. Consult with other nurses to obtain suggestions for improving the approach to care delivery. Senior nurses are often excellent resources because of their experience. Simply changing the care plan is not enough. Implement the new plan, and re-evaluate the client's response to the nursing actions. *Evaluation is continuous.*

On occasion, you will discover unmet client needs during evaluation. This is normal. The nursing process is a systematic, problem-solving approach to individualized client care, but many factors affect each client with health care problems. Clients with the same health care problem are not treated the same way. As a result, you will sometimes make errors in judgement. The systematic use of evaluation provides a way for you to catch these errors. By consistently incorporating evaluation into practice, you will minimize errors and ensure that the client's plan of care is appropriate and relevant.

The evaluation of nursing care is a professional responsibility, and it is a crucial component of nursing care. Evaluation that focuses on a single client's plan of care enables you as a nurse to know the effectiveness of interventions and whether expected outcomes are met. At a system or institutional level, evaluation involves quality improvement and performance improvement activities that focus on the delivery of care provided by an agency or a specific nursing division within an agency. Through the continuous evaluation of care, nurses play a key role in the ongoing improvement of client care.

✲ KEY CONCEPTS

- Evaluation is a step of the nursing process that allows nurses to determine whether nursing interventions are successful in improving a client's condition or well-being.
- During evaluation, the appropriateness of the intervention should be assessed, as should the outcome.

- Evaluation involves two components: an examination of a condition or situation and a judgement as to whether change has occurred.
- During evaluation, apply critical thinking to make clinical decisions and redirect nursing care to best meet clients' needs.
- Evaluation findings are positive when you meet desired outcomes; this enables you to conclude that your interventions were effective.
- When the client's actual response (e.g., behaviours and physiological signs and symptoms) to nursing interventions are compared with expected outcomes established during planning, you determine whether goals of care are met. At this time, you should also determine whether the goals, outcomes, or both were realistic.
- Evaluative measures are assessment skills or techniques that you use to collect data for evaluation.
- It sometimes becomes necessary to collect evaluative measures over time to determine whether a pattern of change exists.
- To interpret evaluative findings, examine the outcome criteria, assess the client's actual behaviour or response, compare the outcome criteria with the actual behaviour or response, and judge the degree of agreement.
- Documentation of evaluative findings allows all members of the health care team to know whether a client is progressing.
- As a result of evaluation, a client's nursing diagnoses, priorities, and interventions sometimes change.

✲ CRITICAL THINKING EXERCISES

1. Mr. Jacko has recently received a diagnosis of asthma and is to be discharged tomorrow. His physician has ordered a metered-dose inhaler for Mr. Jacko to use daily. The client has not used an inhaler before. He asks the nurse, "What do I do at home if I have trouble using this thing?" The nursing diagnosis for Mr. Jacko is *deficient knowledge regarding use of a metered-dose inhaler related to inexperience*. Write a goal and expected outcome for this clinical scenario.

2. Mr. Vicar has been visiting the clinic for more than a month. He visits weekly for follow-up care for a chronic venous stasis ulcer of the left leg. The nurse's note at the time of his first visit contained the following information: "Ulcer with irregular margins, 4 cm wide by 5 cm long, approximately 0.5 cm deep, draining foul-smelling purulent yellowish drainage. Subcutaneous tissue visible. Skin around ulcer, brownish rust in colour. Zinc oxide and calamine gauze applied to ulcer; elastic wrap bandage applied to gauze. Client instructed to return in 1 week." The stated goal is "Wound will demonstrate healing within 4 weeks." As the nurse who is caring for the client on the follow-up visit, what expected outcomes would you anticipate for this goal? What evaluative measures would you use to determine whether the wound is healing?

✲ REVIEW QUESTIONS

1. A nurse caring for a client with pneumonia sits the client up in bed and suctions the client's airway. After suctioning, the client describes some discomfort in his abdomen. The nurse auscultates the client's lung sounds and provides a glass of water for the client. Which of the following is an evaluative measure used by the nurse?
   1. Suctioning the airway
   2. Sitting client up in bed
   3. Auscultating lung sounds
   4. Asking client to describe type of discomfort

2. A nurse caring for a client with pneumonia sits the client up in bed and suctions the client's airway. After the suctioning, the client describes some discomfort in his abdomen. The nurse auscultates the client's lung sounds and provides a glass of water to the client. Which of the following is an appropriate evaluative criterion used by the nurse? (Choose all that apply.)
   1. The client drinks the contents of the water glass.
   2. The client's lungs are clear to auscultation in bases.
   3. The client reports abdominal pain on scale of 0 to 10.
   4. The client's rate and depth of breathing are normal with the head of the bed elevated.

3. The evaluation process, which determines the effectiveness of nursing care, includes five elements, one being interpreting findings. Which of the following is an example of interpretation?
   1. Evaluating the client's response to selected nursing interventions
   2. Selecting an observable or measurable state or behaviour that will reflect goal achievement
   3. Reviewing the client's nursing diagnoses and establishing goals and outcome statements
   4. Matching the results of evaluative measures with expected outcomes to determine client's status

4. A goal specifies the expected behaviour or response that indicates
   1. The specific nursing action was completed
   2. The validation of the nurse's physical assessment
   3. The nurse has made the correct nursing diagnoses
   4. Resolution of a nursing diagnosis or maintenance of a healthy state

5. A client is recovering from surgery for removal of an ovarian tumour. It is one day after her surgery. Because she has an abdominal incision and dressing, the nurse has selected a nursing diagnosis of *risk for infection*. Which of the following is an appropriate goal statement for the diagnosis?
   1. The client will remain afebrile to the time of discharge.
   2. The client's wound will remain free of infection by discharge.
   3. The client will receive ordered antibiotic on time over next three days.
   4. The client's abdominal incision will remain covered with a sterile dressing for two days.

6. Unmet and partially met goals require the nurse to do which of the following? (Choose all that apply.)
   1. Redefine priorities
   2. Continue intervention
   3. Discontinue care plan
   4. Gather assessment data on a different nursing diagnosis
   5. Compare the client's response with that of another client

✳ RECOMMENDED WEB SITES

Center for Nursing Classification & Clinical Effectiveness: www.nursing.uiowa.edu/excellence/nursing_knowledge/clinical_effectiveness/index.htm
The University of Iowa's Center for Nursing Classification & Clinical Effectiveness was established to facilitate ongoing research of the Nursing Interventions Classification (NIC) and Nursing Outcomes Classification (NOC). This Web site provides an overview of the NIC and NOC and offers information about new classification material and publications.

NANDA International: http://www.nanda.org/
Through this Web site, NANDA International provides current information on nursing diagnosis research, publications, support resources, and Internet resources.

Registered Nurses Association of Ontario: Nursing Best Practice Guidelines: http://www.rnao.org
The Registered Nurses Association of Ontario has developed an extensive process for developing best practices guidelines in a variety of areas of clinical nursing. They have received federal and provincial funding for this process, and the results of their work have been made available to all Canadian nurses through this Web site, which lists all current guidelines that have been developed.

16

Documenting and Reporting

Original chapter by Barbara Maxwell, RN, BSN, MS, MSN, CNS

Canadian content written by Maureen A. Barry, RN, MScN

objectives

Mastery of content in this chapter will enable you to:

- Define the key terms listed.
- Describe multidisciplinary communication within the health care team.
- Identify purposes of a health care record.
- Discuss legal guidelines for documentation.
- Identify ways to maintain confidentiality of records and reports.
- Describe six quality guidelines for documentation and reporting.
- Describe the different methods used in record keeping.
- Discuss the advantages of standardized documentation forms.
- Identify elements to include when documenting a client's discharge plan.
- Describe the role of critical pathways in multidisciplinary documentation.
- Identify the important aspects of home care and long-term care documentation.
- Discuss the role of computerized charting and use of electronic health records in documentation.
- Describe the purpose and content of a change-of-shift report.
- Explain how to verify telephone orders.

key terms

media resources

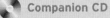 **Web Site**

- Audio Chapter Summaries
- Glossary
- Multiple-Choice Review Questions
- Student Learning Activities
- Weblinks

Companion CD

- Glossary
- Interactive Learning Activities
- Fluids and Electrolytes Tutorial
- Test-Taking Skills

Documentation is anything written or electronically generated that describes the status of a client or the care or service given to that client. Documentation within a client health care record is a vital aspect of nursing practice. Nursing documentation must be accurate, comprehensive, and flexible enough for members of the health care team to retrieve critical data, maintain continuity of care, and track client outcomes, and it must reflect current standards of nursing practice. Information in the client record provides a detailed account of the quality of care delivered to clients. Documentation ensures continuity and quality of care, furnishes legal evidence of care, provides evidence for quality assurance purposes, and constitutes a database for planning future health care (Cheevakasemsook et al., 2006).

Effective documentation can positively affect the quality of life and health outcomes for clients and minimize the risk of errors. Accrediting agencies such as Accreditation Canada (formerly the Canadian Council on Health Services Accreditation) offer guidelines for documentation. However, documentation and reporting practices differ among institutions and jurisdictions and are influenced by ethical, legal, medical, and agency guidelines.

As a member of the health care team, you need to communicate information about clients accurately and in a timely, effective manner. The quality of client care depends largely on caregivers' ability to communicate with one another. All health care professionals require accurate information about clients in order to devise an organized, comprehensive care plan. If the care plan is not communicated to all members of the health care team, care can be fragmented, tasks repeated, and therapies delayed or omitted. Data recorded, reported, or communicated to other health care professionals are confidential, and the confidentiality of these data must be protected.

The health care environment creates many challenges to accurately documenting and reporting client care. Because of the quality of care, the standards of regulatory agencies and nursing practice, and the legal guidelines for nursing practice, documentation and reporting are critical responsibilities of a nurse.

Confidentiality

Whether the transfer of client information occurs through verbal reports, written documents, or electronic transfer, nurses must follow certain principles to maintain confidentiality of information. You are legally and ethically obligated to keep information about clients confidential. You may not discuss a client's examination, observation, conversation, or treatment with other clients or with staff who are not involved in the client's care. Only staff directly involved in a specific client's care have legitimate access to the records. Many clients request copies of their health records, and they have the right to read their records. Each institution has policies for controlling the manner in which records are shared. In most situations, institutions are required to obtain written permission from clients to release medical information.

As a nurse, you are also responsible for protecting records from all unauthorized readers. When nurses and other health care professionals have a legitimate reason to use records for data gathering, research, or continuing education, they must obtain appropriate authorization according to agency policy. Nursing students and faculty may be required to present identification indicating they are authorized to access records. The health care agency stores the records after the treatment ends.

Before the beginning of clinical placements, students and instructors may be required to sign confidentiality agreements with the agencies in question. Students need to understand the practice standards and laws concerning confidentiality. A breach of confidentiality is often a careless rather than a deliberate act. Students need to make sure that client-identifiable information (e.g., files, stickers, information in notebooks, worksheets) is not taken home and is disposed of correctly in a secure bin for shredding. Examples of breaches of confidentiality include accessing information not related to your duties, discussing client information in an inappropriate area such as an elevator or on public transport, revealing to a caller confidential client or coworker details, emailing client information through a public network such as the Internet, and leaving confidential material in a public area. Even after you are no longer on placement at an agency, you are obligated to maintain the confidentiality of clients and coworkers at that agency.

Personal Information Protection and Electronic Documents Act (PIPEDA)

PIPEDA is federal legislation that protects personal information, including health information. *PIPEDA* delineates how private sector organizations may collect, use, or disclose personal information in the course of commercial activities. Individuals have the right to access and request correction of any personal information collected about them as well. *PIPEDA* applies to all organizations engaged in commercial activities unless the federal government exempts an organization or activity in a province with similar legislation. *PIPEDA* is discussed in more detail in Chapter 17.

Multidisciplinary Communication Within the Health Care Team

Client care requires effective communication among members of the health care team. Communication takes place through the client's record or chart and reports.

A client's **record**, or chart, is a confidential, permanent legal documentation of information relevant to a client's health care. Information about the client's health care is recorded after each contact with the client. The record is a continuing account of the client's health care status and is available to all members of the health care team. All health records contain the following information:

- Client identification and demographic data
- Informed consent for treatment and procedures
- Advance directives
- Admission nursing history
- Nursing diagnoses or problems and the nursing or multidisciplinary care plan
- Record of nursing care treatment and evaluation
- Medical history
- Medical diagnosis
- Therapeutic orders
- Progress notes for various health care professions
- Reports of physical examinations
- Reports of diagnostic studies
- Record of client and family education
- Summary of operative procedures
- Discharge plan and summary

Reports are oral, written, or audiotaped exchanges of information between caregivers. Reports commonly compiled by nurses include change-of-shift reports, telephone reports, transfer reports, and incident reports (see "Reporting" section on page 228). A physician or nurse practitioner may call a nursing unit to receive a verbal report on a client's condition and progress. A laboratory submits a written report about the results of diagnostic tests.

Team members communicate information through discussions or conferences (Figure 16–1).For example, a discharge planning conference often involves members of all disciplines (e.g., nursing, social work, dietary, medicine, and physiotherapy), who meet to discuss the client's progress toward established discharge goals. **Consultations** are another form of discussion whereby one professional caregiver gives formal advice about the care of a client to another caregiver. For example, a nurse caring for a client with a chronic wound may need a consultation with a wound care specialist. **Referrals** (an arrangement for services by another care provider), consultations, and conferences must be documented in a client's permanent record so that all caregivers can plan care accordingly.

Purposes of Records

A record is a valuable source of data that is used by all members of the health care team. Its purposes include communication and care planning, legal documentation, education, funding and resource management, research, and auditing–monitoring.

Communication and Care Planning

The record is a means by which health care team members communicate client needs and progress, individual therapies, content of conferences, client education, and discharge planning. The plan of care needs to be clear to everyone reading the chart. The record should be the most current and accurate source of information about a client's health care status.

In the record, always communicate the manner in which you conduct the nursing process with a client. The admitting nursing history and physical assessment are comprehensive and provide baseline data about the client's health status on admission to the facility. These data usually include biographical information (e.g., age and marital status), method of admission, reason for admission, a brief medical–surgical history (e.g., previous surgeries or illnesses), allergies, current medication (prescribed and over-the-counter), the client's perceptions about illness or hospitalization, and a review of health risk factors. Results of a physical assessment of all body systems are either documented in the nursing history or included on a separate form (see Chapter 32).

The medical progress notes should complement nursing process information. The notes detail the physician's or nurse practitioner's findings at the time of assessment. Nurses first refer to the client's health care record for relevant assessment findings so that they can

anticipate the client's status and then conduct an individualized client assessment.

The record provides data that you use to identify and support nursing diagnoses, establish expected outcomes of care, and plan and evaluate interventions. Information from the record adds to your observations and assessment. You do not need to collect information that is already available. If you have reason to believe that the information is inaccurate, information should be verified and appropriate changes made to the client's record.

Legal Documentation

Accurate documentation is one of the best defences against legal claims associated with nursing care (see Chapter 9). From a legal perspective, the purpose of documentation is "always to accurately and completely record the care given to patients, as well as their response to that care" (Monarch, 2007, p. 58). To limit nursing liability, you must clearly document that individualized, goal-directed nursing care, based on the nursing assessment, was provided to a client. The record must describe exactly what happened to a client. Charting should be performed immediately after care is provided. Nursing care may have been excellent, but in a court of law, care not documented is care not provided (Graves Ferrell, 2007). In the health care record, you need to indicate all assessments, interventions, client responses, instructions, and referrals. It is important to complete all documentation on appropriate forms and to be sure that client-identifying information (client's name and identification number) is on every page of documentation.

The Nurses Service Organization (2008) (a medical malpractice, professional liability, and risk management company) identified eight common charting mistakes that can result in malpractice: (1) failing to record pertinent health or drug information, (2) failing to record nursing actions, (3) failing to record the administration of medications, (4) recording on the wrong chart, (5) failing to document a discontinued medication, (6) failing to record drug reactions or changes in the client's condition, (7) transcribing orders improperly or transcribing improper orders, and (8) writing illegible or incomplete orders. Table 16–1 provides guidelines for legally sound documentation.

Education

A client's record contains a variety of information, including diagnoses, signs and symptoms of disease, successful and unsuccessful therapies, diagnostic findings, and client behaviours. By reading the client care record, you can learn the nature of an illness and the client's response to the illness. No two clients have identical records, but patterns of information can be identified in records of clients with similar health problems. With this information, you can identify patterns for various health problems and begin to anticipate the type of care required for a client.

Funding and Resource Management

The client care record shows how health care agencies have used their financial resources. Various tools help monitor the timing and reasons for health team–client interactions. These data are then compared with documented entries on the chart to demonstrate the need for and efficacy of health care resources. In some workload assignment systems, health care interactions and tasks are assigned specified points in relation to time spent with each client.

Research

Statistical data relating to the frequency of clinical disorders, complications, use of specific medical and nursing therapies, recovery from illness, and deaths can be gathered from client records. For example,

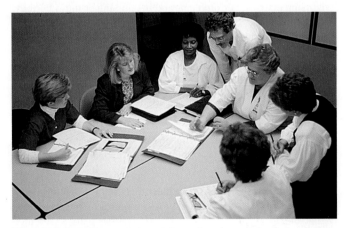

Figure 16-1 Staff communicate information about their clients during a change-of-shift report.

►TABLE 16-1   Legal Guidelines for Recording

Guidelines	Rationale	Correct Action
Do not erase, apply correction fluid to, or scratch out errors made while recording.	Charting becomes illegible: It may appear as if you were attempting to hide information or deface record.	Draw single line through error; write "error," "mistaken entry," "delete," or "void" above it; and sign your name or initials and date. Then record note correctly.
Do not write retaliatory or critical comments about client or care by other health care professionals.	Statements can be used as evidence of non-professional behaviour or of poor quality of care.	Enter only objective descriptions of client's behaviour; direct quotes from client are preferred.
Correct all errors promptly.	Errors in recording can lead to errors in treatment or may imply an attempt to mislead or hide evidence.	Avoid rushing to complete charting; be sure that information is accurate.
Record all facts.	Record must be accurate, factual, and objective.	Be certain entry is factual and thorough; do not speculate or guess. A person reading the documentation should be able to determine that the client was adequately cared for.
Do not leave blank spaces in nurse's notes.	Another person can add incorrect information in spaces.	Chart consecutively, line by line; if space is left, draw line horizontally through it and sign your name at end.
Record all entries legibly and in black ink. Do not use felt-tip pens or erasable ink.	Illegible entries can be misinterpreted, thereby causing errors and lawsuits; felt-tip pen ink smudges or runs when wet and may destroy documentation; erasures are not permitted in client charting. Black ink is more legible when records are photocopied or transferred to microfilm.	Chart legibly in black ink; avoid the use of erasers, correction fluid, and pencils for documentation.
If an order is questioned, record that clarification was sought.	If you perform an order known to be incorrect, you are just as liable for prosecution as the prescriber is.	Do not record, "physician made error"; instead, chart that "Dr. Wong was called to clarify order for analgesic." Include the date and time of phone call, whom you spoke with, and the outcome.
Chart only your own actions.	You are accountable for information you enter into chart.	Never chart for someone else, except for the following situation: If caregiver has left unit for the day and calls with information that needs to be documented, include the date and time of entry, and reference the specific date and time you are referring to and the name of source of information in the entry, and include that the information was provided by telephone.
Avoid using generalized, empty phrases such as "status unchanged" or "had good day."	Such information is too generalized and has no meaning. Specific information about client's condition is missing.	Use complete, concise descriptions of care so that documentation is objective and factual.
Begin each entry with the date and time, and end with your signature and title.	This guideline ensures that correct sequence of events is recorded; signature indicates who is accountable for care delivered.	Do not wait until end of shift to record important changes that occurred several hours earlier; be sure to sign each entry (e.g., Mei Lin, RN).
Avoid "precharting" (documenting an entry before performing a treatment or an assessment or before giving a medication)	Precharting invites error and thus endangers the health and safety of the client; it is also illegal and can constitute falsification of health care records.	Document during or immediately after giving care or after administering a medication.
For computer documentation, keep your password to yourself.	This maintains security and confidentiality.	Once logged on to the computer, do not leave the computer screen unattended. Make sure the computer screen is not accessible for public viewing.

as part of a quality improvement program for clients receiving intravenous therapy, a nurse manager reviews clients' records to investigate the incidence of infection in clients with a specific type of intravenous catheter. This review reveals that the infection rate is increased, and the nurse manager and staff nurses design a new specific method for intravenous catheter care. Once this new intervention is implemented, the manager again reviews clients' records to determine whether the infection rate decreases.

A nurse may use clients' records during a clinical research study to investigate a new nursing intervention. For example, a nurse wants to compare a new method of pain control with a standard pain protocol, by using two groups of clients. The client records provide data on the two types of interventions: the new method and the standard pain control. The nurse researcher collects data from the clients' records that describe the types and doses of analgesic medications used, objective assessment data, and clients' subjective reports of pain relief. The researcher then compares the findings to determine whether the new method was more effective that the standard pain control protocol.

Some data collection activities may be part of the quality improvement practices at an agency, whereas other activities may be actual clinical research studies. Different types of permission must be secured before a researcher can review client records for any type of research study or data analysis. The researcher must be sure that the data collection and analysis adhere to provincial, territorial, and agency policies.

Auditing-Monitoring

A regular review of information in client records helps you evaluate the quality and appropriateness of care. This audit may be either a review of care received by discharged clients or an evaluation of care currently being given. Most Canadian health care agencies have continuous quality improvement programs and teams to monitor and improve the delivery of heath care services. These teams often contain members from across the organization, and they normally perform the self-assessment requirements of Accreditation Canada (see Chapter 11). Nurses or cross-discipline members of a committee monitor or review records throughout the year to determine the degree to which quality improvement standards are met. Deficiencies are explained to the nursing staff so that corrections in policy or practice can be made.

Guidelines for Quality Documentation and Reporting

High-quality documentation and reporting enhance efficient, individualized client care. High-quality documentation and reporting have six important characteristics: They are factual, accurate, complete, current, and organized, and they comply with standards set by Accreditation Canada and by provincial or territorial regulatory bodies.

Factual

A factual record contains descriptive, objective information about what a nurse sees, hears, feels, and smells. An objective description is the result of direct observation and measurement: for example, "BP 80/50, client diaphoretic, heart rate 102 and regular. L. Woo, RPN" (where "BP" stands for "blood pressure"). The use of inferences (e.g., "client appears to be in shock") without supporting factual data is not acceptable because inferences can be misunderstood.

The use of vague terms, such as *appears, seems,* or *apparently,* is not acceptable because these words reflect opinion. For example, the description "the client seems anxious" does not accurately communicate facts and does not inform another caregiver of the details

regarding the behaviours exhibited by the client that led to the use of the word *anxious*. The phrase *seems anxious* is a conclusion without supported facts. Objective documentation includes the observations of the client's behaviours. For example, objective signs of anxiety can include increased pulse rate, increased respirations, and increased restlessness.

When recording subjective data, document the client's exact words within quotation marks whenever possible (e.g., "Client states, 'I feel very nervous and out of control'").

Accurate

The use of exact measurements establishes accuracy. For example, a description such as "Intake, 360 mL of water" is more accurate than "Client drank an adequate amount of fluid." These measurements can later be used as a means to determine whether a client's condition has changed. Charting that an abdominal wound is "5 cm in length without redness, drainage, or edema" is more descriptive than "large wound healing well."

Documentation of concise data should be clear and easy to understand. Avoid the use of unnecessary words and irrelevant detail. For example, the fact that the client is watching TV is relevant only when this activity has relevance to the client's status and plan of care.

Most health care institutions develop a list of standard abbreviations, symbols, and acronyms to be used by all members of the health care team in documenting or communicating client care and treatment. Approved abbreviations and acronyms vary, depending on the type of facility (i.e., long-term versus acute-care facility). Use of an institution's accepted abbreviations, symbols, and system of measures (e.g., metric) ensures that all staff members use the same language in their reports and records. Always use abbreviations carefully to avoid misinterpretation. For example, "od" (every day) can be misinterpreted to mean "O.D." (right eye). If abbreviations are confusing, then to minimize errors, you should spell them out in their entirety.

The Joint Commission on Accreditation of Healthcare Organizations (JCAHO) published a minimum list of dangerous abbreviations that should no longer be used in written medical documents (Karch, 2004). Suggestions include writing "unit" instead of "U"; always using a zero before a decimal point in a decimal fraction (e.g., "0.25 mg"); and not writing a zero alone after a decimal point (e.g., writing "5 mg," not "5.0 mg"). The Institute for Safe Medication Practices (2007) published a more extensive list of error-prone abbreviations, symbols, and dose designations that health care institutions also need to consider adding to their "Do Not Use" lists (see Chapter 34).

Correct spelling demonstrates a level of competency and attention to detail. Many terms can easily be misinterpreted (e.g., *dysphagia* and *dysphasia*). Some spelling errors can also result in serious treatment errors; for example, the names of certain medications, such as *digitoxin* and *digoxin* or *morphine* and *hydromorphone,* are similar and must be transcribed carefully to ensure that the client receives the correct medication.

Record entries must be dated, and a method for identifying the authors of entries must be in place. Therefore, each entry in a client's record ends with the caregiver's full name or initials and status, such as "Holly Lee, RPN." Each time initials are used, the full name and status must previously appear on the same page so that the individual entering initials can be readily identified. A nursing student enters full name, student nurse abbreviation (e.g., "SN" or "NS"), and educational institution: for example, "Henri Gauthier, SN 1 [student nurse, year one], U of S [University of Saskatchewan]."

Records must reflect accountability during the time frame of the entry. Accountability is best accomplished when you chart only your own observations and actions. Your signature holds you accountable for information recorded. If information was inadvertently omitted from the record, it is acceptable for you to ask colleagues to chart information on your behalf after you leave work. The entry needs to clearly show what was done and by whom (e.g., "At 1100 hrs, Sam Roustas, RN, called and reported that at 0800 hrs, morphine sulphate, 5 mg subcutaneous, was administered to client for abdominal pain. F. Khan, R.N.").

You should refer to agency policy before making late entries, correcting errors, or completing an omission. Late entries are often documented by writing the current date and time in the next available space as close to the late entry as possible and writing "late entry for [date and shift]." For adding information to an existing entry, using the current date and time in the next space and adding "addendum to note of [date and time of prior note]" is a good practice.

Complete

The information within a recorded entry or a report must be complete, containing appropriate and essential information. Criteria for thorough communication exist for certain health problems or nursing activities (Table 16–2). Your written entries in the client's health care record describe the nursing care you administer and the client's response. An example of a thorough nurse's note is as follows:

> "1915: Client verbalizes sharp, throbbing pain localized along lateral side of right ankle, beginning approximately 15 minutes ago after twisting his foot on the stairs. Client rates pain as 8 on a scale of 0–10. Pain increased with movement, slightly relieved with elevation. Pedal pulses equal bilaterally. Right ankle circumference 1 cm larger than left. Capillary refill less than 3 seconds bilaterally; right foot warm to touch and pale pink; skin intact on right foot; responds to tactile stimulation on right foot. Ice applied. Percocet 2 tabs (PO) given for pain. Client states pain somewhat relieved with ice, rates pain as 6 on a scale of 0–10. Dr. P. Yoshida notified. Lee Turno, RN."

Current

Timely entries are essential to the client's ongoing care. Documentation should occur during or as soon as possible after the incident or intervention, and events should be described chronologically to reflect a clear record of exactly what happened (College of Nurses of Ontario, 2005). To increase accuracy and decrease unnecessary duplication, many health care agencies use bedside records, which facilitate immediate documentation of information as it is collected from a client.

Flow sheets (described later in this chapter) are a means of entering current information quickly. Portable electronic work stations or secure wall cabinets in client rooms help ensure that client confidentiality is maintained. Nurses often keep notes on a worksheet when caring for several clients, making notes as the care occurs to ensure that entries recorded later in the record are accurate. The following activities and findings should be communicated at the time of occurrence:

- Vital signs
- Administration of medications and treatments
- Preparation for diagnostic tests or surgery
- Change in client's status and who was notified (e.g., nurse practitioner, physician, manager, client's family)
- Admission, transfer, discharge, or death of a client
- Treatment for a sudden change in client's status
- Client's response to treatment or intervention

Health care agencies use military time, a 24-hour system that avoids misinterpretation of "A.M." and "P.M." times (Figure 16–2). Instead of two 12-hour cycles in standard time, the military clock is one 24-hour time cycle. The military clock ends with midnight (2400) and begins with 1 minute after midnight (0001). For example, 10:22 A.M. is 1022 military time; 1:00 P.M. is 1300 military time.

►TABLE 16-2	Examples of Criteria for Reporting and Recording
Topic	**Criteria to Report or Record**
Assessment	
Subjective data	Description of episode in quotation marks; for example, "I feel as if I have an elephant sitting on my chest, and I can't catch my breath."
	Onset, location, description of condition (severity, duration, frequency; precipitating, aggravating, and relieving factors); for example, "The pain in my left knee started last week after I knelt on the ground. Every time I bend my knee, I have a shooting pain on the inside of my knee."
Client behaviour (e.g., anxiety, confusion, hostility)	Onset, behaviours exhibited, precipitating factors, client's verbal response; for example, "Client observed pacing in her room, avoiding eye contact with nurse, and repeatedly stating, 'I have to go home now.'"
Objective data (e.g., rash, tenderness, breath sounds)	Onset, location, description of condition (see "Subjective data" above); for example, "1100 hrs: 2-cm raised pale red area noted on back of left hand."
Nursing Interventions and Evaluation	
Treatments (e.g., enema, bath, dressing change)	Time administered, equipment used (if appropriate), client's response (objective and subjective changes) in comparison with previous treatment; for example, "Client denied pain during abdominal dressing change" or "Client reported severe abdominal cramping during enema."
Medication administration	Immediately after administration, document time when medication is given, preliminary assessment (e.g., pain level, vital signs), client response or effect of medication; for example, "1500: Client reports a 'throbbing headache all over her head.' Rates pain as 6 (scale 0–10). Tylenol 650 mg given PO. 1530: Client reports pain level 2 (scale 0–10) and states 'the throbbing has stopped.'"
Client teaching	Information presented, method of instruction (e.g., discussion, demonstration, videotape, booklet), and client response, including questions and evidence of understanding such as demonstration of correct self-care or change in behaviour.
Discharge planning	Measurable client goals or expected outcomes, progress toward goals, need for referrals.

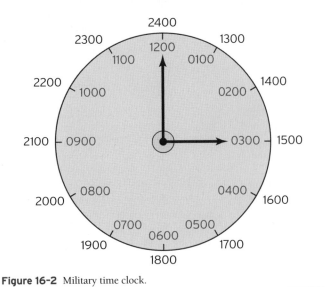

Figure 16-2 Military time clock.

Organized

As a nurse, you want to communicate information in a logical order. For example, an organized note describes the client's pain, the nurse's assessment and interventions, and the client's response. To write notes about complex situations in an organized manner, think about the situation and make notes of what is to be included before you begin to write in the permanent legal record.

Compliant With Standards

Documentation needs to follow standards set by Accreditation Canada and by provincial or territorial regulatory bodies to maintain institutional accreditation and to decrease the risk of liability. Current standards require that all clients who are admitted to a health care institution undergo physical, psychosocial, environmental, and self-care assessments; receive client education; and be provided discharge planning. In addition, criteria for standards stress the importance of evaluating client outcomes, including the client's response to treatments, teaching, or preventive care.

The nursing service department of each health care agency selects a method of documenting client care. The method reflects the philosophy of the nursing department and incorporates the standards of care. Because the nursing process shapes a nurse's approach and direction of care, effective documentation also reflects the nursing process.

Common Documentation Systems

Client data can be recorded in several documentation systems. Each nursing service selects a documentation system that reflects the philosophy of its department. The same documentation system is used throughout a specific agency and may also be used throughout a health care system.

Narrative Documentation

Narrative documentation is the traditional method for recording nursing care. It is simply the use of a story-like format to document information specific to client conditions and nursing care. Narrative charting, however, has many disadvantages, including the tendency to have repetitive information, to be time consuming to complete, and to require the reader to sort through much information to locate desired data.

Problem-Oriented Medical Records or Health Care Records

The **problem-oriented medical record** is a method of documentation that emphasizes the client's problems. Data are organized by problem or diagnosis. Ideally, each member of the health care team contributes to a single list of identified client problems. This assists in coordinating a common plan of care. The problem-oriented medical record has the following major sections: database, problem list, care plan, and progress notes.

Database. The database section contains all available assessment information pertaining to the client (e.g., history and physical examination findings, the nurse's admission history and ongoing assessment, the dietitian's assessment, laboratory reports, and radiological test results). The database is the foundation for identifying client problems and planning care. As new data become available, you revise the database. The database accompanies clients through successive hospitalizations or clinic visits.

Problem List. After analyzing data, health care team members identify problems and make a single problem list. The problems include the client's physiological, psychological, social, cultural, spiritual, developmental, and environmental needs. Team members list the problems in chronological order and file the list in the front of the client's record to serve as an organizing guide for the client's care. Add new problems as they are identified. When a problem has been resolved, record the date of resolution, and highlight the date or draw a line through the problem and its number.

Care Plan. A care plan is developed for each problem by the members of the health care team from each discipline involved in the client's care. Nurses document the plan of care in a variety of formats. In general, these plans of care include nursing diagnoses, expected outcomes, and interventions.

Progress Notes. Health care team members monitor and record the progress of a client's problems (Box 16–1). The information can be expressed in various formats. One method is the **subjective–objective–assessment–plan (SOAP)** charting, involving subjective data (verbalizations of the client), objective data (data that are measured and observed), assessment (diagnosis based on the data), and plan (what the caregiver plans to do). Some institutions add intervention (I) and evaluation (E) (i.e., **SOAPIE**). The logic for SOAP and SOAPIE notes is similar to that of the nursing process: to collect data about the client's problems, draw conclusions, and develop a plan of care. The nurse numbers each SOAP or SOAPIE note and titles it according to the problem on the list.

A second progress note method is the **problem–intervention–evaluation (PIE)** format (see Box 16–1). It is similar to SOAP charting in its problem-oriented nature. However, it differs from the SOAP method in that PIE charting originated in nursing practice, whereas SOAP charting originated from medical records. The PIE format simplifies documentation by unifying the care plan and progress notes. PIE notes differ from SOAP notes because the narrative does not include assessment information. A nurse's daily assessment data appear on flow sheets, preventing duplication of data. The narrative note includes the problem, the intervention, and the evaluation. The PIE notes are numbered or labelled according to the client's problems. Resolved problems are dropped from daily documentation after the nurse's review. Continuing problems are documented daily.

A third progress note format is **focus charting**. It involves use of **data–action–response (DAR) notes**, which include both subjective

➤ BOX 16-1   Examples of Progress Notes Written in Different Formats

Subjective-Objective-Assessment-Plan (SOAP)

01/19/08 Knowledge deficit related to inexperience regarding surgery
1630 hrs

S: "I'm worried about what it will be like after surgery."

O: Client asking frequent questions about surgery.. Has had no previous experience with surgery. Wife present, acts as a support person.

A: Knowledge deficit regarding surgery related to inexperience. Client also expressing anxiety.

P: Explain routine preoperative preparation. Demonstrate and explain rationale for turning, coughing, and deep breathing (TCDB) exercises. Provide explanation and teaching booklet on postoperative nursing care. S. Lazarus, RPN

Problem-Intervention-Evaluation (PIE)

P: Knowledge deficit regarding surgery related to inexperience.

I: Explained to client normal preoperative preparations for surgery. Demonstrated TCDB exercises. Provided booklet to client on postoperative nursing care.

E: Client demonstrates TCDB exercises correctly. Needs review of postoperative nursing care. S. Lazarus, RPN

Focus Charting: Data-Action-Response (DAR)*

D: Client stating, "I'm worried about what it will be like after surgery." Client asking frequent questions about surgery. Has had no previous experience with surgery. Wife present; acts as a support person.

A: Explained to client normal preoperative preparations for surgery. Demonstrated TCDB exercises. Provided booklet to client on postoperative nursing care.

R: Client demonstrates TCDB exercises correctly. Needs review of postoperative nursing care. Client states, "I feel better knowing a little bit of what to expect." S. Lazarus, RPN

*Some agencies also add P (Plan) to make DARP.

---

and objective data, the action or nursing intervention, and the response of the client (i.e., evaluation of effectiveness). One distinction of focus charting is its movement away from charting only problems, which has a negative connotation. Instead, a DAR note addresses client concerns: a sign or symptom, a condition, a nursing diagnosis, a behaviour, a significant event, or a change in a client's condition. Documentation is written in accordance with the nursing process; nurses are encouraged to broaden their thinking to include any client concerns, not just problem areas; and critical thinking is encouraged. The benefits of focus charting are that it incorporates all aspects of the nursing process, highlights the client's concerns, and can be integrated into any clinical setting (*Mosby's Surefire Documentation*, 2006).

Source Records

In a **source record**, the client's chart is organized so that each discipline (e.g., nursing, medicine, social work, respiratory therapy) has a separate section in which to record data. One advantage of a source record is that caregivers can easily locate the proper section of the record in which to make entries. Table 16–3 lists the components of a source record.

➤ TABLE 16-3   Organization of Traditional Source Record

Sections	Contents
Admission sheet	Specific demographic data about client: legal name, identification number, sex, age, birth date, marital status, occupation and employer, health card number, nearest relative to notify in an emergency, religious affiliation, name of attending physician, date and time of admission
Physician's order sheet	Record of physician's orders for treatment and medications, with date, time, and physician's signature
Nurse's admission assessment	Summary of nursing history and physical examination
Graphic sheet and flow sheet	Record of repeated observations and measurements such as vital signs, daily weights, and intake and output
Medical history and examination	Results of initial examination performed by physician, including findings, family history, confirmed diagnoses, and medical plan of care
Nurses' notes	Narrative record of nursing process: assessment, nursing diagnosis, planning, implementation, and evaluation of care
Medication administration record	Accurate documentation of all medications administered to client: date, time, dose, route, and nurse's signature
Progress notes	Ongoing record of client's progress and response to medical therapy and review of disease process completed by physician or nurse practitioner
Health care disciplines' records	Entries made into record by all health care–related disciplines: radiology, social work, laboratories, and so forth
Discharge summary	Summary of client's condition, progress, prognosis, rehabilitation, and teaching needs at time of dismissal from hospital or health care agency

A disadvantage of the source record is that details about a specific problem may be distributed throughout the record. For example, in the case of a client with bowel obstruction, the nurse describes in the nurses' notes the character of abdominal pain and the use of relaxation therapy and analgesic medication. In a separate section of the record, the physician's notes describe the progress of the client's condition and the plan for surgery. The findings of X-ray examinations that reveal the location of the bowel obstruction are in the test results section of the record.

The notes section is where nurses enter a narrative description of nursing care and the client's response (Box 16–2). It is also a section for documenting care that is provided by the physician or nurse practitioner in the nurse's presence. The nurse may record key diagnostic test results from other sections of the record in the nurses' notes if they are of major importance in the care of the client.

Charting by Exception

Charting by exception (CBE) focuses on documenting deviations from the established norm or abnormal findings. This approach reduces documentation time and highlights trends or changes in the client's condition (*Mosby's Surefire Documentation*, 2006). It is a shorthand method for documenting normal findings and routine care on the basis of clearly defined standards of practice and predetermined criteria for nursing assessments and interventions. Clearly defined standards of practice that specify nurses' responsibilities to clients provide the framework for routine care of all clients. With standards integrated into documentation forms, such as predefined normal assessment findings or predetermined interventions, a nurse needs only to document significant findings or exceptions to the predefined norms. In other words, the nurse writes a progress note only when the standardized statement on the form is not met. Assessments are standardized on flow sheets or other forms so that all caregivers evaluate and document findings consistently (Figure 16–3).

Because the standard assessments are located in the chart, client data are already present on the permanent record, and so nurses do not need to keep temporary notes for later transcription, and caregivers have easy access to current data. The assumption with CBE is that all standards are met unless otherwise documented.

> ### ➤ BOX 16-2   Sample Narrative Note

04/03/08

1100 hrs: Client states, "I'm having a hard time catching my breath." Respirations [R], laboured at 32/min; P [pulse] 120; BP 112/70. Oxygen saturation 90% on room air. Client alert and oriented. Client using intercostal muscles during inhalation. Breath sounds auscultated, crackles and wheezes over both lower lobes. Chest excursion equal bilaterally. Elevated head of bed to Fowler's position. Obtained arterial blood gas (ABG) sample at 1045. O_2 started at 2 L/min per nasal prongs as ordered. Remained at bedside to calm client. P. Haske, RN

   1130 hrs: Results of ABGs reported to Dr Stein are pH 7.34; PCO_2 [partial pressure of carbon dioxide] 44 mm Hg; PO_2 [partial pressure of oxygen] 80 mm Hg.

   Client states, "It is easier to breathe now." R 24/min; P 96; BP 110/72. Oxygen saturation 97% on O_2 at 2 L/min per nasal prongs, lips pale pink; capillary refill less than 3 seconds. Crackles and wheezing still audible on auscultation. Client remains in high Fowler's position. P. Haske, RN

When nurses see entries in the chart, they know that something out of the ordinary has been observed or has occurred. For that reason, when changes in a client's condition have developed, it is easy to track them.

When clients' conditions change, it is essential to describe thoroughly and precisely what happens to clients and the actions taken. CBE can pose legal risks if nurses are not diligent in documenting exceptions. This charting method fails to provide a thorough picture of a client's developing condition and does not reflect communication among members of the health care team (*Mosby's Surefire Documentation*, 2006). If nurses rely too heavily on charting standard categories and do not enter exception notes, the client's situation will not be clear. CBE can also be problematic when related documentation forms do not have space allotted for documenting client and family perspectives.

Case Management Plan and Critical Pathways or Care Maps

The **case management** model of delivering care (see Chapter 11) incorporates a multidisciplinary approach to documenting client care. In many organizations, the standardized plan of care is summarized into critical pathways for a specific disease or condition. The **critical pathways** or **care maps** are multidisciplinary care plans that include client health concerns, key interventions, and expected outcomes within an established time frame (Figure 16–4). In a computerized charting system, professionals from many disciplines may access the chart, and this integration of information from the different disciplines can be accessed easily from every computer terminal in the institution at any time. The nurse and other team members such as physicians, nurse practitioners, dietitians, social workers, physiotherapists, and respiratory therapists use the same critical pathway to monitor the client's progress during each shift or, in the case of home care, during every visit.

Critical pathways eliminate the need for nurses' notes, flow sheets, and nursing care plans because the pathway document integrates all relevant information. Unexpected occurrences, unmet goals, and interventions not specified within the clinical pathway time frame are called **variances**. A variance is present when the activities on the clinical pathway are not completed as predicted or the client does not meet the expected outcomes. An example of a negative variance is when a client postoperatively develops pulmonary complications necessitating oxygen therapy and monitoring with pulse oximetry. An example of a positive variance is when a client progresses more rapidly than expected (e.g., use of a Foley catheter may be discontinued a day early). A variance analysis is necessary to review the data for trends and for developing and implementing an action plan to respond to the identified client problems (Box 16–3). In addition, variances may result from changes in the client's health or may occur as a result of other health complications not associated with the primary reason why the client requires care. Once a variance has been identified, the nurse modifies the client's care to meet the needs associated with the variance.

Consensus on the definition and impact of critical pathways is lacking. The pathways were developed to improve the efficiency of care in hospitals and as a cost containment measure to reduce length of hospital stay. According to Dy et al. (2005), critical pathways may be effective only under certain circumstances (e.g., first pathway implemented in a particular practice area or for lesser severity of illness).

PATIENT CARE SERVICES
Interdisciplinary Systems Flowsheet

Key: Initials in Box = Assessment findings meet standards and procedures.
Interventions tolerated or care provided.
* & Initials in Box = Significant finding(s) abnormal or changed.
Document in progress notes.
↓ & Initials in Box = Significant finding(s) has not changed.
√ = Monitored on High Frequency Flow Sheet.

Initial all relevant items. Leave others blank. **Document Clinical Pathway items on Clinical Pathway.**

CLINICAL PATHWAY NAME:

	DATE				
Year					
Month	TIME 24 hr				

NEUROLOGICAL
☐ See pre-existing condition Assessment

Alert & oriented to person, place, time. Behaviour appropriate to situation. Follow simple commands. Verbalization clear and understandable. Pupils equal. Purposeful movement of all extremities and symmetry of strength. Sensation intact. Swallows without choking. **Post Op:** Mild to moderately sedated for first 24 hours. Easy to rouse.

SLEEP
☐ See pre-existing condition Assessment

Patient wakes feeling rested or sleep pattern within patient's norm.

CARDIOVASCULAR
☐ See pre-existing condition Assessment

Regular radial pulse 60 to 100 bpm. No edema, no chest pain, no diaphoresis. No calf tenderness. BP – Systolic 90 – 140. Diastolic 50 – 90 mmHg.

RESPIRATORY
☐ See pre-existing condition Assessment

Respirations quiet, regular, unlaboured, 10 – 20 per min. at rest. Sputum absent or clear. No pallor or cyanosis of nailbeds or mucous membranes. Oximetry as per patient standard. **Auscultation:** Breath sounds clear & audible both lung fields. **BiPAP:** 1=Mask off. 2=Mask on.

Assessment Auscultation
BiPAP
Chest Physio
Tracheotomy Care
Suctioning

PERIPHERAL VASCULAR
☐ See pre-existing condition Assessment

Extremities pink, warm. Sensation present. Peripheral pulses palpable. No limb edema, no calf tenderness. Capillary refill < 3 seconds. **CSM**-Pulses 0=Absent 1+=Weak & Thready 2+=Normal 3+=Full and Bounding. Sensation/movement - (all limbs) Y-Yes N-No

CSM Location: Pulses
Sensation/Movement

Page 1 of 2

INTERDISCIPLINARY SYSTEMS ASSESSMENT FLOWSHEET
Initial all relevant items. Leave others blank.
Document Clinical Pathway items on Clinical Pathway.

CLINICAL PATHWAY NAME:

	DATE				
Year					
Month	TIME 24 hr				

GASTROINTESTINAL
☐ See pre-existing condition Assessment

No nausea, vomiting or pain. Bowel movements within patient's norm. Continent. Abdomen soft. Bowel sounds active in all 4 quadrants. **Post-op:** bowel sounds: Absent – sluggish – normal first 24 hrs. **Post-op:** nausea (scale 0-5). 0=none, 1-2=mild, 3-4=moderate, 5=severe. **Nasogastric drainage:** bile coloured fluid.

Bowel sounds | Hypoactive
| Absent
Nausea Scale
Skin Care Protocol
Nasogastric Drainage (Colour)

GENITOURINARY
☐ See pre-existing condition Assessment Genitalia

Genitalia: No edema, bruising, lesions, abnormal discharge. **Vaginal Flow:** Scant to moderate, light pink to serosanguinous to brownish drainage. No foul odours or bright red bleeding. Few clots may be present. **Bladder:** Able to empty bladder. Output: >30 cc q 1 h. Not distended. Urine clear, yellow to amber, continent. No pain or burning on voiding. **Catheter:** Urinary drainage system patent. Cleansed q shift. Change as per protocol - Δ.

Assessment Vaginal Flow

☐ See pre-existing condition Assessment Bladder

Catheter | ☐ Indwelling ☐ Intermittent
Sitz Bath

MUSCULOSKELETAL/ ADL
☐ See pre-existing condition Assessment

No swelling, tenderness, weakness or muscle spasms. Functional ROM for all joints. **Mobility:** Able to ambulate; steady balance; purposeful gait. Functional ROM for all joints. **Post op:** as ordered. **ADL**=Progressing to optimal level of functioning. **Mobility/ADL Levels:** 1-Total Assistance 2-Maximum Assistance 3-Moderate Assistance 4-Minimum Assistance 5-Supervision Only 6-Independent with Aide 7-Independent.

Mobility
ADL
Activity

PSYCHOSOCIAL DISCHARGE PLANNING

Psychosocial: Has realistic perception of what is happening. Affect appropriate. No mood swings noted. **Discharge Planning:** Plans progressing according to Care Plan.

Assessment: Psychosocial
Discharge Planning

Page 2 of 2

Figure 16-3 Example of a standardized form (in this case, a client care flow sheet) that can be used for charting by exception; predefined normal assessment findings are listed on the form, and the nurse notes when assessment findings are not normal or have changed. ADL, activities of daily living; AP, anteroposterior (film); BiPAP, bilevel positive airway pressure; CSM, circulation, sensation, and movement; ROM, range of motion; subcut, subcutaneous; TPN, total parenteral nutrition. **Source:** Courtesy Queensway-Carleton Hospital (2004), Nepean, Ontario.

PATIENT CARE SERVICES
Interdisciplinary Care Flowsheet

Queensway Carleton Hospital

Key: Initials in Box = Assessment findings meet standards and procedures.
Interventions tolerated or care provided.

* & Initials in Box = Significant finding(s) **abnormal or changed.**
Document in progress notes.

→ & Initials in Box = Significant finding(s) **has not changed.**

√ = Monitored on High Frequency Flow Sheet.

*Initial all relevant items. Leave others blank. **Document Clinical Pathway items on Clinical Pathway.***

CLINICAL PATHWAY NAME:

Year	DATE	
Month	TIME 24 hr	

NUTRITION

Maintaining healthy body weight. Feeds self. No dehydration. **Oral Intake:** Consuming at least 3/4 of prescribed diet. **Swallowing:** No coughing/choking on liquids/solids. **Tube Feed/TPN:** Tolerating prescribed type, rate & amount of feeding. Flush entral tube and change dressing as per protocol. ∆=dressing change

☐ See pre-existing condition Assessment

Assessment: Oral Intake

Assessment: Swallowing

Assessment: Tube Feeding/TPN

INTEGUMENTARY

Skin warm, dry & intact; mucous membranes moist. Able to reposition self. Normal Braden Scale.

☐ See pre-existing condition Assessment

Hygiene

Reposition as per protocol

Pressure support surface: _____

WOUND / ULCER / INCISION

Site: No redness, inflammation. Incision well approximated. Sutures, steristrips, staples intact. D/C=staples, sutures removed. **Stage:** I-red, non-blanchable, II-blister, broken epidermis, III-subcutaneous tissue visible, IV-muscle, bone or tendon exposed, X-black necrotic tissue on wound. **Dressing:** dry and intact. ∆=dressing change. **Drainage:** S=serous, SG=serosanguineous **Amount:** 1=nil, 2=small, 3=moderate, 4=copious.

Site 1: _____
Assessment/Stage

Dressing Type: _____

Drainage

Site 2: _____
Assessment

Dressing Type: _____

Drainage

Site 3: _____
Assessment

Dressing Type: _____

Drainage

Page 1 of 2

INTERDISCIPLINARY CARE FLOWSHEET
Complete and initial all relevant items. Leave others blank.
Document Clinical Pathway items on Clinical Pathway.

CLINICAL PATHWAY NAME:

Year	DATE	
Month	TIME 24 hr	

PAIN / COMFORT

Patient describes pain as nil, mild, or moderate & is satisfied with management.
Pain Scale: 0-10 (none to excruciating)

Location #1
Pain Score
Location #2
Pain Score

Ice/heat

SAFETY

Low risk for falls or wandering. Basic safety precautions in place. Low risk to harm self or others. Restrained as per protocol.

Assessment

Restraint: _____

TEACHING / LEARNING

Verbalizing & understands treatment goals & care needs. Educational goals met as per teaching plan.

Assessment

PERIPHERAL / CENTRAL LINES / SALINE LOCK

Absence of redness, swelling or tenderness at site. IV infusing at prescribed rate. IV site checked as per protocol. Saline lock patent. Flushed as per protocol. ∆=dressing change

Site Assessment
☐Lock ☐Peripheral ☐Central
☐Other ☐S/C line

Site Assessment
☐Lock ☐Peripheral ☐Central
☐Other ☐S/C line

Site Assessment
☐Lock ☐Peripheral ☐Central
☐Other ☐S/C line

DRAINS

Patent & draining as expected. **Drainage:** S=serous, SS=sanguineous, SG=serosanguineous.
P=purulent, B=bile, I=Irrigated
Amount: 1=nil, 2=small, 3=moderate, 4=copious, SH=shortened D/C=discontinued

Type: _____
Location #1:
Type: _____
Location #2:
Type: _____
Location #3:
Type: _____
Location #4:

TRANSURETHRAL PROCEDURES

Urine: C=Clear, P=pink, T=tea coloured, M=moderate sanguineous, SC=Sanguineous with clots, D/C=discontinued.

Bladder — Continuous
Irrigation — Intermittent

Urine Drainage

CHEST TUBE

Patent. Dressing dry and intact. Suction method as ordered. **Drainage:** S=serous, SS=sanguineous SG=serosanguineous, P=purulent.

Assessment

Drainage

CAST SITE

Cast dry and intact; nil-minimal drainage; sensation normal; swelling nil-minimal. Damp 24-48 hours.

Assessment

Damp

Page 2 of 2

Figure 16-3 Continued

The Ottawa | L'Hôpital
Hospital | d'Ottawa

CLINICAL PATHWAY – PLAN CLINIQUE

Hemi-Knee Arthroplasty
Hemi-genou arthroplastie

☐ Civic   ☐ Gen.-Gén.

Addressograph/Plaque

IN PATIENT
5
FLOW SHEET

PAU — Unité pré-admission	Day of Surgery Pre-op — SDA/SDCU — Jour de la chirurgie pré-opératoire
Date: yyaa _____ mm _____ dj _____	Date: yyaa _____ mm _____ dj _____
Critical Path	**Critical Path**

• Assessment & teaching per PAU standard of care and procedure specific education material
• Pre-operative diagnostic testing as per PAU Medical Directive for Pre-Admission Diagnostic Testing for Elective Surgery
 	
Tests
• CBC
• PTT, INR
• Type and screen
 	
Additional Orders
• Social work consult if indicated
• X-ray:
 1) Standing AP of both knees
 2) Lateral and skyline patella view of operative knee
 	
Discharge Planning
• Discuss expected length of stay (LOS)
• Discuss issues that could cause delay of discharge & discuss discharge preparation
• Provide patient with Hemi-Knee Arthroplasty education booklet
	• Assessment and teaching per same day admission standard of care and procedure specific education material.
	
	Tests
	• Glucose meter: for diabetic patient
	• PTT/INR: for patient normally taking warfarin (Coumadin) – Unless normal result obtained after warfarin discontinued per pre-op instructions
	• Electrolytes: for dialysis dependant patient unless acceptable post-dialysis results obtained within 24 h of surgery
	• CBC if autologous blood donor
	
	Additional Orders
	• IV NS at 50 mL/h if IV medications to be given in SDA/SDCU
	  OR
	  If patient is insulin-dependent diabetic: IV D5W @ 100 mL/h
	
	Antibiotics:
	• If No history of allergy to penicillin or to other beta-lactam antibiotics;
	  or
	• History of non-life threatening reaction to penicillin or other beta-lactam antibiotics
	  (eg. rash, diarrhea, stomach upset)
	
	IV Cefazolin *on chart for administration in OR:*
	• 1 g if weight < 60 kg
	• 2 g if weight ≥ 60 kg
	Or
	• If patient has a history of life threatening reaction (hypotension, bronchospasm, urticaria, angioedema) to penicillin or other beta-lactam antibiotics
	
	IV Vancomycin:
	• 1 g if weight < 90 kg (infuse over 60 minutes pre-op)
	• 1.5 g if weight ≥ 90 kg (infuse over 90 minutes pre-op)

Patient Outcomes	**Patient Outcomes**
Patient/Family Teaching • Understands pre-op instructions and events • Understands usual post-op course, plan for pain management, and usual self care measures to prevent post-op complications **Discharge Planning** • Understands usual LOS • Appropriate discharge plan in place or if not suitable discharge plan in place – social work has been consulted	**Patient Teaching** • Adherence with pre-op instructions • Understands usual events/expectations of operative day • Understands usual post-op course, plan for pain management, and usual self care measures to prevent post-op complications
Patient progress corresponds with clinical pathway	**Patient progress corresponds with clinical pathway**

Nursing:
☐ Yes ☐ No Signature: _____
 	
   Time: _____ NTV – circle above, VC
	Nursing:
	☐ Yes ☐ No Signature: _____
	
	   Time: _____ NTV – circle above, VC _____

Variance Codes (VC)

186	Activity variance		**510**	Not discharged by end of pathway – non-medical reason
653	Consult not sent by Day 3		**NTV**	Non-Tracked Variance
492	Not discharged by end of pathway – continued need for acute care		**OFF**	Ordered off clinical pathway

CP 22A (REV 01–2008) (12–2006)   CHART – DOSSIER   © THE OTTAWA HOSPITAL – L'HÔPITAL D'OTTAWA

Figure 16-4 Example of a critical pathway (care map) for a hemi-knee arthroplasty. ALC, alternate level of care; AP (anterior-posterior [film]); APS, acute pain service; CBC, complete blood cell count; CPM, continuous passive motion; D/C, discontinue; DVT, deep vein thrombosis; IHT, interhospital transfer; INR, international normalized ratio; IV D5W, intravenous 5% dextrose in water; IV NS, intravenous normal saline; NPO, nothing by mouth; NVS, neurovascular system; O₂, oxygen; PRN, as needed; PACU, postanaesthesia care unit; PTT, partial thromboplastin time; SDA, same-day admission; SDCU, surgical day care unit; SpO₂, pulse oximetry; VS, vital signs. **Source:** Courtesy The Ottawa Hospital (L'Hôpital d'Ottawa) (2008), Ottawa, Ontario.

Patient(e) _____   Chart No. – N° du dossier _____

Day of Surgery Post-op / PACU Jour de la chirurgie / Post-opératoire / Unité de soins post-anesthésiques		Day of Surgery Post-op Ward Jour de la chirurgie / Post-opératoire / Unité regulière	
Date: yyaa _____ mm _____ dj _____		Date: yyaa _____ mm _____ dj _____	
Critical Path	**Patient Outcomes**	**Critical Path**	**Patient Outcomes**

• SpO$_2$ monitoring and O$_2$ administration per PACU protocol
• VS, assessment, treatment, and teaching per PACU standard of care
 	
Additional Orders
• Bedrest
• NPO to Clear fluids prn
	• Achieves PACU criteria for transfer to Ward	**Assessments/Treatments**
		• VS, NVS, pain q4h x 24 hrs, SpO$_2$
		• Monitor Hemovac drainage
		• Monitor Dressing
		• Monitor Intake & Output
		• Pain management as per APS
		
		Activity
		• Up in chair x 1 _____ initial
		• Ambulate x 1 with assistance, if able _____ initial
		• CPM as ordered (when dressing removed)
		
		Nutrition
		• Diet as ordered
		
		Elimination
		• Catheter as ordered
		
		Patient Teaching
		• Reinforce:
		  - Deep Breathing and Coughing (DB&C)
		  - ankle pumping
		  - positioning of the leg when on back and on side
		• Pain management
		• Ensure patient has Hemi-Knee Arthroplasty booklet
		
		Discharge Planning
		• Per Discharge Preparation indicators
			Pain Control
			• Adequate pain control achieved: Pain ≤ 3 rest, ≤ 5 activity; pain not preventing movement; satisfied with pain control
			
			Activity
			• Demonstrates understanding of positioning
			
			Prevention of DVT
			• Performs ankle exercises
			
			Prevention of Infection
			• Verbalizes importance of adequate hydration
			• Performs DB&C
			
			Patient Teaching
			• Demonstrates:
			  - DB&C
			  - Positioning of leg
			  - Ankle exercises

Patient progress corresponds with clinical pathway	**Patient progress corresponds with clinical pathway**
Nursing: ☐ Yes ☐ No Signature: _____ Time: _____ NTV – circle above, VC _____	**Nursing:** **D** ☐ Yes ☐ No Signature: _____ Initials _____ Time: _____ NTV – circle above, VC _____ **E** ☐ Yes ☐ No Signature: _____ Initials _____ Time: _____ NTV – circle above, VC _____ **N** ☐ Yes ☐ No Signature: _____ Initials _____ Time: _____ NTV – circle above, VC _____

D = 8-12 h day shift	**E** = evening shift, if applicable	**N** = 8-12 h night shift

Variance Codes (VC)

186	Activity variance	**510**	Not discharged by end of pathway – non-medical reason
653	Consult not sent by Day 3	**NTV**	Non-Tracked Variance
492	Not discharged by end of pathway – continued need for acute care	**OFF**	Ordered off clinical pathway

CP 22A (2 – 5)   CHART – DOSSIER   © THE OTTAWA HOSPITAL – L'HÔPITAL D'OTTAWA

Figure 16-4 Continued

Patient(e) _____   Chart No. – N° du dossier _____

Post-op Day 1 — Jour 1 post-opératoire

Date: yyaa _____   mm _____   dj _____

Critical Path	Patient Outcomes

Critical Path

Consults
☐ Outpatient physio   *or*   ☐ Short Term Rehab

Assessments/Treatments
• VS, NVS, pain q4h → q shift, SpO$_2$
• Monitor Intake & Output
• D/C Hemovac
• D/C dressing & change to strip
 – If drainage notify MD
• Pain management as per APS. Discontinue APS modality as per weaning guideline if patient meets criteria

Activity
• DB&C
• Exercise program
• Up in chair x 2 _____ initial, _____ initial
• Ambulate x 2 with assistance: _____ initial, _____ initial
• Assistive devices, specify: _____
• CPM as ordered

Nutrition
• Diet as ordered

Elimination
• Discontinue Foley catheter

Patient Teaching
• Reinforce exercise program
• If patient on Low Molecular Weight Heparin – start self injection teaching
• Pain Management

Discharge Planning
• Equipment needs addressed
• Confirm out-patient physio if applicable
• If patient is not expected to achieve discharge criteria by Post-op Day 2, and meets the criteria for rehab, consult service for transfer
• Discharge plan confirmed with patient / family
 – If transferring to another facility:
  Specify facility _____
• Confirm (✓) arrangements re:
  ☐ Discharge Summary   ☐ Doctor's letter
  ☐ IHT / Nurses letter   ☐ Ambulance booked or transportation arranged
(see last page for rehab criteria)

Patient Outcomes

Patient Teaching
• Verbalizes understanding of "Hemi-Knee Arthroplasty" instructions and exercise program
• Understands the basics of self injection if applicable
• Demonstrates:
 – Proper positioning
 – Understanding of mobility aids

Pain Control
• Adequate pain control achieved:
 Pain ≤ 3 rest, ≤ 5 activity; pain not preventing movement; satisfied with pain control

Activity
• Completes transfer with assistance
• Performs exercises according to self directed program

Prevention of DVT
• Demonstrates appropriate exercises & positioning for prevention of DVT
• Verbalizes understanding of anticoagulant therapy

Patient progress corresponds with clinical pathway

Physiotherapy:
☐ Yes   ☐ No   Signature: _____   Time: _____   NTV – circle above, VC _____

Nursing:
D ☐ Yes   ☐ No   Signature: _____ , Initial _____   Time: _____   NTV – circle above, VC _____

E ☐ Yes   ☐ No   Signature: _____ , Initial _____   Time: _____   NTV – circle above, VC

N ☐ Yes   ☐ No   Signature: _____ , Initial _____   Time: _____   NTV – circle above, VC _____

D = 8-12 h day shift	**E** = evening shift, if applicable	**N** = 8-12 h night shift

Variance Codes (VC)

186	Activity variance	**510**	Not discharged by end of pathway – non-medical reason
653	Consult not sent by Day 3	**NTV**	Non-Tracked Variance
492	Not discharged by end of pathway – continued need for acute care	**OFF**	Ordered off clinical pathway

© THE OTTAWA HOSPITAL – L'HÔPITAL D'OTTAWA   CHART – DOSSIER   CP 22A (3 – 5)

Figure 16-4 Continued

Patient(e) _____   Chart No. – N° du dossier _____

Post-op Day 2 / Discharge Day — Jour 2 post-opératoire / Jour de congé

Date: yyaa _____   mm _____   dj _____

Critical Path	Patient Outcomes

Assessments/Treatments
• VS / NVS q shift, SpO$_2$
• Pain q4h
• Wound care
 	
Activity
• Continue exercise program
• Ambulate x 2
• CPM as ordered
• Assistive devices, specify: _____
• Gait training on stairs if required
 	
Nutrition
• Diet as ordered
 	
Elimination
• Assess for patient's normal bowel pattern
 	
Patient Teaching
• Review physician specific discharge instructions and provide discharge instruction sheet
• Assess patient for knowledge of discharge instructions / Hemi-Knee Arthroplasty precautions
• Review anticoagulant therapy and self injection teaching if applicable
• Review Question and Answer sheet in booklet
• Review pain management plan
 	
Discharge Planning
• Patient to be discharged unless otherwise indicated by physician
• Discharge patient after seen by Physio in p.m., once discharge criteria met
• If unable to discharge today:
  – Verify ALC status if discharge delayed and acute care no longer required
  – Document appropriate delay of discharge variance code
  – Discontinue pathway after Day 2
	Discharge Criteria
	• Patient / family understand post-discharge care and follow-up plan
	• Adequate pain control
	• No clinical evidence of DVT
	• If patient on Low Molecular Weight Heparin – is able to give own injection
	• No clinical signs of infection
	• Adequate bowel function and understands bowel managment plan
	• Appropriate gait aides arranged
	• Ambulates independently with assistive devices
	• Safe on stairs (if needed)
	• Transfers independently with mobility devices
	• Appropriate place to go and support available as required post-discharge

Patient progress corresponds with clinical pathway

Physiotherapy:

☐ Yes ☐ No   Signature: _____   Time: _____   NTV – circle above, VC _____

Nursing:

D ☐ Yes ☐ No   Signature: _____ , Initial _____   Time: _____   NTV – circle above, VC _____

E ☐ Yes ☐ No   Signature: _____ , Initial _____   Time: _____   NTV – circle above, VC _____

N ☐ Yes ☐ No   Signature: _____ , Initial _____   Time: _____   NTV – circle above, VC _____

D = 8-12 h day shift	**E** = evening shift, if applicable	**N** = 8-12 h night shift

Variance Codes (VC)

186	Activity variance	**510**	Not discharged by end of pathway – non-medical reason
653	Consult not sent by Day 3	**NTV**	Non-Tracked Variance
492	Not discharged by end of pathway – continued need for acute care	**OFF**	Ordered off clinical pathway

CP 22A (4 – 5)   CHART – DOSSIER   © THE OTTAWA HOSPITAL – L'HÔPITAL D'OTTAWA

Figure 16-4 Continued

Common Record-Keeping Forms

A variety of forms are specially designed for the type of information that nurses routinely document. The categories within a form are usually derived from institutional standards of practice or guidelines established by accrediting agencies.

Admission Nursing History Forms

A nursing history form is completed when a client is admitted to a nursing care unit. The history form guides the nurse through a complete assessment to identify relevant nursing diagnoses or problems (see Chapter 13). Data on history forms provide baselines that can be compared with changes in the client's condition.

Flow Sheets and Graphic Records

Flow sheets are forms in which nurses can quickly and easily enter assessment data about the client, including vital sign measurements and routine repetitive care actions, such as hygiene measures, ambulation, meals, weights, and safety and restraint checks (Box 16–4). The format of the flow sheet varies in accordance with the agency and the data being recorded. For example, some flow sheets may be used only to record vital sign measurements (often called *graphic records*); others may be more comprehensive (Figure 16–5; note that Figure 16–3 shows a flow sheet that is used for CBE). For flow sheets, a coding system is used for data entry. It is important to fill out all spaces on the flow sheet, even for items that are "not applicable" (for which you can write "N/A"). A blank space can raise doubts about whether an intervention was or was not performed. If an occurrence recorded on the flow sheet is unusual or changes significantly, a focus note is needed (see Box 16–3). For example, if a client's blood pressure becomes dangerously high, the nurse completes a focus assessment and records the findings, as well as action taken, in the progress notes. Flow sheets provide a quick, easy reference for the health care team members in assessing a client's status. Critical care and acute care units commonly use flow sheets for all types of physiological data.

Client Care Summary or Kardex

Many agencies now have computerized systems that provide basic, summative information in the form of a client care summary. This is printed out for each client during each shift. This summary is continually updated and provides the nurse with a current detailed list of orders, treatment, and diagnostic testing. In some settings, a **Kardex** system, a portable "flip-over" file or notebook, is kept at the nurses' station. Most Kardex forms have an activity and treatment section and a nursing care plan section that organize information for quick

> **BOX 16-3**   **Example of Variance Documentation**

A 56-year-old client is on a surgical unit one day after a bowel resection. His temperature is slightly elevated, his breath sounds are decreased bilaterally at the bases of both lobes of the lungs, and he is slightly confused. Ordinarily, one day postoperatively, a client should be afebrile with clear lungs. The following is an example of the variance documentation for this client.

9/23/05
1000 hrs: Breath sounds diminished bilaterally at the bases. T [temperature] 37.8°C; P 92; R 28/min; oxygen saturation 84%. Daughter states he is "confused" and did not recognize her when she arrived a few minutes ago. Oxygen started at 2 L/min via nasal prongs as per standing orders. Will monitor pulse oximetry and vital signs every 15 minutes. Dr. P. Yoshida notified of change in status. Daughter at bedside. R. Balliol, RN

> **BOX 16-4**   **Benefits of Using a Flow Sheet**

- Information is accessible to all members of the health care team.
- Time spent on writing a narrative note is decreased.
- Information is current.
- Errors resulting from transfer of information are decreased.
- Team members can quickly see trends over time.

reference as nurses give change-of-shift reports or make walking rounds. An updated Kardex form eliminates the need for repeated referral to the chart for routine information throughout the day. In many institutions, entries on Kardex forms are made in pencil because of the need for frequent revisions as the client's needs change. In settings in which the Kardex form is a permanent part of the client's record, entries are made in ink. Information commonly found on the client care summary or Kardex form includes the following:

- Basic demographic data (e.g., age, sex, religious affiliation)
- Hospital identification number
- Physician's name
- Primary medical diagnosis
- Medical and surgical history
- Current physician's or nurse practitioner's treatment orders to be carried out by the nurse (e.g., dressing changes, ambulation, glucose monitoring)
- Nursing care plan
- Nursing orders (e.g., education sessions, symptom relief measures, counselling)
- Scheduled tests and procedures
- Safety precautions to be used in the client's care
- Factors related to activities of daily living
- Contact information about nearest relative or guardian or person to contact in an emergency
- Emergency code status
- Allergies

Acuity Records or Workload Measurement Systems

Acuity records (also known as **workload measurement systems**) provide a method of determining the hours of care and staff required for a given group of clients. A client's *acuity level* is based on the type and number of nursing interventions required for providing care in a 24-hour period. The acuity level determined by the nursing care allows clients to be rated in comparison with one another. For example, an acuity system might rate bathing clients from 1 to 5 (1 means client is totally dependent on others for bathing, 5 means client bathes independently). A client who has just undergone surgery and who requires frequent monitoring and extensive care may be listed with an acuity level of 1. On the same continuum, another client awaiting discharge after a successful recovery from surgery has an acuity level of 5. Accurate acuity ratings may also be used to justify overtime and the number and qualifications of staff needed to safely care for clients. The client-to-staff ratios established for a unit depend on a composite gathering of data for the 24-hour interventions that are necessary for each client receiving care.

Standardized Care Plans

Some institutions use **standardized care plans** to make documentation easier for nurses. The plans, based on the institution's standards of nursing practice, are preprinted, established guidelines that are used to care for clients who have similar health problems. After a nursing assessment is completed, the staff nurse identifies the standard care plans that are appropriate for the client. The care plans are

Ottawa–Carleton Hospital Post-Op Flow Sheet

Key to Amount
- – Nil
s – Small
M – Moderate
L – Large
Sc – Scant

Key to Colour
br – Bright Red
dr – Dark Red
b – Brown
dg – Dark Green
lg – Light Green
y – yellow
p – pink

Key to Urine Colour
c – clear
tc – tea colour
p – pink
br – bright red
dr – dark red
rc – red with clots
b – brown

DATE   MONTH   YEAR

TIME

PAIN
- absent/comfortable
- relieved with meds
- meds not effective

CHEST
- clear
- congested
- D B & C
- D B & C with encouragement

ABDOMEN
- soft
- distended

BOWEL SOUNDS
- absent
- sluggish
- normal
- passing flatus

DRESSING
- dry, intact
- reinforced
- amount of drainage (key)
- colour of drainage (key)

DIET
NPO
- sips/ice chips
- fluids
- diet tolerated
- diet not tolerated

Ottawa–Carleton Hospital Post-Op Flow Sheet

Key to Amount
- – Nil
s – Small
M – Moderate
L – Large
Sc – Scant

Key to Colour
br – Bright Red
dr – Dark Red
b – Brown
dg – Dark Green
lg – Light Green
y – yellow
p – pink

Key to Urine Colour
c – clear
tc – tea colour
p – pink
br – bright red
dr – dark red
rc – red with clots
b – brown

DATE   MONTH   YEAR

TIME

AMBULATION
- active exercise in bed
- dangles
- up as ordered
- up and about
- not tolerating activity

URINE
- colour (key)

P.V. LOSS
- colour (key)
- amount (key)

CIRCULATION
- temp. satis.
- temp. unsatis.
- pulses   – present
           – absent
- edema   – absent
           – present
- cyanosis/pallor
- sensation – absent
            – present

DRAINAGE
- N.G. tube
- colour (key)

Figure 16–5 Example of a client care flow sheet. D B & C, deep breathing and coughing; N.G., nasogastric; NPO, nothing by mouth. **Source:** Adapted from Ottawa–Carleton Hospital, 2000. Queensway-Carleton Campus. Nepean, ON: Author.

placed in the client's health care record. The standardized plans can be modified (and changes are noted in ink) to individualize the therapies. Most standardized care plans also allow the nurse to write in specific goals or desired outcomes of care and the dates by which these outcomes should be achieved.

One advantage of standardized care plans is establishment of clinically sound standards of care for similar groups of clients. These standards can be useful when quality improvement audits are conducted. These care plans can help nurses recognize the accepted requirements of care for clients and also improve continuity of care.

The use of standardized care plans is controversial. The major disadvantage is the risk that the standardized plans prevent nurses from providing unique, individualized therapies for clients. Standardized care plans cannot replace the nurse's professional judgement and decision making. In addition, care plans need to be updated on a regular basis to ensure that content is current and appropriate.

Discharge Summary Forms

It is important to prepare clients for an efficient, timely discharge from a health care facility. A client's discharge should also result in desirable outcomes. Multidisciplinary involvement in discharge planning helps ensure that a client leaves the hospital in a timely manner with the necessary resources in place (Box 16–5).

Ideally, discharge planning begins at admission. You need to revise the care plan as the client's condition changes. Remember to involve the client and family members in the discharge planning process so that they have the information needed to return the client home. Discharge information and instructions should include data such as the following:

- Instruction about potential food–drug interactions, nutrition intervention, and modified diets
- Rehabilitation techniques to support adaptation to, or functional independence in, the environment, or both
- Access to available community resources
- Circumstances in which clients should obtain further treatment or follow-up care
- Methods of obtaining follow-up care
- The client's and family's responsibilities in the client's care
- Medication instructions, including the times and reasons to take each medication, the dose, the route, precautions, possible adverse reactions, and information about when and how to get prescriptions refilled

Furthermore, a common standard in nursing practice is to educate clients about the nature of their disease process, its likely progress, and the signs and symptoms of complications.

When a client is discharged from inpatient care, a discharge summary that includes information from members of the health care team is prepared. The summary is given to the client or family or to the home care, rehabilitation, or long-term care agency. Discharge summary forms help make the summary concise and instructive (Figure 16–6). A summary form emphasizes previous learning by the client and family and care that should be continued in any restorative care setting. When given directly to clients, the form may be attached to pamphlets or teaching brochures.

Home Health Care Documentation

As a result of shorter hospitalizations and larger numbers of older adults who require home care services, home health care is expanding. Because clients are leaving acute care settings earlier, increasing numbers of home care clients are presenting in the community setting with more acuity (i.e., sicker). The focus in home health care is on family-centered care and forming a partnership or collaboration with the client and the family to help the client regain health, help the family take over the client's care, or to help accomplish both. Documentation in the home health care system has different implications than in other areas of nursing. Two primary differences are that the majority of the care is performed by the client and family and that the nurse is often teaching and helping the client and family achieve greater independence. Nurses must have astute assessment skills to gather the needed information about changes in the client's health care status. In addition, documentation systems need to provide the entire health care team with the information needed for them to work together effectively (Box 16–6).

In the home care setting, the client is the guardian of the health care record. A hard copy of the health care record is kept in the client's home, and the client is responsible for its safekeeping. Communication is crucial in home care because much of the interaction between health care professionals is conducted virtually by phone or fax over password-protected voice mail or secure fax lines. With the increasing availability of hand-held devices such as **personal digital assistants** and laptop computers or tablets, records can be available in multiple locations, which enables easier access to the multidisciplinary needs that are often associated with home care. Privacy remains a unique challenge in home health care, however, inasmuch as not all member of the health care team have access to secure electronic transmission of confidential material (e.g., as is the case in physicians' offices).

> **BOX 16-5** **Discharge Summary Information**

- Use clear, concise descriptions in client's own language.
- Provide step-by-step description of how to perform a procedure (e.g., home medication administration). Reinforce explanation with printed instructions.
- Identify precautions to follow when the client performs self-care or administers medications.
- Review signs and symptoms of complications that should be reported to the primary care practitioner.
- List names and phone numbers of health care professionals and community resources that the client can contact.
- Identify any unresolved problem, including plans for follow-up and continuous treatment.
- List actual time of discharge, mode of transportation, and who accompanied the client.

> **BOX 16-6** **Home Care Forms for Documentation**

The usual forms used to document home care include the following:
- Assessment forms
- Referral source information or intake form
- Discipline-specific care plans
- Physician's plan of treatment
- Professional order form (e.g., MD, speech language pathologist, specialty nurses)
- Medication administration record
- Clinical progress notes
- Miscellaneous (case conference notes, professional communication forms, private billing forms, insurance company forms)
- Discharge summary

Adapted from Iyer, P. W., & Camp, N. H. (1999). *Nursing documentation: A nursing process approach.* St. Louis: Mosby.

Ottawa–Carleton Hospital
Discharge Protocol

ADMITTING INFORMATION
(Completed by Nurse on Admission)

Admission Date: _____ Doctor: _____ Diagnosis: _____

Support Systems: □ Spouse □ Children □ Friend/Neighbour □ None
□ Other: _____

Community Services: CCAC: □ Nursing □ OT □ PT □ Homemaking
□ GAOT □ Helpline □ Day Hospital □ Meals on Wheels
□ Seniors Support □ Other (describe): _____

If not admitted from home, name of facility: _____

DISCHARGE SUMMARY (Completed on Discharge)
Discharge Date: _____ Time: _____ Level: _____ Quad: _____

Discharge Destination: □ Home alone □ Home with other: _____
□ Facility: _____ □ Informed of DC Date: _____
□ Transfer & Referral Form □ Transportation arranged: _____

Accompanied By: □ Spouse □ Relative/friend □ Alone □ Other: _____

Appliances/Aids: □ None □ Crutches □ Cane □ Walker □ Other: _____

Community Referrals Arranged: CCAC: □ Nursing □ OT □ PT □ Homemaking
□ GAOT □ Helpline □ Day Hospital □ Meals on Wheels
□ Seniors Support □ Other (describe): _____

Outpatient Follow-Up: □ None □ Clinic □ Physician's office □ Other: _____
□ Tests _____

Discharge Medications: □ None   Prescription □ Yes □ No   Teaching □ Yes □ No   Comments: _____

Discharge Teaching Completed: □ Yes □ No   Comments: _____

Incision Assessed: □ Yes □ No □ Not applicable

Patient's Condition on Discharge:
Bladder Function: □ Good □ Fair □ Poor   Independence: □ Good □ Fair □ Poor
Bowel Function: □ Good □ Fair □ Poor   Nutrition: □ Good □ Fair □ Poor
Emotional Status: □ Good □ Fair □ Poor   Skin: □ Good □ Fair □ Poor

Date: _____   Nurse's Signature: _____

KEY: ADL = Activities of Daily Living
CNS = Clinical Nurse Specialist
GAOT = Geriatric Assessment Outreach Team
N/A = Not Applicable
RRT = Registered Respiratory Therapist
ARDU = Alzheimer & Related Disorder Unit
DC = Discharge
LTC = Long-Term Care
OT = Occupational Therapy
Rx = Treatment
CCAC = Community Care Access Centre
Dx = Diagnosis
MRSA = Methicillin-Resistant Staphylococcus Aureus
PT = Physiotherapy
SOB = Short of Breath

CLIENT PROBLEMS (Referral Criteria):
Multidisciplinary Team members to ✓ and date problems applicable to client.

MEDICAL HISTORY
□ Many chronic medical problems Refer: Social Worker CNS (if patient >75 yrs)
□ Many ER visits or hospital admissions Refer: Social Worker
□ Cancer, AIDS/HIV, or terminal illness & client/family needing support Dr. to consider Palliative Care
□ Behavioural or psychological problems Dr. to consider Geriatrician, Psychogeriatric/Psychiatry, ARDU
□ Other (describe)

HEALTH MANAGEMENT
□ Positive MRSA screen Refer: Infection Control
□ Needs stress management training Refer: OT

MEDICATIONS
□ Noncompliant or needs education
□ Uncertain of drug allergy reaction
□ DC medications differ from admission & is taking >6 schedule medications
□ Frequent medication changes or multiple generic brands, numerous herbal preparation Refer: Pharmacist
□ Taking multiple medications (>75 yr) Refer: CNS
□ Other (describe)

RESPIRATORY
□ O2 titration, spirometry
□ Home O2 or home O2 candidate
□ Needs education: disease, devices Candidate for Asthma Clinic Refer: RRT
□ Respiratory problem with mobility restrictions & safety issues Refer: CNS
□ Respiratory deficiency, SOB, difficulty clearing secretions Refer: PT
□ Pneumonia Refer: PT Refer: RRT
□ Other (describe)

ELIMINATION
□ Stoma care problem (any age)
□ Altered bowel function
□ Altered urinary function Refer: CNS
□ Other (describe)

COGNITIVE & SENSORY
□ Cognitive impairment Refer: OT Refer: CNS (if patient >75 yr)
□ Motivational problems Refer: CNS (if patient >75 yr) Refer: OT
□ Other (describe)

SKIN
□ Delayed wound healing
□ Decubitus ulcer, exudating open wound, large burn, nutritional edema
□ Positioning & pressure relief Refer: Dietitian Refer: CNS Refer: OT
□ Limited mobility due to wound on joint Refer: PT Refer: CNS
□ Lymphedema, skin care problem Refer: CNS
□ Other (describe)

PAIN
□ Needs pain/symptom management Dr. to consider Palliative Care
□ Origin is musculoskeletal, articular, neural, gross edema
□ Palliative patient with pain Refer: PT Refer: OT
□ Other (describe)

NUTRITION
□ Dysphagia Refer: Speech Therapy Refer: Dietitian
□ Malnutrition or weight loss
□ Inadequate food intake (prolonged) Special diet
□ Enteral/parenteral nutrition Needs diet intervention/teaching
□ Diabetic — new or uncontrolled Candidate for Diabetes Info. Program Candidate for Lipid Clinic Refer: Dietitian
□ Other (describe)

□ Communication difficulty (recent) Refer: Speech Therapy
□ Other (describe)

MOBILITY
□ Concern for ADL safety/independence
□ Need for wheelchair
□ Meal preparation Refer: OT Refer: Dietitian
□ Restricted/unsafe mobility
□ Severe general weakness/balance difficulties
□ Recent inability to do stairs at home
□ Problem moving in bed or transferring Refer: PT Refer: CNS (if patient >75 yr)
□ Other (describe)

PSYCHOSOCIAL
□ Lives alone and at risk
□ Unable to return to previous living situation
□ Financial concerns for living needs
□ Indications of abuse
□ Needs 24-h supervision
□ Anticipated DC to a facility
□ Sole caregiver for dependent person
□ Caregiver unable to manage Refer: Social Worker Refer: CNS (if patient >75 yr) Refer: OT Refer: Geriatric Day Hospital
□ Other (describe)

SPIRITUAL
□ Fear or anxiety related to Dx or Rx
□ Questioning meaning or purpose of life, self or situation, values & beliefs
□ Non-urgent sacramental care needed Refer: Hospital Chaplain
□ Acute fear or anxiety or grief Urgent sacramental care needed Notify on-call chaplain
□ Other (describe)

Figure 16-6 Example of a discharge summary form. AIDS, acquired immune deficiency syndrome; HIV, human immunodeficiency virus. **Source:** Adapted from Ottawa-Carleton Hospital, 2000. Queensway-Carleton Campus. Nepean, ON: Author.

Long-Term Health Care Documentation

An increasing number of older adults require care in long-term care or residential facilities. Many individuals live in this setting for the rest of their lives and are therefore referred to as **residents** rather than as *clients*. In long-term care settings, nursing personnel face challenges much different from those in acute care settings. Residents' health is often stable, and so daily documentation can be completed on flow sheets. Assessments performed several times a day in acute care settings are required only weekly or monthly in long-term care settings.

Governmental agencies and provincial and territorial laws are instrumental in determining the standards and policies for documentation. Documentation is used to review the levels of care given to and needed by residents in long-term care facilities. Although most long-term care facilities have different documentation systems, these systems are based on the need for a concise, nonduplicating method of documentation and on the importance of nursing documentation in support of evidence-informed practice (Box 16–7).

Computerized Documentation

Many hospitals are using computerized documentation systems or are in the process of transitioning to computerized charting. Current software programs enable nurses to quickly enter specific assessment data, fill in forms with typical entry choices, and enter narrative for unique situations; computer memory is also adequate for large amounts of data, and information can be automatically transferred to different reports. Computers can also help generate nursing care plans and document all facets of client care.

Hand-held devices such as personal digital assistants also have the potential to increase nursing productivity by providing access to clinical and reference material, providing a means for decreasing medication

---

errors, and reducing documentation time (Scordo, Yeager, & Young, 2003). Nurses can document at the client's bedside—at the point of care. **Point-of-care information systems** consist of hand-held devices such as personal digital assistants or computers that nurses bring to the client's bedside.

Nursing Information Systems

A good information system supports the work you do. As a nurse, you need to be able to easily access a computer program, review the client's medical history and physician order, and then go to the client's bedside to conduct a comprehensive assessment. Once you have completed the assessment, you enter data into the computer terminal at the client's bedside and develop a plan of care from the information gathered. Periodically, you will return to the computer to check on laboratory test results and document the therapies you administer. The computer screens and optional pop-up windows make it easy to locate information, enter and compare data, and make changes.

Nursing information systems have two basic designs. The nursing process design is the most traditional. It organizes documentation within well-established formats, such as admission and postoperative assessment, problem lists, care plans, discharge planning instructions, and intervention lists or notes. The nursing process design also includes formats for the following tasks:

- Generation of a nursing worklist that indicates routine scheduled activities related to the care of each client.
- Documentation of routine aspects of client care, such as hygiene, positioning, fluid intake and output, wound care measures, and blood glucose measurements.
- Progress note entries with the use of narrative notes, CBE, and flow sheet charting.
- Documentation of medication administration.

The second design model for a nursing information system is the protocol, or critical pathway, design (Hebda et al., 2005). This design offers a multidisciplinary format to managing information. All health care professionals use a protocol system to document the care that they provide clients. Evidence-informed clinical protocols or critical pathways provide the formatting or design for the type of information that clinicians enter into the system. The information system allows a user to select one or more appropriate protocols for a client. An advanced system merges multiple protocols so that a master protocol, or path, is used to direct client care activities. The system identifies variances of the anticipated outcomes on the protocols as they are charted. This system provides all caregivers the ability to analyze variances and to obtain an accurate clinical picture of the client's progress.

Advantages of a Nursing Information System. Few formal well-designed studies have demonstrated the impact of computerized record systems on nursing practice or client outcomes. Anecdotal reports and descriptive studies suggest that nursing information systems do offer important advantages to nurses in practice. Hebda et al. (2005) outlined some specific advantages of nursing information systems:

- Increased time to spend with clients
- Bettter access to information
- Enhanced quality of documentation
- Reduced numbers of errors of omission
- Reduced hospital costs
- Increased nurse job satisfaction
- Enhanced compliance with accreditation standards
- Development of a common clinical database

> **► BOX 16-7** | **Components of Documentation in Long-Term Care**

Section 1: The Health Care Record
The health care record includes the resident's name and medical number; date and time of admission; change in resident's condition; informed consent; note or discharge summary; incident reporting; monthly summary charting; and type of therapy and treatment time.

Section 2: Resident Assessments and Related Documents
This section consists of the admission record; preadmission assessment; admission assessment; assessment of risk for falls; skin assessment; bowel and bladder assessment; physical restraint assessment; record of self-administration of medication; nutrition assessment; and activities, recreation, or leisure interests.

Section 3: Other Records
Other records include drug therapy records, medication or treatment records, flow sheets or other graphic records, laboratory and special reports, consent forms, acknowledgements and notices, advance directives, and discharge or transfer records.

Security Mechanisms. Computerized documentation has legal risks. Any given person could theoretically access a computer station within a health care agency and obtain information about almost any client. Protection of privacy of information in computer systems is a top priority. As described in Chapter 17, Canada has both provincial and national privacy legislation to protect personal health information in electronic or other form.

In most security mechanisms for information systems, a combination of logical and physical restrictions is used to protect information and computer systems. These measures include the installation of firewalls, antivirus software, and spyware-detection software. A firewall is a combination of hardware and software that protects private network resources (e.g., a hospital's information system) from outside hackers, network damage, and theft or misuse of information. An example of a logical restriction is an automatic sign-off, a mechanism that logs a user off the computer system after a specified period of inactivity on the computer (Hebda et al., 2005).

Physical security measures include the placement of computers or file servers in restricted areas. This form of security may have limited benefit, especially if an organization uses mobile wireless devices such as notebooks, tablet personal computers, or personal digital assistants. Such devices can be easily misplaced or lost, which allows them to be accessed by unauthorized persons. An organization may use motion detectors or alarms with devices to help prevent theft.

One method of authenticating access to automated records is the use of access codes and passwords. A password is a collection of alphanumeric characters that a user types into the computer before he or she can access a program. A user is usually required to enter a password after the entry and acceptance of an access code or user name. A password does not appear on the computer screen when it is typed, nor should it be known to anyone but the user and information systems administrators (Hebda et al., 2005). Efficacious passwords contain combinations of letters, numbers, and symbols that are not easily guessed. When using a health care agency computer system, you must not share your computer password, under any circumstances, with anyone. A secure system requires frequent and random changes in personal passwords to prevent unauthorized persons from tampering with records. In addition, most staff members have access to clients in their work area only. Select staff members (e.g., administrators or risk managers) may be given authority to access all client records.

Handling and Disposal of Information. It is important to keep medical records confidential, but it is equally important to safeguard the information that is printed from the record or extracted for report purposes. For example, you print a copy of a nursing activities worklist to use as a day planner while administering care to clients. You refer to information on the list and hand-write notes to enter later into the computer. Information on the list is considered to be personal health information and must be kept confidential and not left out for view by unauthorized persons. You must destroy anything that is printed when the printed information is no longer needed.

All papers containing personal health information (e.g., client's health care number, date of birth, age, name, or address) must be destroyed if they are not part of the client's health record. Most agencies have shredders or locked receptacles for shredding and later incineration. Be sure you familiarize yourself with the disposal policies for records in the institution where you work.

Clinical Information Systems

Any clinician, including nurses, physicians, pharmacists, social workers, and therapists, will use programs available on a clinical information system. These programs include monitoring systems; order entry systems; and laboratory, radiology, and pharmacy systems. A monitoring system includes devices that automatically monitor and record biometric measurements (e.g., vital signs, oxygen saturation, cardiac index, and stroke volume) in critical care areas and specialty areas. The devices electronically send measurements directly to the nursing documentation systems.

Order entry systems enable nurses to order supplies and services from another department. Such systems eliminate the need for written order forms and expedite the delivery of needed supplies to a nursing unit. The **computerized physician order entry (CPOE)** is one type of order entry system gaining popularity in many larger hospitals. CPOE is a process by which the physician or nurse practitioner directly enters orders for client care into the hospital information system. CPOE can eliminate the issues related to illegible handwriting and transcription errors, prevent duplication, and speed the implementation of ordered diagnostic tests and treatments. It can improve staff productivity and save money. Orders made through CPOE are integrated within the record and sent to the appropriate departments (e.g., pharmacy and radiology). In advanced systems, CPOE is linked to **clinical decision support**, which has a range of computerized tools such as built-in reminders and alerts that help the health care professional select the most appropriate medication or diagnostic test or remind the practitioner about drug interactions, allergies, and the need for subsequent orders. Medication errors and adverse drug-related events can potentially be reduced. Few studies have measured the effects of CPOE with clinical decision support on these variables, however, and more research (especially randomized controlled trials) in this area is needed (Wolfstadt et al., 2008).

The Electronic Health Record

The traditional paper health care record no longer meets the needs of today's health care industry. A paper record is episode oriented, with a separate record for each client visit to a health care agency (Hebda et al., 2005). Key information can be lost from one episode of care to the next, which can jeopardize a client's safety. An **electronic health record (EHR)** is a longitudinal record of client health information accessible online from many separate but interoperable automated systems within an electronic network (Health Canada, 2007; see Chapter 17). A unique feature of an EHR is its ability to integrate all pertinent client information into one record, regardless of the number of times a client enters a health care system.

The development and implementation of an EHR to support effective health care delivery for Canadians is in progress through Canada Health Infoway Inc. (Infoway; Health Canada, 2007). Infoway has set a target of 50% of Canadians to have EHRs by 2010 (Canada Health Infoway, 2007).

Reporting

Nurses communicate information about clients so that all team members can make appropriate decisions about the care of clients. Any verbal report must be timely, accurate, and relevant. Some Canadian hospitals having been using the **situation–background–assessment–recommendation (SBAR)** communication technique to provide "a common and predictable structure to communication" between members of the health care team about a client's care (Leonard et al., 2004, p. 86). The SBAR technique is an attempt to align ways of communicating important information that often necessitates immediate attention, and it fosters a culture of client safety.

Nurses commonly make four types of reports: change-of-shift reports, telephone reports, transfer reports, and incident reports. The SBAR technique (Box 16–8) can be incorporated into a variety of ways of reporting (e.g., a nurse's report to a physician about a critically ill client, change-of-shift reports about individual clients) and can be adapted for use with or by other health care professionals.

Change-of-Shift Reports

At the end of each shift, nurses report information about their assigned clients to the nurses working on the next shift. The purpose of the report is to provide continuity of care among nurses who are caring for a client.

Nurses give a **change-of-shift report** orally in person, by audiotape recording, by writing information on a summary report sheet, or during "walking–planning" rounds at each client's bedside. Oral reports can be given in conference rooms, with staff members from both shifts participating. Oral reports can also take the form of one-to-one reports: for example, a report given by the night nurse to the day nurse. An advantage of oral reports is that they allow staff members to ask questions or clarify explanations. When nurses make rounds, the client and family members also have the opportunity to participate in any decisions. The nurses can see the client together to perform needed assessments, evaluate progress, and discuss the interventions best suited to the client's needs. An audiotape report is given by the nurse who has completed care for the client; this type of report is left for the nurse on the next shift to review. Taped reports can improve efficiency by being recorded before the end of the shift when time is available and by avoiding social conversations between peers. However, it is essential to schedule an opportunity for the incoming nurses to ask questions for clarification after they listen to the taped report.

Because nurses have many responsibilities, it is important to compile a change-of-shift report quickly and efficiently (Table 16–4). An effective report describes clients' health status and tells staff on the next shift exactly what kind of care the clients require. A change-of-shift report should *not* simply be a reading of documented information. Instead, significant facts about clients are reviewed (e.g., condition of wounds, episodes of chest pain) to provide a baseline for comparison during the next shift. Data about clients need to be objective, current, and concise.

An organized report follows a logical sequence. To prepare for the report, the nurse gathers information from worksheets, the client's records, and the care plan. The following is an example of a change-of-shift report:

Background information: Cy Tolan in bed 4, a 32-year-old client of Dr. Lang, is scheduled for a colon resection this morning at 0800 hours. He has had ulcerative colitis for two years with recent bouts of frank bleeding in his stools. He was admitted at 0600 hours this morning with slight abdominal discomfort. This is his first experience with surgery. He knows he may require a colostomy. He has been NPO [had nothing by mouth] since midnight at home.

Assessment: Mr. Tolan mentioned that he was unable to sleep last night. He had many questions about surgery on admission this morning.

Nursing diagnosis: His chief nursing care problems are anxiety related to inexperience with surgery and risk for body image disturbance.

Teaching plan: I talked to him about postoperative routines and answered all his questions. He attended the preoperative admission clinic two weeks ago, but he did not have as many concerns at that time. He stated that he felt less anxious now that he knows what to expect.

Treatments: I started a intravenous infusion of normal saline in his left arm at 125 mL/hr at 0645 hrs.

Family information: His wife came with him this morning and will wait in the surgical waiting room till his surgery is complete.

Discharge plan: Mr. Tolan is a very active person and participates in strenuous sports such as swimming. Mrs. Tolan is concerned about how he might react to a colostomy. I suggest making a referral to the enterostomal therapist early, if the colostomy is performed.

Priority needs: Right now, Mr. Tolan is relaxing in his room. All preoperative procedures have been completed except for his preoperative antibiotic, due on call to the operating room.

A professional demeanour is essential when you give a report about clients or family members. It is often necessary to describe the interactions among clients, nurses, and family members in behavioural terms. Nurses must avoid using judgemental language such as *uncooperative, difficult,* or *bad* when describing such behaviours.

In many settings, unregulated care providers (UCPs) are involved in the change-of-shift report. UCPs are part of the health care team and can contribute more when they also know a client's condition and the nursing team's priorities in care. The nurse can use the report to emphasize to UCPs the tasks that need to be accomplished.

Telephone Reports

Nurses inform physicians of changes in a client's condition and communicate information to nurses on other units about client transfer. The laboratory staff or a radiologist may phone to report results of

---

> **BOX 16-8** **The Situation-Background-Assessment-Recommendation (SBAR) Technique**

When calling the physician, follow the SBAR process as follows:

Situation: What is the situation you are calling about?
- Identify yourself, the unit, the client, and the room number
- Briefly state the problem: what it is, when it started, and the severity

Background: Provide background information related to the situation, including the following:
- The client's health care record
- The admitting diagnosis and date of admission
- A list of current medications, allergies, intravenous fluids, and laboratory tests
- The most recent vital signs
- Laboratory results, with the date and time each test was performed and results of previous tests for comparison
- Other clinical information
- Code status

Assessment: What is your assessment of the situation?

Recommendations: What is your recommendation, or what do you want?

Examples include the following:
- Client to be admitted
- Client to be seen now
- Order to be changed

Source: Joint Commission on Accreditation of Healthcare Organizations. (2005, February). The SBAR technique: Improves communication, enhances patient safety. *Joint Commission Perspectives on Patient Safety, 5*(2), 2.

> **TABLE 16-4**   **Change-of-Shift Reports: Dos and Don'ts**

Dos	Don'ts
Do provide only essential background information about client (i.e., name, sex, age, physician's diagnosis, and medical history).	Don't review all routine care procedures or tasks (e.g., bathing, scheduled changes).
Do identify client's nursing diagnoses or health care problems and their related causes.	Don't review all biographical information already available in written form.
Do describe objective measurements or observations about client's condition and response to health problem, and emphasize recent changes.	Don't use critical comments about client's behaviour, such as "Mrs. Wills is so demanding."
Do share significant information about family members as it relates to client's problems.	Don't make assumptions about relationships between family members.
Do continuously review ongoing discharge plan (e.g., need for resources, client's level of preparation to go home).	Don't engage in idle gossip.
Do relay to staff significant changes in the way therapies are given (e.g., different position for pain relief, new medication).	Don't describe basic steps of a procedure.
Do describe instructions given in teaching plan and client's response.	Don't explain detailed content unless staff members ask for clarification.
Do evaluate results of nursing or medical care measures (e.g., effect of back rub or analgesic administration), and describe results specifically.	Don't simply describe results as "good" or "poor."
Do be clear about priorities to which incoming staff must attend.	Don't force incoming staff to guess what to do first.

diagnostic tests. Telephone reports should provide clear, accurate, and concise information. Information in a telephone report is documented when significant events or changes in a client's condition have occurred. In documenting a phone call, the nurse includes information about when the call was made, who made it (if other than the writer of the information), who was called, to whom information was given, what information was given, and what information was received. An example is as follows: "At 1005 hrs called Dr. Morgan's office; S. Thomas, RN, was informed that Mr. Rush's stat potassium level drawn at 0800 hrs was 3.2. C. Skala, RN."

Telephone or Verbal Orders

A telephone order (often written "TO") involves a physician stating a prescribed therapy over the phone to a registered nurse. A verbal order (often written "VO") may be accepted when the physician has no opportunity to write the order, as in emergency situations. Clarifying for accuracy is important when you accept a physician's orders over the telephone or verbally. You need to verify the order by repeating it clearly and precisely. You are responsible for writing the order on the physician's order sheet in the client's permanent record and signing it. An example is as follows: "1/16/2008, 1920 hrs: acetaminophen 325 mg PO [orally] 2 tabs now and q4h [every four hours] prn [as needed]. TO Dr. Reiss/Carol Skala, RN." The physician later verifies the telephone order legally by signing it within a set time period (e.g., 24 hours). Many telephone orders are given at night or during an emergency and need to be used only when absolutely necessary. In some situations, it may be prudent to have a second person listen to telephone orders. Box 16–9 provides guidelines that can be used to prevent errors when receiving telephone orders and verbal orders.

Transfer Reports

Clients may transfer from one unit to another to receive different levels of care. For example, clients transfer from an intensive care unit or the recovery room to general nursing units when they no longer require intense monitoring. To promote continuity of care, you may give **transfer reports** by phone or in person. When giving a transfer report, you need to include the following information:

- Client's name, age, name of primary physician, and medical diagnosis
- Summary of progress up to the time of transfer
- Client's current health status (physical and psychosocial)
- Client's allergies
- Client's emergency code status
- Client's family support (e.g., spouse or partner, children, parents)

> **BOX 16-9**   **Guidelines for Telephone Orders and Verbal Orders**

- Clearly determine the client's name, room number, and diagnosis.
- Repeat any orders back to the prescribing physician.
- Ask for clarification to avoid misunderstandings.
- Write telephone order ("TO") or verbal order ("VO"), including date and time, name of client, and the complete order, and sign the names of the physician and nurse.
- Follow agency policies; some institutions require telephone (and verbal) orders to be reviewed and signed by two nurses.
- The physician must co-sign the order within the time frame required by the institution (usually 24 hours).

- Client's current nursing diagnoses or problem and care plan
- Any critical assessments or interventions to be completed shortly after transfer (helps receiving nurse to establish priorities of care)
- Need for any special equipment, such as isolation equipment, suction equipment, or traction

After completion of the transfer report, the receiving nurse needs an opportunity to ask questions about the client's status. In some cases, written documentation must include a record of information reported.

Incident Reports

An incident is any event that is not consistent with the routine operation of a health care unit or routine care of a client. Examples of incidents include client falls, needle-stick injuries, a visit by someone who has symptoms of illness, medication administration errors, accidental omission of ordered therapies, and circumstances that led to injury or risk for client injury. Analysis of **incident reports** (also known as *adverse occurrence reports*) helps with the identification of trends in systems and unit operations that justify changes in policies and procedures or the scheduling of in-service seminars. Incident reports are an important part of a unit's quality improvement program and should not be used for punitive purposes (see Chapter 11).

✲ KEY CONCEPTS

- The health care record is a legal document and requires information describing the care that is delivered to a client.
- All information pertaining to a client's health care management that is gathered by examination, observation, or conversation or as a result of treatment is confidential.
- Multidisciplinary communication is essential within the health care team.
- Accurate record keeping requires an objective interpretation of data with precise measurements, correct spelling, and proper use of abbreviations.
- A nurse's signature on an entry in a record designates that particular nurse's accountability for the contents of that entry.
- Any change in a client's condition warrants immediate documentation to keep a record accurate.
- Problem-oriented health care records are organized by the client's health care problems.
- The intent of SOAP, SOAPIE, PIE, and DAR charting is to organize entries in the progress notes according to the nursing process.
- Critical pathways or care maps provide members of the health care team with a way to document their contributions to the client's total plan of care.
- Home care documentation is accessible to a variety of caregivers in the home.
- Long-term care documentation is multidisciplinary. Assessments performed several times a day in the acute care setting are required only weekly or monthly in long-term care.
- Computerized information systems contain information about clients that is organized and easily accessible.
- Protection of the confidentiality of client health information and the security of computer systems should be a top priority.
- The major purpose of the change-of-shift report is to maintain continuity of care.
- When information pertinent to care is communicated by telephone or verbally, the information needs to be verified.
- Incident reports objectively describe any event that is not consistent with the routine care of a client.

✲ CRITICAL THINKING EXERCISES

1. Joseph Vojnovic is an 80-year-old man admitted with a diagnosis of possible pneumonia. He complains of general malaise and a frequent productive cough, worse at night. Vital sign measurements are as follows: blood pressure, 150/90 mm Hg; pulse rate, 92 beats per minute; respiration rate, 22 breaths per minute; and temperature, 38.5°C. During your initial assessment, he coughs violently for 40 to 45 seconds without expectorating. He exhibits wheezes and coarse crackles at both bases of the lungs. He states, "It hurts in my chest when I cough." Differentiate between objective and subjective data in this case example.

2. The nurse positions Mr. Vojnovic in a semi-Fowler's position, encourages him to increase his fluid intake, and gives him acetaminophen (Tylenol), 650 mg PO, as ordered for fever. One hour later, the client is resting in bed. Vital sign measurements are as follows: blood pressure, 130/86 mm Hg; pulse, 86 beats per minute; respiration rate, 22 breaths per minute; and temperature, 37.7°C. He states that he has been able to sleep. His fluid intake over the past hour has been 200 mL of water. Use the given information to write a nurse's progress note in the PIE format.

3. Near the end of your shift, you have identified *fluid volume deficit* as a nursing diagnosis for Mr. Vojnovic. Since his admission, he has had fluid intake of about 600 mL, and his urine output was 300 mL of dark, concentrated urine. His temperature is back up to 38.4°C, his mucous membranes are dry, and he states that he feels very weak. List what should be included in the change-of-shift report.

4. Several days later, after treatment with intravenous antibiotics, Mr. Vojnovic is feeling much better, and preparations are being made for discharge. He is to take cephalexin (Keflex) 500 mg every six hours, for the next 10 days; continue to drink extra fluids; and get extra rest. He lives alone. Although he is generally cooperative, he does not like drinking water or taking pills. He is to make an appointment with his physician for one week from today and should call the physician if symptoms recur. Write a discharge summary that is concise and instructive.

✲ REVIEW QUESTIONS

1. A fellow nursing student is a client in the hospital where you have your clinical placement. You became aware of his admission when you transferred your own client to his unit today. What should you do?
   1. Keep the information to yourself.
   2. Advise a few of his friends so that they can visit him.
   3. Visit him on his unit during your lunch break.
   4. Access his EHR to see if he is well enough for you to visit.

2. A manager is reviewing the nurses' notes in a community client's health care record. She finds the following entry, "Client is difficult to care for, refuses advice for improving appetite." Which of the following suggestions should the manager give to the community health nurse who entered the note?
   1. Avoid rushing when charting an entry.
   2. Use correction fluid to remove the entry.
   3. Draw a single line through the statement and initial it.
   4. Enter only objective and factual information about the client.

3. A client tells the nurse, "I have stomach cramps and feel nauseated." This is an example of which type of data?
   1. Objective
   2. Historical
   3. Subjective
   4. Assessment

4. During your visit to a client's home, your client says, "I do not know what is going on; I cannot get an explanation from my doctor about the results of my test. I want something done about this." Which of the following is the most appropriate documentation of the client's emotional status?
   1. The client has a defiant attitude.
   2. The client appears to be upset with his physician.
   3. The client is demanding and complains frequently.
   4. The client stated he felt frustrated by the lack of information he has received regarding test results.

5. Clients frequently request copies of their health care records. Which of the following statements is true regarding client access to health care records?
   1. Clients have the right to read those records.
   2. Clients are not allowed to read those records.
   3. Only the health care workers have access to the records.
   4. Only the families may read the records.

6. Accurate entries are an important characteristic of good documentation. Which of the following charting entries is most accurately written?
   1. Client ambulated in hall with assistance, exercise well tolerated.
   2. Client ambulated 15 m (50 feet) up and down hall, exercise well tolerated.
   3. Client ambulated 15 m (50 feet) up and down hall with assistance from nurse.
   4. Client ambulated 15 m (50 feet) with assistance from nurse. HR 88 before exercise and HR 94 after exercise.

7. What is the purpose of acuity records?
   1. To guide all nursing care
   2. To document the client admission
   3. To determine hours of care needed
   4. To establish guidelines for client care

8. Match the correct numbered entry with the appropriate SOAP category.

   S   1. Repositioned client on right side. Encouraged client to use patient-controlled analgesia.

   O   2. "The pain increases every time I try to turn on my left side."

   A   3. Acute pain related to tissue injury from surgical incision.

   P   4. Left lower abdominal surgical incision, 3 inches in length, closed, sutures intact, no drainage. Pain noted on mild palpation.

✷ RECOMMENDED WEB SITES

Accreditation Canada: http://www.cchsa.ca
Accreditation Canada (formerly the Canadian Council on Health Services Accreditation) is a national, nonprofit, independent organization whose role is to help health and social service organizations, across Canada and internationally, examine and improve the quality of care and service they provide to their clients through a voluntary external peer review.

Canada Health Infoway: http://www.infoway-inforoute.ca
Canada Health Infoway (Infoway) is a federally funded, independent, not-for-profit organization. Members include the 14 federal, provincial and territorial Deputy Ministers of Health. Infoway has a mandate to accelerate the use of electronic health information systems and EHRs across Canada.

Canadian Nurses Association: Provincial/Territorial Organizations: http://www.cna-aiic.ca/CNA/about/members/provincial/default_e.aspx
This part of the Web site of the Canadian Nurses Association provides links to each provincial and territorial nursing association. Most associations provide information about documentation standards and requirements in their province or territory.

Canadian Nursing Informatics Association: http://cnia.ca/
The Canadian Nursing Informatics Association (CNIA) is affiliated with the Canadian Nurses Association and has been established as the voice for health informatics in Canada. *Nursing informatics* refers to the integration of nursing science, computer science, and information science to document and communicate data and knowledge in nursing practice.

17

Nursing Informatics and Canadian Nursing Practice

Written by Kathryn J. Hannah, RN, PhD,

and Margaret Ann Kennedy, RN, PhD

objectives

Mastery of content in this chapter will enable you to:

- Define the key terms listed.
- Differentiate how nursing informatics differs from routine use of technologies in nursing practice.
- Identify key issues and challenges in managing nursing data in Canada.
- Identify and compare strategies in Canada for identifying and documenting key nursing data.
- Discuss how health information data standards influence nursing practice in Canada.
- Discuss why using the standardized nursing data is important for acknowledging the professional contributions of nursing to health outcomes of Canadians.
- Develop a beginning understanding of the scope of nursing informatics concepts and the ways in which nurses can be involved in nursing informatics.
- Discuss the relationship of national privacy legislation to nursing practice in a digital practice environment.
- Discuss how the national *E-Nursing Strategy* influences current and future nursing practice.

key terms

American Medical Informatics Association (AMIA), p. 243
Canada Health Infoway Inc. (Infoway), p. 236
Canadian Institute for Health Information (CIHI), p. 234
Canadian Nursing Informatics Association (CNIA), p. 243
Canadian Organization for Advancement of Computers in Health (COACH), p. 234
Electronic health record (EHR), p. 234
Health Information: Nursing Components (HI:NC), p. 238
Health Outcomes for Better Information and Care (HOBIC) project, p. 242
International Classification for Nursing Practice® (ICNP®), p. 239

International Council of Nurses (ICN), p. 239
International Health Terminology Standards Development Organisation (IHTSDO®), p. 236
International Medical Informatics Association (IMIA), p. 243
International Medical Informatics Association–Special Interest Group in Nursing Informatics (IMIA-SIGNI), p. 243
Nursing informatics, p. 234
Personal Information Protection and Electronic Documents Act (PIPEDA), p. 241
Standards, p. 236
Systematized NOmenclature of MEDicine—Clinical Terms (SNOMED CT®), p. 236

media resources

evolve Web Site

- Audio Chapter Summaries
- Glossary
- Multiple-Choice Review Questions
- Student Learning Activities
- Weblinks

Companion CD

- Glossary
- Interactive Learning Activities
- Fluids and Electrolytes Tutorial
- Test-Taking Skills

As health care systems respond to an increasingly complex technological environment, long-standing routines and tools are being superseded by strategic, evidence-informed practices that mandate high-quality, timely health information. In an era when complex health care is provided by dynamic multidisciplinary teams, effective nursing documentation is crucial for supporting clinical decision making, as well as for supporting aggregation with documentation from other nurses and clinical disciplines, in enabling optimal client outcomes. Current information needs in health care challenge nurses to identify the elements of their practice that are most critical for consideration in decision making. **Nursing informatics**, a specialty area of nursing practice dedicated to optimal use of technology to support professional practice and enable optimal client outcomes, has responded to this challenge and continues to support the progression of effective nursing practice and documentation.

Hannah et al. (2006) tracked the evolution of technology in health care, noting that since its introduction in the health care sector, nurses have recognized the value of technology to inform effective practice and have fostered technological development in support of client care. Current technological applications include client scheduling and transfer, billing and financial management, diagnostic imaging, laboratory results reporting, order entry applications, pharmacy, client documentation systems, clinical support tools, and resource management applications. Developers of health care software offer integrated suites of applications that incorporate multiple tools for health care facilities or regions, and many health care institutions customize software to meet specific needs. Efforts are under way in every Canadian province and territory to develop a jurisdictional **electronic health record (EHR)**—a longitudinal record of an individual's health status (including diagnosed morbid conditions), diagnostic tests, treatments, and results—that will be interoperable with a pan-Canadian EHR. This movement toward provincial and national EHRs requires that developers or vendors incorporate into their information systems the capacity for interoperability with other vendors' systems so that client information can be communicated to caregivers as clients move across all sectors of the regional, provincial, or national health care delivery system.

However, despite of the vast array of technologies available in current health care, nurses must continue to contextualize technology within the scope of their professional practice. For example, Hannah (2005, p. 48) noted that "the issues for nurses are no longer computers or management information systems, but rather information and information management. The computer and its associated software are merely tools to support nurses as they practise their profession."

Nursing Informatics and the Canadian Health Care System

As the use of technology in health care settings burgeoned, pioneers in nursing informatics recognized that nurses needed to adopt strategically those information technologies that support professional practice. Furthermore, nursing informatics pioneers realized that there was also a need to consider the impact on nurses and nursing workflow of the demands related to using information technology. The term *nursing informatics* was introduced initially by Dr. Marion Ball at the 1983 International Medical Informatics Association (IMIA) Conference in Amsterdam (IMIA, 2004). In the 1980s, nursing informatics emerged as a new nursing specialty in health care information management. Since the 1984 publication of the first text devoted to nursing informatics, by Ball and Hannah, relevant journals and texts have proliferated across Canada and internationally. Hannah et al. (2006) noted that, despite the escalation of technology in health care and the recognition of the importance of nursing informatics, methods for defining and coding nursing contributions to health care outcomes have not been universally accepted, and the persistent absence of such methods is a significant obstacle to the collection of nursing data.

Defining Nursing Informatics

As research, education, and practice continue to inform nursing informatics, and as nursing informatics continues to evolve, definitions have correspondingly evolved. Early definitions of nursing informatics focused on technology and its effective use in practice, whereas current definitions focus more on the role of information management and the role of the nurse as an information manager. Table 17–1 is an overview summary of definitions that reflect the evolving understanding of nursing informatics (Staggers & Bagley Thompson, 2002).

Evolution of Informatics in the Canadian Health Care System

Health informatics encompasses all health care disciplines, and unique informatics knowledge and skills reflect specialties such as medical informatics and nursing informatics. The **Canadian Organization for Advancement of Computers in Health (COACH)**, Canada's Health Informatics Association, defines health informatics as the "intersection of clinical, IM/IT [Information Management/Information Technology] and management practices to achieve better health" (COACH, 2007, p. 7). The importance of informatics was recognized over many years and as the result of dedicated efforts of many professionals. Although other types of informatics practices exist, the focus of this chapter is on nursing informatics.

From the mid-1980s onward, Canada's health information infrastructure experienced numerous evolutions and reconfigurations, all of which had significant implications for nursing. The 1989 Canadian merger of the National Hospital Productivity Improvement Program and the Management Information System Project, which resulted in the Management Information System (MIS) Group, was an important event in Canadian health care information management (Hannah et al., 2006). The MIS Group, according to Hannah et al. (2006), developed guidelines on the collection of data for demographic, statistical, and resource use and consumption purposes. The problem with the MIS data is that, like hospital discharge summaries, this health information was restricted to physician-driven data and contained no clinical nursing data elements. Hannah et al. (2006, p. 89) made the point that "noteworthy, again, is the *total absence* of clinical nursing data."

The *Wilk Report* (National Task Force on Health Information, 1991) had a significant effect on health information in Canada, triggering the 1993 merger of the MIS Group, Hospital Medical Records Institute (HMRI), portions of Statistics Canada, and Health and Welfare Canada to create the **Canadian Institute for Health Information (CIHI)** (Alvarez, 1993; Hannah, 2005). CIHI is the national, independent, and not-for-profit body that records, analyzes, and disseminates essential data and analyses on Canada's health system and the health of Canadians (CIHI, 2007). Although not initially attentive to nursing data, this institution later became more important to several issues directly influencing nursing, including issues related to nursing workforce recruitment and retention.

In response to recommendations issued by the National Forum on Health for a pan-Canadian EHR, the federal government committed an initial $500 million to the development of e-health, which included the EHR, telehealth, and Internet-based health information (Canadian Nurses Association [CNA], 2006a; Hannah, 2005).

> **TABLE 17-1**   **Evolution of Nursing Informatics Definitions**

Focus of Definition	Date	Author	Definition
Information technology	1984; 1994	Ball & Hannah (p. 181); Hannah, Ball, & Edwards (p. 5)	"any use of information technologies by nurses in relation to the care of their patients, the administration of health care facilities, or the educational preparation of individuals to practise the discipline is considered nursing informatics"
	1986	Saba & McCormick (p. 116)	"systems that use computers to process nursing data into information to support all types of nursing activities"
	1990	Zielstorff, Abraham, Werley, Saba, & Schwirian	Central role of technology
	1996	Saba & McCormick (p. 226)	"use of technology and/or a computer system to collect, store, process, display, retrieve, and communicate timely data and information in and across health care facilities that administer nursing services and resources, manage the delivery of patient and nursing care, link research resources and findings to nursing practice, and apply educational resources to nursing education"
	1998	International Medical Informatics Association (IMIA; http://www.imia.org/working_groups/WG_Profile.lasso?-Search=Action&-Table=CGI&-MaxRecords=1&-SkipRecords=15&-Database=organizations&-KeyField=Org_ID&-SortField=workgroup_sig&-)	The integration of nursing, its information, and information management with information processing and communication technology, to support the health of people worldwide
	2000	Ball, Hannah, Newbold, & Douglas (p. 10)	"all aspects of nursing—clinical practice, administration, research and education—just as computing holds the power to integrate all four aspects"
	2001b	Canadian Nurses Association (http:www.cnia.ca/documents/OHIHfinalappendixA.doc)	"the application of computer science and information science to nursing. NI promotes the generation, management and processing of relevant data in order to use information and develop knowledge that supports nursing in all practice domains"
Conceptual	1986	Schwirian (p. 134)	"solid foundation of nursing informatics knowledge [that] should have focus, direction, and cumulative properties"
	1989	Graves & Corcoran (p. 227)	"A combination of computer science, information science, and nursing science designed to assist in the management and processing of nursing data, information, and knowledge to support the practice of nursing and the delivery of nursing care"
	1996	Turley	Development of a NI model which included cognitive science, information science, and computer science
Role centred	1992	American Nurses Association (ANA) Council on Computer Applications in Nursing (p. 1)	"specialty that integrates nursing science, computer science, and information science in identifying, collecting, processing, and managing data and information to support nursing practice, administration, education, and research and to expand nursing knowledge. The purpose of nursing informatics is to analyze information requirements; design, implement and evaluate information systems and data structures that support nursing; and identify and apply computer technologies for nursing"
	1994	ANA (p. 1)	"specialty that integrates nursing science, computer science, and information science in identifying, collecting, processing, and managing data and information to support nursing practice, administration, education, research, and expansion of nursing knowledge. It supports the practice of all nursing specialties, in all sites and settings, whether at the basic or advanced level. The practice includes the development of applications, tools, processes, and structures that assist nurses with the management of data in taking care of patients or in supporting their practice of nursing"

Continued

> **TABLE 17-1** | **Evolution of Nursing Informatics Definitions**   *continued*

| 2002 | Staggers & Bagley Thompson (p. 260) | Nursing informatics is a specialty that integrates nursing science, computer science, and information science to manage and communicate data, information, and knowledge in nursing practice. Nursing informatics facilitates the integration of data, information, and knowledge to support patients, nurses, and other providers in their decision making in all roles and settings. This support is accomplished through the use of information structures, information processes, and information technology |

NI, nursing informatics.

From American Nurses Association. (1994). *The scope of practice for nursing informatics.* Washington, DC: Author.

Canada Health Infoway Inc. (**Infoway**), incorporated in 2001, was a key outcome of the federal, provincial, and territorial partnership (CNA, 2006b). Infoway is a national body with a national mandate to generate consensus on health information standards, to drive forward the national agenda of creating an EHR, and to act as the liaison to international standards development organizations (Canada Health Infoway, 2007). Infoway has experienced significant growth since its inception; by 2008, Infoway had spent approximately $1 billion on electronic health systems in Canada (Canada Health Infoway, 2008a). In 2006, Infoway launched the Standards Collaborative, which is a "Canada-wide coordination function created to support and sustain health information standards in Canada" (Canada Health Infoway, 2008b, p. 4). The global mandate for the Standards Collaborative was endorsed by the federal, provincial, and territorial Ministries of Health to coordinate support for (1) development and implementation, (2) education for general and specific users groups (e.g., information management specialists, programmers, change management and adoption specialists, clinicians), (3) conformance (testing and evaluation), and (4) maintenance of EHR standards developed by Infoway and its jurisdictional partners.

The Standards Collaborative also incorporates nine Standards Collaborative Working Groups (SCWGs), in which clinicians, information technology experts, academics, researchers, and policymakers collaborate to address standards development for health information and systems in Canada. Membership in these groups is voluntary and open to any individual with an interest in contributing to the development of a specific aspect of the EHR. Box 17–1 illustrates the nine SCWGs and their respective focus of attention.

By March 31, 2007, Infoway had approved more than $1 billion, or 85% of its total funding, across all its program areas (Canada Health Infoway, 2008a). At the time of its publication, Infoway had committed more than $33 million to various provincial and territorial initiatives; as a result, in more than 20 projects have been completed or are nearing completion (Canada Health Infoway, 2008b). For example, one implementation project is the Picture Archiving & Communication Systems (PACS) initiative in Nova Scotia, through which diagnostic images are transmitted by computers to local and remote physicians, which enables a much faster response time between assessment and treatment. Projects in various stages of planning, implementation, or completion are recorded in every province in Canada.

The technological advances since the 1970s have directed national attention to the need for timely, secure, and appropriate health information access. Multiple health care and standards development organizations operate to coordinate broad documentation of health information and to monitor the Canadian health care system. You must have both an awareness and understanding of the roles and relevance of each of these entities in relation to your nursing practice.

Standards in Health Informatics

Standards Development in Canada

Standards for health care data are the established and formally endorsed coding protocols for all health information, including coding types of care provided, location of care provision, pharmaceutical ordering and dispensing, and coding for billing messages. A broader meaning for the term *standards* is the standardization of forms of technology, information, or business processes (Canada Health Infoway, 2004). Canada Health Infoway (2008b) noted that standards ensure interoperability by supporting information exchange and identified standards as a critical foundation for the interoperable electronic health record. Additional benefits of standards for various stakeholder groups are identified in Table 17–2.

Standards play a role in shaping health care data in a number of ways. Standards such as the **Systematized NOmenclature of MEDicine—Clinical Terms (SNOMED CT®)**, client registry standards, provider registry standards, diagnostic imaging standards, drug standards, and laboratory messaging and nomenclature standards all influence how nurses document clinical practice and access health data. For example, SNOMED CT (originally developed by the College of American Pathologists, enhanced over time by collaboration with other health care professionals, and currently managed by the **International Health Terminology Standards Development Organisation [IHTSDO®]** in Copenhagen, Denmark) contains clinical terminology used to describe multidisciplinary clinical practice. In addition, standards operate in the background to support consistent packaging or coding of data. These standards include security and consent standards, interoperable EHR technical standards, and interoperable EHR clinical messaging standards.

In Canada, Infoway uses a consistent process to bring standards forward from initiation to conformance, implementation, and maintenance. Two types of needs can trigger the development of a standard. *Technical needs* are generated from gaps in information management; to address these needs, a consistent manner of communicating health data is needed among providers or between institutions or jurisdictions. *Business needs* are identified from analysis of the actual clinical work processes; for example, a particular condition or clinical situation may not be described consistently. Infoway has a three-option process of standards development, in decreasing order of preference: (1) *adopt* an existing standard; (2) *adapt* an existing standard; and (3) *develop* a new standard (Canada Health Infoway, 2008b). Upon adoption, adaptation, or development of a standard, Infoway issues a "Stable for Use" designation to indicate that the standard is ready for limited implementation and testing. Before formal approval, the proposed standard must undergo rigorous evaluation, and testing, as well as demonstrate a

➤ BOX 17-1	Standards Collaborative Working Groups

Standards Collaborative Working Groups (SCWGs)	Scope
SCWG 1: Population Health (Delivery of Care)	Immunization Communicable disease management • Public health case • Public health outbreak • Public health investigations

SCWG 2: Individual Care (Delivery of Care)	Electronic health records (EHRs)
	Shared health record
	• Adverse event
	• Allergy
	• Clinical observations
	• Discharge care summary
	• Health conditions
	   • Care compositions (e.g., encounters and episodes)
	   • Professional services
	   • Referral and referral note
	Health summary records
	Chronic disease management

SCWG 3: Managing the Health System	Claims Client administrative Wait times Secondary use Research Clinical data warehouse
SCWG 4: Medication Management	Prescribing Dispensing Client (drug) queries Drug queries Contraindications
SCWG 5: Labs & Diagnostics	Human laboratory Nonhuman laboratory Diagnostic imaging Diagnostic investigations
SCWG 6: Infostructure & Architecture	Data types Common message element types Message wrappers Common message patterns Broadcast EHR record retrieval Event tracking Queue management (polling) Retract OIDs
SCWG 7: Non-Clinical Registries	Client registry and identification management Provider registry and identification management Location registry and identification management Organization registry and identification management
SCWG 8: IT Privacy & Security Services	Security Privacy Consent User registries (Access & Authentication) *Note: This SCWG does not address privacy and security policy, regulatory issues, or legislation.*
SCWG 9: Terminology Representation & Services	Terminology services HL7 Common terminology servers Terminology models HL7 Vocabulary worksheet

From Canada Health Infoway. (2008b). *Standards Collaborative: Enabling solutions, enhancing health outcomes . . . together* (p. 11). Toronto, ON: Author. HL7, Health Level 7 Standards; OIDS, object identifiers.

consensus among users (balloting). Various international standards form the foundation of pan-Canadian standards:

- Health Level 7 (HL7)
- SNOMED CT®
- Logical Observation Identifier Names and Codes (LOINC®)
- *The Canadian Enhancement of ICD-10 [International Statistical Classification of Diseases and Related Health Problems, 10th Revision]* (ICD-10-CA) (CIHI, 2001)
- Canadian Classification of Health Interventions (CCI)
- Integrating the Healthcare Enterprise (IHE)
- Digital Imaging and Communication in Medicine (DICOM)
- Unified Codes for Units of Measure (UCUM)
- Health Canada Drug Product Database (DPD)

Standardizing Nursing Language

A widely held perception among many nurses is that nursing, as a professional practice, is generally considered invisible in regard to formal and tangible recognition (CNA, 2000; Clark, 1999; Clark & Lang, 1992; Hannah et al., 2006; Marck, 1994; Norwood, 2001; Powers, 2001; Weyrauch, 2002). Clark (1999, p. 42) observed that despite its being the largest group of health care clinicians, nursing was invisible in health policy decisions, in descriptions of health care, and in contracts and service specifications.

Clark and Lang (1992, p. 109), in their assessment of the invisibility of nursing, noted that nurses cannot control what cannot be named, stating that "if we cannot name it, we cannot control it, finance it, teach it, research it, or put it into public policy." According to the stance of Clark and Lang (1992) and other scholars (such as Graves & Corcoran, 1989; Werley, 1988), giving nursing visibility requires a standardized language to reflect what nursing is and what nursing does. Clark (1999, p. 42) advocated for a standardized nursing language, using the argument that ". . . without a language to express our concepts we cannot know whether our understanding of their meaning is the same, so we cannot communicate them with any precision to other people." More recently, the argument has shifted from the issue of visibility to the value and necessity of client safety and professionals' accountability, along with accurate data for system and clinical evaluation. Adopting a standardized nursing language is urgent, as the pan-Canadian interoperable EHR moves forward and information management further enables evidence-informed practice.

Health Information: Nursing Components

Before a standard nursing language is adopted, the most important data elements required for effective nursing decision making and evaluation must be identified. The minimum number of essential nursing data elements are referred to as a *minimum nursing data set*. In Canada, the process of capturing nursing data was led by the Alberta Association of Registered Nurses (AARN) in 1992. This provincial nursing body, in conjunction with the CNA, hosted a national conference focused on generating and validating a Canadian nursing minimum data set (NMDS) (Giovannetti et al., 1999). The Canadian version of an NMDS is known as **Health Information: Nursing Components (HI:NC)**. The CNA (2000, p. 5)

► TABLE 17-2	Benefits of Standards for Stakeholder Groups
Stakeholder Group	**Benefits of Standards in Health Care Data**
Clients	• Reduced repetition of health information • Accessible personal health history • Improved coordination of care • Reduced duplication of tests and procedures • Improved health outcomes
Providers	• Timely access to health data • Availability of more reliable health information • Reduced duplication of efforts • Shorter response time between assessment and treatment • Improved quality and consistency of care resulting from enhanced information access • Enhanced client outcomes
Service delivery organizations	• Reuse of solutions, benefiting from lessons learned and change management strategies • Greater breadth of data to use for evaluating outcomes • Enhanced ability to work collaboratively with other organizations or jurisdictions • Increased confidence in products when suitability for use is determined
Educators	• Support for curriculum design that is aligned with accreditation process • Increased value of data for educational purposes • Enabling of educators and students to understand the health informatics environment at early stages of education • Enhanced ability to extract data, such as best practice guidelines, from published sources
Researchers	• Availability of higher quality data • Reduced time to prepare data for use • Comprehensive data sets • Improved ability to monitor and assess health outcomes and determinants

Adapted from Hannah, K. J. (2005). Health informatics and nursing in Canada. *Healthcare Information Management and Communications, 19*(3), 45–51. Reprinted by permission of Healthcare Computing and Communications Canada, Inc.

described HI:NC as the "most important pieces of data about the nursing care provided to the client during a health care episode." Since 1992, the majority of Canadian nurses have agreed that HI:NC is composed of five categories of elements: client status, nursing interventions, client outcomes, nursing resource intensity, and primary nurse identifier (AARN, 1994; CNA, 2000, 2001a). Table 17–3 presents the HI:NC definitions.

Chapter 16 provides an overview of computerized nursing documentation. Many clinical information systems incorporate the HI:NC into the architecture or design of the nursing system. This enables capture of the most significant nursing data. Computerized nursing documentation systems continue to evolve, and their design relies on an underlying philosophy of documentation. For example, many systems do not encourage narrative documentation; instead, they provide checklists of common activities and encourage exception charting. This issue is further discussed in Chapter 16.

International Classification for Nursing Practice®

In 2001, the CNA endorsed the **International Classification for Nursing Practice (ICNP®)** "for use in Canada as a foundational classification system for nursing practice in Canada" (CNA, 2001b, p. 1). This endorsement was renewed in 2006 (CNA, 2006a). The **International Council of Nurses (ICN)**—an international federation of countries representing national nursing organizations that advances professional nursing practice, advocates for effective health policy, and enhances health globally—developed the ICNP in response to concerns regarding the visibility of nursing contributions in health care and calls for standardization of nursing data for comparability and analysis, as well as for evidence-informed practice. ICN proposed the use of a single unified nomenclature to represent nursing practice; ICNP is the only unified international terminology for recording nursing practice. The goals were to capture nursing practice across practice settings, cultures, languages, and geographical settings, as well as to ensure that professionals who used this new terminology could communicate electronically with the numerous nursing terminologies already in use in information systems and software. Initially endorsed in 1989 by resolution at the ICN's nineteenth quadrennial conference (ICN, 2005), the Alpha version of the ICNP® was released in 1995. Version 1.0 was released in 2005 and is substantively different from previous iterations (Alpha, Beta, Beta 2): To unify all previous ICNP® axes, it comprises seven axes with associated terms for describing nursing practice (Figure 17–1).

ICNP® is used to generate statements of nursing diagnoses, nursing actions, and nursing outcomes, in which terms arranged in a hierarchical order are used (Figure 17–2), and in catalogues (or subsets) of previously combined terms. Catalogues comprise nursing data subsets of diagnoses, actions, and outcomes specific to various practice areas or specialties (such as wound care) and continue to be developed. To begin catalogue development, nurses select a health care topic on the basis of the needs of clients. The organization of the catalogue content would be determined by the nurses as ICNP® diagnoses, outcomes, and interventions are identified. ICN (2005) suggested that catalogues can fill a practical need in building health information systems with all the benefits of being part of a unified nursing language.

As stated earlier, the Canadian Nurses' Association endorsed ICNP® as the terminology of choice for documenting professional nursing practice in Canada (CNA, 2001b, 2006a). Although Canada Health Infoway, in consultation with various stakeholder groups, adopted SNOMED CT® as the terminology of choice for the pan-Canadian EHR, ICNP® remains the preferred terminology for nursing. ICN, which holds the intellectual property rights to ICNP®, is in discussions with SNOMED CT® to identify means of linking the two standardized clinical terminologies to ensure that nursing practice is accurately documented.

As illustrated in Figure 17–1, Version 1.0 of ICNP® is constructed with seven axes: Focus, Judgement, Means, Action, Time, Location, and Client. Table 17–4 lists definitions for each axis and examples of terms. According to ICNP® requirements, both nursing diagnoses and nursing outcomes *must* contain a term from the Focus axis and the Judgement axis and may include terms from additional axes as needed to fully describe the phenomenon of attention. Nursing

► TABLE 17-3	Health Information: Nursing Components
Nursing Component	**Definition**
Client status	A label for the set of indicators that reflect the phenomena for which nurses provide care, relative to the health status of clients (McGee, 1993). Although client status is similar to nursing diagnosis, the term *client status* is preferred because it represents a broader spectrum of health and illness. The common label *client status* is inclusive of input from all disciplines. The summative statements referring to the phenomena for which nurses provide care (i.e., nursing diagnosis) are merely one aspect of client status at a point in time, in the same way as medical diagnosis.
Nursing interventions	Purposeful and deliberate health-affecting interventions (direct and indirect), based on assessment of client status, which are designed to bring about results which benefit clients (Alberta Association of Registered Nurses [AARN], 1994).
Client outcome	A "client's status at a defined point(s) following health care [affecting] intervention" (Marek & Lang, 1993). It is influenced to varying degrees by the interventions of all care providers.
Nursing intensity	"Refers to the amount and type of nursing resource used to [provide] care" (O'Brien-Pallas & Giovannetti, 1993).
Primary nurse identifier	A single unique, lifetime identification number for each individual nurse. This identifier is independent of geographic location (province or territory), practice sector (e.g., acute care, community care, public health), or employer.

From Hannah, K. J. (2005). Health informatics and nursing in Canada. *Healthcare Information Management and Communications, 19*(3), 49.

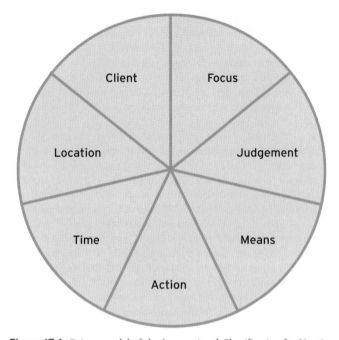

Figure 17-1 7-Axes model of the International Classification for Nursing Practice (ICNP®), Version 1.0. **Source:** From International Council of Nurses. (2005). *International Classification for Nursing Practice®, Version 1.0.* (p. 29). Geneva, Switzerland: Author. Reproduced with permission of the International Council of Nurses © 2005.

Interventions *must* include a term from the Action axis and the Target axis, and may include additional terms from other axes as necessary. ICN (2005) described a "Target term" as a term originating in any axis except the Judgement axis.

The format of these nursing diagnosis statements may not correspond with those identified in previous chapters. These statements may not be used literally in daily verbal communication among nurses; they will be used for nursing documentation in the EHR to enable aggregation. The following examples reflect the core details for coding key nursing data in the EHR:

Nursing diagnosis: *Decreasing level of pain in right knee joint*
- *Pain* is from the Focus axis.
- *Decreasing level* is from the Judgement axis.
- Both *right* and *knee joint* are from the Location axis.

Nursing intervention: Analgesic injected
- *Injected* and *injecting* are from the Action axis.
- *Analgesic* is from the Means axis.

Nursing outcome: Sputum decreased
- *Sputum* is from the Focus axis.
- *Decreased* is from the Judgement axis.

As with all languages, development of ICNP® is continuous, and research is under way in many countries (Boxes 17–2 and 17–3). Version 1.0 is subjected to ongoing evaluation to refine and enhance terms, catalogues, and translations.

Canadian Privacy Legislation

Although both provincial standards of practice and the CNA (2008a) *Code of Ethics* address confidentiality, you also need to be aware of Canadian privacy legislation that also affects nursing practice and the protection of client data. Even as you fulfill the standards of practice, it is possible to violate privacy legislation. Canadians recognize this risk of privacy violation, and "two thirds of Canadian citizens believe that personal health information is one of the most important areas in need of protection under privacy laws" (Roch, 2008, p. 8). Although privacy legislation varies between provinces, you must develop a working knowledge of the relevant legislation, both provincial and national.

Two federal legislative acts address the privacy of personal information. These include the *Privacy Act* (Government of Canada,

Figure 17-2 Hierarchical structure of the International Classification for Nursing Practice (ICNP®), Version 1.0. **Source:** From Hierarchical structure of International Council of Nurses Version 1.0. Reproduced with permission of the International Council of Nurses © 2005.

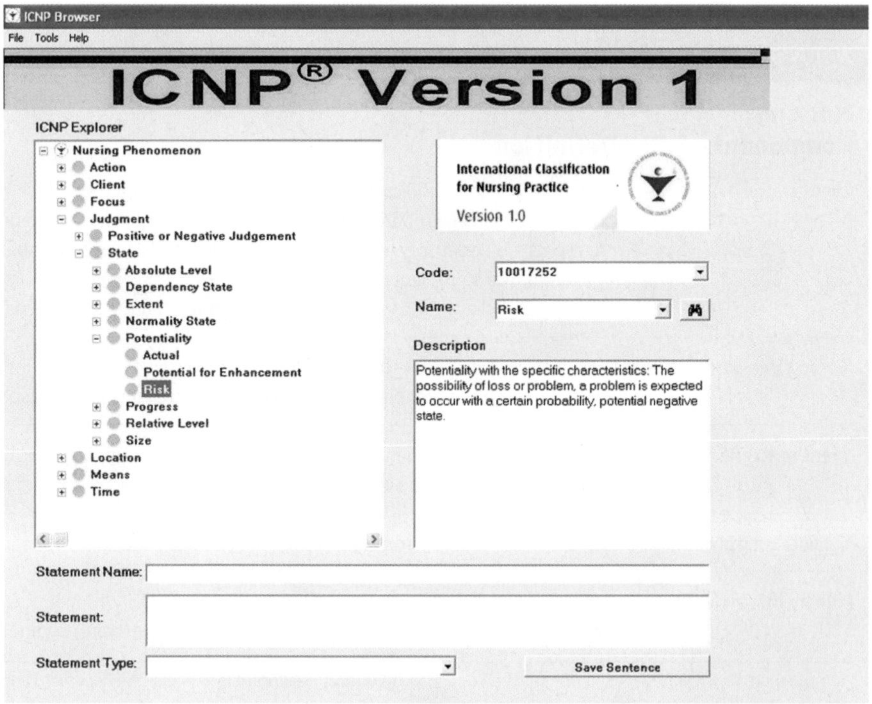

►TABLE 17-4	Definitions and Examples of Terms in ICNP® Version 1	
Axis	**Definition**	**Sample Terms**
Focus	The area of attention relevant to nursing	*Elder abuse, sputum, air, child labour law*
Judgement	Clinical opinion or determination related to the focus of nursing practice	*High, enhanced, partial, risk*
Means	A manner or method of accomplishing an intervention	*Wound drainage bag, nebulizer, bed rail, cardiac monitor*
Action	An intentional process applied to or performed by a client	*Violence prevention, explaining, listening, resuscitating*
Time	The point, period, interval, or duration of an occurrence	*Rarely, chronic, discharge, intermittent*
Location	Anatomical or spatial orientation of a diagnosis or intervention	*Chest wall, distal, residential building, supine, intravenous route*
Client	Subject to which a diagnosis refers and who is the recipient of an intervention	*Extended family, community, adolescent, older adult, infant*

Adapted from International Council of Nurses. (2005). *International Classification for Nursing Practice®, Version 1.0* (p. 29). Geneva, Switzerland: Author. Reproduced with permission of the International Council of Nurses © 2005.

1983) and the ***Personal Information Protection and Electronic Documents Act (PIPEDA)*** (Government of Canada, 2004). Both acts identify specific limitations to the disclosure of personal information, whether in electronic or other forms. Regardless of the practice setting or mode, you are professionally and ethically obligated to protect all personal information of clients in your care. Knowledge of these two pieces of federal privacy legislation can help you uphold the standards of practice and *Code of Ethics.*

According to the *Privacy Act*, Section 8.1, "Personal information under the control of a government institution shall not, without the consent of the individual to whom it relates, be disclosed by the institution . . . ." (Government of Canada, 1983). The *PIPEDA* is federal legislation governing the disclosure of personal health information in any electronic environment. This act extends the *Privacy Act* by addressing specific risks associated with electronic data collection, storage, retrieval, and communication. *PIPEDA* addresses personal health information specifically and identifies *personal health information,* with regard to any individual, whether living or deceased, as having any of the following meanings (Government of Canada, 2004, Section 1.2):

1. Information concerning the physical or mental health of the individual
2. Information concerning any health care service provided to the individual
3. Information concerning the donation by the individual of any body part or any bodily substance of the individual or information derived from the testing or examination of a body part or bodily substance of the individual
4. Information that is collected in the course of providing health care services to the individual
5. Information that is collected incidentally to the provision of health care services to the individual

Furthermore, *PIPEDA* restricts the disclosure of personal information to only the most stringent of conditions, such as law enforcement requirements (Government of Canada, 2004, Division 1, Section 7.3). You must exercise diligence in examining and adhering to these pieces of legislation in your professional nursing practice. Chapter 16 explores how *PIPEDA* applies to specific nursing documentation.

✳ BOX 17-2   RESEARCH HIGHLIGHT

Evaluating Standardized Nursing Terminology

Nursing data have not been included in national data repositories for a variety of reasons, including the lack of a single nursing terminology to describe nursing practice. Consequently, health care decisions have been made in the absence of valuable nursing data. The need for a standardized nursing language stimulated the development of the ICNP®. Testing was necessary to evaluate the representational capacity of this terminology for Canadian nursing practice. Kennedy (2005) examined the effectiveness of the ICNP® in representing the contributions of nursing care to health care outcomes in Canada. The ICNP® was used to code retrospective nursing data extracted from client records originating in acute care, in-patient mental health, home health care, and long-term care practice settings. In spite of a wide variation in documentation practices,

ICNP® achieved matches with a significant majority of nursing data, thereby confirming the utility of ICNP® for documenting nursing practice in Canada.

Representing Nursing Practice

ICNP® represents Canadian nursing practice with high accuracy. Variations and gaps in nursing documentation practices are further evidence of the need for standardized terminology to ensure that at least minimum nursing data are recorded.

References: Kennedy, M. A. (2005). *Packaging nursing as politically potent: A critical reflexive cultural studies approach to nursing informatics.* Unpublished doctoral dissertation, University of South Australia, Adelaide, Australia; Kennedy, M. A., & Hannah, K. J. (2007). Representing nursing practice: Evaluating the effectiveness of a nursing classification system. *Canadian Journal of Nursing Research, 39*(7), 58–79.

> **BOX 17-3**   **Creating Canadian Nursing History**

The C-HOBIC Initiative

The CNA launched a multiprovince project in 2007, in collaboration with the provinces of Ontario, Saskatchewan, Manitoba, and Prince Edward Island, with financial contribution from Canada Health Infoway. This project focused on collecting information reflecting evidence-informed, nursing-sensitive client outcomes (CNA, 2008b). Drawing on the work of the original **Health Outcomes for Better Information and Care (HOBIC) project**, the Canadian Health Outcomes for Better Information and Care (C-HOBIC) project (http://www.cna-aiic.ca/c-hobic/about/default_e.aspx) implements a standardized nursing documentation approach for capturing, analyzing, and reporting nursing-sensitive outcomes for acute care, complex continuing care, long-term care, and home care.

The C-HOBIC project addresses gaps in health information related to the contribution of nursing care to client outcomes and also addresses the need for standardized nursing data to be included in client admission and discharge summaries. The C-HOBIC project is a systematic approach to gathering nursing content that is documented with a standardized clinical terminology, ICNP®, and coded in a format suitable for inclusion in the EHRs being developed or implemented by the participating provinces. C-HOBIC provides an opportunity for Canadian nurses to make substantive contributions to the ongoing development of ICNP® through research that adds new terms or concepts to ICNP®. One particular component of

the C-HOBIC project was the mapping of outcomes concepts to the ICNP® Version 1.0.

Mapping challenges provided an immediate opportunity for Canadian nurses to contribute to the iterative development of ICNP® by proposing multiple new terms and a catalogue of precombined terms for inclusion in ICNP® that are uniquely Canadian and reflect C-HOBIC concepts. The mapping was validated at a national forum (Kennedy, 2008; Kennedy et al., 2008) that included C-HOBIC partners, nursing informatics experts, nurse educators, nurse researchers, representatives from government ministries, policy institutions and practice environments, and two international ICNP® experts.

In total, 96 concepts were addressed in the mapping aspect of the C-HOBIC project: 58 HOBIC concepts were matched and validated as C-HOBIC terms; 13 HOBIC concepts were partially mapped to ICNP®, and a new term was required in ICNP® in order to fully communicate the original concept in C-HOBIC; 24 concepts did not match and new C-HOBIC terms were proposed for inclusion in ICNP®; and only one HOBIC concept ("Activity did not occur") could not be mapped to ICNP®. In addition, two HOBIC ordinal scales (for pain scale and for the number of falls) were retained for use in C-HOBIC. Consensus by the group was achieved for all concepts, terms and issues. Critical next steps include the creation of the C-HOBIC catalogue by ICNP® and the establishment of a Nursing Terminology Working Group.

National E-Nursing Strategy

The CNA (2006b) released the *E-Nursing Strategy for Canada* to direct the coordinated integration of technology into Canadian nursing practice. The strategy addresses both medium- and long-term targets, with the overall goal of improving both nursing practice and outcomes for clients. This strategy is intended to completely integrate information and communication technologies (ICT) in such a way that the "e" in *e-nursing* is no longer required; ICT will simply be another tool that nurses use in their practice (CNA, 2006b). The CNA (2006b, p. 4) identified seven key outcomes that are projected to emerge from the *E-Nursing Strategy*. These include:

1. Nurses will integrate ICT into their practice to achieve desirable client outcomes.
2. Nurses will have the required information and knowledge to support their practice.
3. Human resources planning will be facilitated.
4. New models of nursing practice and health services delivery will be supported.
5. Nursing groups will be well connected.
6. ICT will improve the quality of nurses' work environments.
7. Canadian nurses will contribute to the global community of nursing.

Three fundamental directions for CNA's *E-Nursing Strategy* were developed among working groups and from national feedback: access, competencies, and participation. *Access* to quality ICT in the practice environment is imperative if Canadian nurses are to realize the full benefits of technology in their practices. The CNA (2006b) noted that health care organizations have a responsibility to ensure that nurses have connectivity—tools such as computers, mobile technology (e.g., laptops, personal digital assistants wireless technology), as well as resource databases and Internet resources—that will support professional practice.

The CNA (2006b) encouraged nurses to develop *Competencies* in the application of ICT and recommended that such competencies be part of both undergraduate and graduate level nursing programs. Just as you have a responsibility to develop competencies in performing a variety of client care tasks, such as assessments and treatments, it is also your responsibility to develop and maintain competencies in technological applications that support information management in professional practice.

Many examples of innovative nursing practice incorporating ICT are evident in Canada. Two such examples are the mobile wound assessment program used by the Victorian Order of Nurses and the standardized assessment approaches currently being integrated in the Local Health Integration Network in Ontario. Goodwin et al. (2008) combined telemedicine and telemonitoring with client education and peer supports in assisting chronically ill clients to stay at home in rural Ontario. Without this program, these clients would have had to travel for care provision and would have potentially experienced more frequent hospitalizations, loss of independence, and significantly less self-care. Tracey (2008) described how a standardized assessment approach is in pilot testing at two sites. This pilot format will ultimately replace six different assessment forms; therefore, data collection will be more systematic and the capacity for data aggregation and analysis will be greater.

The CNA (2006b, p. 12) identified *Participation* as including strategic partnerships with nurses in clinical practice; with employers and administrators; with federal, provincial, and territorial ministries; with nursing organizations (professional associations, regulatory bodies, educational groups, and unions); and with educators and researchers. The concept of partnership has far-reaching consequences: With effective partnerships, you can contribute to the selection and design of information technology applications, as well as to educational programs. For example, many health care institutions and agencies have clinical committees that collaborate with information technology experts in the design and selection of electronic documentation systems. Especially as a novice nurse, you have both the knowledge and the opportunity to contribute insights into which information management systems are user friendly or present unexpected challenges. It is also helpful to have this type of clinician involvement when the system requires revision or adaptation. Even small changes can sometimes have significant impact on the capture of appropriate nursing data and on how other nurses view the system. Without partnerships, however, you, and all nurses, risk being excluded from decision making and risk being required to use systems that are selected without valuable clinician contributions.

The Canadian Nurses Portal is a key component of the *E-Nursing Strategy*. The portal was initially funded from a grant from the First Nations and Inuit Health Branch (FNIHB) of Health Canada (CNA, 2006c). The nursing portal, now known as NurseONE, enables you to register, create a personal profile, and customize use of the site's tools and resources. NurseONE provides such services as the following:

- Professional links (resources with clinical or professional orientation)
- Professional development (including resources for continuing competence, online and continuing education, and career development)
- Library (access to numerous articles and publications)
- NurseConnect (use of the portal to create discussion groups among individual subscribers)

Resources available to subscribers include activities for conducting self-assessments, creating individualized learning plans, and developing an online professional portfolio. You can also track current news and nursing information, receive updates and alerts on items of interest, access educational opportunities, and search for practice support on the NurseONE site. This site will continue to develop over time and provides a centralized professional nursing forum for Canadian nurses. You should sign up today!

Clinician Engagement and Informatics Communities

Many Canadian and international health informatics communities offer exciting opportunities for participation: support, educational programs, and networking opportunities. Of most importance, these communities always welcome new members who are interested in advancing informatics. As noted throughout this chapter, involving clinicians in the selection, design, and revision of technology is crucial. As a professional, you have both an obligation and a right to be involved in issues that affect your professional practice and your work environment.

Many informatics organizations have specific strategies to foster clinician engagement or encourage clinicians to become involved; however, literature on the topic of clinician engagement is scarce. Mercer (2008) promoted involvement through five questions (the "5 Ws"): (1) What is it? (2) Who should be involved? (3) Why is it important? (4) Where does it fit? (5) When should clinicians get involved? Mercer advocated immediate involvement and in any clinical environment.

The CNA is the national professional body representing Canadian nurses. The CNA's mandate of supporting professional nursing practice also includes supporting the integration of nursing informatics in Canada. The CNA has issued many position statements and professional guidelines to support all nurses as technology has become increasingly integrated into Canadian practice environments. The CNA provides an excellent starting point from which you can explore nursing informatics in Canada.

The **Canadian Nursing Informatics Association (CNIA)** is the national special interest group dedicated to the advancement of nursing informatics in Canada. CNIA is designated as a group affiliated with the CNA. Also affiliated with COACH, CNIA is the Canadian nursing representative to the **International Medical Informatics Association–Special Interest Group in Nursing Informatics (IMIA-SIGNI)**. Originally functioning as a special interest group within COACH, this group disbanded in 2000 and resumed as the CNIA (CNIA, 2000). This group was agreed to include the following mandates (CNIA, 2000):

- To provide nursing leadership for the development of nursing and health informatics in Canada
- To establish national networking opportunities for nurse informaticians
- To facilitate informatics educational opportunities for all nurses in Canada
- To engage in international nursing informatics initiatives
- To act as a nursing advisory group in matters of nursing and health informatics

Since being founded, the CNIA has hosted successful national nursing informatics conferences, launched a national online journal (*Canadian Journal of Nursing Informatics*), provided educational offerings, and advocated for the advancement of nursing informatics in Canada.

As noted earlier in this chapter, COACH is another organization dedicated to promoting health informatics within the Canadian health system through education, information, networking, and communication. COACH was formed in 1975 by software developers and health care clinicians (COACH, 2008). Their original focus was to support effective use information technology and systems among Canadian health institutions by sharing ideas and efforts. This focus has expanded to include the effective use of health information for decision making.

COACH's multidisciplinary membership encompasses more than 1300 individuals, including health care executives, physicians, nurses and allied health care professionals, researchers and educators, chief information officers, information managers, technical experts, consultants, and information technology vendors (COACH, 2008). Member organizations include health care service delivery agencies, government and nongovernment agencies, consulting firms, commercial providers of information and telecommunications technologies, and educational institutions.

In addition to the previous groups, you can also contribute your clinician perspective to the various SCWGs sponsored by Infoway. These groups, as noted previously in this chapter, are open and voluntary in nature, which means that you need only express your interest; you do not need to be nominated or elected as a member. You will be welcomed to any SCWG or multiple groups. Participating in these SCWGs not only supports your professional practice but also offers you an opportunity for professional development and mentoring. Many experienced nurses are currently involved in advisory groups of the Standards Collaborative, but the SCWGs consistently need and solicit clinician engagement.

Many international informatics organizations exist, in which you can be involved. These include the **American Medical Informatics Association (AMIA)**, the **International Medical Informatics Association (IMIA)**, and the Health Informatics Society of Australia (HISA), all of which host special interest groups in nursing informatics. You can be involved at every level of information management in health care. Your challenge and your opportunity are to decide how your interest and energy can be best used.

In addition to the formal organizations that you may consider joining, numerous informal communities are devoted to nursing informatics and creating dialogue among nurses. You may decide to explore a variety of informal communities or social entities, including the following:

- Blogs: These are online diaries generally sponsored by individuals, which are occasionally interactive but typically present only the thoughts or opinions of the blog's sponsor.
- Wikis: These are Web pages that are interactive and allow subscribers to modify or contribute to the content. Subscribers are able to use any Web browser. Wikis also allows users to incorporate hyperlinks and use a simplified language to create new pages and linkages rapidly.
- Listserv and discussion groups: These are e-mail distributions lists. Many nursing informatics sites allow and encourage you to subscribe to the listserv or discussion groups so that you can receive regular contact and updates in regard to content, activities, or networking opportunities. These tools also allow you to ask questions, post messages, and network with colleagues.
- Social networks: Communities such as MySpace and Facebook allow subscribers to join groups of individuals who are interested in shared interests and activities. These Web-based communities include a variety of ways in which subscribers may communicate, including chat, messaging, e-mail, blogs, video, voice chat, file sharing, discussion groups, and message boards.

The value of interest in informal networking cannot be underestimated; however, you should not depend on these types of forums for consistent, professional, and credible health informatics information. Some sites may offer highly professional informatics advice or information; unfortunately, no standard exists with regard to either content or process. Many sites offer only personal or anecdotal commentary and may provide misleading information, which can create liability if used in your professional practice. Consequently, you must critically evaluate the content of these informal sites and groups to determine the validity of the content, the credibility of the organization or group, and the intent of the networking tool. The most effective way to obtain reliable and authoritative information is through formalized organizations that are committed to the professional advancement of informatics.

❋ CRITICAL THINKING EXERCISES

1. You are making a presentation to a group of nursing peers. Your task is to lead the selection of an electronic documentation tool. How do you prepare your peers for evaluation discussions preceding the selection decision? What factors do you consider when determining what are the most important pieces of nursing documentation to record?

2. During the course of documenting an admission assessment, you note that your client has in the past been admitted to a psychiatric unit. One of your colleagues is a neighbour of the client and asks you to share whether this client has a psychiatric history. Your colleague is not providing care to the client today or tomorrow. How do you respond to this inquiry? What pieces of legislation do you consider in making a decision?

❋ REVIEW QUESTIONS

1. What changes that occurred in the health care system since the 1950s have led to the recognition of nursing informatics?

2. What factors are behind the need for standardized nursing documentation?

3. How is standardized nursing terminology being used in Canada?

4. How does privacy legislation influence nursing practice in Canada?

5. How can nurses implement the *E-Nursing Strategy?*

6. What nursing or health informatics communities are available to nurses?

❋ RECOMMENDED WEB SITES

American Medical Informatics Association (AMIA): http://www.amia.org/
AMIA is a national association in the United States and is dedicated to the adoption and advancement of technology in health care.

American Medical Informatics Association–Nursing Informatics: http://www.amia.org/mbrcenter/wg/ni/
The American Medical Informatics Association–Nursing Informatics is a special interest group within the American Medical Informatics Association. This group is focused on the advancement of informatics as it relates specifically to American professional nursing practice.

Canada Health Infoway: http://www.infoway-inforoute.ca/
Canada Health Infoway is Canada's national not-for-profit body that generates consensus on health information standards, drives forward the national agenda of creating an EHR, and acts as the liaison to international standards development organizations.

Canadian Nursing Informatics Association (CNIA): http://cnia.ca/intro.htm
The Canadian Nursing Informatics Association is Canada's national body with a mission to advance nursing informatics in Canada. CNIA is also the publisher of the *Canadian Journal of Nursing Informatics.*

Canadian Organization for Advancement of Computers in Health (COACH): http://www.coachorg.com/
COACH is a Canadian not-for-profit association that is dedicated to the effective integration of technology in health care. This association is one of the largest informatics associations in Canada and includes members from all health care disciplines.

Health Informatics Society of Australia (HISA): http://www.hisa.org.au/
HISA is the national not-for-profit association for advancing informatics in Australia.

Health Informatics Society of Australia–Nursing Informatics: http://www.hisa.org.au/nursing
The Health Informatics Society of Australia–Nursing Informatics is a special interest group within the Health Informatics Society of Australia. This group is focused on the advancement of informatics as it relates specifically to professional nursing practice in Australia.

International Medical Informatics Association (IMIA): http://www.imia.org/
IMIA is an international not-for-profit association and is dedicated to the adoption and advancement of technology in health care.

International Medical Informatics Association–Nursing Informatics: http://www.imia.org/working_groups/WG_Profile.lasso?-Search=Action&-Table=CGI&-MaxRecords=1&-SkipRecords=15&-Database=organizations&-KeyField=Org_ID&-SortField=workgroup_sig&-SortOrder=ascending&type=wgsig
The International Medical Informatics Association–Nursing Informatics is a special interest group within the International Medical Informatics Association. This group is focused on the advancement of nursing informatics with international implications.

NurseONE: http://www.nurseone.ca/
The NurseONE site is one of the outcomes of the Canadian Nurses Association's *E-Nursing Strategy.* This site offers nurses a diverse array of educational tools, professional practice supports, and networking opportunities.

18

Communication

Original chapter by Jeri Burger, RN, PhD

Canadian content written by Nancy C. Goddard, RN, BScN, MN, PhD

Communication is a lifelong learning process for the nurse. Nurses are intimately involved with clients and their families from birth to death. It is important to build therapeutic communications for this journey. Nurses must communicate effectively with people under stress. They must function as client advocates and as members of interdisciplinary teams, other members of which often have different priorities for client care. Nurses must also be able to communicate their own needs to avoid burnout and to continue providing effective care within a high-stress environment (Balzer Riley, 2004). Despite the competing demands on nurses' time and despite current technological complexity, it is the intimate nurse–client connection that makes the difference in the quality of care and in the meaning of the illness experience for both (Balzer Riley, 2004). Therefore, nurses must be competent in a variety of communication techniques in order to develop and maintain therapeutic relationships. Effective communication promotes collaboration and interdisciplinary teamwork, helps ensure that ethical and legal responsibilities and professional practice standards are met, and contributes to positive client outcomes. It is an essential element of professional nursing practice (Apker et al., 2006). Ineffective communication may lead to poor client outcomes, increases in adverse incidents, and decreases in professional credibility. The Conference Board of Canada considers communication and interpersonal relationship skills to be crucial for successful employment and the establishment of healthy work environments (Devito et al., 2005).

The qualities, behaviours, and therapeutic communication techniques described in this chapter characterize professionalism in helping relationships. Although the term *client* is often used, the same principles can be applied in communicating with any person, in any nursing situation.

Communication and Interpersonal Relationships

At the core of nursing care are therapeutic interpersonal relationships based on caring, mutual respect, and dignity. Communication is the means to establish these helping–healing relationships. Because all behaviour communicates, and all communication influences behaviour, nurses must become experts in communication if they are to provide effective care.

The nurse's ability to relate to other people—to take initiative in establishing and maintaining a relationship, to be authentic, and to respond appropriately to the other person—is a crucial aspect of interpersonal communication. Effective interpersonal communication also requires a sense of mutuality, a belief that the nurse–client relationship is a partnership and that both partners are equal participants. Mutuality requires that both participants respect each other's autonomy and value system and are committed to the client's well-being (Arnold & Boggs, 2007). Nurses honour the fact that people are complex and ambiguous beings. Often, more is communicated than is at first apparent, and client responses are not always what you might expect. It is helpful for nurses to purposefully focus on shared problem solving and on positive client outcomes and to develop a mutual vision of hope and shared responsibility for health care outcomes (Grover, 2005).

According to one perspective of human relationships, energy fields permeate and connect all beings. Although the use of energy to heal is relatively new concept in Western cultures, it has long existed in Eastern cultures. Healers in early cultures treated their clients holistically and often focused on the concept of balancing energy within each human being to maintain health (McCaffrey & Fowler, 2003).

Therefore, it is not surprising that nurses often perceive a strong sense of connection to other people within a helping relationship. Most nurses embrace the profession's view of people as holistic beings and have experienced synergy in human interactions. When clients and nurses work together, they accomplish much more.

Therapeutic communication occurs within a healing environment between a nurse and a client (Arnold & Boggs, 2007). Nurses know that attitudes and emotions are easily transmitted and can be communicated intentionally or unintentionally. Every nuance of posture, every small expression and gesture, every word chosen, every attitude held—all have the potential to hurt or heal. Because thought patterns (positive or negative), intention, and behaviour directly influence human energy fields and therefore health, nurses have a tremendous ethical responsibility to do no harm to people entrusted to their care. Communication must be respected for its potential power and not carelessly misused to hurt, manipulate, or coerce clients. Good communication empowers clients and enables them to know themselves and make their own choices, which is an essential aspect of the healing process. Nurses have the opportunity to create positive outcomes for themselves, their clients, and their colleagues through therapeutic communication.

Developing Communication Skills

Gaining expertise in communication, as in any aspect of nursing, requires both an understanding of the communication process and reflection about your personal communication experiences. Developing good critical thinking skills enables the most effective communication. You can draw on theoretical knowledge about communication and integrate this knowledge with previously learned knowledge gained through personal experience. You can interpret messages received from other people, analyze their content, make inferences about their meaning, evaluate their effect, explain the rationale for communication techniques used, and self-examine personal communication skills (Balzer Riley, 2004).

Other qualities of good critical thinking are also important to the communication process. Curiosity, perseverance, creativity, self-confidence, independence, fairness, integrity, and humility are useful in approaching a problem. Curiosity motivates you to learn more about a person, and clients are more likely to communicate with nurses who express an interest in them. Perseverance and creativity are necessary for identifying innovative solutions. Self-confidence enables you to more readily establish interpersonal helping-trust relationships and conveys competence in the professional role. A sense of independence enables you to take the risk of communicating ideas about nursing interventions even though colleagues may question your suggestions. An attitude of fairness enables you to listen to both sides in any discussion: You are able to recognize when your opinions conflict with those of the client, to review positions objectively, and to decide how to communicate to reach mutually beneficial decisions. Integrity prompts you to communicate responsibly and ask for help if you are uncertain or uncomfortable with any aspects of client care. Humility is necessary for you to recognize and communicate the need for more information before a decision can be made (Paul & Elder, 2001). In summary, critical thinking that is based on established nursing practice standards and a professional code of ethics promotes effective communication and facilitates high-quality client care.

Interpersonal communication may be challenging because it is based on an individual's perception of received information and is therefore subject to misinterpretation. **Perception** is based on information acquired through the five senses of sight, hearing, taste, touch, and smell (Stuart & Laraia, 2005). It is a process of mentally organizing and interpreting sensory information to arrive at a meaningful conclusion. An individual's culture, education, and personal background also influence perception. Critical thinking can help nurses overcome **perceptual biases**, which are human tendencies that interfere with accurately perceiving and interpreting messages from other people. People often assume that others would think, feel, act, react, and behave as they themselves would in similar circumstances. People tend to distort or ignore information that goes against their expectations, preconceptions, or stereotypes (Beebe et al., 2004). By thinking critically about personal communication habits, you will learn to control these tendencies and become more effective in interpersonal relationships.

As communication skills develop, competence in the nursing care process also grows. You need to integrate communication skills throughout the nursing care process as you collaborate with clients and members of the health care team to achieve goals (Box 18–1). Communication skills are used to gather, analyze, and transmit information and to accomplish the work of each step of the process. Assessment, diagnosis, planning, implementation, and evaluation all depend on effective communication among nurse, client, family, and other members of the health care team. Although the nursing care process is a reliable framework for client care, it does not work well unless you master the art of effective interpersonal communication.

The nature of the communication process requires nurses to constantly make decisions about what, when, where, why, and how to convey messages to other people. Decision making is always contextual: The unique features of any situation influence the nature of the decisions made. For example, the importance of following a prescribed diet will be explained differently to a client with a newly diagnosed medical condition than to a client who has repeatedly chosen not to follow diet restrictions. Effective communication techniques are easy to learn, but their application is more difficult. Deciding which techniques best fit each unique nursing situation is challenging. Communication about specific diagnoses such as cancer or end-of-life conditions and dealing with client and family emotions can be challenging, and some nurses struggle to cope with their own reactions and emotions (Sheldon et al., 2006).

Throughout this chapter, brief clinical examples guide you in the use of effective communication techniques. Situations that challenge nurses' decision-making and communication skills and call for careful consideration of therapeutic techniques often involve the styles of individuals described in Box 18–2. Because the best way to acquire skill is through practice, it is useful for you to discuss and role-play these scenarios before experiencing them in the clinical setting. Consider that clients, family, nurse colleagues, unregulated care providers, physicians, or other members of the health care team might be involved, and decide which communication techniques might be most effective.

Levels of Communication

Nurses use different levels of communication in their professional role. The nurse's communication skills need to include techniques that reflect competence in each level.

> **BOX 18-1   Communication Throughout the Nursing Care Process**

Assessment

Verbal interviewing and history taking

Visual and intuitive observation of nonverbal behaviour

Documentation of visual, tactile, and auditory data during physical examination

Written medical records, diagnostic test results, and literature review

Nursing Diagnosis

Intrapersonal analysis of assessment findings

Validation of health care needs and priorities through verbal discussion with client

Handwritten or electronic documentation of nursing diagnosis

Planning

Interpersonal or small-group planning sessions with health care team

Interpersonal collaboration with client and family to determine implementation methods

Written documentation of expected outcomes

Written or verbal referral to members of the health care team

Implementation

Delegation and verbal discussion with health care team

Verbal, visual, auditory, and tactile health teaching activities

Provision of support through therapeutic communication techniques

Contact with other health care resources

Written documentation of client's progress in medical record

Evaluation

Acquisition of verbal and nonverbal feedback

Comparison of actual and expected outcomes

Identification of factors affecting outcomes

Modification and update of care plan

Verbal or written explanation, or both, of revisions of care plan to client

---

> **BOX 18-2   Challenging Communication Styles of Clients**

- Silent, withdrawn; do not express any feelings or needs
- Sad, depressed; have slow mental and motor responses
- Angry, hostile; do not listen to explanations
- Uncooperative; resent being asked to do something
- Talkative, lonely; want someone with them all the time
- Demanding; want someone to wait on them or meet their requests
- Ranting and raving; blame nursing staff unfairly for their misfortunes or difficulties
- Sensory impaired; cannot hear or see well
- Verbally impaired; cannot articulate needs or desires
- Gossiping; violate confidentiality and cause friction
- Mentally handicapped; are frightened and distrustful
- Confused, disoriented; are bewildered and uncooperative
- Foreign-born; speak very little of the dominant culture's language
- Anxious, nervous; cannot cope with what is happening
- Grieving, crying; have sustained a major loss
- Screaming, kicking (toddlers); want their parents
- Flirtatious, sexually inappropriate
- Loud, obscene; cause disturbances or violate rules

Intrapersonal Communication

Intrapersonal communication, also known as *self-talk* or *inner thought,* is a powerful form of communication that occurs within an individual. It is exemplified in one's thinking (Beebe et al., 2004). People's thoughts strongly influence perceptions, feelings, behaviour, and self-concept; thus, it is important for you to be aware of the nature and content of your thinking. Nurses and clients use intrapersonal communication to develop self-awareness and a positive self-concept that can facilitate self-expression and improve health and self-esteem by replacing negative thoughts with positive assertions. Another type of intrapersonal communication, self-instruction, can provide a mental rehearsal for difficult tasks or situations.

Interpersonal Communication

Interpersonal communication is one-to-one interaction between the nurse and another person that often occurs face to face. It is the level most frequently used in nursing situations and is the crux of nursing practice. It takes place within a social context and includes all the symbols and cues used to give and receive meaning.

Sometimes messages are received differently than the messenger intended. Nurses work with people who have different opinions, experiences, values, and belief systems; therefore, meaning must be validated or mutually negotiated between participants. Meaningful interpersonal communication results in exchange of ideas, problem solving, expression of feelings, decision making, goal accomplishment, team building, and personal growth.

Transpersonal Communication

Transpersonal communication is interaction that occurs within a person's spiritual domain. Interest in the influence of religion and spirituality has increased dramatically since the 1980s and much has been written to promote nurses' understanding of the role spirituality plays in facilitating health care and coping ability (Burkhardt & Nagai-Jacobson, 2002; Taylor, 2002). Many people use prayer, meditation, guided reflection, religious rituals, or other means to communicate with their "higher power." Nurses who value the importance of human spirituality often use this form of communication with clients and for themselves. Nurses have a moral and ethical responsibility to assess clients' spiritual needs and to intervene to meet those needs.

Small-Group Communication

Small-group communication is interaction that occurs when a small number of people meet together and share a common purpose. This type of communication is usually goal directed and requires an understanding of group dynamics. When nurses work on committees, lead client support groups, form research teams, or participate in client care conferences, they are using a small-group communication process. For small groups to function effectively, members must feel accepted, comfortable in sharing ideas and thoughts openly and honestly, able to actively listen to other group members and consider possible alternative viewpoints (Sully & Dallas, 2005).

Public Communication

Public communication is interaction with an audience. Nurses have opportunities to speak with groups of consumers about health-related topics, present scholarly work to colleagues at conferences, or lead classroom discussions with peers or students. Public communication requires special adaptations in eye contact, gestures, and voice inflection and the use of media materials to communicate messages effectively. Effective public communication increases audience knowledge about health-related topics, health care issues, and other issues important to the nursing profession.

Basic Elements of the Communication Process

Communication is an ongoing, dynamic, and multidimensional process. Its basic elements are illustrated in Figure 18–1 and described in the following paragraphs. This simple model represents a very complex process, but it helps identify its essential components. Nursing situations have many unique aspects that influence the nature of communication and interpersonal relationships. In the professional role, you use critical thinking to focus on each aspect of communication so that interactions can be purposeful and effective.

Referent

The **referent** motivates one person to communicate with another. In a health care setting, sights, sounds, odours, time schedules, messages, objects, emotions, sensations, perceptions, ideas, and other cues trigger communication. The nurse who knows the stimulus that triggered communication is able to develop and organize messages more efficiently and better perceive meaning in another person's message. For example, a client's request for help prompted by difficulty breathing triggers a different nursing response than does a request prompted by boredom.

Sender and Receiver

The **sender** is the person who encodes and delivers the message, and the **receiver** is the person who receives and decodes the message. The sender puts ideas or feelings into a form that can be transmitted and is responsible for accuracy and emotional tone. The sender's message acts as a referent for the receiver, who is responsible for attending to, decoding, and responding to the sender's message. Sender and receiver roles are fluid and change back and forth as people interact; sometimes sending and receiving even occur simultaneously. The more the sender and receiver have in common and the closer their

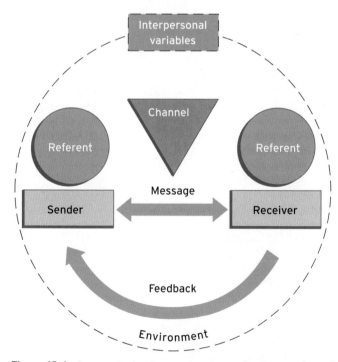

Figure 18-1 Communication is an active process between sender and receiver.

relationship is, the more likely they will accurately perceive one another's meaning and respond accordingly.

Messages

The **message** is the content of the communication. It contains verbal, nonverbal, and symbolic expressions of thoughts or feelings that are transmitted from the sender to the receiver (Arnold & Boggs, 2007). Personal perceptions sometimes distort the receiver's interpretation of the message. Two nurses can provide the same information and yet convey very different messages according to their personal communication styles. One nurse can send the same message to two people and be understood differently by each. You can send effective messages by expressing yourself clearly, directly, and in a manner familiar to the receiver. By watching the listener for nonverbal cues that suggest confusion or misunderstanding, you can determine whether the message needs to be clarified. Communication can be difficult when participants have different levels of education and experience. "Your incision is well approximated without purulent drainage," means the same as "Your wound edges are together, and you have no signs of infection," but the latter is easier to understand. You must be sure clients are able to read before you send messages in writing.

Channels

Channels are means of conveying and receiving messages through visual, auditory, and tactile senses. Facial expressions send visual messages, spoken words travel through auditory channels, and touch traverses tactile channels. The more channels the sender uses to convey a message, the more clearly the message is usually understood. For example, when teaching about insulin self-injection, the nurse talks about and demonstrates the technique, gives the client printed information, and encourages hands-on practice with the vial and syringe. Nurses use verbal, nonverbal, and mediated (technological) communication channels. They send and receive information in person, by informal or formal writing, over the telephone or pager, by audiotape and videotape, through fax and electronic mail, and through electronic online interactive and information sites.

Feedback

Feedback is the message returned by the receiver. It indicates whether the meaning of the sender's message was understood by the receiver. Senders need to seek verbal and nonverbal feedback to ensure that good communication has occurred. To be effective, the sender and receiver must be sensitive and open to each other's messages, clarify the messages, and modify behaviour accordingly. In a social relationship, both participants assume equal responsibility for seeking openness and clarification, but in the nurse–client relationship, this responsibility is primarily the nurse's.

Interpersonal Variables

Interpersonal variables are characteristics within both the sender and receiver that influence communication. Perception is one such variable that provides a uniquely personal view of reality that is informed by the person's expectations and experiences. People sense, interpret, and understand events differently. A nurse might say, "You have been very quiet since your family left. Is something on your mind?" One client might perceive the nurse's question as showing caring and concern; another might perceive the nurse as being intrusive. Other interpersonal variables include educational and developmental levels, sociocultural backgrounds, values and beliefs, emotions, gender, physical health status, and roles and relationships. Variables associated with illness, such as pain, anxiety, and medication effects, can also affect nurse–client communication (Feldman-Stewart et al., 2005).

Environment

The **environment** is the setting for sender–receiver interaction. For effective communication, the environment should meet participants' needs for physical and emotional comfort and safety. Noise, temperature extremes, distractions, and lack of privacy or space create confusion, tension, and discomfort. Environmental distractions are common in health care settings and interfere with messages sent between people; therefore, nurses must try to control the environment as much as possible to create favourable conditions for effective communication.

Forms of Communication

Messages are conveyed verbally, nonverbally, concretely, and symbolically. As people communicate, they express themselves through words, movements, voice inflection, facial expressions, and use of space. These elements work in harmony to enhance a message, or they conflict with one another to contradict and garble the message.

Verbal Communication

Verbal communication entails the use of spoken or written words. Verbal language is a code that conveys specific meaning through a combination of words. The most important aspects of verbal communication are discussed as follows.

Vocabulary. Communication is unsuccessful if senders and receivers cannot decode each other's words and phrases. When a nurse cares for a client who speaks another language, the services of an interpreter may be necessary. Even those who speak the same language use subcultural variations of certain words: *dinner* may mean a noon meal to one person and the last meal of the day to another. Medical jargon (technical terminology used by health care professionals) may sound like a foreign language to clients and should be used only with other members of the health care team. Children have more limited vocabularies than do adults and may use special words to describe bodily functions or a favourite blanket or toy. Teenagers often use words in unique ways that are unfamiliar to adults.

Denotative and Connotative Meaning. A single word can have several meanings. Individuals who use a common language share the denotative meaning: *Baseball* has the same meaning for everyone who speaks English, but *code* denotes cardiac arrest primarily to health care professionals. The connotative meaning is the shade or interpretation of a word's meaning influenced by the thoughts, feelings, or ideas that people have about the word. Families who are told that a loved one is "in serious condition" may believe that death is near, but to nurses *serious* may simply describe the nature of the condition. You need to select words carefully, avoiding terms that can be easily misinterpreted, especially when explaining a client's medical condition or therapy. Even a much-used phrase such as "I'm going to take your vital signs" can be unfamiliar to an adult or frightening to a child.

Pacing. Messages are conveyed more successfully when sent at an appropriate speed or pace. Speak slowly enough to enunciate clearly. Talking rapidly, using awkward pauses, or speaking slowly and deliberately can convey an unintended message. Long pauses and rapid shifts to another topic may give the impression that you are hiding the truth. Pacing is improved by thinking before speaking and by developing awareness of the cadence of your speech.

Intonation. Tone of voice dramatically affects the meaning of a message. Depending on intonation, even a simple question or statement can express enthusiasm, anger, concern, or indifference. To avoid sending unintended messages, be aware of your tone of voice. For example, clients may interpret a nurse's tone of voice as condescending, and further communication may be inhibited. A client's voice tone often provides information about his or her emotional state or energy level.

Clarity and Brevity. Effective communication is simple, brief, and direct. Fewer words result in less confusion. You achieve clarity by speaking slowly, enunciating clearly, and using examples to make explanations easier to understand. Repeating important parts of a message also clarifies communication. Phrases such as "you know" or "OK?" at the end of every sentence detract from clarity. Brevity is achieved by using short sentences and words that express an idea simply and directly. "Where is your pain?" is much better than "I would like you to describe for me the location of your discomfort."

Timing and Relevance. Timing is critical in communication. Even though a message is clear, poor timing can limit its effectiveness. For example, you should not begin routine teaching when a client is in severe pain, is in emotional distress, or is distracted by pressing matters. Often the best time for interaction is when a client expresses an interest in communicating. If messages are relevant or important to the situation at hand, they are more effective. When a client is facing emergency surgery, discussing the risks of smoking is less relevant than explaining preoperative procedures.

Nonverbal Communication

Nonverbal communication makes use of all five senses and refers to transmission of messages that do not involve the spoken or written word. Researchers have estimated that approximately 7% of meaning is transmitted by words, 38% is transmitted by vocal cues, and 55% is transmitted by body cues. Nonverbal communication serves to accent, complement, contradict, regulate, repeat, or substitute for verbal messages (Devito et al., 2005). Nonverbal communication is unconsciously motivated and therefore reflects a person's intended meaning more accurately than do spoken words (Stuart & Laraia, 2005). When verbal and nonverbal communication are incongruous, the receiver usually "hears" the nonverbal message as the true message.

All kinds of nonverbal communication are important, but interpreting them is often difficult. Sociocultural background is a major influence on the meaning of nonverbal behaviour. Nonverbal messages between people of different cultures are easily misinterpreted. Because the interpretation of nonverbal behaviour is subjective, it is important to check its perceived meaning (Adler et al., 2004). Assessing nonverbal messages is an important nursing skill (Grover, 2005).

Personal Appearance. Personal appearance includes physical characteristics, facial expression, manner of dress and grooming, and adornments. These factors help communicate physical well-being, personality, social status, occupation, religion, culture, and self-concept. First impressions are largely based on appearance. Nurses learn to develop a general impression of client health and emotional status through appearance, and clients develop a general impression of the nurse's professionalism and caring in the same way.

Posture and Gait. Posture and gait are forms of self-expression. The ways that people sit, stand, and move reflect attitudes, emotions, self-concept, and health status. For example, an erect posture and a quick, purposeful gait communicate a sense of well-being and confidence. Leaning forward conveys attention. A slumped posture and a slow, shuffling gait may be indicative of depression, illness, discomfort, or fatigue.

Facial Expression. The face is the most expressive part of the body. Facial expressions convey emotions such as surprise, fear, anger, happiness, and sadness. Some people have an expressionless face, or flat affect, which reveals little about what they are thinking or feeling. An inappropriate affect is a facial expression that does not match the content of a verbal message: for example, smiling when describing a sad situation. People are sometimes unaware of the messages their expressions convey. For example, a nurse may frown in concentration while doing a procedure and the client may interpret this as anger or disapproval. Clients closely observe nurses. Consider the impact a nurse's facial expression might have on a person who asks, "Am I going to die?" The slightest change in the eyes, lips, or facial muscles will reveal the nurse's feelings. Although it is hard to control all facial expression, try to avoid showing shock, disgust, dismay, or other distressing reactions in the client's presence.

Eye Contact. People signal readiness to communicate through eye contact. In European and American cultures, maintaining eye contact during conversation shows respect and willingness to listen. Eye contact also allows people to closely observe one another. Lack of eye contact may indicate anxiety, defensiveness, discomfort, or lack of confidence in communicating. However, people from some Asian and Aboriginal cultures consider eye contact intrusive, threatening, or harmful, and they minimize or avoid its use. Eye movements can also communicate feelings and emotions. Standing above a person (looking downward) conveys authority, whereas interacting at the same eye level indicates equality in the relationship. Rising to the same eye level as an angry person communicates self-assertion.

Gestures. Gestures emphasize, punctuate, and clarify the spoken word. Gestures alone carry specific meanings, or they create messages with other communication cues. A finger pointed toward a person may communicate several meanings, but when accompanied by a frown and stern voice, the gesture conveys an accusation or a threat. Pointing to an area of pain may be more accurate than verbally describing the location.

Sounds. Sounds such as sighs, moans, groans, or sobs also communicate feelings and thoughts. When combined with other nonverbal communication, sounds help send clear messages. Sounds can be interpreted in several ways: sighing often suggests boredom or anxiety, moaning may convey pleasure or suffering, and crying may communicate happiness, sadness, or anger. You need to validate such nonverbal messages with the client in order to interpret them accurately.

Territoriality and Personal Space. Territoriality is the need to gain, maintain, and defend one's right to space. Territory is important because it provides people with a sense of identity, security, and control. Territory can be distinguished and made visible to other people, as with a fence around a yard or a curtain around a bed in a hospital room. Personal space, however, is invisible and individual, and it travels with the person. During interpersonal interaction, people maintain varying distances between each other, depending on their culture, the nature of their relationship, and the situation. When personal space becomes threatened, people respond defensively and communicate less effectively. Specific situations dictate whether the interpersonal distance between nurse and client is appropriate. Nurses often must move into clients' territory and personal space because of the nature of caregiving. Before entering into a client's personal space, it is essential that you prepare both your client and the environment. By explaining to your client what you will do and preparing the environment for particular nursing interventions, your client will recognize a shift toward the establishment of a therapeutic interaction. You need to convey confidence, gentleness, and respect for privacy, especially when your actions will require intimate contacts or involve a client's vulnerable zone. Box 18–3 provides examples of nursing actions within zones of personal space (Stuart & Laraia, 2005) and zones of touch.

Symbolic Communication

Good communication requires awareness of **symbolic communication**, the verbal and nonverbal symbolism used to convey meaning. Art and music are forms of symbolic communication that nurses use to enhance understanding and promote healing. Lane (2006) found that creative expressions such as art, music, and dance have a healing effect on clients. Clients reported decreased pain and greater joy and hope.

Metacommunication

Metacommunication is a broad term that refers to all factors that influence how a message is perceived by other people (Arnold & Boggs, 2007). It is communication *about* communication (Devito et al., 2005) that reflects the relational aspects of messages (Adler et al., 2004) and helps people better understand what has been communicated. For example, a nurse observes a young client holding his body rigidly erect, and his voice is sharp as he says, "Going to surgery is no big deal." The nurse replies, "You say having surgery doesn't bother you, but you look and sound tense. I'd like to help." Awareness of the tone of the verbal response and the nonverbal behaviour may result in further exploration of the client's feelings and concerns.

Professional Nursing Relationships

The nurse's application of knowledge, understanding of human behaviour and communication, and commitment to ethical behaviour all contribute to the formation of professional relationships. Having a philosophy based on caring and respect for other people will help you be more successful in establishing professional relationships.

Nurse-Client Helping Relationships

Helping relationships are the foundation of clinical nursing practice. In such relationships, the nurse assumes the role of professional helper and comes to know the client as an individual who has unique health care needs, human responses, and patterns of living. The relationship is therapeutic, promoting a psychological climate that facilitates positive change and growth. Therapeutic communication allows clients to achieve their health care–related goals and attain optimal personal growth (Arnold & Boggs, 2007). It includes an explicit time frame and a goal-directed approach, and confidentiality is an expected feature. The nurse establishes, directs, and takes responsibility for the interaction, and the client's needs take priority over the nurse's needs. The relationship is also characterized by the nurse's nonjudgemental acceptance of the client. Acceptance conveys a willingness to hear a message or to acknowledge feelings. It does not mean you always agree with the client or approve of the client's decisions or actions. A helping relationship between nurse and client does not just happen; you create it through care, skill, and the development of trust.

The nurse–client helping relationship is characterized by a natural progression of four goal-directed phases: preinteraction, orientation, working, and termination phases (Box 18–4). These phases often begin before the nurse meets the client and continue

---

> **BOX 18-3**   **Zones of Personal Space and Touch**

Zones of Personal Space

Intimate Zone (0 to 45 cm)
Holding a crying infant
Performing physical assessment
Bathing, grooming, dressing, feeding, and toileting a client
Changing a client's dressing

Personal Zone (45 cm to 1 m)
Sitting at a client's bedside
Taking the client's nursing history
Teaching an individual client
Exchanging information with health care staff at change of shift

Social Zone (1 to 4 m)
Participating in client care rounds
Sitting at the head of a conference table
Teaching a class for clients with a specific disease
Conducting a family support group session

Public Zone (4 m and greater)
Speaking at a community forum
Testifying at a legislative hearing
Lecturing to a class of students

Zones of Touch

Social Zone (permission not needed)
Hands, arms, shoulders, back

Consent Zone (permission needed)
Mouth, wrists, feet

Vulnerable Zone (special care needed)
Face, neck, front of body

Intimate Zone (great sensitivity needed)
Genitalia, rectum

---

until the caregiving relationship ends. Even a brief interaction is characterized by an abbreviated version of these four phases. For example, the student nurse gathers client information to prepare in advance for caregiving, meets the client and establishes trust, accomplishes health care–related goals through use of the nursing care process, and says goodbye at the end of the shift or when the client leaves the unit.

Socializing is an important initial component of interpersonal communication. It helps people get to know one another and relax. It is easy, superficial, and not deeply personal, whereas therapeutic interactions are often more difficult, intense, and uncomfortable. A nurse often uses social conversation to lay a foundation for a closer relationship: "Hi, Mr. Simpson. I hear it's your birthday today. Happy birthday!" A friendly, informal, and warm communication style helps establish trust, but nurses must get beyond social conversation to talk about issues or concerns affecting the client's health. During social conversation, clients may ask personal questions about the nurse's family, place of residence, and so forth. Students often wonder whether it is appropriate to reveal such information. The skillful nurse uses judgement about what to share and provides minimal information or deflects such questions with gentle humour and refocuses conversation back to the client.

► BOX 18-4   Phases of the Helping Relationship

Pre-interaction Phase

Before meeting the client, the nurse accomplishes the following tasks:

- Reviews available data, including the medical and nursing history
- Talks to other caregivers who may have information about the client
- Anticipates health care concerns or issues that may arise
- Identifies a location and setting that will foster comfortable, private interaction with the client
- Plans enough time for the initial interaction

Orientation Phase

When the nurse and client meet and get to know one another, the nurse accomplishes the following tasks:

- Sets the tone for the relationship by adopting a warm, empathetic, caring manner
- Recognizes that the initial relationship may be superficial, uncertain, and tentative
- Expects the client to test the nurse's competence and commitment
- Closely observes the client and expects to be closely observed by the client
- Begins to make inferences and form judgements about client messages and behaviours
- Assesses the client's health status
- Prioritizes the client's problems and identifies the client's goals
- Clarifies the client's and nurse's roles
- Negotiates a contract with the client that specifies who will do what
- Lets the client know when to expect the relationship to be terminated

Working Phase

When the nurse and client work together to solve problems and achieve goals, the nurse accomplishes the following tasks:

- Encourages and helps the client to express feelings about his or her health
- Encourages and helps the client to explore own feelings and thoughts
- Provides information that the client needs to understand and change behaviour
- Encourages and helps the client to set goals
- Takes actions to meet the goals set with the client
- Uses therapeutic communication skills to facilitate successful interactions
- Uses appropriate self-disclosure and confrontation

Termination Phase

During the ending of the relationship, the nurse accomplishes the following tasks:

- Reminds the client that relationship termination is near
- Evaluates goal achievement with the client
- Reminisces about the relationship with the client
- Separates from the client by relinquishing responsibility for his or her care
- Facilitates a smooth transition for the client to other caregivers as needed

Creating a therapeutic environment depends on the your ability to communicate, comfort, and help clients meet their needs. Comfort is crucial in the practice of nursing. Therapeutic interactions increase feelings of personal control by helping clients feel secure, informed, and valued. Optimizing personal control facilitates emotional comfort, which minimizes physical discomfort and promotes recovery (Williams & Irurita, 2006) (Box 18-5).

In a therapeutic relationship, nurses often encourage clients to share personal stories, which are called *narrative interactions*. Through narrative interactions, such as reminiscing with clients, you begin to understand the context of clients' lives and learn what is meaningful to the clients from their perspective (Shattell & Hogan, 2005). For example, a nurse asked a client to tell about a time in his life when he had to make a hard decision. The client related the following story:

"When I was a young man, I worked on the family farm. An uncle died and left me some money. All of a sudden, I could afford to go to college, but Dad didn't want me to go because he needed me there. I had to decide whether to stay or go, and it was real hard because at first I just wanted to get away. I talked to our preacher, and he said it was up to me, to pray about it and do what my heart told me to. So I stayed. Oh, I've thought from time to time what I might have made of myself, but I never regretted it. I had a good life in farming."

From this brief story, the nurse understood that it was important to the client to put his family's needs above his personal desires and that seeking spiritual guidance was an important component of his decision making. This same information may not have been

✳ BOX 18-5   EVIDENCE-INFORMED PRACTICE GUIDELINE

Emotional Comfort

Evidence Summary

In a study by Williams and Irurita (2006), recently hospitalized clients described emotional comfort as a pleasant positive feeling and state of relaxation that resulted from therapeutic interactions. Clients described emotional discomfort as unpleasant negative feelings and tension. Personal control over the situation contributed to emotional comfort. Therapeutic interactions helped the client achieve control and were associated with emotional comfort. Clients perceived a positive link between emotional comfort and recovery.

Application to Nursing Practice

- Clients perceive a connection between the mind and body.
- Increased emotional comfort increases physical comfort and enhances recovery.
- Nurse–client therapeutic interactions improve the client's emotional and physical comfort.
- By using therapeutic communication to increase the client's perceived control of the situation and the environment, nurses increase the client's comfort.

References: Williams, A. M., & Irurita, V. F. (2006). Emotional comfort: The patient's perspective of a therapeutic context. *International Journal of Nursing Studies, 43*(4), 405–415.

revealed had the nurse used a standard history that usually elicits only short answers.

Collaboration between nurses and clients builds relationships and is based on principles of mutual gain and respect. It reflects a desire to satisfy the needs of both parties (Dubrin & Geerinck, 2006). Collaborative communication promotes personal responsibility, enables self-expression, and strengthens the client's problem-solving ability.

Nurse-Family Relationships

Many nursing situations, especially those in community care and home care settings, require the nurse to form helping relationships with entire families. The same principles that guide one-to-one helping relationships also apply when the client is a family unit; however, communication within families requires additional understanding of the complexities of family dynamics, needs, and relationships (see Chapter 20).

Nurse-Health Care Team Relationships

Nurses function in roles that require interaction with multiple members of the health care team. Many elements of the nurse–client helping relationship also apply to collegial relationships, which focus on accomplishing the work and goals of the clinical setting. Communication in such relationships may be geared toward team building, facilitating group process, collaboration, consultation, delegation, supervision, leadership, and management (see Chapter 11). You need a variety of communication skills, including presentational speaking, persuasion, group problem solving, providing performance reviews, and writing business reports.

Social and therapeutic interactions are needed between the nurse and members of the health care team to build morale and strengthen relationships within the work setting. Everyone has interpersonal needs for acceptance, inclusion, identity, privacy, power and control, and affection (Stewart & Logan, 2005). Nurses need friendship, support, guidance, and encouragement from one another to cope with the many stressors imposed by the nursing role and must extend the same caring communication used with clients to build positive relationships with colleagues and coworkers.

Nurse-Community Relationships

Many nurses form relationships with community groups by participating in local organizations, volunteering for community service, or becoming politically active. In a community-based practice, you must be able to establish relationships with their community to be an effective agent for change (see Chapter 4). Understanding the importance of community-oriented, population-focused nursing practice and developing the skills to practise it are crucial in attaining a leadership role in health care, regardless of the practice setting (Stanhope & Lancaster, 2004). Through neighbourhood newsletters, public bulletin boards, newspapers, radio, television, and electronic information sites, you can share information and discuss issues important to community health care.

Elements of Professional Communication

Professional appearance, demeanour, and behaviour are important in establishing your trustworthiness and competence. They communicate the impression that you have assumed the professional helping role, are clinically skilled, and are focused on the client. Nothing harms the professional image of nurses as much as an individual nurse's inappropriate appearance or behaviour.

A health care professional is expected to be clean, neat, well-groomed, conservatively dressed, and free of scent and odour. Visible tattoos and body piercings other than ear piercings are not acceptable in the professional setting. Professional behaviour should reflect warmth, friendliness, confidence, and competence. Professionals speak in a clear well-modulated voice, use good grammar, listen to other people, help and support colleagues, and communicate effectively. Being punctual, organized, well-prepared, and equipped for the responsibilities of the nursing role also communicate professionalism.

Courtesy

Common courtesy is part of professional communication. To practise courtesy, say hello and goodbye to clients, knock on doors before entering, and use self-introduction. A courteous nurse will also state his or her purpose, address people by name, say "please" and "thank you" to members of the health care team, and apologize for inadvertently causing distress. When a nurse is discourteous, he or she is perceived as rude or insensitive. Such behaviour sets up barriers between nurse and client and causes friction among members of the health care team.

Use of Names

Self-introduction is important. Failure to give a name, indicate status (e.g., student nurse, registered nurse, or licensed practical nurse), or acknowledge the client creates uncertainty about the interaction and conveys a lack of commitment or caring. Making eye contact and smiling at other people communicates recognition. Addressing other people by name conveys respect for human dignity and uniqueness. Because using last names is respectful in most cultures, nurses usually use the client's last name in the initial interaction, but they may use the first name in subsequent interactions at the client's request. It is important to ask other people how they would like to be addressed and to honour their preferences. Using first names is appropriate for infants, young children, confused or unconscious clients, and close colleagues. Terms of endearment such as "honey," "dear," "Grandma," or "sweetheart" are not appropriate; they may be perceived as disrespectful. The use of plural pronouns such as "we" when referring to clients implies a loss of independence and may be interpreted as condescending (Williams et al., 2004). Referring to a client by diagnosis, room number, or another attribute is demeaning and implies that you do not care enough to know the client as an individual.

Trustworthiness

Trust entails relying on someone without doubt or question. Being trustworthy means helping other people without hesitation. To foster trust, you need to communicate warmth and demonstrate consistency, reliability, honesty, integrity, competence, and respect. Sometimes it is not easy for a client to ask for help. Trusting another person involves risk and vulnerability, but it also fosters open, therapeutic communication and enhances the expression of feelings, thoughts, and needs. Without trust, a nurse–client relationship rarely progresses beyond social interaction and superficial care. Avoid dishonesty. Knowingly withholding key information, lying, or distorting the truth violates both legal and ethical standards of practice. Maintaining confidentiality and protecting a client's privacy are also important aspects of professional behaviour. Sharing personal information or gossiping about other people communicates the message that you cannot be trusted and damages interpersonal relationships.

Autonomy and Responsibility

Autonomy is the ability to be self-directed and independent in accomplishing goals and advocating for other people. Professional nurses make choices and accept responsibility for the outcomes of their actions (Townsend, 2005). They take initiative in solving problems and communicate in a manner that reflects the importance and purpose of the therapeutic interaction (Arnold & Boggs, 2007). It is also important to recognize the client's autonomy because people who seek health care are often concerned about losing control of decisions regarding how they live.

Assertiveness

Assertive communication allows individuals to act in their own best interests without infringing on or denying the rights of other people (Devito et al., 2005). Assertiveness conveys self-assurance and respect for other people (Stuart & Laraia, 2005).

Nurses teach assertiveness skills to other people as a means of promoting personal health. Assertive people express feelings and emotions confidently, spontaneously, and honestly. They make decisions and control their lives more effectively than do nonassertive individuals. They can deal with criticism and manipulation by other people and learn to say "no," set limits, and resist other people's efforts to impose guilt.

Assertive responses are characterized by feelings of security, competence, power, optimism, and professionalism. They are good tools for dealing with criticism, change, negative conditions in personal or professional life, and conflict or stress in relationships. Assertive responses often contain "I" messages, such as "I want," "I need," "I think," and "I feel."

Communication Within the Nursing Care Process

In the following sections, the focus of the nursing care process is on providing care for clients who need special assistance with communication. However, the section on implementation contains examples of therapeutic communication techniques that are appropriate strategies for use in any interpersonal nursing situation.

❖Assessment

Assessment of a client's ability to communicate includes gathering data about the many contextual factors that influence communication. The word *context* refers to all the parts of a situation that help determine its meaning. A context includes all the environmental factors that influence the nature of communication and interpersonal relationships. This includes the participants' internal factors and characteristics, the nature of their relationship, the situation prompting communication, the environment, and the sociocultural elements present (Beebe et al., 2004). Box 18–6 lists the contextual factors that influence communication. Understanding these contextual factors helps you make sound decisions during the communication process.

Physical and Emotional Factors

Assessing the psychophysiological factors that influence communication is especially important. Many altered health states and human responses limit communication. People with hearing or visual impairments have fewer channels through which to receive messages

---

> **BOX 18-6** | **Contextual Factors That Influence Communication**

Psychophysiological Context

This refers to the internal factors that influence communication:

- Physiological status (e.g., pain, hunger, weakness, dyspnea)
- Emotional status (e.g., anxiety, anger, hopelessness, euphoria)
- Growth and development status (e.g., age, developmental tasks)
- Unmet needs (e.g., safety or security; love or belonging)
- Attitudes, values, and beliefs (e.g., meaning of illness experience)
- Perceptions and personality (e.g., optimistic or pessimistic, introverted or extroverted)
- Self-concept and self-esteem (e.g., positive or negative)

Relational Context

This refers to the nature of the relationship between the participants:

- Social, helping, or working relationship
- Level of trust between participants
- Level of caring expressed
- Level of self-disclosure between participants
- Shared history of participants
- Balance of power and control

Situational Context

This refers to the reason for the communication:

- Information exchange
- Goal achievement
- Problem resolution
- Expression of feelings

Environmental Context

This refers to the physical surroundings in which communication takes place:

- Privacy level
- Noise level
- Comfort and safety level
- Distraction level

Cultural Context

This refers to the sociocultural elements that affect the interaction:

- Educational level of participants
- Language and self-expression patterns
- Customs and expectations
- Media influences

(see Chapter 48). Facial trauma, laryngeal cancer, tracheostomy, or endotracheal intubation often prevents movement of air past vocal cords or mobility of the tongue, which results in inability to articulate words. An extremely breathless person must use oxygen to breathe rather than speak. People with aphasia after a stroke or in late-stage Alzheimer's disease often cannot understand or form words. People with delirium cannot focus attentively, and those with dementia often cannot make sense of what is being said. Certain mental illnesses such as psychoses or depression cause clients to demonstrate flight of ideas (words do not keep up to rapidly changing thoughts), constant verbalization of the same words or phrases, a loose association of ideas, or slowed speech pattern. People who are highly anxious are sometimes unable to perceive environmental stimuli or hear explanations. Unresponsive or heavily sedated people cannot send or respond to verbal messages.

Review of the client's medical record helps provide relevant information about the client's ability to communicate. Through the health history and physical examination, you document physical barriers to speech, neurological deficits, and pathophysiological conditions that affect hearing or vision. Reviewing the client's medication record is also important. For example, opiates, antidepressants, neuroleptics, hypnotics, or sedatives may cause a client to slur words or use incomplete sentences. The nursing progress notes may reveal other factors that contribute to communication difficulties, such as the absence of family members who could provide more information about a confused client.

Assessment should include communicating directly with clients to provide information about their ability to attend to, interpret, and respond to stimuli. If clients have difficulty communicating, it is important to assess the effects of the problem. Clients who cannot communicate effectively will often have difficulty expressing their needs and responding appropriately to the environment. A client who is unable to speak is at risk for injury unless the nurse identifies an alternative communication method. If barriers make it difficult to communicate directly with the client, then family or friends become important sources of information about the client's communication patterns and abilities.

Developmental Factors

Aspects of a client's growth and development also influence nurse–client interactions. For example, an infant's self-expression is limited to crying, body movement, and facial expression, whereas most older children express their needs more directly, through speech and specific actions such as pointing. Nurses adapt communication techniques to the special needs of infants and children. Communication with children and their parents requires special considerations. It is important to include the parents, child, or both as sources of information about the child's health, depending on the child's age. If a young child is given toys or other distractions, parents can give you their full attention. Children are especially responsive to nonverbal messages, and sudden movements, loud noises, or threatening gestures can be frightening. Children often prefer to initiate interpersonal contacts and, like adults, do not like adults to stare or look down at them. A child who has received little environmental stimulation may have delayed language development, which makes communication more challenging.

Age also influences communication. Age alone does not determine an adult's capacity for communication. However, approximately 12% of Canadians aged 65 and older have speech or hearing disorders that limit self-expression or their ability to understand other people (Canadian Association of Speech–Language Pathologists and Audiologists, n.d.). Although many older adults have some form of communication barrier, you need to communicate with them on an adult level to avoid being perceived as patronizing or condescending (Williams et al., 2004). Box 18–7 highlights tips for communicating with older adults who have communication needs and barriers. These tips can be applied to all clients with communication problems.

Sociocultural Factors

Culture is a blueprint for thinking, feeling, behaving, and communicating. Nurses need to be aware of the typical patterns of interaction that characterize various cultures. For example, most Inuit and First Nations peoples value privacy, respect, and silence. Whereas Canadians of European descent are more open and willing to discuss private family matters, Aboriginal Canadians may be reluctant to reveal personal or family information to strangers. Personal information is often conveyed indirectly through storytelling. For example, Hutterite colonies, which form a large portion of the rural Canadian population, have a hierarchical social order, and elders make decisions that affect all community members. For the Hutterites, taking individual responsibility for health care–related choices would not be consistent with communalism and their culture (Fahrenwald et al., 2001). Awareness of such cultural values will facilitate communication between you and your clients (see Chapter 10).

Foreign-born people may not speak or understand English or French. Those who speak a second language often experience difficulty with self-expression or language comprehension. To practise cultural sensitivity in communication, you must understand that people of different cultures use different degrees of eye contact, personal space, gestures, voice modulation, pace of speech, touch, silence, and meaning of language. Make a conscious effort to avoid interpreting messages from your own cultural perspective and to consider communication within the context of the client's background. Do not stereotype, patronize, or make fun of other cultures. Lack of knowledge by both nurses and clients about each other's cultural background and expectations frequently leads to feelings of anxiety, doubt, embarrassment, anger, and frustration (Spence, 2001). Language and cultural barriers prevent effective communication and not only are frustrating but also may lead to delayed or inappropriate care. Developing cultural competence increases understanding between clients and health care professionals and promotes positive client outcomes.

Gender

Gender is another factor that influences how people think, act, feel, and communicate. Male and female communication patterns tend to differ, which can sometimes create barriers to effective communication (Beebe et al., 2004). Boys and men tend to use less verbal communication but are more likely to initiate conversations and address issues directly. Girls and women tend to disclose more personal information, use more active listening, and respond in ways that encourage continued conversation. A male nurse might say to his colleague, "Help me turn Jeremy." A female nurse might say, "Jeremy needs to be turned," expecting her colleague to understand the implied request for help.

To practise gender sensitivity in communication, recognize the differences in male and female communication patterns to avoid misinterpreting messages sent by someone of the opposite gender. Avoid conversations with sexual overtones, gender-denigrating jokes, and male–female stereotyping.

✳ BOX 18-7   FOCUS ON OLDER ADULTS

Tips for Improved Communication With Older Adults Who Have Communication Needs or Barriers

- Capture the client's attention before speaking.
- Check for hearing aids and glasses.
- Introduce yourself.
- Choose a quiet, well-lit environment, and minimize visual and auditory distractions.
- Face the client, and use facial expressions and gestures as needed.
- Amplify your voice if necessary, but do not shout because it distorts sound and your facial expression could be misinterpreted. Speak clearly at a moderate rate.
- Allow time for the client to respond. Do not assume the client is being uncooperative if the client makes no response or a delayed response.
- Give clients time to ask questions and clarify responses.
- Whenever possible, ask a family member or caregiver to join you and the client in the room. Such people are usually most familiar with the client's communication patterns and can assist in the communication process.

❖Nursing Diagnosis

Most individuals experience difficulty with some aspect of communication. People who are free of illness or disability may lack skills in attending, listening, responding, and self-expression. Often, you will direct your care toward individuals who experience more serious communication impairments.

The primary nursing diagnostic label used to describe the client with limited or no ability to communicate verbally is *impaired verbal communication*. This is the state in which the ability to receive, process, transmit, and use symbols is decreased or absent (Doenges et al., 2005). Defining characteristics include the inability to articulate words, inappropriate verbalization, difficulty forming words, and difficulty in comprehending, which the nurse clusters together to form the diagnosis. This diagnosis is useful for a wide variety of clients with special problems and needs related to communication, such as impaired perception, reception, and articulation. Although a client's primary problem may be impaired verbal communication, the associated difficulty in self-expression or altered communication patterns may also contribute to other nursing diagnoses:

- Anxiety
- Social isolation
- Ineffective coping
- Compromised family coping
- Powerlessness
- Impaired social interaction

The related (contributing) factors for a nursing diagnosis focus on the causes of the communication disorder. In the case of impaired verbal communication, these are physiological, mechanical, anatomical, psychological, cultural, or developmental in nature. Accuracy in the identification of related factors is necessary so that you can select interventions that can effectively resolve the diagnostic problem. For example, the diagnosis of *impaired verbal communication related to cultural difference* (Ukrainian heritage) would be managed very differently than the diagnosis of *impaired verbal communication related to deafness*.

❖Planning

Once you have identified the nature of the client's communication dysfunction, you must consider several factors as you design the nursing care plan. Motivation is a factor in improving communication, and clients often must be encouraged to try different approaches. It is especially important to involve the client and family in decisions about the plan of nursing care to determine whether suggested methods are acceptable. Make sure that basic comfort and safety needs are met before you introduce new communication methods and techniques, and allow plenty of time for practice. Participants must be patient with themselves and with each other when learning new skills if communication is to be effective. When the focus is on practising communication, it is best to arrange for a quiet, private place that is free of distractions such as television or visitors. Communication aids, such as a writing board for a client with a tracheostomy or a special call system for a paralyzed client, enhance communication.

Goals and Outcomes

The primary goal of nursing interventions is to facilitate the development of trust between the client and members of the health care team. It is important to identify expected outcomes for all clients, particularly when impaired communication is a concern. Outcomes are specific and measurable and provide the means to determine whether the broader goal is met. For example, outcomes for the client might be as follows:

- The client initiates conversation about diagnosis or health care problem.
- The client is able to attend to appropriate stimuli.
- The client conveys clear and understandable messages with family members and members of the health care team.
- The client expresses increased satisfaction with the communication process.

At times, you will care for well clients whose difficulty in sending, receiving, and interpreting messages interferes with healthy interpersonal relationships. In this case, impaired communication may be contributing to other nursing diagnoses such as *impaired social interaction* or *ineffective coping*. In such cases, you need to plan interventions to help your clients improve their communication skills. For example, you could model effective communication techniques and provide feedback regarding the client's communication. Role-play helps clients rehearse situations in which they have difficulty communicating. Expected outcomes for a client in this situation might include demonstrating the ability to appropriately express needs, feelings, and concerns; communicating thoughts and feelings more clearly; engaging in appropriate social conversation with peers and staff; and increasing feelings of autonomy and assertiveness.

Setting of Priorities

It is essential for the nurse to always be available for communication so that the client is able to express any pressing needs or problems. This may involve an intervention as simple as keeping a call light within reach for a client restricted to bed or providing a communication augmentative device for the client to use (e.g., message board, Braille keyboard). When you plan to have lengthy interactions with a client, it is important to address physical care priorities (i.e., pain or elimination needs) first, so that the client is comfortable and the discussion is not interrupted.

Continuity of Care

To ensure an effective care plan, you may need to collaborate with other members of the health care team who have expertise in communication strategies. Speech therapists help clients with aphasia, interpreters are often needed for clients who speak a foreign language, and psychiatric nurse specialists help angry or highly anxious clients communicate more effectively.

❖Implementation

In carrying out any care plan, nurses use communication techniques that are appropriate for the client's individual needs. Before learning how to adapt communication methods to help clients with serious communication impairments, it is necessary to learn the communication techniques that serve as the foundation for professional communication. It is also important to understand techniques that create barriers to effective interaction.

Therapeutic Communication Techniques

Therapeutic communication techniques are specific responses that encourage the expression of feelings and ideas and convey acceptance and respect. By learning these techniques, you develop awareness of the variety of nursing responses available for use in different situations. Although some of the techniques seem artificial at first, skill and comfort in using them increase with practice. Tremendous satisfaction will result from the development of therapeutic relationships and achievement of desired client outcomes.

Active Listening.
Active listening means to be attentive to what the client is saying both verbally and nonverbally. Active listening enhances trust and facilitates client communication because it demonstrates acceptance and respect for the client. Several nonverbal skills facilitate attentive listening. They can be identified by the acronym *SOLER* (Townsend, 2005):

S: *Sit* facing the client. This posture indicates that you are there to listen and are interested in what the client is saying.

O: Keep an *open* posture (i.e., keep arms and legs uncrossed). This posture suggests that you are receptive ("open") to what the client has to say. A "closed" position may convey a defensive attitude, possibly invoking a similar response in the client.

L: *Lean* toward the client. This posture indicates that you are involved and interested in the interaction.

E: Establish and maintain intermittent *eye contact*. This behaviour conveys your involvement in and willingness to listen to what the client is saying. Absence of eye contact or shifting of the eyes indicates that you are not interested in what the client is saying.

R: *Relax*. It is important to communicate a sense of being relaxed and comfortable with the client. Restlessness communicates a lack of interest and also conveys a sense of discomfort that may extend to the client.

Sharing Observations.
Nurses make observations by commenting on how the client looks, sounds, or acts. Stating observations often helps the client communicate without the need for extensive questioning, focusing, or clarification. This technique helps start a conversation with quiet or withdrawn people. Do not state observations that might anger, embarrass, or upset the client, such as telling someone "You look a mess!" Even if such an observation is made with humour, the client can become resentful.

Sharing observations differs from making assumptions, which means drawing unwarranted conclusions about the client without validating them. Making assumptions puts the client in the position of having to contradict the nurse. Examples might include the nurse interpreting fatigue as depression or assuming that untouched food indicates lack of interest in meeting nutritional goals. Making observations is a gentler and safer technique: "You look tired," "You seem different today," or "I see you haven't eaten anything."

Sharing Empathy.
Empathy is the ability to emotionally and intellectually understand another person's reality, to accurately perceive unspoken feelings, and to communicate this understanding to the other person (Devito et al., 2005). Empathy is expressed when you reflect understanding of the other person's feelings. Cultivating an ability to empathize requires patience, a sense of curiosity, and a willingness to understand a client's viewpoint (Larson & Yao, 2005). Such empathic understanding requires you to be both sensitive and imaginative, especially if you have not had similar experiences. Although nurses are not always empathic, it is an important goal to work toward, a key to unlocking concern and communicating support for other people. Statements reflecting empathy are highly effective because they indicate that you heard the emotional content, as well as the factual content, of the communication. Empathy statements are neutral and nonjudgemental and help establish trust in difficult situations. For example, to an angry client who has limited mobility after a stroke, you might say, "It must be very frustrating to know what you want to do and not be able to do it."

Sharing Hope.
You must recognize that hope is essential for healing, and you must learn to communicate a "sense of possibility" to other people. Appropriate encouragement and positive feedback are important in fostering hope and self-confidence and for helping people achieve their potential and reach their goals. You can instill hope by commenting on the positive aspects of the other person's behaviour, performance, or response. Sharing a vision of the future and reminding clients of their internal resources and coping abilities also strengthens hope. You can reassure clients that many kinds of hope exist and that meaning and personal growth can arise from illness experiences. For example, you might say to a client discouraged about a poor prognosis: "I believe you will find a way to face your situation, because I have seen your courage and creativity in the past."

Sharing Humour.
Humour is an important but underused resource in nursing interactions. Research suggests that a sense of humour is a useful coping strategy for clients, health care professionals, and families (Wanzer et al., 2005) and an essential communication tool for nurses (Dziegielewski et al., 2004). Humour has been shown to have positive effects on both a person's psyche and physiology. Laughter signifies positive events to people and contributes to feelings of togetherness, closeness, and friendliness (Balzer Riley, 2004). Shulman and Haugo (2003) noted that humour positively influences the immune system by decreasing levels of stress-related hormones that suppress immune function and by increasing numbers of defensive immune cells. Humour fosters feelings of power and security, creates nurturing environments, provides a means for expressing empathy, and facilitates social bonding, intimacy, and conflict resolution. Chauvet and Hofmeyer (2006) found that humour also promoted health and well-being, strengthened social connections, enhanced communication, and fostered resilience and coping abilities. Humour is a social lubricant that facilitates therapeutic communication and interpersonal interactions. It reduces tension, increases trust, promotes social bonding, improves self-esteem, stimulates creativity, and broadens one's perspectives, thereby permitting cognitive reframing of difficult situations (Dziegielewski et al., 2004.

Today it is common for nurses to care for clients from different cultures. When nurses interact with clients who do not have a full grasp of the language, it is important to realize that their clients may misunderstand or misinterpret jokes and statements that are meant to be humorous. It is also important to recognize that when either a nurse or a client tries to speak in another language, mistakes can sometimes occur.

Health care professionals sometimes use negative humour after difficult or traumatic situations as a way to deal with extreme tension and stress. This coping humour has a high potential for misinterpretation as lack of caring by people not involved in the situation. For example, student nurses are sometimes offended and wonder how staff can laugh and joke after unsuccessful resuscitation efforts. When nurses use coping humour within earshot of clients or their loved ones, great emotional distress can result.

Sharing Feelings.
Emotions are subjective feelings that result from thoughts and perceptions. Feelings are not right, wrong, good, or bad, although they may be pleasant or unpleasant. If individuals do not express their feelings, stress and illness may worsen. You can help clients express their emotions by making observations, acknowledging feelings, encouraging communication, giving them permission to express "negative" feelings, and modelling healthy emotional self-expression. At times, clients direct anger or frustration prompted by their illness toward nurses, who should not take such expressions personally. Acknowledging clients' feelings demonstrates empathy

and communicates that you listened to and understood the emotional aspects of their illness situation.

When you care for clients, you must be aware of your own emotions because feelings are difficult to hide. Students may wonder whether it is helpful for nurses to share their feelings with clients. Sharing emotion makes nurses seem more human and often brings people closer. It is appropriate to share feelings of caring, or even cry with other people, as long as you are in control of the expression of those feelings and do so in a way that does not burden the client or break confidentiality. Clients are perceptive and can sense a nurse's emotions. It is usually inappropriate to discuss negative personal emotions such as anger or sadness with clients. A social support system of colleagues is helpful, and employee assistance programs, peer group meetings, and the use of interdisciplinary teams such as social work and pastoral care provide other means for nurses to safely express feelings away from clients.

Using Touch. In today's fast-paced technical environments, nurses are required more than ever to bring the sense of caring and human connection to their clients (see Chapter 19). Touch is one of the nurse's most potent forms of communication. Touch conveys many messages, such as affection, emotional support, encouragement, tenderness, and personal attention. Comfort touch, such as holding a hand, is especially important for vulnerable clients who are experiencing severe illness with its accompanying physical and emotional losses. Nurses often use touch with older people to provide comfort and reassurance (Gleeson & Timmins, 2004), to convey caring and consolation, to add emphasis to explanations, and to convey empathy in situations when speaking might break a mood (Arnold & Boggs, 2007). It is important for nurses to abide by cultural norms when interacting with clients from other cultures (Figure 18–2).

Students may initially find giving intimate care stressful, especially when caring for clients of the opposite gender. Students learn to cope with intimate contact by changing their perception of the situation. Because much of what nurses do involves touching, you must learn to be sensitive to other people's reactions to touch and use it wisely. Touch should be as gentle or as firm as needed and delivered in a comforting, nonthreatening manner. In certain situations, you must withhold touch, for example, when interacting with highly suspicious or angry people who may respond negatively or even violently when touched.

Using Silence. It takes time and experience to become comfortable with silence. Most people have a natural tendency to fill silences with words, but sometimes silences serve the need for time for the nurse and client to observe one another, sort out their feelings, think about how to say things, and consider what has been communicated. Silence prompts some people to talk. Silence allows clients to think and gain insight into their situations. In general, you should allow the client to break the silence, particularly when the client has initiated it (Stuart & Laraia, 2005).

Silence is particularly useful when people are confronted with decisions that require much thought. For example, silence may help a client gain confidence needed to share the decision to refuse medical treatment. Silence also allows the nurse to pay particular attention to nonverbal messages such as worried expressions or loss of eye contact. Remaining silent demonstrates the nurse's patience and willingness to wait for a response when the other person is unable to reply quickly. Silence may be especially therapeutic during times of profound sadness or grief (Box 18–8).

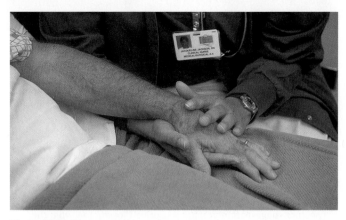

Figure 18-2 The nurse uses touch to communicate.

Providing Information. Providing relevant information that the client needs or wants to know empowers the client to make informed decisions, experience less anxiety, and feel safe and secure. It is also an integral aspect of health teaching. Hiding information from clients is not usually helpful, particularly when they are seeking it. If a physician withholds information, you need to clarify the reason with the physician. Clients have a right to know about their health status and what is happening in their environment. Information of a distressing nature needs to be communicated with sensitivity, at a pace appropriate to what the client can absorb, and in general terms at first: "John, your heart sounds have changed from earlier today, and so has your blood pressure. I'll let your doctor know." It is important to provide information that enables clients to understand what is happening and what to expect: "Ms. Evans, John is getting an echocardiogram right now. This test uses painless sound waves to create a moving picture of his heart structures and valves and should tell us what is causing his murmur."

✳ BOX 18-8   NURSING STORY

Communication With a Dying Client

A young third-year nursing student who was assigned to care for a dying client came to me, as her nursing instructor, to discuss her assignment. The student nurse appeared to be anxious and distraught and was tearful. She requested a change of assignment and, when asked why she felt she needed to be moved, she stated: "I just don't know what I'm supposed to be *doing* with her. She is asking for her family, but they aren't here. She's dying and I just don't know what to do to *help* her." I asked the student what she was doing while she was in the room and she said: "I'm just sitting there holding her hand and listening to her when she's awake. She really isn't talking much, and she drifts off to sleep a lot, but she's afraid of being left alone, so I'm just holding her hand and letting her know I'm there, even when she's sleeping; that way she'll know she's not alone whenever she wakes up. I make sure she's comfortable but I don't know what else she needs. I'm just not *doing* anything." As I looked into her tear-filled eyes, I simply asked her: "So, what makes you think you aren't doing anything?" Communication involves so much more than dialogue. In this case, communication involved very little verbal interaction; it involved active listening, shared empathy, comfort care, gentle touch, silence, presence, and "being with," as the student compassionately accompanied the client through her final stage of life and assisted with her transition into death.

Clarifying. To check whether understanding is accurate, restate an unclear or ambiguous message to clarify the sender's meaning or ask the other person to rephrase it, explain further, or give an example of what he or she means. Without clarification, you may make invalid assumptions and miss valuable information. Despite efforts at paraphrasing, you sometimes will still not understand the client's message and should let the client know that this is the case: "I'm not sure I understand what you mean by 'sicker than usual.' What is different now?"

Focusing. Focusing centres on key elements or concepts of a message. If conversation is vague or rambling or if clients begin to repeat themselves, focusing is a useful technique. Do not use focusing if it interrupts clients while they are discussing an important issue. Rather, use focusing to guide the direction of conversation to important areas: "We've talked a lot about your medications, but let's look more closely at the trouble you're having in taking them on time."

Paraphrasing. Paraphrasing is restating another person's message more briefly in your own words. Through paraphrasing, you let the client know you are actively involved in the search for understanding. Practice is required to paraphrase accurately. If the meaning of a message is changed or distorted through paraphrasing, communication becomes ineffective. For example, a client may say, "I've been overweight all my life and never had any problems. I can't understand why I need to be on a diet." Paraphrasing this statement by saying, "You don't care if you're overweight or not," is incorrect. It would be more accurate to say, "You're not convinced you need a diet because you've stayed healthy."

Asking Relevant Questions. Nurses ask relevant questions to seek information needed for decision making. You should ask only one question at a time and fully explore one topic before moving to another area. During client assessment, questions should follow a logical sequence and proceed from general to more specific. Open-ended questions allow the client to take the conversational lead and introduce pertinent information about a topic. For example, "What's your biggest concern at the moment?" Focused questions are used when more specific information is needed in an area: "How has your pain affected your life at home?" Allow clients to fully respond to an open-ended question before asking more focused questions. Closed-ended questions elicit "yes," "no," or one-word responses: "How many times a day are you taking pain medication?" Although they are helpful during assessment, they are generally less useful during therapeutic exchanges.

Asking too many questions is sometimes dehumanizing. Seeking primarily factual information does not allow you or your client to establish a meaningful relationship or deal with important emotional issues. It is a way to ignore uncomfortable areas in favour of more comfortable, neutral topics. A useful exercise is to try conversing without asking the other person a single question. By giving general leads ("Tell me about it."), making observations, paraphrasing, focusing, providing information, and so forth, you may discover important information that would have remained hidden if communication were limited primarily to questions.

Summarizing. Summarizing is a concise review of key aspects of an interaction. Summarizing brings a sense of satisfaction and closure to an individual conversation and is especially helpful during the termination phase of a nurse–client relationship. By reviewing a conversation, participants focus on key issues and add additional relevant information as needed. Beginning a new interaction by summarizing a previous one helps the client recall topics discussed and shows the client that you have analyzed the communication. Summarizing also clarifies expectations, as in this example of a nurse manager who has been working with a dissatisfied employee: "You've told me a lot of reasons about why you don't like this job and how unhappy you've been. We've also come up with some possible ways to make the situation better, and you've agreed to try some and let me know if any of them help."

Self-Disclosure. Self-disclosures are subjectively true, personal experiences about the self that are intentionally revealed to another person. This is not therapy for the nurse; rather, it shows clients that you understand and that their experiences are not unique. You may choose to share experiences or feelings that are similar to those of the client and emphasize both the similarities and differences. This kind of self-disclosure is indicative of the closeness of the nurse–client relationship and involves a particular kind of respect for the client. It is offered as an expression of genuineness and honesty and is an aspect of empathy (Stuart & Laraia, 2005). Self-disclosure should be relevant and appropriate and made to benefit the client. Self-disclosure should be used sparingly so that the client remains the focus of the interaction: "That happened to me once, too. I was devastated . . . . I went for counselling, and it really helped. What are your thoughts about seeing a counsellor?"

Confrontation. To confront someone in a therapeutic way, you help the other person become more aware of inconsistencies in his or her feelings, attitudes, beliefs, and behaviours (Stuart & Laraia, 2005). This technique improves client self-awareness and helps the client recognize growth and deal with important issues. Confrontation should be used only after you have established a trusting relationship with the client, and it requires gentleness and sensitivity: "You say you've already decided what to do, but you're still talking a lot about your options."

Nontherapeutic Communication Techniques

Certain communication techniques hinder or damage professional relationships. These specific techniques are referred to as *nontherapeutic* or *blocking* and will often cause recipients to activate defences to avoid being hurt or negatively affected. Nontherapeutic techniques tend to discourage further expression of feelings and ideas and may engender negative responses or behaviours in other people.

Asking Personal Questions. Asking personal questions that are not relevant to the situation but simply to satisfy your curiosity (e.g., "Why don't you and John get married?") is not appropriate professional communication. Such questions are invasive and unnecessary. If clients wish to share private information, they will. To learn more about the client's interpersonal roles and relationships, ask a question such as "How would you describe your relationship with John?"

Giving Personal Opinions. When you provide a personal opinion (e.g., "If I were you, I'd put your mother in a long-term care facility"), it takes decision making away from the client. It inhibits spontaneity, stalls problem solving, and creates doubt. Personal opinions differ from professional advice. At times, clients need suggestions and help to make choices. Suggestions should be presented to clients as options because the final decision rests with the client. Remember that the problem and its solution belong to the client. A much better response is "Let's talk about what options are available for your mother's care."

Changing the Subject. When another person is trying to communicate something important, changing the subject (e.g., "Let's not talk about your problems with the insurance company. It's time for your walk") is rude and shows a lack of empathy. It tends to block further communication, and the sender then withholds important messages or fails to openly express feelings. Thoughts and spontaneity are interrupted, ideas become tangled, and information provided may be inadequate. In some instances, changing the subject serves as a face-saving manoeuvre. If this happens, reassure the client that you will return to his or her concerns: "After your walk, let's talk some more about what's going on with your insurance company."

Automatic Responses. Stereotypes (e.g., "Older adults are always confused" or "Administration doesn't care about the staff") are generalized beliefs held about people. Making stereotyping remarks about other people reflects poor nursing judgement and can threaten nurse–client or nurse–team relationships. A cliché is a generalizing comment such as "You can't win them all" that tends to belittle the other person's feelings and minimize the importance of his or her message. These automatic phrases communicate that you are not taking concerns seriously or responding thoughtfully. Another kind of automatic response is parroting, repeating what the other person has said, word for word. Parroting is easily overused and is not as effective as paraphrasing. If the client says something that takes you by surprise, responding simply "Oh?" will give you time to think.

A nurse who is excessively task oriented automatically makes the task or procedure the entire focus of interaction with clients, missing opportunities to communicate with them as individuals and meet their needs. Task-oriented nurses are often perceived as cold, uncaring, and unapproachable. When you first perform technical tasks, you may have difficulty integrating therapeutic communication because of your need to focus on the procedure. In time, you will learn to integrate communication with high-visibility tasks and accomplish several goals simultaneously.

False Reassurance. When a client is seriously ill or distressed, you may be tempted to offer hope to the client with statements such as "Don't worry, everything will be all right"; "You'll be fine"; or "You have nothing to worry about." When a client is reaching for understanding, false reassurance discourages open communication. Offering reassurance not supported by facts or based in reality does more harm than good. Although you may be attempting to be kind, such reassurance has the secondary effect of helping you avoid the client's distress, tends to block conversation, and discourages further expression of feelings. A more facilitative nursing response is "It must be difficult not to know what the surgeon will find. What might be helpful to you at this time?"

Sympathy. Sympathy is concern, sorrow, sadness, or pity felt for the client generated by personal identification with the client's needs (Grover, 2005). Sympathy is a subjective vision of another person's viewpoint that prevents a clear perspective of the issues confronting that person. If you over-identify with the client (e.g., "I'm so sorry about your mastectomy; it must be terrible to lose a breast"), you will lose objectivity and be unable to effectively help the client work through his or her situation (Arnold & Boggs, 2007). Although sympathy is a compassionate response to another's situation, it is not as therapeutic as empathy. Your own emotional issues may prevent effective problem solving and impair your judgement. A more empathetic approach is "The loss of a breast is a major change. How do you think it will affect your life?"

Asking for Explanations. You may be tempted to ask your client to explain why he or she believes, feels, or has acted in a certain way (e.g., "Why are you so anxious?"). Clients frequently interpret "why" questions as accusations or think you already know the reason and are simply testing them. "Why" questions tend to interrupt clients' descriptions of their feelings and experience and cause them to refocus their energy into intellectual or defensive responses (Shattell & Hogan, 2005). Regardless of your motivation, "why" questions can cause resentment, insecurity, and mistrust. If you require additional information, it is best to phrase your questions to avoid using the word "why": "You seem upset. What's on your mind?" is more likely to help the anxious client to communicate.

Approval or Disapproval. Do not impose your personal attitudes, values, beliefs, and moral standards on other people while in the professional helping role (e.g., "You shouldn't even think about assisted suicide; it's not right"). Other people have the right to speak their minds and make their own decisions. Judgemental responses often contain terms such as *should, ought, good, bad, right,* and *wrong.* Agreeing or disagreeing conveys the subtle message that you are making value judgements about the client's decisions. Approving implies that the behaviour being praised is the only acceptable one. Often the client shares a decision not in an effort to seek approval but to provide a means to discuss feelings. On the other hand, disapproving implies that the client needs to meet your expectations or standards. Instead, help clients explore their own beliefs and decisions. The nursing response "I'm surprised you're considering assisted suicide; tell me more" gives the client a chance to express ideas or feelings without fear of being judged.

Defensive Responses. Becoming defensive in response to criticism (e.g., "No one here would intentionally lie to you") implies that the other person has no right to an opinion. The sender's concerns are ignored when you focus on the need for self-defence, defence of the health care team, or defence of other people. When clients express criticism, it is important to listen to what they have to say. Listening does not imply agreement. To discover reasons for the client's anger or dissatisfaction, you must listen uncritically. By avoiding defensiveness, you can defuse anger and uncover deeper concerns: "It sounds as if you believe people have been dishonest with you. That must make it difficult for you to trust anyone."

Passive or Aggressive Responses. Passive responses (e.g., "Things are bad, and I can't do anything about it") serve to avoid conflict or sidestep issues. They reflect feelings of sadness, depression, anxiety, powerlessness, and hopelessness. Aggressive responses (e.g., "Things are bad, and it's all your fault") provoke confrontation at the other person's expense and reflect feelings of anger, frustration, resentment, and stress. When nurses lack assertiveness skills, they may also use triangulation, complaining to a third party rather than confronting the problem or expressing concerns directly to the source. This lowers team morale and draws other people into the conflict situation. Assertive communication is a far more professional approach to take.

Arguing. Challenging or arguing against perceptions (e.g., "How can you say you didn't sleep a wink, when I heard you snoring all night long?") denies that they are real and valid to the other person. They imply that the other person is lying, misinformed, or uneducated. Skillful nurses give information or present reality in a way that avoids argument: "You feel as if you didn't get any rest at all last night, even though I thought you slept well because you seemed peaceful when I checked your room during the night."

Adapting Communication Techniques for the Client With Special Needs

With Canada's steadily aging population, increasing numbers of clients have visual, hearing, and speech impairments or other difficulties communicating. Interacting effectively with clients who have conditions that impair communication requires special thought and sensitivity. Such clients benefit greatly when you adapt communication techniques to their unique circumstances or developmental level. For example, if you are caring for a client with impaired verbal communication related to cultural differences, you can provide a table of simple words in the client's language. You and the client can use the table to help communicate about basic needs such as food, water, toileting, pain relief, sleep, and so forth. Similar techniques can be used with clients suffering with aphasia or some dementias (Goldfarb & Santo Pietro, 2004). Research findings suggest that many of the difficulties in communicating with clients with severe communication impairment arise from the lack of an understandable nurse–client communication system.

Clients who are deaf or hard of hearing have the greatest risk for miscommunication with health care professionals (Meador & Zazove, 2005). For some people, being deaf may seem worse than being blind because being blind isolates people from things but being deaf isolates people from other people. In a study of people who were deaf or hard of hearing, findings suggested that one of the most important actions of the nurse was to ask the client how best to communicate with him or her (Iezzoni et al., 2004).

You need to direct nursing actions toward meeting the goals and expected outcomes identified in the plan of care, addressing both the communication impairment and its contributing factors. Box 18–9 lists many methods available to encourage, enhance, restore, or substitute

---

> **BOX 18-9** Communicating With Clients Who Have Special Needs

Clients Who Cannot Speak Clearly (Aphasia, Dysarthria, Muteness)
Listen attentively, be patient, and do not interrupt.
Ask simple questions that require "yes" or "no" answers.
Allow time for understanding and response.
Use visual cues (e.g., words, pictures, and objects) when possible.
Allow only one person to speak at a time.
Do not shout or speak too loudly.
Encourage the client to converse.
If you have not understood the client, let him or her know.
Collaborate with a speech therapist as needed.
Use communication aids:
- Pad and felt-tipped pen or Magic Slate
- Communication board with commonly used words, letters, or pictures denoting basic needs
- Call bells or alarms
- Sign language
- Use of eye blinks or movement of fingers for simple responses ("yes" or "no")

Clients Who Are Cognitively Impaired
Reduce environmental distractions while conversing.
Capture client's attention before you speak.
Use simple sentences, and avoid long explanations.
Ask one question at a time.
Allow time for the client to respond.
Be an attentive listener.
Include family and friends in conversations, especially in topics known to the client.

Clients Who Are Hearing Impaired
Check for the presence of hearing aids and glasses.
Reduce environmental noise.
Get the client's attention before you speak.
Face the client so that your mouth is visible.
Do not chew gum.
Speak at normal volume; do not shout.
Rephrase rather than repeat, if your message is misunderstood.
Provide a sign language interpreter if this is indicated.

Clients Who Are Visually Impaired
Check for use of glasses or contact lenses.
Identify yourself when you enter room, and notify client when you leave room.
Speak in a normal tone of voice.
Do not rely on gestures or nonverbal communication to convey messages.
Use indirect lighting, avoiding glare.
Use at least 14-point print.

Clients Who Are Unresponsive
Call the client by name during interactions.
Communicate both verbally and by touch.
Speak to the client as though he or she can hear.
Explain all procedures and expected sensations.
Provide orientation to person, place, and time.
Avoid talking about client to other people in his or her presence.
Avoid saying things that the client should not hear (e.g., gossip or speculations about client's condition).
Always assume that clients can hear and understand everything said at their bedside.

Clients Who Do Not Speak English
Speak to the client in a normal tone of voice (shouting may be interpreted as anger).
Establish a method for the client to signal a desire to communicate (call light or bell).
Provide an interpreter (translator) as needed.
Avoid using family members, especially children, as interpreters.
Develop communication board, pictures, or cards.
Translate words from the English list into the client's native language for the client to make basic requests.
Ensure that a dictionary (English–French, English–Cree, and so forth) is available if client can read.

for verbal communication. You must be sure that the client is physically able to use the chosen method and that it does not cause frustration by being too complicated or difficult.

Because nursing care of the older adult is ideally provided through an interdisciplinary model, your primary goal is to establish a reliable communication system that is easily understood by all members of the health care team. Effective communication involves adapting to any special needs resulting from sensory, motor, or cognitive impairments that are present. You can also encourage older adults to share life stories and reminisce about the past, which has a therapeutic effect and increases their sense of well-being. Avoid sudden shifts from topic to topic. It is helpful to include the client's family and friends and to become familiar with the client's favourite topics for conversation.

❖Evaluation

To determine whether the plan of care has been successful, both the nurse and the client evaluate the client's communication outcomes. You need to evaluate nursing interventions to determine what strategies or interventions were effective and what changes in the client's situation resulted because of the interventions. For example, if using a pen and paper proves frustrating for a nonverbal client whose handwriting is shaky, you need to revise the care plan to include use of a picture board instead. If expected outcomes are not met or progress is not satisfactory, you need to determine what factors influenced the outcomes and then modify the plan of care.

You can evaluate the effectiveness of your own communication by videotaping practice sessions with peers, making process recordings, and analyzing written records of your verbal and nonverbal interactions with clients. Process recording analysis reveals faults in personal communication techniques, so that you can improve their effectiveness. Box 18–10 contains a sample communication analysis of such a record. Analyzing a process recording enables you to evaluate the following:

- Determine whether the nurse encouraged openness and allowed the client to "tell his or her story," expressing both thoughts and feelings.
- Identify any missed verbal or nonverbal cues or conversational themes.
- Examine whether nursing responses blocked or facilitated the client's efforts to communicate.
- Determine whether nursing responses were positive and supportive or superficial and judgemental.
- Examine the type and number of questions that were asked.
- Determine the type and number of therapeutic communication techniques used.
- Discover any missed opportunities to use humour, silence, or touch.

Evaluation of the communication process helps you gain confidence and competence in interpersonal skills. Becoming an effective communicator greatly increases your professional satisfaction and success. No skill is more basic, and no tool more powerful, than communication.

> **BOX 18-10** **Sample Communication Analysis**

NURSE: Good morning, Mr. Simpson. [*Smiles and approaches bed, holding clipboard*]
- Acknowledging by name, social greeting to begin conversation

CLIENT: What's good about it? [*Arms crossed over chest, frowning, with a direct stare*]
- Nonverbal signs of anger

NURSE: You sound unhappy. [*Pulls up chair and sits at bedside*]
- Sharing observation, nonverbal communication of availability

CLIENT: You'd be unhappy, too, if nobody would answer your questions. [*Angry tone of voice, challenging expression*]
- Further expression of feelings, facilitated by nurse's accurate observation

NURSE: This hospital has a fine staff, Mr. Simpson. I'm sure no one would intentionally keep information from you.
- Feeling threatened and being defensive: a nontherapeutic technique

CLIENT: All right, then: Why wouldn't that girl tell me what my blood sugar was?

NURSE: I'm not sure. If I were you, I'd forget about it and get a fresh start.
- Giving advice and using cliché, which is nontherapeutic; would have been better to acknowledge that client had a right to know the information

NURSE: I'm going to test your blood sugar levels in a minute, and I'll tell you the results. [*Performs test*] Your blood sugar level was 20.
- Providing information, demonstrating trustworthiness

CLIENT: That's up pretty high, isn't it? [*Worried facial expression*]
- Feeling very concerned about test results

NURSE: [*Nods; long pause*]
- Nonverbal affirmation, use of silence to allow client time to absorb information and gather thoughts

CLIENT: I'm so afraid complications will set in because my blood sugar is high. [*Stares out window*]
- Feeling free to express deeper concerns, which are hard to face

NURSE: What kinds of things are you worried about?
- Open-ended question to elicit information

CLIENT: I could lose a leg, as my mother did. Or go blind. Or have to live hooked up to a kidney machine for the rest of my life.

NURSE: You've been thinking about all kinds of things that could go wrong, and it adds to your worry not to be told what your blood sugar is.
- Summarizing to let client "hear" what he has communicated

CLIENT: I always think the worst. [*Shakes head in exasperation*]
- Expressing insight into his "inner dialogue"

NURSE: I'll pass along to the technician that it's OK to tell you your blood sugar levels. And later this afternoon, I'd like us to talk more about some things you can do to help avoid these complications and set some goals for controlling your blood sugar. [*Stands up, keeps looking at client*]
- Providing information, encouraging collaboration and goal setting; giving nonverbal cue that conversation is nearing end

CLIENT: OK, I'll see you later.

✳ KEY CONCEPTS

- Communication is a powerful therapeutic tool and an essential nursing skill used to influence other people and achieve positive health care outcomes.
- Communication involves the entire human being: body, mind, emotions, and spirit.
- Critical thinking facilitates communication through creative inquiry, focused self-awareness and awareness of other people, purposeful analysis, and control of perceptual biases.
- Nurses consider many contexts and factors influencing communication when making decisions about what, when, where, how, why, and with whom to communicate.
- Nurses use intrapersonal, interpersonal, transpersonal, small-group, and public interaction to achieve positive change and health goals.
- Communication is most effective when the receiver and sender accurately perceive the meaning of each other's messages.
- Message transmission is influenced by the sender's and receiver's physical and developmental status, perceptions, values, emotions, knowledge, sociocultural background, roles, and environment.
- Effective verbal communication requires appropriate vocabulary, intonation, clear and concise phrasing, proper pacing of statements, and proper timing and relevance of a message.
- Nonverbal communication often conveys the true meaning of a message more accurately than verbal communication.
- Helping relationships are strengthened when the nurse demonstrates caring by establishing trust, empathy, autonomy, confidentiality, and professional competence.
- Effective communication techniques are facilitative and tend to encourage the other person to openly express ideas, feelings, or concerns.
- Ineffective communication techniques are inhibitive and tend to block the other person's willingness to openly express ideas, feelings, or concerns.
- The nurse must blend social and informational interactions with therapeutic communication techniques so that other people can explore feelings and manage health issues.
- Older adult clients with sensory, motor, or cognitive impairments require the adaptation of communication techniques to compensate for their loss of function and special needs.
- Clients with impaired verbal communication require special consideration and alterations in communication techniques to facilitate the sending, receiving, and interpreting of messages.
- Desired outcomes for clients with impaired verbal communication include increased satisfaction with interpersonal interactions, the ability to send and receive clear messages, and attending to and accurately interpreting verbal and nonverbal cues.

✳ CRITICAL THINKING EXERCISES

1. Ms. Mary Goodrunning, an Aboriginal Canadian of Chipewyan descent, must learn how to manage her diabetes mellitus and self-administer insulin injections. What communication techniques could you use to help her?

2. Jan, a nurse colleague of Mary Ellen, is having difficulty interacting assertively with Dr. Fielding, a physician who has an abrupt, intimidating communication style. Jan frequently complains of tension headaches, pent-up anger, and crying easily. What can Mary Ellen do to help Jan?

3. Mr. Hess, a client with Parkinson's disease living at a long-term care facility, has a stiff, expressionless face as a result of his disease. He sits slumped in a recliner chair all day and seems lost in his own world, rarely looking at or interacting with anyone. When he does talk, he mumbles in a soft voice, and his words are difficult to understand. What nursing interventions could you use to establish a helping–healing relationship with Mr. Hess?

4. Ms. Velma Eberhard, a member of a Hutterite colony in western Canada, is considering whether she should have her two young children immunized before they begin attending school. What communication techniques could you use to help her decide, and what traps must you avoid in such a situation?

5. Ms. Esther Simons, a client who is receiving palliative care, confides in you that she feels overwhelmed with the number of issues she must attend to, now that she's facing the possibility of death. She says, "My thoughts are all over the place. I don't know where to start." What communication techniques, based on the critical thinking model, can you use to help her at this point?

✳ REVIEW QUESTIONS

1. Communication is not about the message that was intended but rather the message that was received. The statement that best helps explain this is as follows:
   1. Clear communication can ensure the client will receive the message intended.
   2. Sincerity in communication is the responsibility of the sender and the receiver.
   3. Attention to personal space can minimize misinterpretation of communication.
   4. Contextual factors, such as attitudes, values, beliefs, and self-concept, influence communication.

2. As a nurse, you would demonstrates active listening by
   1. Agreeing with the client
   2. Repeating everything the client says to clarify
   3. Assuming a relaxed posture, establishing eye contact, and leaning toward the client
   4. Smiling and nodding continuously throughout the interview

3. During the orientation phase of the helping relationship, you might
   1. Discuss the cards and flowers in the room
   2. Work together with the client to establish goals
   3. Review the client's history to identify possible health concerns
   4. Use therapeutic communication to manage the client's confusion

4. If you are working with a client who has expressive aphasia, it would be most helpful for you to
   1. Ask open-ended questions
   2. Speak loudly and use simple sentences
   3. Allow extra time for the client to respond
   4. Encourage a family member to answer for the client

5. The statement that best explains the role of collaboration with other members of the health care team for the client's plan of care is that the professional nurse
    1. Collaborates with colleagues and the client's family to provide combined expertise in planning care
    2. Consults the physician for direction in establishing goals for clients
    3. Depends on the latest literature to complete an excellent plan of care for clients
    4. Works independently to plan and deliver care and does not depend on other staff for assistance

6. "I'm not sure I understand what you mean by 'sicker than usual.' What is different now?" This statement reflects the therapeutic technique of
    1. Paraphrasing
    2. Providing information
    3. Clarifying
    4. Focusing

7. "We've talked a lot about your medications, but let's look more closely at the trouble you're having in taking them on time." In this situation, you would be using the therapeutic technique of
    1. Paraphrasing
    2. Providing information
    3. Clarifying
    4. Focusing

8. As a nursing student, you give yourself positive messages regarding your ability to do well on a test. This type of communication is
    1. Public
    2. Intrapersonal
    3. Interpersonal
    4. Transpersonal

9. When working with an older adult, you should remember to avoid
    1. Touching the client
    2. Shifting from subject to subject
    3. Allowing the client to reminisce
    4. Asking the client how he or she feels

10. You should consider zones of personal space and touch when caring for clients. If you are taking the client's nursing history, you should be
    1. 0 to 45 cm from the client
    2. 45 cm to 1 m from the client
    3. 1 to 4 m from the client
    4. 4 m or farther from the client

✳ RECOMMENDED WEB SITES

American Sign Language Browser:
http://www.commtechlab.msu.edu/sites/aslweb/browser.htm
This Web site provides an English and manual alphabet and dictionary, a brief history of sign language, and links to other relevant Web sites.

Communicative Disorders Assistant Association of Canada:
http://www.cdaac.ca/links.htm
This Web site provides links to various Canadian and international resources for people with conditions that affect communication.

Hutterites and Peaceful Societies:
http://www.hutterites.org/organizationStructure.htm;
http://www.peacefulsocieties.org/Society/Hutter.HTML
Both of these Web sites provide links to articles and resources about Hutterite culture and social organization.

Jest for the Health of It!: http://www.jesthealth.com
This Web site provides links to articles and resources about using therapeutic humour in nursing practice.

Medscape: http://www.medscape.com/px/urlinfo
Medscape is a resource for physicians and nurses that requires a one-time registration (free of charge) and offers links to current literature on numerous health care topics. Enter "Communication" in the search frame, and the site will list current articles on communication in health care.

National Institute on Deafness and Other Communication Disorders: http://www.nidcd.nih.gov/
Part of the National Institutes of Health (NIH) in the United States, the National Institute on Deafness and Other Communication Disorders (NIDCD) is mandated to conduct and support biomedical and behavioural research and research training in the normal and disordered processes of hearing, balance, smell, taste, voice, speech, and language.

19

Caring in Nursing Practice

Original chapter by Anne G. Perry, RN, EdD, FAAN

Canadian content written by Cheryl Sams, RN, BScN, MSN

media resources

evolve Web Site

- Audio Chapter Summaries
- Glossary
- Multiple-Choice Review Questions
- Student Learning Activities
- Weblinks

Companion CD

- Glossary
- Interactive Learning Activities
- Fluids and Electrolytes Tutorial
- Test-Taking Skills

Caring is central to nursing practice, and it is of great importance because of today's hectic health care environment. The demands, pressure, and time constraints in the health care environment leave little room for caring practice; as a result, nurses and other health care professionals may become cold and indifferent to clients' needs (Watson 2006a). Cara (2003) believed that the current health care climate, with its emphasis on restructuring, threatens to dehumanize client care. She stressed that the nursing profession must ensure that caring continues to be a strong force within all areas of nursing: in the clinical, administrative, educational, and research fields. Increasing use of technological advances for rapid diagnosis and treatment often causes nurses and other health care professionals to perceive their relationship with the client as relatively unimportant. Technological advances become dangerous without a context of skillful and compassionate care. Caring practices and expert knowledge that are at the heart of competent nursing practice must be valued and embraced (Benner & Wrubel, 1989; Lesniak, 2005). When you engage clients in a caring and compassionate manner, you learn that the therapeutic gains in the health and well-being of your clients are enormous.

Think about your own experiences of being ill or having a problem that necessitated health care intervention. Then consider the following two scenarios, and select the situation that you believe most successfully demonstrates a sense of caring.

A nurse enters a client's room, greets the client warmly while touching the client lightly on the shoulder, makes eye contact, sits down for a few minutes, and asks about the client's thoughts and concerns. The nurse listens to the client's story, looks at the intravenous solution being administered, briefly examines the client, and then checks the vital sign summary on the bedside computer screen before departing the room.

A second nurse enters the client's room, looks at the intravenous solution being administered, checks the vital sign summary sheet on the bedside computer screen, and acknowledges the client but never sits down or touches the client. The nurse makes eye contact from above while the client is in the vulnerable horizontal position. The nurse asks a few brief questions about the client's symptoms and then leaves.

The first scenario depicts the nurse in specific acts of caring. The nurse's calm presence, parallel eye contact, attention to the client's concerns, and physical closeness all express a client-centred, comforting approach. In contrast, the second scenario is task-oriented and expresses a sense of indifference to the client's concerns. During times of illness or when a person seeks the professional guidance of a nurse, caring is essential in helping the individual reach positive outcomes.

Theoretical Views on Caring

Caring is a universal phenomenon influencing the ways in which people think, feel, and behave in relation to one another. Since the time of Florence Nightingale, nurses have studied caring from a variety of philosophical and ethical perspectives. A number of nursing scholars developed theories about caring because of its importance to the practice of nursing. This chapter does not detail all of the theoretical positions on caring, but it helps you understand why caring is at the heart of your ability to work with all clients in a respectful and therapeutic way.

Caring Is Primary

Benner (1984) and Benner and Wrubel (1989) offered nurses a rich, holistic understanding of nursing practice and caring through the interpretation of expert nurses' stories. After listening to nurses' stories and analyzing their meaning, Benner described caring as the essence of professional nursing practice. The stories revealed the nurses' behaviour and decisions that expressed caring. *Caring* means concern about a person, events, projects, and things (Benner & Wrubel, 1989). It is a word for being connected.

Caring reflects what matters to a person; it describes a wide range of involvements, from parental love to friendship, from caring for one's work to caring for one's pet, to caring for and about one's clients. Benner and Wrubel (1989, p. 1) noted, "Caring creates possibility." Personal concern for another person, an event, or a thing provides motivation and direction for people to care. Caring as a framework has practical implications for transforming nursing practice (Boykin et al., 2003). Caring is an inherent feature of nursing practice whereby nurses help clients recover from illness, give meaning to that illness, and maintain or re-establish connection with other people. Caring helps nurses identify successful interventions, and this concern then guides future caregiving.

Each individual client has a unique background of experiences, values, and cultural perspectives. As you acquire more experience, you learn that caring helps you focus on the clients for whom you are caring. Caring facilitates your ability to understand a client, which enables you to recognize a client's problems and to find and implement individualized solutions.

In addition to their work in understanding caring, Benner and Wrubel (1989) described the relationship between health, illness, and disease. Health is not the absence of illness, nor is illness identical to disease (see Chapter 1 for further information). Health is a state of being that people define in relation to their own values, personality, and lifestyle. Health exists along a continuum. Illness is the experience of loss or dysfunction, whereas disease is the manifestation of an abnormality at the cellular, tissue, or organ level. Some clients have a disease (e.g., arthritis or diabetes) but do not experience the sense of being ill or a decrease in function. Some individuals do not seek health care until they experience a disruption, loss, or concern. For example, a client who has had diabetes for a number of years may not sense being ill until the disease causes serious visual impairment, which threatens the ability to work. Illness therefore has meaning only within the context of the person's life.

Because illness is the human experience of loss or dysfunction, any treatment or intervention given without consideration of its meaning to an individual is likely to be worthless. Expert nurses understand the difference between health, illness, and disease. Through caring relationships, you learn to listen to clients' stories about their illness so that you obtain an understanding of the meaning of illness to them. With this understanding, you provide therapeutic, client-centred care.

The Essence of Nursing and Health

From a **transcultural** perspective, Leininger (1978) described the concept of care as the essence and the central, unifying, and dominant domain that distinguishes nursing from other health disciplines. Care is an essential human need, necessary to the health and survival of all individuals. Care, unlike cure, assists an individual or group in improving a human condition. Acts of caring are the nurturant and skillful activities, processes, and decisions to assist people in ways that are empathetic, compassionate, and supportive. An act of caring is dependent on the needs, problems, and values of the client. Leininger's studies of numerous world cultures have revealed that care helps protect, develop, and nurture people and enable them to survive. Care is vital to recovery from illness and to the maintenance of healthy life practices in all cultures.

Leininger (1988) stressed the importance of understanding cultural caring behaviours and other **cultural aspects of care**. Event though caring is a universal phenomenon, the expressions, processes, and patterns of caring vary among cultures (Box 19–1). Caring is very personal, and thus expressions of caring differ for each client. For caring to be effective and meaningful to clients, you need to learn culturally specific behaviours and words that reflect human caring in different cultures. Refer to Chapter 10 for more information on culture and ethnicity.

Transpersonal Caring

Clients and their families should receive high-quality human interaction with nurses. Unfortunately, many of the conversations occurring between clients and their nurses are brief and disconnected. According to Watson's (1979, 1988, 2008) theory of caring (a holistic nursing model), a conscious intention to care promotes healing and wholeness (Hoover, 2002). This intention is complementary to conventional science and modern nursing practices. The theory integrates human caring processes with healing environments, incorporating the life-generating and life-receiving processes of human caring and healing for both nurses and their clients (Watson, 2006b). The theory describes a consciousness that allows nurses to raise new questions about what it means to be a nurse, what it means for a client to be ill, and how caring and healing should take place. Transpersonal caring theory rejects the disease orientation of health care and stresses care as more important than cure (Watson, 1988). Instead of focusing on the client's disease and its treatment by conventional means,

transpersonal caring explores inner sources of healing to protect, enhance, and preserve a person's dignity, humanity, wholeness, and inner harmony.

In Watson's (2006b) view, caring is almost spiritual. Caring preserves human dignity in the technological, cure-dominated health care system. The emphasis is on the nurse–client relationship, as well as the caring relationship. During a single caring moment between the nurse and client, the nurse and client may communicate to each other on a level deeper than simple verbal exchange. There may be a sense of connection between the one cared for and the one caring. Caring on a deep, interpersonal level can promote healing (Watson 2006b). Application of Watson's caring model may enhance your caring practices. The model is **transformative** because the relationship influences both the nurse and the client, for better or for worse (Hoover, 2002). Watson further developed her caring science theory, described in her 2008 book. Her carative factors are now called *carative processes* and are outlined in Table 19–1. Evidence-informed material that enhances caring is described in Box 19–2.

Swanson's Theory of Caring

In an effort to develop a theory of caring applicable for nursing practice, Swanson (1991) studied clients and professional caregivers. Three different groups were interviewed: women who miscarried, parents and health care professionals in a neonatal intensive care unit, and socially at-risk mothers who had received long-term, public health intervention. All groups were interviewed before, during, or after labour and delivery of a child and had experienced the phenomenon of caring. Researchers asked each subject questions regarding how they experienced caring in their situation. After analyzing the stories and descriptions of the three research groups, Swanson developed a theory of caring, whereby caring consists of five categories or processes: knowing, "being with," "doing for," enabling, and maintaining belief (Table 19–2).

Swanson's (1991) contributions are valuable in providing direction for how to develop useful and effective caring strategies. Each of the caring processes are crucial in making positive differences in clients' health and well-being outcomes. Thus, research findings used to develop the theory are useful in guiding clinical nursing practice. For example, Swanson (1999) tested the effects of caring-based counselling on women's emotional well-being in the first year after the miscarriage. Caring-based counselling was significant in reducing women's depression and anger, particularly during the first four months after the miscarriage.

The Human Act of Caring

Roach (1997) also focused on the integration of caring and spirituality in her "human act of caring" theory. She was requested by the Canadian Nurses Association (CNA) in 1977 to develop the first Canadian code of ethics for Canadian nurses. This first code was based on her caring theory, which comprised five concepts: compassion, competence, confidence, conscience, and commitment (Table 19–3). This foundational work set the stage for a value-based code that has been updated over time but continues to retain Roach's caring principles as the framework (Storch, 2007). The CNA (1997) *Code of Ethics* was revised and published in the summer of 2008.

Pusari (1998) applied Roach's theory in work with people with life-threatening illnesses. She proposed that Roach's caring elements be extended to include the concepts of courage, culture, and communication; thus, the theory would be more holistic. These eight concepts incorporate physical, psychological, emotional, spiritual, and cultural components to guide nurses as they provide comprehensive and individualistic care.

✳ BOX 19-1 CULTURAL ASPECTS OF CARE

Nurse Caring Behaviours

As a nurse, you must provide caring behaviours that are based on clients' cultural values and beliefs. Although the need for human caring is universal, its application is based on cultural norms. For example, providing time for family presence is often more valuable to traditional Asian families than is nursing presence. Using touch to convey caring sometimes crosses cultural norms. Sometimes gender-congruent caregivers or the client's family need to provide caring touch. In some cultures, maintaining eye contact while listening to the client is considered disrespectful.

Implications for Practice

- Know the client's cultural norms for caring practices.
- Know the client's cultural practices regarding end-of-life care. In some cultures, it is considered insensitive to tell the client that he or she is dying.
- Determine whether a member of the client's family or cultural group is the most appropriate resource for presence or touching.
- Determine the need for gender-congruent caregivers.
- Avoid the use of idioms because they can often create misunderstanding between the caregiver and the client or family.
- Know the client's cultural practices regarding the removal of life support.

Data from Galanti, G. A. (2004). *Caring for patients from different cultures* (3rd ed.). Philadelphia, PA: University of Pennsylvania Press; and Watson, J. (2006). Caring theory as an ethical guide to administrative and clinical practices. *Nursing Administration Quarterly, 30*(1), 48–55.

►TABLE 19-1   **Watson's Carative Processes**

Carative Factors or Caritas Processes	Description
Humanistic–altruistic values	Practising loving-kindness and equanimity for self and others
Instilling or enabling faith and help	Being authentically present: enabling, sustaining, and honouring deep belief system and subjective world of self and others
Cultivating sensitivity to oneself and others	Cultivating one's own spiritual practices; deepening self-awareness, going beyond "ego-self"
Developing a helping–trusting, human caring relationship	Promoting and supporting a relationship that is characterized by trust, authenticity, helping and caring
Promoting and accepting expression of positive and negative feelings	Being present to and supportive of the expression of positive and negative feelings, recognizing both as important to a deep, interpersonal connection between self and person being cared for
Systematic use of scientific (creative) problem-solving process	Creatively using self and all ways of knowing, being, and doing as part of the caring process (engaging in artistry of caring–healing practices)
Providing for a supportive, protective, or corrective mental, social, spiritual environment	Creating healing environment at all levels: physical and nonphysical, whereby wholeness, beauty, comfort, dignity, and peace are potential (being or becoming the environment)
Assisting with the gratification of human needs	Reverentially and respectfully assisting with basic needs; holding an intentional, caring consciousness of touching and working with the embodied spirit of another; honouring a sense of unity within oneself; allowing for spirit-filled connection
Allowing for existential–phenomenological dimensions	Being open-minded and attending to spiritual, mysterious, unknown existential dimension of life, death, and suffering: "allowing for a miracle"

Adapted from Watson, J. (2008). *Nursing: The philosophy and science of caring* (rev. ed., p. 31). Boulder, CO: University Press of Colorado. Reprinted by permission of University Press of Colorado.

The Moral and Ethical Bases of Responsive Nurse–Client Relationships

Tarlier (2004), a Canadian author, presented another perspective on the principle of caring as a foundational nursing concept: that the concept of caring has not been well defined and that the nursing ethic of caring must be empirically shown to make a difference in client outcomes. For the nursing profession, it is important to provide evidence that caring is tied to a broader ethical knowledge base.

A personal moral sense that is shared by other people needs to be agreed on as a principle and integrated specifically into the

---

✳BOX 19-2   **EVIDENCE-INFORMED PRACTICE GUIDELINE**

Enhancing Caring

Evidence Summary

Caring facilitates healing and improves client satisfaction with nursing care. However, does the instructional process influence human caring? Do nurse educators present instructional methods that improve students' caring practices? In Hoover's (2002) study, undergraduate nursing students attended a 15-week educational module on nursing as human caring. The purpose of the module was to improve students' understanding of caring practice and to thus make them more caring practitioners. Researchers interviewed the students before and after completing the module to understand the effect of this module on their caring practices. For example, they asked students about factors that facilitate and impede their caring practices. The students reported an increase in self-awareness in regard to (1) connecting in relationships with self and others, (2) finding purpose and meaning in life, and (3) clarifying values. Several students spoke of becoming more tolerant of others, recognizing each person's uniqueness, and appreciating a person's perspectives. By recognizing themselves as caring persons, the students gained meaning in their lives. Many were able to report a great deal of satisfaction in recognizing that they were caring persons and how nursing allowed them to express that characteristic. Students worked through the emotional issues and practical constraints, which allowed them to grow spiritually and connect with clients at a deeper level. Finally, students also expressed an enhanced appreciation of what they valued.

Application to Nursing Practice

- Increasing knowledge and understanding of caring helps nurses begin to understand clients' worlds and to change their approach to nursing care.
- The use of caring in nursing practice encourages a more holistic approach to nursing care.
- As nurses use caring, they get to know their clients and therefore better meet their needs.
- The caring model involves closeness, commitment, and involvement in the nurse–client relationship.

From Hoover, J. (2002). The personal and professional impact of undertaking an educational module on human caring. *Journal of Advanced Nursing, 37*(1), 79–86.

► **TABLE 19-2** **Swanson's Theory of Caring**

Caring Process	Definitions	Subdimensions
Knowing	Striving to understand an event as it has meaning in the life of the other person	Avoiding assumptions about the life of the other person Centring on the one cared for Seeking cues
"Being with"	Being emotionally present for the other person	Engaging the self or both the self and the other person "Being there" Conveying ability Sharing feelings
"Doing for"	Doing for (assisting) the other person with actions that he or she would do for himself or herself if it were at all possible	Not burdening Comforting Anticipating Performing skillfully Protecting
Enabling	Facilitating the other person's passage through life transitions (e.g., birth, death) and unfamiliar events	Preserving dignity Informing and explaining Supporting and allowing Focusing Generating alternatives
Maintaining belief	Sustaining faith in the other person's capacity to get through an event or transition and face a future with meaning	Validating and giving feedback Believing in and holding in esteem Maintaining a hope-filled attitude Offering realistic optimism Spending extra effort to help the other person

From Swanson, K. M. (1991). Empirical development of a middle-range theory of caring. *Nursing Research, 40*(3), 161–166.

discipline of nursing and the nursing ethical knowledge base. Tarlier (2004) put forward the idea of responsive nurse–client relationships that are conceptualized in the nursing literature. Responsive relationships are based on respect, trust, and mutuality. These relationships can tie together theory, ethical knowledge, and clinical outcomes and strengthen the nursing ethical knowledge base.

Summary of Theoretical Views

Nursing caring theories have common themes. Caring is highly relational. Caring relationships open up possibilities (e.g., for comfort, touch, and solace) or close them down (Benner, 2004). The nurse and the client enter into a relationship that is much more than one person simply "doing tasks for" another. A mutual give-and-take

► **TABLE 19-3** **The Human Act of Caring**

Compassion	• Way of living born out of an awareness of one's relationship to all living creatures • Engendering a response of participation in the experience of another • A sensitivity to the pain and brokenness of the other; a quality of presence that allows one to share with and make room for the other
Competence	• State of having the knowledge, judgement, skills, energy, experience, and motivation required to respond adequately to the demands of one's professional responsibilities
Confidence	• Quality that fosters trusting relationships • Goals of service rendered within an environment and under conditions of mutual trust and respect
Conscience	• State of moral awareness • Compass directing one's behaviour according to the moral fitness of things
Commitment	• Complex affective response characterized by a convergence between one's desires and one's obligations and by a deliberate choice to act in accordance with them

From Roach, S. (1992). *The human act of caring. A blueprint for the health professions.* Ottawa, ON: Canadian Hospital Association.

develops as nurse and client begin to know and care for one another. In his own experience with cancer, sociologist Arthur Frank (1998) noted that what he wanted when he was ill was a mutual relationship with persons who were also clinicians and clients. It was important for Frank to be seen as one of two fellow human beings, not the dependent client being cared for by the expert technical clinician.

Caring seems highly invisible at times when a nurse and client enter a relationship of respect, concern, and support. The nurse's empathy and compassion become a natural part of every client encounter. The absence of caring, however, is very obvious. For example, if the nurse shows lack of interest or chooses to avoid a client's request for help, the nurse's inaction quickly conveys an uncaring attitude. Benner and Wrubel (1989, p. 14) related the story of a clinical nurse specialist who learned from a client what caring is all about: "I felt that I was teaching him a lot, but actually he taught me. One day he said to me (probably after I had delivered some well-meaning technical information about his disease), 'You are doing an OK job, but I can tell that every time you walk in that door you are walking out.'" In this nurse's story, the client perceived that the nurse was simply going through the motion of teaching and showed little caring toward the client. Clients quickly sense nurses' failure to empathize with them.

As a nurse is being caring, the client senses commitment on the part of the nurse and is willing to allow the nurse to gain an understanding of the client's experience of illness. In a study of oncology clients' descriptions of their nursing care, Radwin et al. (2005, p. 166) found that clients characterized a caring nurse as one who would "quietly try to care for every need I had" and "be there when you need them" versus "treat[ing] you like a number or a case rather than a person." Thus, you become a coach and partner rather than a detached provider of care.

Imagine the situation in which a nurse is working with a client who recently received a diagnosis of diabetes mellitus and who must learn to administer daily insulin injections. In this scenario, the nurse's caring behaviour might be enabling. When a nurse practises enabling, the client and nurse work together to identify treatment alternatives and resources. The nurse enables the client to understand diabetes management, and the nurse supports the client in progressing through self-care activities.

Another common theme in caring is to understand the context of the client's life and illness. It is difficult to demonstrate caring without gaining an understanding of who the other person is and that person's perception of his or her illness. By exploring the following questions with the client, you can begin understanding the client's perception of illness: "How was your illness first recognized?" "How do you feel about the illness?" "How does the illness affect your daily life practices?" Knowing the context of a client's illness helps you choose and individualize interventions that will actually help the client. This approach is more successful than simply selecting interventions on the basis of the client's symptoms or the disease process.

Client's Perceptions of Caring

Swanson's (1991) theory of caring is a foundation for understanding the behaviours and processes that characterize caring. Other researchers have also studied caring from clients' perceptions (Table 19–4). Identifying nurse behaviours that clients perceive as caring helps nurses understand what clients expect of them as caregivers. Clients continue to value nurses' effectiveness in performing tasks; however, clients clearly also value the affective dimension of nursing care (Williams, 1997): establishing a reassuring presence, recognizing

an individual as unique, and being attentive to the client. Each client has a unique background of experiences, values, and cultural perspectives; however, understanding common behaviours that clients associate with caring helps you learn to express caring in practice.

The study of clients' perceptions is important because health care emphasizes client satisfaction. What clients experience in their interactions with institutional services and health care professionals, and what they think of that experience, determines how clients use the health care system and how they can benefit from it (Gerteis et al., 1993; Mayer, 1986). When clients believe that health care professionals are sensitive, sympathetic, compassionate, and interested in them as people, they usually become active partners in the plan of care (Attree, 2001). Williams (1997) studied the relationship between clients' perceptions of four dimensions of caring and their satisfaction with nursing care. Clients in the study indicated that they were more satisfied when they perceived nurses to be caring. Radwin (2000) found that oncology clients associated excellent nursing care with attentiveness, partnership, individualization, rapport, and caring. As institutions look to improve client satisfaction, creating a caring environment is a necessary and worthwhile goal. Client's satisfaction with nursing care is an important factor in their decision to return to a hospital.

As a new clinical practitioner, you must account for how clients perceive caring and the best approaches to providing care. To start, consider behaviours associated with caring and consider an individual client's perceptions and unique expectations. Clients and nurses frequently differ in their perceptions of caring (Mayer, 1987; Wolf et al., 2003). For example, consider the situation in which your client is fearful of having an intravenous catheter inserted, and you are still a novice at catheter insertion. Instead of giving a lengthy description of the procedure to relieve the client's anxiety, you decide the client will benefit more if you obtain assistance from a skilled staff member. Understanding clients' perceptions helps you select caring approaches that are most appropriate to the clients' needs.

Ethic of Care

Caring is a moral imperative. Through caring for others, human dignity is ultimately protected, enhanced, and preserved. Watson (1988) suggested that caring, as a moral ideal, provides the stance from which a nurse intervenes. This stance ensures the practice of ethical standards for good conduct, character, and motives. Chapter 8 explores the importance of ethics in professional nursing. The term *ethic* refers to the ideals of right and wrong behaviour. In any client encounter, a nurse needs to know what behaviour is ethically appropriate. An **ethic of care** ensures that nurses do not make decisions solely on the basis of intellectual or analytical principles. Instead, an ethic of care places caring at the centre of decision making. For example, consider whether placing a disabled relative in a long-term care facility is truly caring.

An ethic of care is concerned with relationships between people and with a nurse's character and attitude toward others. Nurses who function according to an ethic of care are sensitive to unequal relationships that can lead to an abuse of one person's power over another, intentional or otherwise. In health care settings, clients and families are often on unequal footing with professionals because of the client's illness, lack of information, regression caused by pain and suffering, and unfamiliar circumstances. According to an ethic of care, the nurse is the client's advocate, solving ethical dilemmas by attending to relationships and by recognizing each client's uniqueness as a human being.

> **TABLE 19-4**   **Comparison of Research Studies Exploring Clients' Perceptions of Nurse Caring Behaviour**

Wolf et al. (2003) Clients With Cardiac Conditions	Male Clients	Attree (2001): General Medical Clients and Families	Chang et al. (2005): Clients With Cancer
Managing equipment skillfully	Being physically present so that client feels valued	Checking up on client	Being accessible to client and family
Being perceptive and compassionate	Returning voluntarily without being called	Being compassionate and patient	Providing comfort
Being physically present	Making client feel comfortable, relaxed, and secure	Demonstrating sensitivity and sympathy	Being trustworthy
Using a soft, gentle voice	Attending to comfort and needs of client before performing tasks	Using a calm, gentle, and kind approach	Anticipating client and family needs
Returning to client voluntarily without being asked	Using a kind, soft, pleasant, gentle voice and attitude		
Providing comfort and security			
Helping reduce pain			

Caring in Nursing Practice

It is impossible to prescribe ways that will guarantee whether or when a nurse becomes a caring professional. Experts disagree as to whether caring is teachable or fundamentally a way of being. Cook and Cullen (2003) wrote about the importance of teaching caring as an integral part of a nursing curriculum. In order for the value of caring to be internalized by the student nurse, caring behaviours must be demonstrated, and clinical opportunities to practise these behaviours must be built into the program. Caring models are essential to help in the development of a student's capacity to care (Roach, 1992). For example, Watson's nursing model has been adopted by many nursing programs in which the concept of caring is integrated throughout the curriculum.

For people who view caring as a normal part of their lives, caring is a product of their cultures, values, experiences, and relationships with other people. Persons who do not experience care in their lives often find it difficult to act in caring ways. As nurses deal with health and illness in their practice, their ability to care grows. Nursing behaviours that show caring include providing presence, a caring touch, and listening in each encounter with clients.

Providing Presence

Providing **presence** is to have a person-to-person encounter that conveys closeness and a sense of caring. Fredriksson (1999) explained that presence involves "being there" and "being with." "Being there" is not only physical presence but also communication and understanding. The interpersonal relationship of "being there" seems to depend on the fact that a nurse is attentive to the client (Cohen et al., 1994). You offer this type of presence to the client with the purpose of achieving some goal, such as support, comfort, or encouragement, to diminish the intensity of unwanted feelings or for reassurance (Fareed, 1996; Pederson, 1993).

"Being with" is also interpersonal. It means being available and at your clients' disposal (Pederson, 1993). If clients accept the nurse, they will invite the nurse to see and share their vulnerability and suffering. One person's human presence never leaves another person unaffected (Watson, 2003). The nurse then enables the client to articulate his or her feelings and to understand himself or herself in a way that leads to identifying solutions, seeing new directions, and making choices (Gilje, 1997).

By establishing presence—through eye contact, body language, voice tone, listening, and having a positive and encouraging attitude—you create openness and understanding. The message conveyed this way is that the client's experience matters to you (Swanson, 1991). Establishing presence with a client enhances your ability to learn from the client, which enhances nursing care.

It is especially important to establish presence when clients are experiencing stressful events or situations. Awaiting a physician's report of test results, preparing for an unfamiliar procedure, and planning to return home after serious illness are just a few examples of events in the course of a person's illness that can create unpredictability and dependency on health care professionals. Your presence can help calm a client's anxiety and fear in such situations. Giving reassurance and thorough explanations about a procedure, remaining at the client's side, and coaching the client through the experience all convey caring, which is invaluable to the client's well-being.

Touch

Clients face situations that can be embarrassing, frightening, and painful. Whatever the feeling or symptom, clients look to nurses for **comfort**. Touch is one comforting approach in which the nurse communicates concern and support.

Touch is relational and leads to a connection between nurse and client. Touch involves contact (physical) and noncontact touch. Contact touch involves obvious skin-to-skin contact, whereas noncontact touch refers to eye contact. It is difficult to separate the two. Both are described within three categories: task-orientated touch, caring touch, and protective touch (Fredriksson, 1999).

Nurses use task-orientated touch when performing a task or procedure. The skillful and gentle performance of a nursing procedure conveys security and a sense of competence. An expert nurse learns that any procedure is more effective when administered carefully and with consideration for any client concern. For example, if a client is anxious about a procedure such as an insertion of a nasogastric tube, the nurse provides comfort through full explanation of the procedure and what the client will feel. The nurse then assures the client that the procedure will be performed safely, skillfully, and successfully. This assurance is conveyed in the way that supplies are prepared, the client is positioned, and the nasogastric tube is gently manipulated and inserted. Throughout the procedure, the nurse talks quietly with the client to provide reassurance and support.

Caring touch is a form of nonverbal communication that successfully influences a client's comfort and security, enhances self-esteem, and improves reality orientation (Boyek & Watson, 1994). The nurse can express this caring touch by holding a client's hand, by giving the client a back massage, by gently positioning a client, or by participating in a conversation. When using a caring touch, the nurse is making a connection with showing acceptance of the client (Tommasini, 1990).

Protective touch is a form of touch that protects the nurse, the client, or both. The client views it either positively or negatively. The most obvious form of protective touch is in preventing an accident, such as holding and bracing the client to avoid a fall. This protects the client. Sometimes a nurse withdraws from a client or distances himself or herself when he or she is unable to tolerate suffering or needs to escape from a tense situation. This protects the nurse but elicits negative feelings in a client (Fredriksson, 1999).

Because touch conveys many messages, it must be used with discretion. Touch itself is a concern when crossing cultural boundaries of either the client or the nurse (Benner, 2004). Clients generally permit task-orientated touch because most individuals give nurses and doctors authority to enter their personal space to provide care. However, exceptions can exist because of clients' cultural backgrounds. You should understand whether clients are accepting of touch and how they interpret your intentions.

Listening

Caring involves an interpersonal interaction that is much more than two people simply talking back and forth. In a caring relationship, the nurse establishes trust, opens lines of communication, and listens to the client (Figure 19–1). Listening is key because it conveys the nurse's full attention and interest. Listening includes "taking in" what a client says, as well as interpreting and understanding what is the client is saying and conveying that understanding to the person talking (Kemper, 1992). Listening to the meaning of what a client says helps create a mutual relationship. True listening leads to truly

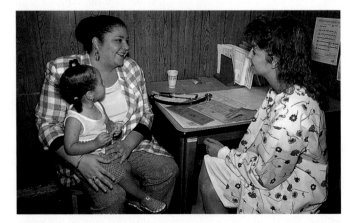

Figure 19-1 Nurse listening to a client.

knowing and responding to what really matters to the client and family (Boykin et al., 2003).

When an individual becomes ill, he or she usually has a story to tell about the meaning of the illness. Any critical or chronic illness affects all of a client's life choices and decisions and sometimes the individual's identity. Being able to tell that story helps the client deal with the distress of illness. Thus, a story needs a listener. Frank (1998) described his own feelings during his experience with cancer, saying that he needed a health care professional's gift of listening in order to make his suffering a relationship between them instead of an iron cage around him. He needed to be able to express what he needed when he was ill. The personal concerns that are part of a client's illness story are what is at stake for the client. Caring through listening enables the nurse to be a participant in the client's life.

To listen effectively, listeners need to silence themselves (Fredriksson, 1999). Fredriksson described silencing one's mouth and also one's mind: that is, to silence one's own thoughts that might distract from fully listening to a client. It is important to remain intentionally silent and to concentrate on what the client has to say. You need to be able to give clients your full, focused attention as they tell their stories.

When an ill person chooses to tell his or her story, it involves reaching out to others. Telling the story implies a relationship that can develop only if the clinician exchanges his or her stories as well. Frank (1998) argued that professionals do not routinely take seriously their own need to be known as part of a clinical relationship. Yet, unless the professional acknowledges this need, the relationship is not reciprocal; it is only an interaction (Campo, 1997). The clinician is pressured to know as much as possible about the client, but this pressure isolates the clinician from the client. In contrast, in knowing and being known, each supports the other (Frank, 1998).

Through active listening, you begin to truly know the client and what is important to him or her (Bernick, 2004). Learning to listen to a client is sometimes difficult. It is easy to become distracted by tasks at hand, colleagues shouting instructions, or other clients waiting to have their needs met. However, the time you take to listen is worthwhile both in the information gained and in the strengthening of the nurse–client relationship. Listening involves paying attention to the individual's words and tone of voice and understanding his or her perspective. Chapter 18 provides more detailed information on the art of communication. By observing the expressions and body language of the client, you will find cues to help assist the client in exploring ways to achieve a greater sense of peace and well-being.

Knowing the Client

One of the five caring processes described by Swanson (1991) is knowing the client. This concept comprises both your understanding of a specific client's situation and your subsequent selection of interventions (Radwin, 1995). Knowing develops over time as you learn the clinical conditions within a specialty and the behaviours and physiological responses of clients. Intimate knowing helps you respond to what really matters to the client (Bulfin, 2005). To know a client means that you avoid assumptions, focus on the client, and engage in a caring relationship with the client so that you can detect information and cues that facilitate critical thinking and clinical judgements (see Chapter 8 for further details on nursing values and ethics). Knowing that the client is at the core of the process, you use this process to make clinical decisions. By establishing a caring relationship, you develop the understanding that helps you better know the client as a unique individual and choose the most appropriate and helpful nursing therapies.

The caring relationships that you develop over time, coupled with your growing knowledge and experience, enable you to detect changes in a client's clinical status. Expert nurses develop this ability to detect such changes almost effortlessly. Clinical decision making, perhaps the most important nursing responsibility, involves various aspects of knowing the client: responses to therapies, routines, and habits; coping resources; physical capacities and endurance; and body typology and characteristics (Tanner et al., 1993). The experienced nurse knows additional facts about his or her clients, such as their experiences, behaviours, feelings, and perceptions (Radwin, 1995). When you make clinical decisions accurately in the context of knowing a client well, client outcomes are improved. Swanson (1999b) noted that when nurses base care on knowing the client, the clients perceived care as personalized, comforting, supportive, and healing.

The most important thing for a beginning nurse to recognize is that knowing a client is more than simply gathering data about the client's clinical signs and condition. Success in knowing the client depends on the relationship you establish. To know a client is to enter into a caring, social process that results in "bonding," whereby the client comes to feel known by the nurse (Lamb & Stempel, 1994). The bonding then enables the relationship to evolve into "working" and "changing" phases so that you can help the client become involved in his or her care and accept help when needed (Bulfin, 2005).

Spiritual Caring

Spiritual health occurs when a person finds a balance between his or her own life values, goals, and belief systems and those of others (see Chapter 28 for more information on spiritual health). Human beings have physical, emotional, spiritual, and psychological dimensions. An individual's beliefs and expectations do have effects on his or her physical well-being.

Establishing a caring relationship with a client involves an interconnectedness between the nurse and the client. This interconnectedness is why Watson (1979, 2006a, 2006b, 2008) described the caring relationship in a spiritual sense. Spirituality offers a sense of connection intrapersonally (connected with oneself), interpersonally (connected with others and the environment), and transpersonally (connected with an unseen higher power). In a caring relationship, the client and the nurse come to know one another so that the relationship becomes one of healing through the following actions:

- Mobilizing hope for the client and for the nurse
- Finding an interpretation or understanding of illness, symptoms, or emotions that is acceptable to the client
- Assisting the client in using social, emotional, or spiritual resources

Family Care

Each individual experiences life through relationships with others. Thus, caring for an individual does not occur in isolation from that person's family. It is important for you as a nurse to know the family almost as thoroughly as they know the client (Figure 19–2). The family is an important resource. Success with nursing interventions often depends on the family's willingness to share information about the client, their acceptance and understanding of therapies, whether the interventions fit with the family's acceptance and understanding of therapies, whether the interventions fit with the family's daily practices, and whether the family supports and provides the therapies recommended.

Many nurse caring behaviours are perceived as most helpful by families of clients with cancer (Box 19–3). Ensuring the client's well-being and helping the family become active participants in the client's care are critical for family members. These behaviours, although specific to families of clients with cancer, are useful for developing a caring relationship with all families. Begins a relationship by learning who makes up the client's family and what family members' roles are

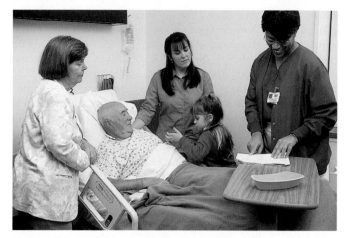

Figure 19-2   The nurse discusses the client's health care needs with the family.

in the client's life. Showing the family care and concern for the client creates an openness that then enables a relationship to form with the family. Caring for the family takes into consideration the context of the client's illness and the stress it imposes on all members. Chapter 20 contains more material on family nursing.

The Challenge of Caring

Assisting individuals during a time of need is the reason that many people enter the field of nursing. When nurses are able to affirm themselves as caring individuals, they reinforce a meaning and purpose to their lives (Benner, 2004; Hoover, 2002). Caring is a motivating force for people to become nurses, and it becomes the source of satisfaction when nurses know they have made a difference in their clients' lives.

It is becoming more of a challenge to care in today's health care system. Being a part of the helping professions is difficult and demanding. Nurses are torn between the human caring model and the task-oriented biomedical model and institutional demands that consume their practice (Watson & Foster, 2003). The time that nurses can spend with clients is diminishing, which makes it much

---

► **BOX 19-3**   **Nurse Behaviours Perceived by Families as Caring**

- Being honest
- Giving clear explanations
- Keeping family members informed
- Trying to make the client comfortable
- Showing interest in answering questions
- Providing necessary emergency care
- Assuring the client that nursing services will be available
- Answering family members' questions honestly, openly, and willingly
- Allowing the client to do as much for himself or herself as possible
- Teaching the family how to keep the client physically comfortable

Data from Brown, C. L., Holcomb, L., Maloney, J., Naranjo, J., Gibson, C., & Russell, P. (2005). Caring in action: The patient care facilitator role. *International Association for Human Caring Journal, 9*(3), 51–58; Mayer, D. K. (1986). Cancer patients' and families' perceptions of nurse caring behaviors. *Topics in Clinical Nursing, 8*(2), 63–69; and Radwin, L. (2000). Oncology patients' perceptions of quality nursing care. *Research in Nursing & Health, 23*(3), 179–190.

harder to know their clients. Too often, clients are perceived as just cases, and their real needs are either overlooked or ignored. The nature of caring is undermined by reliance on technology, reliance on cost-effective health care strategies, and efforts to standardize and refine work processes. These factors can lead to an increased risk of burnout from the stress and inability to fully practice professional standards that include caring behaviours. In addition, it is very important that student and novice nurses are supported in their efforts to be client focused.

The CNA has partnered with the Canadian Council on Health Services Accreditation, Health Canada's Office of Nursing Policy, and other important stakeholders to research, develop, and promote quality of worklife indicators (CNA, 2002). These fundamental indicators are designed to help organizations improve the health of their work environments. Healthy work environments are important for implementing client-focused care, preventing burnout, and preserving the practice of caring. Providing safe, compassionate, competent, and ethical care is a hallmark of the new CNA (2008) *Code of Ethics*.

The Registered Nurses Association of Ontario (2006) developed a guideline for nursing best practices that is informed by evidence about how to provide client-centred care. This guideline includes practice, education, organization, and policy recommendations that can help the individual nurse, educational organizations, and health care organizations implement client-centred care and integrate the ethic of caring into practice.

If health care is to make a positive difference in their lives, human beings cannot be treated like machines or robots. Instead, health care must become more humanized. Nurses play an important role in making caring behaviours an integral part of the health care delivery. First, nurses must make caring a part of the philosophy and environment in the workplace. By incorporating care concepts into standards of nursing care, nurses establish the guidelines for professional conduct. Finally, during day-to-day practice with clients and families, nurses need to be committed to caring and be willing to establish the relationships necessary for personal, competent, compassionate, and meaningful nursing care.

✳ KEY CONCEPTS

- Caring is at the heart of a nurse's ability to work with people in a respectful and therapeutic way.
- Caring is always specific and relational for each nurse–client encounter.
- For caring to be effective and meaningful to clients, nurses must learn culturally specific behaviours and words that reflect human caring in different cultures.
- Because illness is the human experience of loss or dysfunction, any treatment or intervention given without consideration of its meaning to the individual is likely to be worthless.
- Swanson's theory of caring includes five caring processes: knowing, "being with," "doing for," enabling, and maintaining belief.
- Roach's caring theory comprises five concepts: compassion, competence, confidence, conscience, and commitment.
- Caring involves a mutual give-and-take that develops as nurse and client begin to know and care for one another.
- It is difficult to demonstrate caring to clients without gaining an understanding of who they are and their perception of their illness.
- Presence involves a person-to-person encounter that conveys closeness and a sense of caring that involves "being there" and "being with" clients.
- Research has shown that touch, both contact and noncontact, includes task-orientated touch, caring touch, and protective touch.

- The skillful and gentle performance of a nursing procedure conveys security and a sense of competence in the nurse.
- Listening includes interpreting and understanding what is said.
- Knowing the client is at the core of the process by which nurses make clinical decisions.
- A nurse demonstrates caring by helping family members become active participants in a client's care.

✳ CRITICAL THINKING EXERCISES

1. Mrs. Lowe is a 52-year-old client being treated for lymphoma (cancer of the lymph nodes) that occurred 6 years after lung transplantation. Mrs. Lowe is discouraged about her current health status and a lot of what she describes as muscle pain. The unit where Mrs. Lowe is receiving care has a number of very sick clients and is short-staffed.
   a. You enter her room to perform a morning assessment and find Mrs. Lowe crying. How are you going to use caring practices to help Mrs. Lowe, knowing that you have only begun your tasks for the day?
   b. When you listened to Mrs. Lowe, she explained that her muscle pain was very bothersome and it was worse particularly when she was alone. Both you and Mrs. Lowe determine that an injection for her pain would be beneficial. In what way are you caring when you administer the injection to Mrs. Lowe?
   c. Mrs. Lowe seems more comfortable and is crying less. What else can you do for Mrs. Lowe?

2. During your next clinical practicum, select a client to talk with for at least 15 to 20 minutes. Ask the client to tell you about his or her illness:
   a. What do you believe the client was trying to tell you about his or her illness?
   b. Why was it important for the client to share his or her story?
   c. What did you do that made it easy or difficult for the client to talk with you? What did you do well? What could you have done better?
   d. Would you rate yourself a good listener? How can you listen better?

✳ REVIEW QUESTIONS

1. A nurse hears a colleague tell a student nurse that she never touches the clients unless she is performing a procedure or doing an assessment. The nurse tells the colleague that
   1. She does not touch the clients either
   2. Touch is a type of verbal communication
   3. Using touch is never a problem
   4. Touch forms a connection between nurse and client

2. Of the five caring processes, "knowing" the client is best described as
   1. Anticipating the client's cultural preference
   2. Determining the client's physician preferences
   3. Gathering task-oriented information during assessment
   4. Establishing an enhanced understanding of the client's needs

3. Helping a new mother through the birthing experience demonstrates which of the five caring behaviours?
   1. Knowing
   2. Enabling
   3. "Doing for"
   4. "Being with"
   5. Maintaining belief

4. Mr. Kline is fearful of upcoming surgery and a possible cancer diagnosis. He discussed his love for the Bible with Jada, his nurse, and she recommends a favourite Bible verse. Another nurse tells Jada that spiritual caring has no place in nursing. Jada replies:
   1. "Spiritual care should be left to a professional."
   2. "You are correct; expressions of spirituality are a personal decision."
   3. "Nurses should not force their spiritual beliefs on clients."
   4. "Healing can be promoted by assisting the client in using spiritual resources."

5. A number of strategies have potential for creating work environments that enable nurses to demonstrate more caring behaviours. Some of these include
   1. Increases in working hours
   2. Increases in monetary gain
   3. Flexibility, autonomy, and improvements in staffing
   4. Increases in physicians' input concerning nursing functions

6. A nurse demonstrates caring by helping family members
   1. Become active participants in care
   2. Provide activities of daily living
   3. Remove themselves from personal care
   4. Make health care decisions for the client

7. Listening is not only "taking in" what a client says; it also includes
   1. Incorporating the views of the physician
   2. Correcting any errors in the client's understanding
   3. Injecting the nurse's personal views and statements
   4. Interpreting and understanding what the client means

8. Presence involves a person-to-person encounter that
   1. Enables clients to care for themselves
   2. Provides personal care to a client
   3. Conveys a closeness and sense of caring
   4. Describes being in close contact with a client

9. By considering the clients' perceptions of caring, nurses are better able to
   1. Understand what clients expect of them as caregivers
   2. Be more efficient in performing tasks
   3. Provide continuity of care
   4. Establish nursing priorities

✳ RECOMMENDED WEB SITES

International Association for Human Caring:
http://www.humancaring.org
The focus of this Web site is to advance nursing and other related disciplines in the knowledge of caring and caring theory. This site provides access to the *International Journal for Human Caring,* a well-recognized journal that details research on caring.

Nursing as Caring:
http://www.nursingascaring.com/index.html
This Web site describes current research, development, practice, and education projects related to the theory of "nursing as caring." It also lists a bibliography of publications on the subject of caring.

20

Family Nursing

Written by Lorraine M. Wright, RN, PhD, Maureen Leahey, RN, PhD,

and Francis Loos, RN, MN, CNCC(C)

Based on the original chapter by Anne G. Perry, RN, EdD, FAAN

media resources

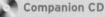 **Web Site**

- Audio Chapter Summaries
- Glossary
- Multiple-Choice Review Questions
- Student Learning Activities
- Weblinks

Companion CD

- Glossary
- Interactive Learning Activities
- Fluids and Electrolytes Tutorial
- Test-Taking Skills

The family continues to be a central institution in Canadian society. The role of the family in health care has been evolving. In the early twentieth century, visiting public health nurses and private duty nurses worked closely with family members while providing nursing care in the client's home. After World War II and the implementation of Medicare, most nursing services were provided in hospitals rather than in homes. As a result, families were generally excluded from their relatives' nursing care, and physicians and nurses were considered to be the final authorities to determine what was best for the client (Canadian Nurses Association [CNA], 1997). Since the 1970s, however, families and health care professionals have been forging more collaborative relationships, in which families' needs and contributions are taken into consideration.

Today, nurses strive to provide *family-centred care,* also known as *family nursing.* **Family nursing** is based on the assumption that every person, regardless of age, is a member of some type of family form and that individuals are best understood within the context of the family. A change in one family member, such as an illness or health condition, affects the other family members. Family nursing promotes, supports, and provides for the well-being and health of the family and individual family members (Astedt-Kurki et al., 2002). Nurses are responsible for first understanding the makeup (configuration), structure, and coping capacity of the family and then building on the family's relative strengths and resources (Feeley & Gottleib, 2000). Studies have shown that when nurses and families establish meaningful relationships, families are better able to manage the illness, and nurses gain greater clinical confidence and job satisfaction (Leahey et al., 1995). The goal of family nursing is to help the family and its individual members achieve and maintain optimal health throughout and beyond the illness experience. Family nursing is the focus of the future across all practice settings and is emphasized in all health care environments.

What Is a Family?

Defining *family* may initially appear to be a simple undertaking. However, different definitions have resulted in heated debates among social scientists and legislators. The family can be defined as a biological entity, as a legal entity, or as a social network with personally constructed ties and ideologies. To some clients, family may include only people who are related by marriage, birth, or adoption.

Other clients consider aunts, uncles, close friends, cohabiting people, and even pets as family. Families are as diverse as the individuals that compose them, and clients may have deeply ingrained values about their families that must be respected. Thus, **family** is defined as a set of relationships that each client identifies as family or as a network of individuals who influence each other's lives, regardless of whether actual biological or legal ties exist. In other words, each person has an individual definition of who or what constitutes family (Baumann, 2006).

Your personal beliefs do not have to coincide with those of the client. To provide individualized care, you must understand that families have many forms and have diverse cultural and ethnic orientations. In addition, no two families are alike; each has its own strengths, weaknesses, resources, and challenges (Bell et al., 2001). However, some general characteristics of a family include future obligations and caregiving functions, such as protection, nourishment, and socialization of its members (Stuart, 1991).

Current Trends in the Canadian Family

Although the institution of the family remains strong, the family itself is changing. You should be aware of current trends and social factors that affect the structure and function of the family. The following information about current family trends is based on data from Statistics Canada's 2001 and 2006 censuses (Statistics Canada, 2002, 2003a, 2003b, 2004, 2007a, 2007b, 2007c, 2007d, 2007e).

Family Forms

Family forms are patterns of people considered by family members to be included in the family (Box 20–1). Although all families have some common characteristics, each family form has unique problems and strengths. You need to keep an open mind about what constitutes a family so that potential resources and concerns are not overlooked.

The proportion of "traditional" families (married parents and their biological children) has been declining since about 1980, whereas the proportions of common-law and lone-parent families have been increasing (Figure 20–1). The number of couples without children at home is also increasing: In 1981, 32% of married and common-law

---

► BOX 20-1   Family Forms

Traditional Nuclear Family
Consists of a mother and father (married or common-law) and their children

Extended Family
Includes the nuclear family and other relatives (perhaps grandparents, aunts, uncles, cousins)

Step-Family
Formed when at least one child in a household is from a previous relationship of one of the parents

Blended Family
Formed when both parents bring children from previous relationships into a new, joint living situation or when children from the current union and children from previous unions are living together

Lone-Parent Family
Consists of one parent (either father or mother) and one or more children. The lone-parent family is formed when one parent leaves the nuclear family because of death, divorce, or desertion or when a single person decides to have or adopt a child.

Other Family Forms
These relationships include married and common-law couples without children, "skip-generation" families (grandparents caring for grandchildren), "nonfamilies" (adults living alone), and same-sex couples (with or without children).

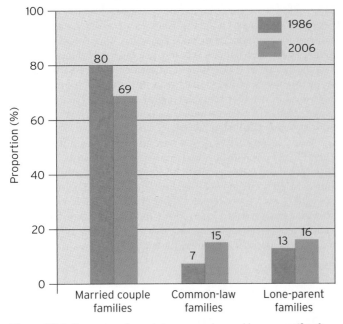

Figure 20-1 Proportion of married, common-law, and lone-parent families, 1986 and 2006. **Source:** Adapted from Statistics Canada. (2007, September 12). *2006 Census: Families, marital status, households, and dwelling characteristics.* Retrieved October 20, 2008, from www.statcan.ca/Daily/English/070912/d070912a.htm

couples had no children living at home; by 2001, this number had risen to 37%. This increase is partly a result of lower fertility rates, couples' delay in having children, and increased life expectancy, which is resulting in greater numbers of older couples with independent adult children (Statistics Canada, 2002).

Divorce rates have increased dramatically since the 1950s, and although the rate seems to be dropping, it is now estimated that 38% of Canadian marriages will end in divorce (Statistics Canada, 2004). Most divorced people eventually remarry, which results in blended families with complex sets of relationships among step-parents, stepchildren, half-brothers and half-sisters, and extended family members. When transitioning to a blended family, parents must deal with sometimes hostile or upset reactions of the children, the extended families, and an ex-spouse. Parents also must address the new family organization, including roles and relationships.

Same-sex couples define their relationships in family terms. According to the 2006 census, same-sex couples accounted for 0.6% of all couples, and 16.5% of these couples were married. Some families of same-sex couples include children, through adoption, through artificial insemination, or from prior relationships. About 16% of female couples and 3% of male couples have children (Statistics Canada, 2007b).

Grandparents are also increasingly taking responsibility for raising their grandchildren. In 2001, about 1% of all grandparents were living with their grandchildren without either of the children's parents involved (Statistics Canada, 2003a). This parenting responsibility is most often a consequence of legal intervention when parents are deemed unfit or renounce their parental obligations.

The proportion of teenagers who give birth has declined steadily since 1980, probably as a result of increased sex education, the availability of contraceptives, and the use of abortion (Dryburgh, 2000). Nevertheless, adolescents who give birth are now more likely to raise their children themselves than to place the children for adoption (The Vanier Institute of the Family, 2000). A teenage pregnancy tends to have health and social conse-

quences for the baby and mother and often severely strains family relationships and resources. In addition, these families are at increased risk for continued poverty. Child-bearing often interrupts the mother's education, thereby limiting her employment opportunities. Many adolescent parents—already struggling with the normal tasks of development and identity—must also accept a responsibility for which they may not be ready physically, emotionally, socially, or financially.

Marital Roles

Marital roles are also more complex as families increasingly comprise two wage earners. The majority of mothers—both wives and lone mothers—work outside the home; more than 75% of mothers with children older than 6 years are in the workforce (The Vanier Institute of the Family, 2000). Balancing employment and family life creates a variety of challenges in terms of child care and household work. Concerns that maternal employment is detrimental for children are unsubstantiated (Harvey, 1999). However, finding high-quality substitute child care is a major issue for parents. Managing household tasks can also be a major challenge. Both the management of household tasks and parenting responsibilities can vary substantially from family to family. Fathers are now expected to participate more fully in day-to-day parenting responsibilities.

Economic Status

In 2000, the median annual income of Canadian families was about $67,600. The median annual income for lone-parent households is $30,000 (Statistics Canada, 2007e). In fact, in 2000, about 13% of all families had low annual income, and almost half (46%) of all lone-parent families with children younger than 18 years had low annual incomes (Statistics Canada, 2003b). Distribution of wealth greatly affects the capacity to maintain health. Low educational preparation, poverty, and decreased amounts of support magnify each other's impact on sickness in the family and increase the amount of sickness in the family.

Aboriginal Families

Aboriginal families are the fastest growing group with children younger than 24 years. They are undergoing substantial changes while trying to maintain their traditional structure and function. Aboriginal families, in their multigenerational form, consist of a network of grandparents, parents, children, aunts, uncles and cousins. Each member has obligations to the family. Children are held in high esteem and are expected to be treated gently and protected from harm (Castellano, 2002).

Aboriginal peoples include First Nations, Métis, and Inuit. The number of individuals of Aboriginal origin increased 54% (and at six times the growth rate of other groups) between 1996 and 2006 (Statistics Canada, 2007c). Half of the Aboriginal population lives in urban areas, in comparison with 80% of the non-Aboriginal population. In the non-Aboriginal population, the median age is 40 years; in contrast, the median age of Aboriginal people is 27 years. Therefore, approximately half (48%) of Aboriginal people are younger than 24 years, in comparison with 31% of non-Aboriginal people. In addition, life expectancy is shorter and fertility rates are higher among Aboriginal peoples (Statistics Canada, 2007d).

Aboriginal families thus tend to be larger, be younger, and contain more diverse family members than do non-Aboriginal families. Their needs must be considered on an individual basis as more Aboriginal peoples move to urban centres and fewer remain in traditional living arrangements. Each group of Aboriginal peoples has its own traditions, relationships, and functions. The Calgary Family Assessment Model is well suited for evaluating these individual situations.

Family Caregivers

The fastest growing age group in Canada is 80 years of age and older. One per seven Canadians is a senior citizen. The growth in this group is projected to accelerate in 2011 as baby boomers turn 65 years old. Life expectancy is 82.5 years for women and 77.7 years for men (Statistics Canada, 2007a). This aging of the population has affected family life cycle, especially the middle generation. Often, family members serve as informal caregivers for older adults and other persons with disabilities. The majority of these caregivers are women, and they frequently provide 10 hours or more of unpaid assistance per week (The Vanier Institute of the Family, 2000). Family caregiving involves the routine provision of services and personal care activities for a family member by spouses, siblings, or children. Caregiving activities might include personal care (bathing, feeding, or grooming), monitoring for complications or side effects of medications, instrumental activities of daily living (shopping or housekeeping), and ongoing emotional support.

Whenever an individual becomes dependent on another family member for care and assistance, both the caregiver and the care recipient are under significant stress. The caregiver must continue to meet the demands of his or her normal lifestyle (e.g., raising children, working full time, or dealing with personal problems or illness). In many cases, older adult children care for their parents or older relatives. Although family caregivers often find that providing care has many rewards, they usually also have to balance caregiving with career and other family responsibilities. This group frequently must make major adjustments to integrate the challenges and time commitments of caring for a family member with their own lives (Hunt, 2003). Caregivers' physical and emotional health may suffer, as may their careers and family relationships (The Vanier Institute of the Family, 2000). Box 20–2 provides a list of family nursing gerontological concerns.

The Family and Health

The family is the primary social context in which health promotion and disease prevention take place (Box 20–3). The health of the family is influenced by many factors (e.g., its relative position in society, economic resources, and geographical boundaries). The family's beliefs, values, and practices also strongly influence health-promoting behaviours of its members (Hartrick, 2000). In turn, the health status of each individual influences how the family unit functions and its ability to achieve goals. When the family functions satisfactorily to meet its goals, its members tend to feel positive about themselves and their family. Conversely, when they do not meet goals, families view themselves as ineffective.

Good health may not be highly valued in some families; in fact, detrimental practices may be accepted. In some cases, a family member may provide mixed messages about health. For example, a parent may continue to smoke while telling children that smoking is "bad" for them. Family environment is crucial because health behaviour reinforced in early life has a strong influence on later health practices. In addition, the family environment can be a crucial factor in an individual's adjustment to a crisis. Although illness can strain relationships, research indicates that family members have the potential to be a primary force for coping.

Attributes of Healthy Families

In his classic work, Hill (1958/2003) noted that it is possible to explain the reactions of crisis-proof and crisis-prone families. A crisis-proof, or effective, family is able to integrate the need for stability with the need for growth and change. This type of family has a flexible structure that

✱ BOX 20-2   FOCUS ON OLDER ADULTS

- The nurse must consider caregiver strain; caregivers are usually either spouses, who may also be older adults and whose own physical stamina may be declining, or middle-age children, who often have other responsibilities.
- Older families have a different social network than do younger families because friends and same-generation family members may have died or have been ill themselves. The nurse may need to look for social support within the community and within the client's religious affiliation.
- Greater physical health impairment increases the risk of depression in older adults.
- As in the other stages of life, members of older families need to work on developmental tasks (see Chapter 25).
- Abuse of older adults in families occurs across all social classes. Family members and family caregivers are the most frequent abusers. Unexplained bruises and skin trauma should not be ignored by health care professionals.

allows adaptable performance of tasks and acceptance of help from outside the family system. The structure is flexible enough to allow adaptability but not so flexible that the family lacks cohesiveness and a sense of stability. An effective family has control over the environment and exerts influence on the immediate environment of home, neighbourhood, and school. A crisis-prone, or ineffective, family may lack or believe it lacks control over these environments.

Health promotion researchers have focused on the stress-moderating effect of hardiness and resiliency as factors that contribute to long-term health. Family **hardiness** has been defined as the internal strengths and durability of the family unit and is characterized by a

✱ BOX 20-3   FOCUS ON PRIMARY HEALTH CARE

Community health nurses meet families in a wide variety of settings and have many opportunities to use holistic family nursing practices. Nursing duties in health promotion include neonatal assessments, bereavement visits, school health care, occupational health care, substance abuse programs, palliative care, infusion clinics, home care, and numerous other clinical encounters.

When family nursing care is implemented, health promotion interventions are needed to improve or maintain the physical, social, emotional, and spiritual well-being of the family and its members (Ford-Gilboe, 2002). Individual members and the total family are encouraged to reach their optimal levels of wellness. Identifying attributes that contribute to health and resilience in families has been a focus of ongoing research since at least the 1970s. "Strong" families that adapt to expected transitions and unexpected crises and change tend to be characterized by clear communication among members, good problem-solving skills, a commitment to each other and to the family unit, and a sense of cohesiveness and spirituality (Svavarsdottir et al., 2000; also see Chapter 28). Health promotion programs aimed at enhancing these attributes are available for families and children in many communities. You must be aware of family-oriented community offerings so that families can be referred as needed. Health promotion behaviours that you need to encourage are often tied to the developmental stage of the family, such as programs for the child-bearing family about adequate prenatal care.

sense of control over the outcome of life, a view of change as beneficial and growth producing, and an active rather than passive orientation in adapting to stressful events (McCubbin et al., 1996). A hardy family can transcend long periods and inevitable lifestyle changes. Family **resiliency** is the ability to cope with expected and unexpected stressors: role changes, developmental milestones, and crises. The goal of the family is not only to survive the challenge but also to thrive and grow as a result of the newly gained knowledge. Resources and techniques that a family or individuals within the family use to maintain health can demonstrate a family's level of resiliency (Black & Lobo, 2008; Svavarsdottir et al., 2000).

Family Nursing Care

Nursing practice is enhanced by a family-centred approach. Nurses should examine family patterns, relationships, and interactions when they consider how a health problem or illness affects a family and how a family affects a health problem or illness. A nurse's relationship with the family has a significant influence on client and family functioning (Leahey & Harper-Jaques, 1996). A positive collaborative relationship with family members must be based on mutual respect and trust (Figure 20–2).

To begin working with families, you must have a scientific knowledge base in family theory and an adequate knowledge base in family nursing. Although health care systems in the past tended to emphasize the individual, a family focus is now needed in order to be able to safely discharge clients to the care of the family or community settings. The current emphasis on home nursing care provides another opportunity for family nursing care.

Family nursing care can be described as focusing either on family as context or on family as client. The choice of approach used depends on the situation and the abilities of the nurse.

Family as Context

When considering the family as context, you focus either on the individual client within the context of his or her family or on the family with the individual as context (CNA, 1997). The approach that you use is related to the clinical setting, the clinical problem, and realistic and practical considerations. An example of the first approach is the situation in which a nurse interviews a man with heart disease, asking the man's wife about the family's diet and possible family stressors. The wife's abilities to support her husband's efforts at changing eating patterns and use of stress management techniques are also assessed. The main focus is on the health of the client within the environment of the family. An example of the second approach is the situation in which a community health nurse interviews the adult daughter of a woman with multiple sclerosis, discussing how the daughter is coping with her mother at home. Family members may need direct interventions themselves.

With both approaches, you assess the extent to which the family provides the individual's basic needs. Family members should be considered valuable resources. They can provide you with information about how they have been helping the client maintain health and manage health problems. When clients are unable to communicate, families can provide important information about the client and indicate the client's wishes. All nurses should be competent at considering the family as context. Even if you do not have an opportunity to involve the family directly, you should still consider the client as a member of a family.

Family as Client

When the family as client is the approach, you focus on the entire family: its processes and relationships (e.g., parenting or family caregiving). The focus of nursing assessment is usually on family patterns and interactions among family members rather than on individual characteristics. The nursing process concentrates on the extent to which these patterns and processes are consistent with achieving and maintaining family and individual health. Nursing practice that focuses on family as client is also known as *family systems nursing,* and it usually requires an in-depth knowledge of family dynamics and family systems theory. Therefore, nurses who specialize in family systems nursing usually have extensive clinical practice skills and a postgraduate degree. Dealing with complex family system problems often requires an interdisciplinary approach. You must always be aware of the limits of nursing practice and make referrals when appropriate. When you view the family as the client, you aim to support communication among all family members. This support ensures that the family remains informed of the nurse's intent and progress in providing health care. Often you must support conflict resolution between family members so that each member can confront and resolve problems in a healthy way. You also help family members use the external and internal resources that are necessary. Ultimately, your aim is to help the family achieve optimal function.

Assessing the Needs of the Family: The Calgary Family Assessment Model

Family assessment is essential in providing adequate family care and support. To help families adjust to acute and chronic illness, nurses need to understand the family unit, what the illness means to the family members, what the illness means to family functioning, how the family has been affected by the illness, and the support that the family requires (Neabel et al., 2000). Box 20–4 lists the particular features of families who should be considered for a family assessment. During an assessment, the nurse, client, and family collaboratively engage in conversation to systematically collect information and reflect on issues important to the client's well-being at this particular time.

The **Calgary Family Assessment Model (CFAM)** can be used by nurses to perform a thorough family assessment (Wright & Leahey, 2005). It has received wide recognition, and faculties and schools of nursing around the world have adopted it. The International Council of Nurses recognizes it as one of the four leading family assessment models in the world (Schober & Affara, 2001). The CFAM focuses on

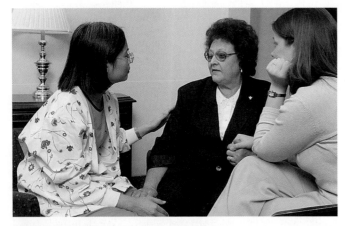

Figure 20-2 Nurse (*left*) and family members.

three major categories of family life: the structural dimension, the developmental dimension, and the functional dimension. Each category has several subcategories; however, not all subcategories are relevant to all families (Figure 20–3). You must decide, on a family-by-family basis, which subcategories are relevant at each time. Using too many subcategories may result in an overwhelming amount of data; using too few may yield insufficient data, which can distort a family's strengths, problems, or both. The model can be consulted during discussions about family issues.

Structural Assessment

The structural dimension of the family includes the following:

- Internal structure: the people who are included in the family and how they are connected to each other
- External structure: the relationships the family has with people and institutions outside the family
- Context: the whole situation or background relevant to the family

Internal Structure. The internal structure of the family—its composition and connections among family members—can be further divided into six subcategories: family composition, gender, sexual orientation, rank order, subsystems, and boundaries.

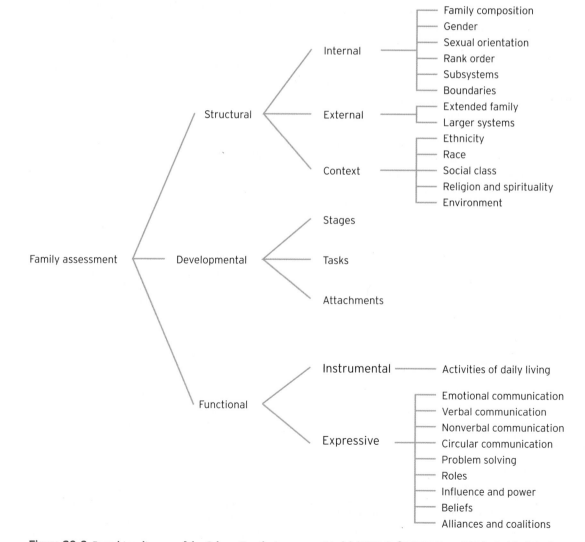

Figure 20-3 Branching diagram of the Calgary Family Assessment Model (CFAM). **Source:** From Wright, L. M., & Leahey, M. (2005). *Nurses and families: A guide to family assessment and intervention* (4th ed., p. 68, Fig. 3-1). Philadelphia: F. A. Davis.

Family Composition. *Family composition* refers to the individual members who form the family. The family composition is not limited to the traditional, nuclear family; it may include any of the various family forms discussed earlier (see Box 20–1). It is important to note whether any recent additions or losses in the family composition have occurred.

Questions to Ask the Family.
- Who is in your family?
- Does anyone else live with you: for example, grandparents, boarders?
- Has anyone recently moved out, married, or died?
- Can you think of anyone else who is like a family member but is not biologically related?

Gender. *Gender* is the set of beliefs about or expectations of masculine and feminine behaviours and experiences. These beliefs are fundamental to male and female relationships and are influenced by culture, religion, and family. It is useful to understand how male and female members of a particular family may view the world differently.

Questions to Ask the Family.
- How have your parents' ideas about masculinity and femininity affected your own?
- Do you have expectations of your children on the basis of their gender?
- Is the division of labour in your family based on gender roles?

Sexual Orientation. *Sexual orientation* refers to heterosexual, homosexual, bisexual, or transgendered orientation (see Chapter 27). Heterosexism, a belief that male–female bonding is the only legitimate type of bonding, is a form of bias that can affect families and health care professionals. Discrimination on the basis of sexual orientation continues to be a problem. Unless it is particularly relevant to the client or family's presenting concern, you do not usually ask questions about sexual orientation, but you are careful to avoid stereotyping or making assumptions when you ask general questions.

Rank Order. The order of children by age and gender is called *rank order*. The birth order, gender, and distance in age between siblings are important factors to consider because they may influence roles and behaviours. Also important is the child's characteristics and the family's idealized "program" for the child (going to school, college, university, work, getting married, and so forth).

Questions to Ask the Family.
- How many children are in your family?
- What are the ages of the children?
- Do you have expectations for the oldest that are different from those for the younger children?

Subsystems. *Subsystems* are smaller groups of relationships within a family. Subsystems can be created on the basis of generation, interests, skills, or gender. For example, a family could have a sibling subsystem, a husband–wife subsystem, and a parent–child subsystem. Each family member usually belongs to several subsystems, and in each subsystem, they play a different role, use different skills, and have a different level of power. For example, a teenager behaves differently with her younger sister than she does with her father. Adapting to the demands of different subsystems is a necessary skill for each family member.

Questions to Ask the Family.
- What are your family's subgroups?
- Do frequent disagreements occur among and between subgroups?
- If your family had more or fewer subgroups, what effect do you think that might have?

Boundaries. *Boundaries* define family subsystems and distinguish one subsystem from another. They influence how members participate in each subsystem. For example, a child in a parent–child subsystem may be given certain responsibilities and power but is not be expected to be involved with family decision making. Boundaries can be weak, rigid, or flexible, and they change over time as family members age or are gained or lost.

Questions to Ask the Family.
- Whom do you talk with when you feel happy?
- Whom do you talk with when you feel sad?
- Does the family have any "unwritten" rules about topics that are never to be discussed with someone outside of the family?

External Structure. *External structure* refers to the connections that family members have to persons outside the family. Two subcategories of external structure exist: extended family and larger systems.

Extended Family. *Extended family* includes the family of origin, the current generation, and steprelatives. How each member sees himself or herself as an individual, yet also as part of the family, should be critically assessed. You should note whether family members make many references to the extended family during the interview.

Questions to Ask the Family.
- Where do your parents live?
- How often do you have contact with them and your brothers and sisters?
- Which family members do you see or speak with regularly?
- To which relatives are you closest?

Larger Systems. *Larger systems* are groups with whom the family has meaningful contact. Groups include health care organizations, work, religious affiliations, school, friends, and social agencies such as public welfare, child welfare, foster care, and courts. Usually, contact with such larger systems is helpful. However, some families have difficult relationships with individuals from these groups, which can create stress for the family.

Questions to Ask the Family.
- What agency professionals are involved with your family?
- How many agencies regularly interact with you?
- How is this involvement helpful or unhelpful?

Context. *Context* refers to the situation or background relevant to the family. A family can be viewed in the context of ethnicity, race, social class, religion and spirituality, and environment.

Ethnicity. *Ethnicity,* which is the concept of a family's cultural and ethnic heritage is an important influence on family interaction. Ethnicity often influences a family's function, structure, perspectives, values, health beliefs, and philosophies (see Chapter 10). Cultural and ethnic heritage can affect, for example, religious practices, child-rearing practices, recreational activities, and nutrition. Members of one ethnic group may subscribe to differing beliefs, traditions, and restrictions, even within the same generation.

Questions to Ask the Family.
- Do you think of your family as having a strong ethnic identity?
- Has your ethnic background influenced your health care?
- Could you tell me about ethnic traditions you practise?
- How are your practices similar to or different from those suggested by our health care clinic?

Race. *Race* (biological characteristics such as skin and hair colour) influences individual and group identification and is closely connected to ethnicity. Family members' interactions among themselves and with health care professionals are influenced by racial attitudes, stereotypes, and discrimination. If ignored, these influences can harm the nurse and family's relationship.

Questions to Ask the Family.
- If you and I were of the same race, would our conversation be different?
- If so, how?

Social Class. *Social class* is shaped by education, income, and occupation. Each class has its own values, lifestyles, and behaviours that influence family interaction and health care practices.

Questions to Ask the Family.
- What is your job, and how many hours a week do you work?
- Does anyone in the family work shifts?
- How does that influence your family functioning?
- What level of education have you completed?
- Does your family have economic problems at this time?

Religion and Spirituality. Family members' spiritual or religious beliefs, rituals, and practices can influence their ability to cope with or manage an illness or health concern (Wright, 2004). Spirituality is often an underused resource in family work (see Chapter 28).

Questions to Ask the Family.
- Are you involved in a church, temple, mosque, or synagogue?
- Would you discuss a family problem with anyone from your place of worship?
- Do you consider your spiritual beliefs a resource?

Environment. The family *environment* refers to the larger community, neighbourhood, and home. Environmental factors that may affect family functioning include availability or lack of adequate space and of access to schools, day care, recreation, and public transportation.

Questions to Ask the Family.
- What are the advantages and disadvantages of living in your neighbourhood?
- What community services does your family use?
- What community services would you like to learn about?

Structural Assessment Tools. The CFAM encourages you to create genograms and ecomaps to help document and understand the structure of a family and its contact with outside individuals and organizations. A **genogram** is a sketch of the family structure and relevant information about family members (Figure 20–4). Some agencies have genogram forms, but genograms can also be sketched on other forms, such as admission forms or Kardex cards. The genogram becomes part of the documentation about the client and family. In some facilities, the information is collected on admission and then hung at the client's bedside, serving as a visual reminder to all health care professionals involved with the client to think about the family. An **ecomap** is a sketch of the family's contact with persons outside the family (Figure 20–5). The family members who share the household are depicted in the centre of the ecomap, and various important extended family members or larger systems are sketched in to show their relationship to the family.

You should draw genograms and ecomaps for families with whom you will be involved for more than one day. Information for brief genograms and ecograms can be gleaned from family members during the structural assessment. The most essential information for genograms includes data about ages, occupation or school grade, religion, ethnicity, and current health status of each family member. For a brief genogram, you focus only on information that is relevant to the family and the health problem.

Developmental Assessment

Families, like individuals, change and grow over time. Although each family is unique, all families tend to go through certain stages that require family members to adjust, adapt, and change roles. Each developmental stage presents challenges and includes tasks that need to be completed before the family can successfully move on to the next stage. Family development is more than the concurrent development of children and adults. It is the interaction between an individual's development and the phase of the family developmental life cycle that can be significant for family functioning. Therefore, in addition to understanding family structure, you should understand the developmental life cycle of each family.

In their model of family life stages, McGoldrick and Carter (1982; Carter & McGoldrick, 1999) described the emotional aspects of lifestyle transition and the changes and tasks necessary for the family to proceed developmentally (Table 20–1). You can use this model to promote behaviours to achieve essential tasks and help families prepare for transitions. The model presented in Table 20–1, however, does not address diverse family forms, such as blended families, lone-parent families, families without children, or common-law partners.

Functional Assessment

A *functional assessment* focuses mainly on how family members interact and behave toward each other. You assess how family members function by closely observing their interactions. Family functioning consists of two subcategories: instrumental and expressive functioning.

Instrumental Functioning. *Instrumental functioning* refers to the normal activities of daily living such as preparing meals, eating, sleeping, and attending to health needs. For families with health problems, these activities often become a challenge. Roles may change as family members cope with a relative's illness and disability.

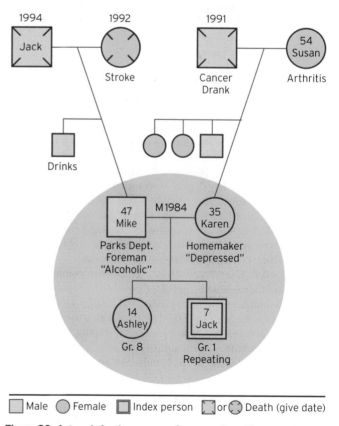

Figure 20-4 Sample family genogram. **Source:** Adapted from Wright, L. M., & Leahey, M. (2000). *Nurses and families: A guide to family assessment and intervention* (3rd ed., p. 90, Fig. 3-9). Philadelphia: F. A. Davis.

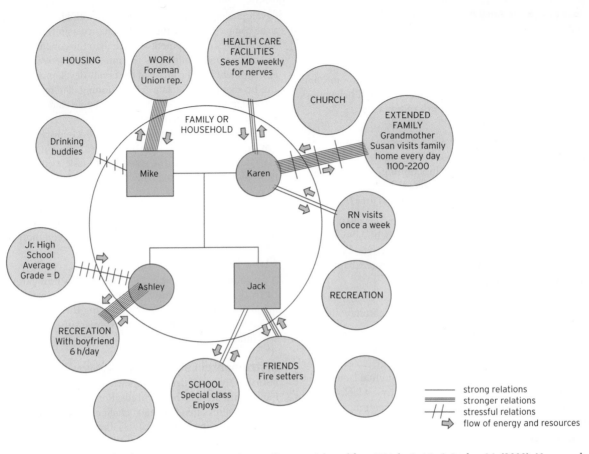

Figure 20-5 A sample family ecomap. RN, registered nurse. **Source:** Adapted from Wright, L. M., & Leahey, M. (2000). *Nurses and families: A guide to family assessment and intervention* (3rd ed., p. 96). Philadelphia: F. A. Davis.

Questions to Ask the Family.
- Who is usually responsible for housekeeping and child care?
- Do other family members help with these tasks?
- Does anyone in the family require help with activities of daily living?
- Who usually provides this help?

Expressive Functioning. *Expressive functioning* refers to the ways in which people communicate. Illness and disability often alter expressive functioning within the family. A diagnosis may cause intense feelings of anxiety or grief, both within the person being diagnosed and within other family members. You should encourage families to explore their understanding of illness and how it affects their lives. Ten subcategories of expressive functioning exist: emotional, verbal, nonverbal, and circular communication; problem solving; roles; influence; beliefs; and alliances and coalitions.

Emotional Communication. Emotional communication encompasses the range and types of feelings that are expressed by the family. Most families express a wide range of feelings. However, families with problems often have rigid patterns with a narrow range of emotional expression. For example, a family coping with a father's diagnosis of cancer may be consumed with anxiety and not express optimism or hope for the future. Family roles and gender may affect emotional expression.

Questions to Ask the Family.
- How can you tell when each member of your family is happy, sad, or under stress?
- How do you express happiness, sadness, or stress?

Verbal Communication. You should observe a family's **verbal communication,** focusing on the meaning of the words in terms of the relationship. Is communication among family members clear and direct, or is it vague and indirect? You should also ask family members their opinions about how well the family communicates.

Questions to Ask the Family.
- Which family member communicates most clearly?
- How might your family members communicate with each other more effectively?

Nonverbal Communication. **Nonverbal communication** consists of messages conveyed without words, including body language, eye contact, gesturing, crying, and tone of voice.

Questions to Ask the Family.
- How do you think your daughter feels when your son rolls his eyes while she's talking?
- Who shows the most distress when talking about your dad's drinking?

Circular Communication. **Circular communication** refers to communication between family members that is reciprocal; that is, each person influences the behaviour of the other. Circular communication can be adaptive or maladaptive. For example, an adaptive communication pattern occurs when a parent comforts a child because the child cries. Because the parent responds to the child, the child feels safe and secure. An example of a maladaptive communication pattern is when a parent criticizes a teenager for not phoning home. The teenager is angry for being criticized and avoids the

> **TABLE 20-1**   Stages of the Family Life Cycle

Family Life Cycle Stage	Emotional Process of Transition: Key Principles	Changes in Family Status Required to Proceed Developmentally
Between families: unattached young adult	Accepting parent–offspring separation	Differentiation of self in relation to family of origin Development of intimate peer relationships Establishment of self in work
Joining of families through marriage: newly married couple	Commitment to new system	Formation of marital system Realignment of relationships with extended families and friends to include spouse
Family with young children	Accepting new generation of members into system	Adjusting marital system to make space for children Taking on parental roles Realignment of relationships with extended family to include parenting and grandparenting roles
Family with adolescents	Increasing flexibility of family boundaries to include children's independence	Shifting of parent–child relationships to permit adolescents to move into and out of system Refocus on midlife material and career issues Beginning shift toward concerns for older generation
Launching children* and moving on	Accepting multitude of exits from and entries into family system	Renegotiation of marital system as dyad Development of adult-to-adult relationships between grown children and their parents Realignment of relationships to include in-laws and grandchildren Dealing with disabilities and death of parents (grandparents)
Family in later life	Accepting shifting of generational roles	Maintaining own or couple functioning and interests in the face of physiological decline; exploration of new familial and social role options Support for more central role for middle generation Making room in system for older adults' wisdom and experience Supporting older generations without overfunctioning for them Dealing with loss of spouse, siblings, and other peers, and preparation for own death; life review and integration

From McGoldrick, M., & Carter, E. (1982). The stages of the family life cycle. In Walsh, F. (Ed.), *Normal family processes* (pp. 375–398). New York: Guilford Press.
*Enabling children to move out of the family home.

parent. Because the teenager avoids the parent, the parent becomes angrier and criticizes more.

Questions to Ask the Family.
- You mentioned that your teenager does not phone home. What do you do then?
- How do you think that affects her?

Problem Solving. **Problem solving** refers to how a family thinks about actions to take to resolve difficult situations.

Questions to Ask the Family.
- Who first notices problems?
- How does your family tend to deal with problems?
- Is one member more proactive than others about solving problems?

Roles. **Roles** are established patterns of behaviour for family members, often developed through interactions with others. Formal roles include those of mother, husband, friend, and so forth. Informal roles can include, for example, those of "the softy," "the angel," or "the scapegoat."

Questions to Ask the Family.
- Who is the "good listener" in your family?
- Who is "the angel"?

Influence. **Influence** refers to methods of affecting or controlling another person's behaviour. Influence may be instrumental (the use of privileges as reward for behaviour; e.g., the promise of candy, computer time), psychological (the use of communication to influence behaviour; e.g., praise, admonishment), or corporal (the use of body contact; e.g., hugging, hitting).

Questions to Ask the Family.
- What method does your mom use to get you to go to bed at the right time?
- How does your grandma get your brother to attend school when he refuses?

Beliefs. **Beliefs** are individual- and family-held fundamental ideas, values, opinions, and assumptions (Wright et al., 1996). Beliefs influence behaviour and how the family adapts to illness. For example, if a family believes that vaccinations may cause long-term disabilities, the parents may decline vaccinating an infant.

Questions to Ask the Family
- What do you believe is the cause of your husband's depression?
- What do you believe would be the effect on your chronic pain if you choose to participate in that treatment?

Alliances and Coalitions. Alliances and coalitions involve the directionality, balance, and intensity of relationships among family members or between families and nurses.

Questions to Ask the Family.
- If the children are playing well together, who would be most likely to get them to start fighting?
- Who would stop them from fighting?

Family Intervention: The Calgary Family Intervention Model

After the assessment, you need to intervene to help families meet their needs. A range of family nursing interventions can be offered to families. Some, such as parent education and caregiver support, are general; others are specific and require therapeutic communication and family interviewing skills. The ultimate goal is to help family members discover solutions that reduce or alleviate emotional, physical, and spiritual suffering. Whether caring for a client with the family as context or directing care to the family as client, nursing interventions aim to increase family members' abilities in certain areas, to remove barriers to health care, and to perform actions that the family cannot perform for itself. You guide the family in problem solving, provide practical services, and convey a sense of acceptance and caring by listening carefully to family members' concerns and suggestions.

You must tailor your interventions to each family and the chosen domain of family functioning. You must remember that each family is unique. In addition, you can only offer interventions to the family; you should not instruct or insist on a particular kind of change or way of family functioning.

The **Calgary Family Intervention Model (CFIM)** is a companion to the CFAM and can be used as a guide for family interventions (Wright & Leahey, 2005). The CFIM focuses on promoting and improving family functioning in three domains: cognitive (thinking), affective (feeling), and behavioural (doing). Interventions may affect functioning in any or all of the three domains. For example, when a clinic nurse informs a wife that her husband, who has amyotrophic lateral sclerosis, is still capable of large gross motor movement, the nurse can suggest that he help with chores in the house, such as bringing the laundry upstairs. This intervention challenges the wife's thinking that her husband was incapable of work, influences the wife to feel less depressed over her husband's declining physical capacity, and leads the wife to change her behaviour by including her husband when performing other household chores.

The CFIM recommends many nursing practices that promote family functioning, including asking interventive questions, offering commendations, providing information, validating emotional responses, encouraging illness narratives, supporting family caregivers, and encouraging respite.

Asking Interventive Questions

One of the simplest but most effective ways that nurses can help families is by engaging in conversations with families and asking them questions. Questions lead the family to reflect on their situation, clarify their opinions and ideas, and understand how they are affected by their family member's illness or condition. By hearing their own responses to questions, family members can better understand themselves and each other and perhaps discover new solutions. Interventive questions also elicit information important to the nurse.

Interventive questions are of two types: linear and circular (Tomm, 1987, 1988). **Linear questions** elicit information about a client or family. They explore a family member's descriptions or perceptions of a problem. For example, when exploring a couple's perceptions of their daughter's anorexia nervosa, you could begin with linear questions: "When did you notice that your daughter had changed her eating habits?" "Has she been hospitalized in the past for this problem?" These questions inform you of the daughter's eating patterns and illuminate family perceptions or beliefs about eating patterns.

Circular questions help determine changes that could be made in a client's or family's life. They help explain a problem. For example, with the same family, you could ask, "Who is most worried about Cheyenne's anorexia?" or "How does Mother show that she's worrying the most?" Circular questions help you understand relationships between individuals, beliefs, and events, and they elicit valuable information to help create change. In this way, circular questions often help clients make new cognitive connections, paving the way for changes in family behaviours. Whereas linear questions may imply that you know what is best for the family, circular questions facilitate change by inviting the family to discover their own answers. Linear questions tend to target specific "yes" or "no" answers, thereby limiting the options for the family: for example, "Have you tried time out to discipline your three-year-old?" An alternative circular question might be "Which type of discipline seems to work best for your three-year-old?" Several types of circular questions exist, and each can affect the cognitive, affective, and behavioural domains. These types include difference questions, behavioural effect questions, hypothetical or future-oriented questions, and triadic questions (Wright & Leahey, 2005; Table 20–2).

Offering Commendations

Families do not always view their own system as one that has inherently positive components. You can help the family become aware of its own unique strengths, thereby increasing its potential and capabilities. A **commendation** is a statement that emphasizes the strengths or abilities of the family. While spending time with the family, you may observe many instances in which the family displays positive attributes. It is important to acknowledge these to the family so that they can appreciate their own strengths. By commending a family's strengths and competencies, you can offer family members a new view of themselves. You should look for patterns of behaviour to commend, rather than a single occurrence. For example, you may say, "Your family is showing much courage in living with your wife's cancer for five years" or "I'm very impressed with how the family worked together during the crisis." Families coping with chronic, life-threatening, or psychosocial problems frequently feel hopeless in their efforts to overcome or live with the illness. Therefore, you should offer as many truthful commendations as possible. In a study of families experiencing chronic illness, families reported that the nursing team's commendations were "an extremely important facet of the process" (Robinson, 1998).

Family strengths include clear communication, adaptability, healthy child-rearing practices, support and nurturing among family members, and the use of crisis for growth. You can help the family focus on these strengths instead of on its problems and weaknesses.

Providing Information

Families need information from health care professionals about developmental issues, health promotion, and illness management, especially if the illness is complex (Levac et al., 2002; Robinson, 1998). Accurate and timely information is essential for the family to make decisions and cope with difficult situations. One of the roles

> **TABLE 20-2** **Types of Circular Questions**

| | Examples to Elicit Change | | |
Purpose of Question	**Cognitive Domain**	**Affective Domain**	**Behavioural Domain**
Difference Question Explores differences between people, relationships, time, ideas, or beliefs	What is the best advice given you about supporting your son with AIDS? What is the worst advice?	Who in the family is most worried about how AIDS is transmitted?	Which family member is best at getting your son to take his medication on time?
Behavioural Effect Question Explores connections between how one family member's behaviour affects other members	What do you know about the effect of life-threatening illness on children?	How does your son show that he is afraid of dying?	What could you do to show your son that you understand his fears?
Hypothetical/Future-Oriented Question Explores family options and alternative actions or meanings in the future	What do you think will happen if these skin grafts continue to be painful for your son?	If your son's skin grafts are not successful, what do you think his mood will be? Angry? Resigned?	When will your son engage in treatment for his contractures?
Triadic Question Question posed to a third person about the relationship between two other people	If your father were not drinking daily, what would your mother think about his receiving treatment for alcoholism?	What does your father do that makes your mother less anxious about his condition?	If your father were willing to talk with your mother about solutions to his addiction, what do you think he might say?

Adapted from Wright, L. M., & Leahey, M. (2000). *Nurses and families: A guide to family assessment and intervention* (3rd ed., pp. 162–163). Philadelphia: F. A. Davis.
AIDS, acquired immunodeficiency syndrome.

you will need to adopt is that of an educator. Health education is a process by which information is exchanged between nurse and client. Family and client needs for information may be elicited through direct questioning, but they are generally far more subtle. You may recognize, for example, that a new father is fearful of cleaning his newborn's umbilical cord stump or that an older woman is not using her cane safely. Respectful communication is required. Often, you can express your need for information subtly: "I notice you are trying to not touch the umbilical cord stump; I see that a lot with other new parents" or "You use the cane the way I did before I was shown a way to keep from falling or tripping over it; do you mind if I show you?" When you assume a humble position instead of coming across as an authority on the subject, this attitude often decreases the client's defences and invites the client to listen without feeling embarrassed.

Validating or Normalizing Emotional Responses

Validation of intense emotions can alleviate a family's feelings of isolation and loneliness and help family members make the connection between a family member's illness and their own emotional response. For example, after a diagnosis of a life-shortening illness, families frequently feel powerless or frightened. It is important for you to validate these strong emotions as normal and to reassure families that they will adjust and learn new ways to cope.

Encouraging Illness Narratives

Too often, clients and family members are encouraged to talk only about medical aspects of their illness rather than emotional aspects. An **illness narrative** is the person's story of how the illness affects his or her whole being, including emotional, intellectual, social, and spiritual dimensions. Hearing the person's illness narrative helps you

understand the person's strengths and challenges. This information enables you to offer commendations of the client's abilities. Many people also find that the telling of their story helps them better understand themselves, their experience, and their family's experience.

The need to communicate what it is like to live with individual, separate experiences, particularly the experience of illness, is powerful in human relationships (Nichols, 1995; Wright, 2004). Frequently, nurses believe that listening entails an obligation to "fix" whatever concerns or problems are raised. However, showing compassion and offering commendations are usually more therapeutic or helpful than is offering solutions to problems (Bohn et al., 2003; Hougher Limacher, 2003; Hougher Limacher & Wright, 2003; Moules, 2002).

Encouraging Family Support

You can enhance family functioning by encouraging and assisting family members to listen to each other's concerns and feelings. This assistance can be particularly useful if a family member is embracing some constraining beliefs when a loved one is dying or has died (Wright & Nagy, 1993). For example, a family may believe that talking with the ill person about death and dying would hasten the person's death.

Supporting Family Caregivers

Family members are often afraid of becoming involved in the care of an ill member without a nurse's support. One way you can best provide family care is through supporting family caregivers. Without adequate preparation or support, caregiving can be stressful, causing a decline in the health of the caregiver and the care receiver or even the development of abusive relationships.

Despite its demands, caregiving can be a positive and rewarding experience (Picot et al., 1997). Whether it is one spouse caring for the other or a child caring for a parent, caregiving is an interactional process. The interpersonal dynamics between family members influence the ultimate quality of caregiving. Thus, you can play a key role in helping family members develop better communication and problem-solving skills needed for successful caregiving.

Researchers have identified variables, such as caregiver and care recipient expectations of one another, that influence caregiving quality. Carruth (1996) studied the concept of **reciprocity,** in which care recipients acknowledge the importance of the caregiver's help, which contributes to a caregiver's perception of self-worth. When the caregiver knows that the care recipient appreciates his or her efforts and values the assistance provided, the caregiving relationship is healthier and more satisfying. When caregiver and client solve problems together, overprotection or oversolicitous behaviour can be avoided. Clients feel in control of their care and responsible for care decisions. The caregiver also feels very positive and enjoys the caregiving experience (Isaksen et al., 2003).

Encouraging Respite

Nurses should encourage respite for caregivers, who may feel guilty about needing or wanting to withdraw, even temporarily, from the caregiving role. Caregivers may not recognize their needs for respite. Sometimes an ill person may be encouraged to accept another person's temporary assistance so that family members can take a break. Whatever the situation, you should remember that each family's need for respite varies.

Providing care and support for family caregivers often involves using available family and community resources for respite. A caregiving schedule is useful when all family members participate, when extended family members share any financial burdens posed by caregiving, and when distant relatives send cards and letters communicating their support. However, it is imperative for you to understand the relationship between potential caregivers and care recipients. If the relationship is not a supportive one, community services may be a resource for both the client and family.

Use of community resources might include locating a service required by the family or providing respite care so that the family caregiver has time away from the care recipient. Services that may be beneficial to families include caregiver support groups, housing and transportation services, food and nutrition services, housecleaning, legal and financial services, home care, hospice, and mental health resources. Before referring a family to a community resource, it is crucial that you understand the family's dynamics and know whether support is desired or welcomed. Often a family caregiver resists help, feeling obligated to be the sole source of support to the care recipient. You must be sensitive to family relationships and help caregivers understand the normality of caregiving demands.

Interviewing the Family

Once you have a clear conceptual framework for assessment and intervention, you can begin to learn the competencies and skills needed to conduct family interviews. Family interviews follow the same basic principles as any client interview (see Chapter 13). However, family interviews can be more complex because more people are involved. You must develop keen perceptual, conceptual, and executive skills. *Perceptual skills* refer to the ability to make relevant observations. In family interviewing, the nurse must observe multiple interactions and relationships simultaneously. *Conceptual skills* constitute the ability to formulate observations of the entire family and give meaning to those observations. Remember, however, that observations and subsequent judgements are subjective and not conclusive. Executive skills are the actual therapeutic interventions that you carry out in an interview. These therapeutic interventions elicit responses from family members and are the basis for further observations and conceptualizations. During an interview, you monitor responses from a client and family to form opinions and concepts about therapeutic interventions. The type of therapeutic intervention that you provide depends on your clinical expertise and experience in working with families.

Table 20–3 lists four stages of a family interview and the executive skills that might be used during each stage. By using the skills presented in Table 20–3, you can engage a family to assess, explore, and identify strengths and problems. You can also decide to intervene or refer the family to another health professional. These skills should not necessarily be applied to all families. You should tailor the interview to each family's individual context.

It is important to realize that not all family interviews are formal, lengthy processes. Even if you do not have the time to organize a formal family interview, you can still engage the family in productive, therapeutic conversation. Every conversation between you and client or family members improves communication and understanding, and no conversation is trivial. Therapeutic conversations can be as short as one sentence or as long as time allows. All conversations, regardless of time, have the potential to unite the family (Hougher Limacher & Wright, 2003; McLeod, 2003). Even brief interviews, or conversations, have tremendous healing potential because they offer families the opportunity to acknowledge and affirm their problems and seek solutions (Hougher Limacher, 2003; Moules, 2002; Tapp, 2001).

The integration of task-oriented client care with interactive, purposeful conversation distinguishes a time-effective interview (taking less than 15 minutes; Box 20–5). Providing information and involving the family in decision making are integral parts of the process. You should search for opportunities to engage in purposeful conversations with families, which may include the following:

- Routinely inviting families to accompany the client to the unit, clinic, or hospital
- Routinely including families' participation in the admission procedure
- Routinely inviting families to ask questions
- Acknowledging the client and family's expertise in managing the health problem at home
- Routinely consulting clients and families about their ideas regarding treatment and discharge

> **TABLE 20-3** Family Interviewing Skills for Nurses Using the CFAM and CFIM

Perceptual and Conceptual Skills

You understand the following:

Executive Skills

You might do the following:

Stage 1: Engagement

1. An individual family member is best understood in the context of the family.

2. Involvement of partners, parents, or both helps you obtain a broad view of the family and increase engagement among its members.

3. Providing structure to the interview reduces anxiety and increases engagement, especially during times of crisis.

4. Family members are most comfortable talking about the structural aspects of the family.

---

1. Invite to the first interview all family members who are concerned about or involved in the problem.

2. Try to involve partners, parents, or both in initial sessions.

3. Explain the purpose, length, and structure of the interview to family members, and ask whether they have any questions about the interview.

4. Introduce yourself, and ask family members to share their names, ages, work or school information, number of years married, and so forth.

Stage 2: Assessment

1. The CFAM can be used to understand family dynamics.

2. A detailed description and history of the presenting problem are important.

3. The presenting problem is often related to other concerns in the family. For example, a child's outbursts may be related to a family conflict.

4. Noting differences generates more specific information:
   - Clarifying *differences between individuals* reveals information about family functioning.
   - Clarifying *differences between relationships* reveals information about family structure.
   - Clarifying *differences between family members or in relationships* at various times reveals information about family development.

5. The information obtained from the family assessment is used to create a list of strengths and problems. Strengths and problems may be present in the structural, functional, or developmental dimensions of family life. For example:
   - Structural: adjusting to lone parenthood
   - Developmental: adjusting to children's leaving home
   - Functional: reacting to a family-held belief, such as "Father would be displeased with us for still crying about his death"

6. Some problems are beyond the scope of the nurse's competence. Referral is necessary when medical symptoms have not been fully assessed or when longstanding emotional or behavioural problems exist.

7. An extensive inquiry into the most pressing problems is necessary before you intervene.

8. Assessment is complete when you have obtained sufficient information to clearly understand the presenting problem.

---

1. Explore the components of the structural, developmental, and functional aspects of the CFAM to assess strengths and problem areas. Not all components of the CFAM need to be explored if they are not relevant to the situation.

2. Ask family members, including children, to explain their understanding of the presenting problem: "How do you see the problem?"

3. Explore with the family whether other problems or concerns connected to the presenting problem exist.

4. Inquire about differences between individuals, relationships, and points in time. For example:
   - Ask the child, "Who is better at getting you to do those things in the evening, your mother or father?"
   - "Do your father and Ingo fight more or less than your father and Hannah do?"
   - "Do you worry more, less, or the same about your husband's health since his heart attack?"

5. State to the family your understanding of its strengths and problems, and ask whether you are correct. After verifying them with the family, record your conclusions. For example:
   - "I've identified your being a newly single parent and also having to cope with your children's leaving home as your two major concerns. Have I understood this correctly?"

6. Tell the family members whether you will continue to work with them on problems or will refer them to another professional. (If you refer them, proceed to Stage 4, Termination.) For example:
   - "Now that I have a more complete understanding of your concerns, I think it is necessary to have your son examined by a pediatrician."

7. Ask the family members which issue they think is most important, and then explore it in depth. If the family members cannot agree, discuss the lack of consensus. For example:
   - "About which of the problems we have discussed today are you most concerned?"

8. State your understanding of the problem or problems to the family members, and obtain their commitment to work on a specific problem.

Continued

➤ **TABLE 20-3**   Family Interviewing Skills for Nurses Using the CFAM and CFIM   *continued*

Perceptual and Conceptual Skills	Executive Skills
You understand the following:	You might do the following:

Stage 3: Intervention

Perceptual and Conceptual Skills	Executive Skills
1. Families have problem-solving abilities. Families not only possess the capability to change but also the capability to identify and implement solutions.	1. Encourage family members to explore possible solutions to problems. For example: • "You've mentioned that your mother is critical of herself. What do you think she could do to feel more positive?"
2. Interventions are focused on the cognitive, affective, and behavioural domains of functioning, as described in the CFIM. It is not always necessary to design interventions for all domains simultaneously.	2. Plan interventions to influence one or all of the domains of functioning described in the CFIM. For example: • Cognitive: invite the family to think differently. • Affective: encourage different affective expressions. • Behavioural: ask the family to perform new tasks.
3. Lack of information can inhibit the family's problem-solving abilities. With additional information, many families can provide their own creative and unique solutions to problems.	3. Provide information to the family that will support further problem solving. For example: • Ask the family members whether they would like to hear about some typical reactions a three-year-old has to a new baby. This intervention targets cognitive functioning.
4. Persistent, intense emotions can block the family's problem-solving abilities. • Families who experience predominantly negative emotions such as sadness or anger are often unable to deal with problems until the emotional constraint is removed.	4. When appropriate, validate family members' emotional responses. For example: • A son who is suppressing grief may need confirmation that the grieving process is normal. This intervention targets the affective functioning.
5. Suggestions of specific tasks often provide new ways for family members to behave in relation to one another.	5. Assign tasks aimed at improving family functioning. For example: • Suggest that the mother and daughter spend one evening a week together in a common activity. This intervention influences behavioural functioning.

Stage 4: Termination
A. If Consultation or Referral Is Necessary

Perceptual and Conceptual Skills	Executive Skills
1. Families appreciate additional professional resources when problems are complex.	1. Refer individuals, family members, or both for consultation or ongoing treatment. For example: • "I think that your family needs professional input beyond what I can offer. Therefore, I would like to refer you to the learning centre."

B. If Family Interviewing With the Nurse Continues

Perceptual and Conceptual Skills	Executive Skills
1. Evaluating the family interviews at regular intervals is important.	1. Collaborate with family members about the current status of problems, and initiate termination when sufficient progress is made.
2. Interviews over a prolonged period can foster excessive dependency. The nurse must be careful to not inadvertently encourage dependency.	2. If necessary, mobilize other supports for the family, and begin to initiate termination by decreasing the frequency of sessions. You can inadvertently provide "paid friendship" unless other supports, such as partner, friends, or relatives, are available.
3. Recognizing family members' constructive efforts to solve problems is helpful.	3. Commend family members' positive efforts to resolve problems, regardless of whether you think significant improvement has occurred. For example: • "Your family has made tremendous efforts to find ways to care for your aging father at home and still attend to your children's needs."
4. Individuals and families appreciate backup support in times of stress.	4. If appropriate, extend an invitation for further meetings if problems recur or if the family wants consultation.

CFAM, Calgary Family Assessment Model; CFIM, Calgary Family Intervention Model.

Adapted from Wright, L. M., & Leahey, M. (2000). *Nurses and families: A guide to family assessment and intervention* (3rd ed., pp. 195–202). Philadelphia: F. A. Davis.

✳ BOX 20-5 ▸ NURSING STORY

Using Family Interviewing Strategies to Introduce Information, Commend Family Strengths, and Identify Family Needs

Mr. S., 82 years old, was re-admitted today with a diagnosis of severe congestive heart failure. He had suffered a myocardial infarction three months ago. He is accompanied by his daughter Jean, who lives nearby. Jean tells you that other family members are on their way from three hours out of town. Jean tells you that her sister, her brother, and their spouses and children do not really understand how sick her father is. Because the physician can offer Mr. S. only medical management of his congestive heart failure, Jean recognizes that her father's condition is terminal. Jean has also expressed some concern about the level of understanding and acceptance of this situation by other family members. The nurse plans to meet with the whole family when they arrive.

During the nurse's admission assessment of Mr. S., he indicated that he did not want any heroic measures taken to maintain his life and that both his doctor and Jean knew about his wishes. Mr. S. is severely short of breath, receiving high-flow oxygen, and requires diuretics three times daily and doses of morphine as needed to remain even slightly comfortable. He is also taking antiarrhythmic, antihypertensive, and beta-blocking medications to maintain a heart rate of 50 to 70 bpm, and his blood pressure is about 90/60 mm Hg. Despite the antiarrhythmic medications, he has bouts of atrial fibrillation with pounding in his chest. His heart rate can speed up to 150 to 180 bpm, and he turns ashen in colour. The heart rate drops back to 50 to 70 bpm after a few minutes, although he says these episodes are becoming more frequent. His physician has written "do not resuscitate" orders, which include no intubation, no defibrillation, and only comfort measures.

Mr. S.'s other children Mark and Sue, their spouses, and four preteenage children join Jean to meet with the nurse. The nurse engages the family by drawing a genogram to determine who is in the family and their relationships to one another. Then the nurse uses questioning strategies to determine what the family knew previously about Mr. S.'s condition. In response to the question "Who best understands Mr. S.'s condition?" both Mark and Sue indicate that Jean was most knowledgeable. The nurse then asks Mark, "If I asked Sue what she knew about Mr S.'s condition, what would she say?" Mark believes that because Sue talks to her father weekly, she can describe how he is doing and what is wrong with him. The nurse asks Jean what she understands about her father's illness. Jean explains that her father has had heart failure. She indicats that the drugs do not seem to be working very well, her dad is "getting worse," and he does not want "anything else done." On the last visit with the physician at his office, Mr. S. had told

the physician that if his condition deteriorated, he did not want to receive further lifesaving treatment.

The nurse then asks Mark and Sue to explain what they understand about congestive heart failure. Both seem to have an adequate understanding of the condition. When asked who best understands what Mr. S. meant by "not wanting anything more done," Mark replies that when they were working on the farm together, his father expressed on a number of occasions that he did not want to be kept alive by artificial means and that unless he was feeling good, he would "rather be dead." Sue indicates that she had talked to her dad a couple of times about his wishes regarding terminal care. The nurse commends the family for their closeness and their knowledge of Mr. S.'s condition. The nurse indicates that the family appears to understand the situation very well.

The nurse asks the family, "Who is having the most difficulty accepting the situation?" The family responds that Mark is, inasmuch as he seems to have been in the least contact with Mr. S. Mark responds that "although it's hard, I'll be O.K." because he knows that "this is the way my dad wants it."

The nurse includes the children in the discussion by asking, "Who is most concerned that Grandpa may not get well?" The two older children indicate that their parents had explained that Grandpa might not get well and that this might be their last chance to see him. The nurse asks the two younger children, "Who will have the most difficult time visiting Grandpa?" and "What would you need to know to feel better about visiting Grandpa?" The responses to the questions indicate that the two younger children would have the most trouble visiting, and they need to know how their grandfather looks and whether he will recognize them. The nurse responds to both questions with information about Mr. S.'s appearance and cognitive state.

The nurse continues exploring the need for support over the next while and whether the family can do other things for each other. The brief interview with the family provides Jean with information about the knowledge and acceptance levels of other members of the family. The family acknowledges Jean's burden in taking Mr. S. to appointments and helping him because she lives close by. The family demonstrates that they can support each other and would need little additional support. The family believes that if they need anything, they would feel comfortable asking the nursing staff. The nursing staff continues to explore the family's response to Mr. S.'s situation and helps prepare them for the time ahead.

Additional interviews are used to explore the family's understanding of the dying process, to provide information, and to promote support for the children.

✳ KEY CONCEPTS

- Family members influence one another's health beliefs, practices, and status.
- The concept of family is highly individual; thus, you should base care on the client's definition of family rather than on an inflexible definition of family.
- Family nursing care requires that nurses continually examine the current trends in the Canadian family and its health care implications.
- A healthy, resilient family is able to integrate the need for stability with the need for growth and change. The family can be viewed as context, in which you focus either on the individual client within the context of his or her family or on the family with the individual as context, or the family can be viewed as client (family systems nursing), in which you focus on family interactions.
- The CFAM is a conceptual framework that guides you in assessing the structural, developmental, and functional aspects of the family.
- Genograms and ecomaps are structural assessment tools that provide you with a pictorial image of the family's structure and relation to outside influences.
- Family members as caregivers are often spouses who may be either older adults themselves or adult children trying to work full time, care for aging parents, and enable children to move out of the home (launch children) successfully.
- Illness and disability often alter expressive functioning and communication within the family.
- The CFIM is a companion to the CFAM that guides you in implementing family interventions; it is focused on improving family functioning in three domains: cognitive (thinking), affective (feeling), and behavioural (doing).
- One of the simplest and most effective ways that you can help families is by asking them interventive questions.
- Offering commendations is important because they encourage the family to recognize their strengths and competencies.
- Other nursing interventions to help the family include providing information, validating emotional responses, encouraging clients to provide illness narratives, supporting family caregivers, and encouraging respite for family caregivers.
- Family caregiving is an interactional process that occurs within the context of the relationships among its members.
- Family interviews require you to have perceptual, conceptual, and executive skills; interviews may be formal and lengthy or casual and brief.

✳ CRITICAL THINKING EXERCISES

1. Kathy is a palliative care nurse working with a family of four: Wai-Ling, a 45-year-old single mother; her adolescent sons, Chun and Wang; and Heng, her 76-year-old mother, who is in the last stages of terminal breast cancer. The family has lived together for 10 years, ever since they immigrated to Canada from Hong Kong. Heng helped Wai-Ling parent Chun and Wang and supported Wai-Ling when her husband died five years ago. Wai-Ling has decided to care for her mother in the family's home until Heng dies. Kathy will assist this family in achieving their goal. Kathy has just had in-service training in using CFAM.

   a. What parts of the CFAM should Kathy use when assessing the family's needs?
   b. How can Kathy help the family achieve their goal of caring for their aging family member at home?
   c. How can Kathy determine this family's strengths, suffering, and resources?
   d. What cultural aspects are important to consider for a family who has immigrated to Canada and is now facing the death of a loved one?

2. Dan and Kim divorced seven years ago, and neither has remarried. They have three daughters, aged 10, 12, and 14. At the time of the divorce, Dan was HIV-positive, and has remained so for five years. Kim has had repeated tests and remains HIV-negative. Dan is responding to therapy slowly. Kim and Dan share parenting responsibilities and have a friendly relationship. They have decided it would be easier for the family to live together again so that Dan can actively participate in his children's lives without placing caregiver demands on Kim when the extended family visits overnight. Kim also wants to care for her former husband.

   a. What family development tasks are important to assess for this family as the members attempt to reunite?
   b. How should the nurse determine what support services the family needs?
   c. What assessment questions would be useful to ask in order to assess how the illness is affecting this family? Do family members have any signs of emotional, physical, or spiritual suffering?

3. Mr. and Mrs. Baillargeron, both in their early 50s, are the youngest members of large families. They work full-time and have two teenage children. Both sets of their parents are in their 80s and have chronic health problems. All of their siblings live farther away.

   a. How can the nurse help Mr. and Mrs. Baillargeron access resources to aid in caring for their parents and maintain the responsibilities of their own family unit?
   b. What developmental tasks does this family have?
   c. What kinds of questions can you ask to assess the family's emotional and verbal communication (found in CFAM's functional assessment category)?

✳ REVIEW QUESTIONS

1. The nurse must think of family as
   1. Parents and their children
   2. People related by marriage, birth, or adoption
   3. The nuclear family and aunts, uncles, grandparents, and cousins
   4. A set of relationships that the client identifies as family

2. The client is remarried, and her two children from a previous marriage live in the same household. Her husband's children visit on the weekend. This is an example of
   1. A nuclear family
   2. A blended family
   3. An extended family
   4. An alternative family

3. Which of the following is *not* a current trend?
   1. The proportion of couples without children at home is increasing.
   2. The proportion of "traditional" families is declining.
   3. The proportions of common-law and lone-parent families are increasing.
   4. The proportion of teenagers giving birth has increased steadily.

4. The primary social context in which health promotion and disease prevention take place is
   1. At educational institutions
   2. From friends and colleagues
   3. From physicians and nurses
   4. In the family

5. Two factors that contribute to the long-term health of a family are
   1. Structure and function
   2. Caregiving and reciprocity
   3. Hardiness and resiliency
   4. Context and system

6. When nurses view the family as client, their primary focus is on the
   1. Health and development of an individual member existing within a specific environment
   2. Family process and relationships
   3. Family relational and transactional concepts
   4. Family within a system

7. Asking a client "Who is in your family?" helps you assess
   1. Internal structure
   2. External structure
   3. Context
   4. Instrumental functioning

8. According to the CFAM, emotional communication is a subcategory of
   1. Instrumental functioning
   2. Development
   3. Internal structure
   4. Expressive functioning

9. "What do you think when your husband won't visit your son in the hospital?" is an example of a circular question. Asking the family circular questions is an effective way to
   1. Facilitate change by inviting the family to discover their own answers
   2. Encourage family members to be caregivers
   3. Validate their emotional responses
   4. Target specific "yes" or "no" answers

10. During a family interview, the nurse can
    1. Educate the family
    2. Enforce change
    3. Engage a family to assess, explore, and identify strengths and problems
    4. Establish roles

✳ RECOMMENDED WEB SITES

The Vanier Institute of the Family: http://www.vifamily.ca
The Vanier Institute of the Family was established in 1965 under the patronage of Governor General Georges P. Vanier and Madame Pauline Vanier. It is a national voluntary organization dedicated to promoting the well-being of Canadian families through research, publications, education, and advocacy. This Web site provides links to numerous publications related to important trends and issues affecting Canadian families, including a link to an online publication of *Profiling Canada's Families*.

21

Client Education

Original chapter by Amy M. Hall, RN, BSN, MS, PhD

Canadian content written by Nancy A. Edgecombe,

RN-NP, BN, MN, PhD

Client education is one of the most important roles for nurses in any health care setting. Clients and family members have the right to health education so that they can make informed decisions about their health care and lifestyle. Shorter hospital stays, increased demands on nurses' time, increase in numbers of clients with acute conditions, the severity of these acute conditions, and the increase in numbers of chronically ill clients emphasize the importance of high-quality client education. Initial client education often takes place in the hospital while clients are in the highly stressful acute stage of their illness and may not be completed at the time of discharge. Hospitals need to have clear guidelines to provide for follow-up. Client education helps ensure continuity of care as clients move from one health care setting to another. Nurses often clarify information provided by physicians and other health care professionals and may become the primary source of information for people adjusting to health problems (Falvo, 2004). In primary health care settings, nurses are often the main source of information about health promotion and illness prevention (Box 21–1).

The general public has become more assertive in seeking knowledge, understanding health, and finding resources available within the health care system. Nurses need to assist clients in navigating the vast amount of information available to them, through all forms of media. The Internet and other forms of technology (telehealth, e-health) provide nurses and clients with vast amounts of information, some reliable and some not. Clients need guidance regarding the selection of current and reliable resources. Nurses must be able to discuss with clients the criteria for evaluating sources for validity and reliability. The teaching material provided by nurses must honour copyright rules and must reference both written information and illustrations that are used to support client learning.

You need to be mindful of the increasing emphasis on "scientific" evidence and the diminished focus on other kinds of evidence of the efficacy or effectiveness of therapeutic interventions. You need to have a broad perspective of what constitutes meaningful evidence to support the significance of testimonials, lived experiences, and other ways of knowing. Because critical thinking is essential in nursing care, you need to be mindful that knowledge is limited, beliefs change, and conclusions are temporary. A well-designed, comprehensive teaching plan that meets a learner's needs can reduce health care costs, improve quality of care, help clients gain optimal wellness, and increase independence (Bastable, 2006).

Goals of Client Education

The goal of client education is to assist individuals, families, or communities in achieving optimal health (Edelman & Mandle, 2006). Education is a main tool of primary health care; it helps individuals, families, and communities maintain and improve their health, reduces hardship, helps contains health care costs, and enables people to take control of their own health (Canadian Nurses Association, 2003). Client education has three main goals (Box 21–2):

- Maintaining and promoting health and preventing illness
- Restoring health
- Optimizing quality of life with impaired functioning

Maintaining and Promoting Health and Preventing Illness

In the home, clinic, or other community health care setting, you provide information and skills that people need to maintain and improve their health (see Box 21–2). For example, in prenatal classes, nurses teach expectant parents about fetal development and physical and psychological changes during pregnancy. They also teach about the importance of healthy food choices, exercise, and avoiding substances that might harm the fetus. Greater knowledge can result in better health. When clients become more health conscious, they are more likely to seek early diagnosis of health problems (Redman, 2007).

Restoring Health

Many clients seek information and skills that will help them regain or maintain their health (see Box 21–2). However, clients who find it difficult to adapt to illness may be more passive. You learn to identify barriers to learning, to recognize clients' willingness to learn, and to help motivate interest in learning (Redman, 2007).

The family can be a vital part of a client's return to health and may need to know as much as the client. If you exclude the family from a teaching plan, conflicts may arise. For example, if the family does not understand a client's need to regain independent function, their efforts may encourage dependency and slow recovery. You should assess the client–family relationship before involving the family in a teaching plan (see Chapter 20).

✳ BOX 21-1   **FOCUS ON PRIMARY HEALTH CARE**

Educating Clients in Order to Promote Health and Prevent Disease

Promotion of health through prevention of disease is an important goal of primary health care. Nurses can help prevent many diseases (e.g., cardiovascular disease) by teaching clients about preventive actions and lifestyle change. Clients need to know about risk factors and how they can avoid or reduce their risk of developing the disease. To teach clients effective health practices, nurses need to be aware of the evidence in the literature and to apply this to counselling clients. They can also help clients make lifestyle changes by helping interpret the meaning of the evidence.

In order to communicate information successfully, nurses need to use simple, clear, and nontechnical language that clients can understand and develop a rapport with clients so that clients are able to receive and act on the information. Characteristics of a positive relationship with the client include empathic understanding, genuineness, intimacy and reciprocity, respect for the client's right to control lifestyle, and mutual trust.

Because clients may face serious barriers to making lifestyle changes, nurses need to carry out an assessment to determine the readiness for behaviour change and the feasibility of carrying out the change. To determine whether meaningful lifestyle change is possible for clients, nurses must understand principles of learning and behavioural change theories.

Clients need to develop an awareness of their own behaviour, a process that can be enhanced by self-monitoring. When clients can identify areas of difficulty and determine how these can be addressed, goals can be set collaboratively to ensure that clients are able to change their behaviour. Breaking down long-term goals into shorter term goals tends to enhance self-efficacy and client satisfaction. Focusing on behaviour change rather than physiological outcomes is recommended because the former is within the control of the client. Once the client identifies a goal, feedback is given to support the client in the process of achieving the goal. Social support from family or friends can be a positive influence in helping clients achieve their goals.

From Burke, L. E., & Fair, J. (2003). Promoting prevention: Skill sets and attributes of health care providers who deliver behavioural interventions. *Journal of Cardiovascular Nursing, 18*(4), 256–266.

> **BOX 21-2** **Topics for Health Education**

Health Maintenance and Promotion and Illness Prevention

Educate clients about:

First aid

Avoidance of risk factors (e.g., smoking, alcoholism)

Stress management

Typical growth and development patterns

Proper hygiene

Required immunizations

Prenatal care and normal child-bearing

Nutrition

Exercise

Safety (in home and health care setting)

Screening for common conditions (e.g., blood pressure, poor vision, cholesterol level)

Behaviour modification to change risky behaviours (e.g., quitting smoking, treatment for substance abuse)

Restoration of Health

Educate clients about:

Client's disease or condition

Anatomy and physiology of body system affected by disease or condition

Cause of disease

Origin of symptoms

Expected effects on other body systems

Prognosis

Limitations on function

Rationale for treatment

Medications

Tests and therapies

Nursing measures

Surgical intervention

Expected duration of care

Hospital or clinic environment

Hospital or clinic staff

Long-term care implications

Methods for client's participation in care

Limitations imposed by disease or surgery

Optimizing Quality of Life When Functions Are Impaired

Educate clients about:

Home care

Medications

Intravenous therapy

Diet

Activity

Self-help devices

Rehabilitation of remaining function

Physiotherapy

Occupational therapy

Speech therapy

Prevention of complications

Knowledge of risk factors

Implications of noncompliance with therapy

Environmental alterations

Self-help and support groups

Coping With Impaired Functioning

Some clients must learn to cope with permanent health alterations. For example, a client who loses the ability to speak after surgery of the larynx must learn new ways to communicate. A client with severe heart disease must learn to modify risk factors that might cause further heart damage. After the client's needs are identified and the family has displayed willingness to help, you teach family members to assist the client with health care management (e.g., giving medications through gastric tubes and performing passive range-of-motion exercises).

Teaching and Learning

Teaching is an interactive process that promotes learning. Teaching and learning generally begin when a person identifies a need for knowing or acquiring an ability to do something. A nurse-teacher provides information that prompts the client to engage in activities that lead to a desired change (Box 21–3). Teaching is most effective when it addresses the learner's needs, learning style, and capacity. The teacher assesses these needs by asking questions, observing the client, and determining the client's interests. With successful teaching, clients can learn new skills or change existing attitudes (Redman, 2007).

Role of the Nurse in Teaching and Learning

Nurses have an ethical responsibility to teach their clients about health enhancement (Redman, 2005, 2007). The Canadian Nurses Association's (2008) *Code of Ethics* indicates that clients have the right to make informed decisions about their care. The information that clients need to make such decisions must be accurate, complete, and relevant to their needs. You should anticipate clients' needs for information on the basis of their overall condition (physical, mental, emotional, spiritual), identified risks, and interdisciplinary treatment plans. Nurses often clarify information provided by physicians and other health care professionals and may become the primary source of information for adjusting to health problems (Bastable, 2006).

Clients and their families often ask nurses for health information. It is easy to identify the need for teaching when clients request information. However, in some cases, the need for information may be less apparent. You must observe and listen carefully to determine clients' needs for information and learning. When you value education and ensure that your clients learn necessary information, clients are better prepared to assume health care responsibilities. To be an effective educator, you must do more than just pass on facts; you must determine what clients need to know, find time when they are ready to learn, and evaluate the impact of client education on client outcomes (Bastable, 2003, 2006; Redman, 2007).

Teaching as Communication

Effective teaching depends on effective communication (see Chapter 18). To be a good teacher, you must listen empathetically, observe astutely, and speak clearly. Many intrapersonal variables—including attitudes, values, culture, emotions, and knowledge—influence both the nurse's and client's styles and approaches. Both you and the client and are also affected by the client's motivation and ability to learn, which depend on physical and psychological health, education, developmental stage, and previous knowledge.

Domains of Learning

Learning occurs in three domains: cognitive (understanding), affective (attitudes), and psychomotor (motor skills); (Bloom, 1956). Any topic to be learned may involve one domain, all domains, or any combination of the three. For example, clients with diabetes must

✳ BOX 21-3   RESEARCH HIGHLIGHT

The Effectiveness of Nurse-Directed Client Education

Research Focus

Clients living with heart failure need education about their diagnosis and related care to prevent multiple hospitalizations and promote optimal functioning.

Research Abstract

Kutzleb and Reiner (2006) wanted to know whether clients who participated in a nurse-directed client education program (the treatment group) had fewer admissions to the hospital, were more knowledgable about self-management, and had better quality of life and functional ability than did clients who did not participate (the control group). Clients in the treatment group were evaluated by a medical physician with a subspecialty in cardiology. The cardiac clinical nurse specialists performed physical assessments and taught the clients the importance of weighing themselves daily and recording the weights. An educational booklet outlining behaviours for successfully managing heart failure was provided to the clients and their families. The clinical nurse specialists also provided individualized counselling and telephone follow-up between monthly clinic visits. The clients in the control group saw a cardiologist every three

months in a cardiology clinic and received standardized care. Both groups completed a quality-of-life survey and a walking test to measure functional status. The results of this study revealed no actual difference in functional capacity between the two groups. However, the group that received nurse-directed client education program reported greater quality of life and a positive correlation between quality of life and functional capacity.

Research Highlights

- Nurse-directed client education about lifestyle choices and exercise enhanced quality of life in clients with heart failure.
- Cardiac clinical nurse specialists who collaborated with physicians successfully managed clients with heart failure in the outpatient setting.
- Improving quality of life enhanced the perception of functional capacity in clients with heart failure.
- Clients who receive nurse-directed client education improved their ability to manage their diet and medication.

References: Kutzleb, J., & Reiner, D. (2006). The impact of nurse-directed patient education on quality of life and functional capacity in people with heart failure. *Journal of the American Academy of Nurse Practitioners, 18*(3), 116–123.

learn how diabetes affects the body and how to control blood glucose levels for better health (cognitive domain). They must also learn to accept the chronic nature of diabetes by learning positive coping mechanisms (affective domain). Finally, many clients with diabetes must learn to test their blood glucose levels at home. This requires learning how to use a glucose meter (psychomotor domain). By understanding each learning domain, you can select appropriate teaching methods (Box 21–4).

Cognitive Learning

Cognitive learning includes all intellectual behaviours and requires thinking (Bastable, 2003). In the hierarchy of cognitive behaviours, the simplest behaviour is acquiring knowledge, whereas the most complex is evaluation. Cognitive learning includes the folowing:

- Knowledge: the learning of new facts or information and the ability to recall them

➤ BOX 21-4   Appropriate Teaching Methods Based on Domains of Learning

Cognitive

Discussion (One-on-One or Group)

May involve nurse and one client or nurse with several clients
Promotes active participation and focuses on topics of interest to client
Facilitates peer support
Enhances application and analysis of new information

Lecture

Is more formal method of instruction because it is teacher controlled
Helps learner acquire new knowledge and gain comprehension

Question-and-Answer Session

Is designed specifically to address client's concerns
Assists client in applying knowledge

Role Play and Discovery

Encourages client to actively apply knowledge in controlled situation
Promotes synthesis of information and problem solving

Independent Projects (e.g., Computer-Assisted Instruction) and Field Experience

Assists client to assume responsibility for learning at own pace
Promotes analysis, synthesis, and evaluation of new information and skills

Affective

Role Play

Encourages expression of values, feelings, and attitudes

Discussion (Group)

Enables client to acquire support from other people in group
Encourages client to learn from other people's experiences
Promotes responding, valuing, and organizing

Discussion (One-on-One)

Facilitates discussion of personal, sensitive topics of interest or concern

Psychomotor

Demonstration

Provides presentation of procedures or skills by nurse
Encourages client to model nurse's behaviour
Allows nurse to control questioning during demonstration

Practice

Enables client to perform skills by using equipment in a controlled setting
Allows repetition

Return Demonstrations

Enables client to perform skill as nurse observes
Provides excellent source of feedback and reinforcement

Independent Projects and Games

Require teaching method that promotes adaptation and initiation of psychomotor learning
Enable learner to use new skills

- Comprehension: the ability to understand the meaning of learned material
- Application: the use of abstract, newly learned ideas in a practical situation
- Analysis: the breaking down of information into organized parts
- Synthesis: the ability to apply knowledge and skills to produce a new whole
- Evaluation: a judgement of the worth of information given for a specific purpose

Affective Learning

Affective learning concerns expressions of feelings and acceptance of attitudes, opinions, or values. Values clarification (see Chapter 8) is an example of affective learning. The simplest behaviour in the affective learning hierarchy is receiving, and the most complex is characterizing (Krathwohl et al., 1964).

- Receiving: the willingness to attend to another person's words
- Responding: active participation through listening and reacting verbally and nonverbally
- Valuing: attachment of worth to an object, concept, or behaviour, demonstrated by the learner's actions
- Organizing: development of a value system by identifying and organizing values and resolving conflicts
- Characterizing: action and response with a consistent value system

Psychomotor Learning

Psychomotor learning involves acquiring skills that require the integration of mental and muscular activity, such as the ability to walk or to use an eating utensil. The simplest behaviour in the hierarchy is perception and the most complex is origination (Rankin & Stallings, 2005; Redman, 2007).

- Perception: awareness of objects or qualities through the use of sense organs.
- Set: a readiness (mental, physical, or emotional) to take a particular action.
- Guided response: the performance of an act under the guidance of an instructor, involving imitation of a demonstrated act
- Mechanism: a higher level of behaviour by which a person gains confidence and skill in performing a behaviour that is more complex or involves several more steps than does a guided response
- Complex overt response: the smooth and accurate performance of a motor skill that requires a complex movement pattern
- Adaptation: the ability to change motor response when unexpected problems occur
- Origination: use of existing psychomotor skills and abilities to perform a highly complex motor act that involves creating new movement patterns

Basic Learning Principles

Before nurses can teach, they must understand how people learn. Learning depends on the learning environment and on the individual's ability to learn, learning style, and motivation to learn. Learning takes place both in formal learning sessions, which involve planned learning activities, and in teachable moments, which allow you to spontaneously take advantage of teaching opportunities as they occur in the day-to-day contact with the client.

Learning Environment

Client education takes place in a variety of settings: the client's home, community centres, classrooms, and hospital rooms. The ideal environment for learning is a well-lit, well-ventilated room with appropriate furniture and a comfortable temperature. A quiet setting with few distractions and interruptions helps concentration. You can provide privacy even in a busy hospital by closing cubicle curtains or taking the client to a quiet spot. In the home, a bedroom might separate the client from household activities. If the client desires, family members or significant others may share in discussions. However, some clients may be reluctant to discuss their illness when other people, even close family members, are in the room. An ideal environment is not always achievable, however, and rather than miss a teachable moment, you can adapt the environment as much as possible to provide privacy and minimize distractions.

Ability to Learn

The ability to learn depends on emotional, intellectual, and physical capabilities and on developmental stage. If a client's learning ability is impaired, you should modify or postpone teaching activities.

Emotional Capability. Emotions can aid or prevent learning. Mild anxiety may help a person focus. However, stronger levels of anxiety can be incapacitating, creating an inability to attend to anything other than to relieve the anxiety. The prospect of change makes many people anxious. Seriously ill people, who are faced with multiple losses, may be extremely anxious and distressed. Nurses must be sensitive to a client's level of anxiety. If a person is incapacitated by anxiety, you need to find a way to alleviate the anxiety. This may mean teaching relaxation techniques before attempting to teach a task or a procedure.

Intellectual Capability. Clients have different levels of intellectual ability. You must assess the client's knowledge and intellectual level before beginning a teaching plan. For example, measuring liquid or solid food portions requires the ability to perform mathematical calculations. Reading a medication label or discharge instructions requires reading and comprehension skills. Following directions when performing self-care in accordance with limitations requires comprehension and application skills.

Physical Capability. The ability to learn often depends on physical health. To learn psychomotor skills, a client must possess the necessary strength, coordination, and sensory acuity. You should not overestimate the client's physical ability. The following physical attributes are necessary for learning psychomotor skills:

- Size (height and weight adequate for performing the task or using the equipment, such as crutch walking)
- Strength (ability of the client to follow a strenuous exercise program)
- Coordination (dexterity needed for complicated motor skills, such as using utensils, changing a bandage, or opening a medication container)
- Sensory acuity (visual, auditory, tactile, gustatory, and olfactory resources needed to receive and respond to messages taught)

Any physical condition (e.g., pain, fatigue, or hunger) that depletes energy also impairs the ability to learn. For example, a client in a weakened state who has just spent hours undergoing diagnostic tests is likely to be too fatigued to learn. Nurses must assess the client's energy level by noting the client's willingness to communicate, the degree of activity initiated, and the client's responsiveness to questions. You may halt teaching if the client needs rest.

Developmental Stage. Age and stage of development affect the ability to learn (Box 21–5). Without proper biological, motor, language, and personal–social development, many types of learning cannot take place.

> **BOX 21-5**   **Teaching Methods Based on Client's Developmental Capacity**

Infant
Maintain consistent routines (e.g., feeding, bathing).
Hold infant firmly while smiling and speaking softly, to convey sense of trust.
Have infant touch different textures (e.g., soft fabric, hard plastic).

Toddler
Use play to teach procedure or activity (e.g., handling examination equipment, applying bandage to doll).
Offer picture books that describe a story of children in a hospital or clinic.
Use simple words such as "cut" instead of "laceration," to promote understanding.

Preschooler
Use role-playing, imitation, and play to make learning fun.
Encourage questions and offer explanations; use simple explanations and demonstrations.
Encourage several children to learn together through pictures and short stories about how to perform hygiene.

School-Age Child
Teach necessary psychomotor skills. (Complicated skills, such as learning to use a syringe, may take considerable practice.)
Offer opportunities to discuss health problems and answer questions.

Adolescent
Help adolescent learn about feelings and need for self-expression.
Collaborate with adolescent on teaching activities.
Let adolescent make decisions about health and health promotion (safety, sex education, substance abuse).
Use problem solving to help adolescent make choices.

Young or Middle-Aged Adult
Encourage participation in teaching plan by setting mutual goals.
Encourage independent learning.
Offer information so that adult can understand effects of health problem.

Older Adult
Teach when client is alert and rested.
Involve adult in discussion or activity.
Focus on wellness and the person's strength.
Use approaches that enhance sensorially impaired client's reception of stimuli (see Chapter 48).
Keep teaching sessions short.

Learning in Children. As a child matures, intellectual growth progresses from concrete to abstract. Therefore, information should be understandable, and the expected outcomes should be realistic and based on the child's developmental stage. Developmentally appropriate teaching aids should also be used (Figure 21–1).

Adult Learning. Many adults are independent, self-directed learners. However, they may become dependent in new learning situations. Adults typically learn more successfully when they are encouraged to use past experiences to solve problems. Adult clients and nurses should collaborate on educational topics and goals. Needs or issues that are important to the adult should be addressed early in the teaching–learning process. Ultimately, adults must accept responsibility for changing their own behaviours. Assessing what the adult client currently knows, teaching what the client wants to know, and setting mutual goals will improve the outcomes of care and education (Bastable, 2003).

Learning Style and Preference
People have different learning styles. Everyone processes information differently by seeing and hearing, reflecting and acting, reasoning logically and intuitively, and analyzing and visualizing. Some people are visual learners; they learn best by watching. Audiovisual presentations and visual demonstrations often work best for this type of learner. Other people are kinesthetic learners; they learn best when they are able to manipulate tools and find out how they work. Some people learn by taking detailed notes; others prefer to only listen. Some people need to be engaged in activities and discussion in order to learn effectively. Others may be too shy to enjoy this type of learning and prefer to learn from an orderly, structured presentation.

Environmental, social, emotional, psychological, and physical stimuli affect people differently. Some people prefer complete silence in the learning environment, whereas others prefer background sounds. Some prefer to learn in a group; others, on their own. Different people prefer different times of the day for learning experiences.

When developing teaching plans, you should assess the favoured learning style and preferences of the client. With groups, it may not be possible to address every client's preferences. However, including a combination of approaches to meet multiple learning styles can ensure that most people's learning preferences are met (Bastable, 2006). When the client is having difficulty with learning, you should consider a change to accommodate a different learning style.

Motivation to Learn
Motivation is a person's desire or willingness to learn, and it influences a person's behaviour (Redman, 2007; Box 21–6). If a person is not ready or does not want to learn, learning is unlikely to occur. The stimuli for motivation vary between individuals and may be social, task mastery, or physical in nature. *Social motives* reflect a need for connection, social approval, or self-esteem. For example, the motivation to exercise may be linked to the social aspects of the exercise activities (Heading, 2008). *Task mastery motives* are driven by desire for achievement. For example, a high school student with diabetes begins to test blood glucose levels and determine insulin dosages before leaving home and establishing independence. The

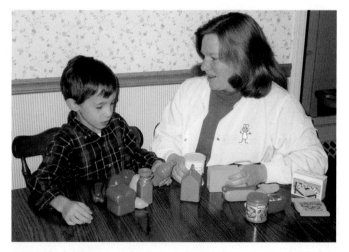

Figure 21-1 The nurse uses developmentally appropriate food models to teach healthy eating behaviours to the school-aged child.

desire to live independently and manage the disease provides the motivation to master the task or skill. After succeeding at a task, a person is usually motivated to achieve more. *Physical motives* come from a desire to maintain and improve health. Clients motivated by the need to survive or overcome hardship are often more motivated than those who wish merely to improve their health (Rankin & Stallings, 2005). For example, a client who has undergone a leg amputation may be extremely motivated to learn to use assistive devices, whereas a client who is overweight but otherwise healthy may not be motivated to exercise.

❋ BOX 21-6   NURSING STORY

"To Take or Not to Take"

In preparation for a trip to Vietnam and Cambodia, Mr. and Mrs. Bennet visited a travel clinic, which recommended that they update their immunization (diphtheria-pertussis-tetanus, hepatitis A, typhoid) and take antimalarial drugs for the Cambodia portion of the trip (atovaquone/proguanil [Malarone], one pill daily starting one day before stay and continuing during stay and one week after). When they came in for their immunizations, they expressed some concerns about taking the antimalarial drugs. They had been talking to friends who told them these antimalarial drugs had severe side effects and caused hallucinations. They had investigated several Internet sites that their friends had recommended; these sites indicated that antimalarial drugs were not required for where they were going. Mrs. Bennet e-mailed the Cambodian Consulate in Canada and was told that malaria was not a concern where they were going.

Assessment
- Concerned about health but received mixed messages about the need for antimalarial drugs.
- Concerned about serious side effects of drugs.
- Motivated to learn.

Plan
- Discussed with Mr. and Mrs. Bennet criteria for evaluating Web sites for health information (author, age, conflict of interest, whether evidence informed rather than opinion based)
- Provided list of known travel health sites (Health Canada; World Health Organization; US Centers for Disease Control and Prevention)
- Identified other measures to reduce risk of contracting malaria (using mosquito repellent, limiting time outside at night, staying in air-conditioned rooms or mosquito nets, wearing protective clothing)
- Discussed various drugs used for malaria and the incidence and types of side effects
- Explored the risk of not taking medication and implications of contracting malaria
- Identified other resources of information (travel agents, pharmacists)

Outcome
Mr. and Mrs. Bennet visited several reliable sources on the Internet and talked to their pharmacist. They identified several strategies to minimize exposure to mosquitoes on their travels. Mr. Bennet learned that the risk of side effects from the Malarone was minimal and decided to take the drug. Mrs. Bennet also recognized that the risk for side effects was minimal; however, because of her concern about those side effects, she decided not to take the Malarone. She was more comfortable taking the risk because she understood that if she developed a high fever and flu-like illness at any time up to a year after the trip, she had to seek immediate medical attention.

Many people do not adopt new health behaviours or change unhealthy behaviours unless they perceive a disease as a threat, overcome barriers to changing health practices, and see the benefits of such changes (Pender et al., 2006). Thus, a client with lung disease may continue to smoke. An obese client may worsen a heart condition by refusing to follow a low-fat diet.

Motivation and Social Learning Theory. Health education often involves changing people's attitudes and values. Change can occur only when education plans and interventions are based on sound learning theories. A number of theories address the complex client education process (Bastable, 2003; Redman, 2007). One of these is **social learning theory**, which helps educators understand learners and develop interventions that enhance motivation and learning (Bandura, 2001; Bastable, 2003; Saarmann et al., 2002).

When people believe that they can execute a particular behaviour, they are more likely to perform the behaviour consistently and correctly (Bandura, 1997). *Self-efficacy*, a social learning theory concept, is a person's perceived ability to successfully complete a task. Beliefs about self-efficacy arise from four sources: verbal persuasion, vicarious experiences, enactive mastery experiences, and physiological and affective states (Bandura, 1997). Understanding these sources lets nurses develop appropriate interventions. For example, a nurse teaching a boy with asthma to use an inhaler expresses positive reinforcement (verbal persuasion). The nurse then demonstrates how to use the inhaler (vicarious experience). The boy uses the inhaler (enactive mastery experience). As the boy's wheezing and anxiety decrease from using the inhaler, the nurse gives him positive feedback, which further enhances his confidence to use the inhaler (physiological and affective states). Interventions such as these enhance perceived self-efficacy, which in turn improves the achievement of desired outcomes.

Motivation and Transtheoretical Model of Change. Health education may involve changes in behaviour. Behavioural change is often challenging and difficult. It involves a process that occurs over time through a series of stages. By identifying the client's stage of change and focusing learning activities to match the client's stage, you faciliate the learner's motivation to change and his or her transition from one stage to the next. Five stages have been identified and used in smoking cessation activities (DiClemente et al., 1991; Prochaska & DiClemente, 1992):

- Precontemplation: is unaware of need for change and has no intention of changing behaviour
- Contemplation: is aware of need for change and intends to change behaviour sometime in the future
- Preparation: alters behaviour in minor ways with the intention to make substantive changes in the immediate future
- Action: modifies behaviour and experiences in order to make sustainable change
- Maintenance: focuses on not reverting to previous behaviour and on solidifying new behaviours

Integrating the Nursing and Teaching Processes

The nursing and teaching processes are related (Redman, 2007) and usually take place concurrently. Like the nursing process, the teaching process requires assessment, nursing diagnosis, planning, implementation, and evaluation. However, the processes are not exactly the same: The nursing process is broader. For example, determining a client's health needs requires assessing all data sources. The teaching process is focused on data sources that reveal the client's learning needs, willingness and ability to learn, and available teaching resources. Table 21–1 compares the teaching and nursing processes.

The teaching process requires assessment. The client's ability to learn, motivation, and needs should be assessed and analyzed. A diagnostic statement specifies the information or skills that the client requires. You set specific **learning objectives** (i.e., what the learner will be able to do after successful instruction) and implement the teaching plan by using teaching and learning principles to ensure that the client acquires knowledge and skills. Finally, the teaching process requires an evaluation of learning; this evaluation is based on learning objectives.

❖Assessment

During assessment, you determine the client's health care needs (see Chapter 13). The client may reveal a need for health care information, or you may identify a need for education. Learning needs identified by both the client and the nurse determine the content to be learned. By performing an effective assessment, you can individualize instruction for each client (Wingard, 2005). Ask specific questions to assess a client's unique learning needs (Box 21–7).

Learning Needs

Most clients can identify at least some of their own learning needs. Effective questioning and assessment tools help you determine a client's perceived learning needs. By listening carefully and using open-ended and closed-ended questions (see Chapter 18), nurses can often find out what a client's needs are. Because a client's health status is dynamic, assessment is an onging activity. Assess the following:

- Information or skills needed by the client to perform self-care and to understand the implications of a health problem. (Health care team members anticipate learning needs related to specific health problems. For example, you teach an adolescent boy to perform testicular self-examination.)
- Client's experiences that influence the need to learn.
- Information that the family members or significant others require to support the client's needs. (The amount of information needed depends on the exent of the family's role in helping the client.)

Ability to Learn

The ability to learn can be impaired by many factors, including body temperature, electrolyte levels, oxygenation status, and blood glucose level. Several factors may influence a client at one time. You assess the client's ability to learn by considering the following:

- Physical strength, movement, dexterity, and coordination (you determine the client's ability to perform skills)
- Sensory deficits that may affect the ability to understand or follow instruction (see Chapter 48)
- Reading level (reading level can be difficult to assess because functional illiteracy is often easy to conceal; one way to assess a client's reading level and level of understanding is to ask the client to read instructions from a teaching brochure and then explain its meaning)
- Developmental level (developmental level influences teaching approaches [see Box 21–5])
- Cognitive function (cognitive function includes memory, knowledge, association, and judgement)

Motivation to Learn

You ask questions that identify a client's motivation level, which help you determine whether the client is prepared and willing to learn. You assesses the client's motivation by studying the following:

- Behaviour (e.g., attention span, tendency to ask questions, memory, and ability to concentrate during the teaching session)
- Health beliefs and perception of a health problem and the benefits and barriers to treatment (e.g., you ask a client with coronary

▶ TABLE 21-1	**Comparison of the Nursing and Teaching Processes**	
Basic Steps	**Nursing Process**	**Teaching Process**
Assessment	Collect data about client's physical, psychological, social, cultural, developmental, and spiritual needs from client, family, diagnostic tests, medical record, health history, learning style, and literature.	Gather data about client's learning needs, motivation, ability to learn, and teaching resources from client, family, learning environment, medical record, health history, and literature.
Nursing diagnosis	Identify appropriate nursing diagnoses based on assessment findings, including deficits.	Identify client's learning needs on basis of three domains of learning.
Planning	Develop individualized care plan. Set diagnosis priorities on the basis of client's immediate needs. Collaborate with client on care plan.	Establish learning objectives, stated in behavioural terms. Identify priorities regarding learning needs. Collaborate with client on teaching plan. Identify type of teaching method to use.
Implementation	Perform nursing care therapies. Include client as active participant in care. Involve family or significant other in care as appropriate.	Implement teaching methods. Actively involve client in learning activities. Include family or significant other in participation as appropriate.
Evaluation	Identify success in meeting desired outcomes and goals of nursing care. Alter interventions as indicated when goals are not met.	Determine outcomes of teaching–learning process. Measure client's ability to achieve learning objectives. Reinforce information as needed .

> **BOX 21-7** Nursing Assessment Questions

Ask Clients

What do you want to know?

What do you know about your illness and your treatment plan?

How does (or will) your illness affect your current lifestyle?

What barriers currently exist that are preventing you from managing your illness the way you would like to manage it?

What cultural or spiritual beliefs do you have regarding your illness and the prescribed treatment?

What experiences have you had that are similar to what you are experiencing now?

Together we can choose the best way for you to learn about your disease. How can I best help you?

What role do you believe your health care professional should take in helping you manage your illness or maintain health?

When you learn new information, do you prefer to have the information given to you in pictures or written down in words?

When you give someone directions to your house, do you tell the person how to get there, write out the instructions, or draw a map?

How involved do you want your family to be in the management of your illness?

Ask Family Members

When are you available to help, and how do you plan to help your loved ones?

Your spouse needs some help. How do you feel about learning how to assist him [her]?

artery disease, "Explain how heart disease will affect you over time. What is the value of eating a low-fat diet?")
- Perceived ability to complete a required healthy behaviour
- Desire to learn
- Attitudes about health care professionals (e.g., role of client and nurse in making decisions, such as your asking, "In what way can I best help you?")
- Knowledge of information to be learned (the client must play an active role in seeking health-related information)
- Pain, fatigue, anxiety, or other physical symptoms that can interfere with the ability to maintain attention and participate (in acute care settings, a client's physical condition can easily detract from learning)
- Sociocultural background (a client's beliefs and values about health and various therapies may be influenced by sociocultural norms or tradition [see Chapter 10]; educational efforts can be especially challenging when clients and educators do not speak the same language)
- Learning style preference (clients who learn better by seeing and hearing may benefit from a video; clients who learn best by reasoning logically and intuitively may learn better if presented with written material that they can analyze and discuss with others)

Teaching Environment

You assess the following factors when choosing a teaching environment:

- Distractions or persistent noise (a quiet area should be set aside for teaching)
- Comfort of the room, including ventilation, temperature, lighting, and furniture
- Room facilities and available equipment

Resources for Learning

Assessment of resources includes a review of available teaching tools. If a client requires family support, you evaluate the readiness and ability of family and friends to learn to care for the client, and you review resources in the home. You assess the following:

- Client's willingness to have family members involved in the teaching plan and care (information about the client's health care is confidential unless the client chooses to share it)
- Family members' perceptions and understanding of the client's illness and its implications (family members and clients' perceptions should match; otherwise, conflicts may arise in the teaching plan)
- Family's willingness and ability to participate in care (family members must be responsible, willing, and able to assist in care activities, such as bathing or administering medications)
- Resources in the home (these resources include health care equipment and a suitable rearrangement of rooms)
- Teaching tools, including brochures, audiovisual materials, or posters. Printed material should present current and easy-to-understand information that matches the client's reading level.

❖Nursing Diagnosis

After assessing the client's ability and need to learn, you interpret data to form an accurate diagnosis. This diagnosis ensures that teaching will be goal directed and individualized. If a client has several learning needs, the nursing diagnoses guide priority setting. By classifying diagnoses according to the three learning domains, you can focus on subject matter and teaching methods. Examples of nursing diagnoses that indicate a need for education include the following:

- *Ineffective health maintenance*
- *Health-seeking behaviours*
- *Impaired home maintenance*
- *Deficient knowledge*
- *Ineffective therapeutic regimen management*
- *Ineffective community therapeutic regimen management*
- *Ineffective family therapeutic regimen management*

When health care problems can be managed through education, the diagnostic statement is *deficient knowledge*. For example, an older adult may be unable to manage a medication regimen because of the number of medications that must be taken at different times of the day. Education may improve the client's ability to schedule and take the medications.

Some nursing diagnoses also indicate that teaching is inappropriate. You may identify conditions that hinder learning (e.g., nursing diagnosis of pain or activity intolerance). In these cases, you should delay teaching until the nursing diagnosis is resolved or the health problem is controlled.

❖Planning

After identifying a client's learning needs and making a nursing diagnosis, you develop a teaching plan, set goals and expected outcomes, and work with the client to select a teaching method (Box 21–8). Expected outcomes or learning objectives determine which teaching strategies and approaches are appropriate. Client participation is essential.